Useful Units in Radiology

SI Prefixes

Factor	Prefix	Symbol
10^{18}	Exa	E
10^{15}	Peta	P
10^{12}	Tera	T
10^{9}	Giga	G
10^{6}	Mega	M
10^{3}	Kilo	k
10^{2}	Hecto	h
10^{1}	Deca	da
10^{-1}	Deci	d
10^{-2}	Centi	c
10^{-3}	Milli	m
10^{-6}	Micro	μ
10^{-9}	Nano	n
10^{-12}	Pico	p
10^{-15}	Femto	f
10^{-18}	Atto	a

SI Base Units

Quantity	Name	Symbol
Length	Meter	m
Mass	Kilogram	kg
Time	Second	s
Electric current	Ampere	A

SI Derived Units Expressed in Terms of Base Units

Quantity	SI UNIT Name	SI UNIT Symbol
Area	Square meter	m^2
Volume	Cubic meter	m^3
Speed, velocity	Meter per second	m/s
Acceleration	Meter per second squared	m/s^2
Density, mass density	Kilogram per cubic meter	kg/m^3
Current density	Ampere per square meter	A/m^2
Concentration (of amount of substance)	Mole per cubic meter	$mole/m^3$
Specific volume	Cubic meter per kilogram	m^3/kg

Special Quantities of Radiologic Science and Their Associated Special Units

Quantity	CUSTOMARY UNIT Name	CUSTOMARY UNIT Symbol	SI UNIT Name	SI UNIT Symbol
Exposure	roentgen	R	air kerma	Gy_a
Absorbed dose	rad	rad	gray	Gy_1
Effective dose	rem	rem	seivert	Sv
Radioactivity	curie	Ci	becquerel	Bq
Multiply	R	by 0.01	to obtain	Gy_a
Multiply	rad	by 0.01	to obtain	Gy_t
Multiply	rem	by 0.01	to obtain	Sv
Multiply	Ci	by 3.73×10^{10}	to obtain	Bq
Multiply	R	by 2.583×10^{-4}	to obtain	C/kg

RADIOLOGIC SCIENCE
for TECHNOLOGISTS

PHYSICS, BIOLOGY, AND PROTECTION

NINTH EDITION

RADIOLOGIC SCIENCE for TECHNOLOGISTS

PHYSICS, BIOLOGY, AND PROTECTION

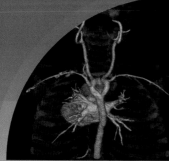
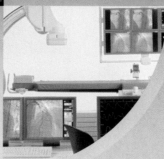

Stewart Carlyle Bushong, ScD, FACR, FACMP

Professor of Radiology Science
Baylor College of Medicine
Houston, Texas

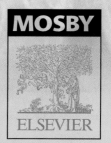

MOSBY

ELSEVIER

11830 Westline Industrial Drive
St. Louis, Missouri 63146

Library of Congress Control Number 2007942686

Publishing Director: Andrew Allen
Publisher: Jeanne Wilke
Senior Developmental Editor: Rebecca Swisher
Publishing Services Manager: Pat Joiner-Myers
Senior Project Manager: Karen M. Rehwinkel
Design Direction: Julia Dummitt

Printed in Canada

Last digit is the print number: 9 8 7 6 5 4 3 2 1

Reviewers

David Armstrong, BS, MEd, RT(R)
Program Director
Pearl River Community College
Hattiesburg, Mississippi

Alberto Bello, Jr., MEd, RT(R)(CV)
Radiologic Technology Program Director
Danville Area Community College
Danville, Illinois

Donna Caldwell, MEd, RT(R)(CV)
Assistant Professor
Arkansas State University
State University, Arkansas

Marilyn H. Carter, BS, RT(R), ARRT
Program Coordinator, Radiologic Technology
Southeast Arkansas College
Pine Bluff, Arkansas

John H. Clouse, MSR, RT(R)
Associate Professor of Radiography
Owensboro Community and Technical College
Owensboro, Kentucky

Edward J. Goldschmidt, Jr., MS, DABMP
Medical Physicist
Cooper Health System
Camden, New Jersey

Sergeo Guilbaud, BS, RT(R)
Education Director
Long Island College Hospital
Brooklyn, New York

Brenda Hassinger, MS, RT(R)(M), ARRT
Program Coordinator, Radiography Program
Hagerstown Community College
Hagerstown, Maryland

Terri Hinson, BS, RT(R)(T), ARRT
Instructor
University of Arkansas for Medical Sciences
Little Rock, Arkansas

Robert Hughes, BGS, RT(R)
Program Director
Nebraska Methodist College
Omaha, Nebraska

James Neal Johnston, PhD, RT(R)(CV)
Assistant Professor
Midwestern State University
Wichita Falls, Texas

Barbara A. Koontz, MA, RT(R)(M)
Radiography Program Manager
Polk Community College
Winter Haven, Florida

Nina Kowalczyk, MS, RT(R)(QM)(CT), FASRT
Clinical Instructor
Ohio State University
Columbus, Ohio

Michael J. Kudlas, BS, RT(R)(QM)
Director, Radiography Program
Associate Professor of Radiology
Mayo Clinic of Medicine
Jacksonville, Florida

Angela M. Lambert, MS, RT(R)
Assistant Professor
Bluefield State College
Bluefield, West Virginia

Sandra H. Lanza, BS, RT(R)(M)(QM)
Clinical Coordinator
Brevard Community College
Cocoa, Florida

Tricia D. Leggett, MSEd, RT(R)(QM)
Radiologic Technology Program Director
Assistant Professor
Zane State College
Zanesville, Ohio

Penelope Logsdon, MA, RT(R)
Radiography Program Director
Elizabethtown Community and Technical College
Elizabethtown, Kentucky

Galen Miller, RT(R), BS
Clinical Coordinator, Radiography Program
Mid Michigan Community College
Harrison, Michigan

Gloria Jean Mongelluzzo, MEd, RT(R)(M)
Program Director
Conemaugh Memorial Medical Center
Johnstown, Pennsylvania

Joe P. Nolen, MEd, RT(R)
Clinical Coordinator
University of Arkansas for Medical Sciences
Area Health Education Center—Southwest
Texarkana, Arkansas

Mimi Polczynski, MSEd, RT(R)(M)(CT)
Radiology Program Director
Kaskaskia College
Centralia, Illinois

Timothy J. Skaife, RT(R), MA
Program Director, Radiography
National Park Community College
Hot Springs, Arkansas

Ian Thompson, FNZIMRT, DHA (Massey) DCR
Specialist Lecturer
Universal College of Learning
Palmerston North, New Zealand

Jonathan White, BSRT(R), BS (Radiology)
Instructor, Diagnostic Imaging
Northern Virginia Community College
Springfield, Virginia

Paul Wilder, BS, RT(R)(T), ARRT
Program Director
Central New Mexico Community College
Albuquerque, New Mexico

Christine E. Wiley, MEd, RT(R)(M)
Radiologic Technology Program Director
North Shore Community College
Danvers, Massachusetts

Ray Winters, MS, RT(R)(CT)
Chair, Radiologic Sciences Department
Arkansas State University
State University, Arkansas

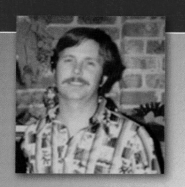

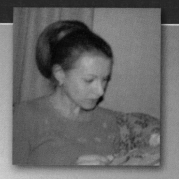

*N*o medical physicist has been as fortunate as I
over these past four academic decades.
My success would have been so shallow
if not for the support, encouragement, and friendship
of these two wonderful people
to whom I dedicate this 9th Edition.
Thanks you two for the great ride.

NOW

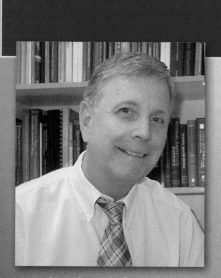

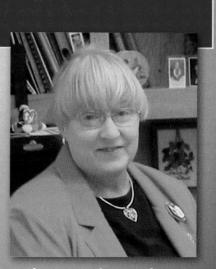

Benjamin Ripley Archer

Sharon Briney Glaze

This Book is also Dedicated to My Friends Here and Gone:

Abby Kuramoto
Bailey Schroth (†)
Bailey Spaulding
Bandit Davidson (†)
Bella Bushong
Belle Davidson
Boef Kuipers (†)
Brittney Prominski
Brownie Hindman (†)
Brutus Payne (†)
Buffy Jackson (†)
Butterscotch Bushong (†)
Casper Miller (†)
Cassie Kronenberger (†)
Chandon Davis (†)
Chester Chase (†)
Choco Walker (†)
Coco Winsor
Cookie Lake (†)
Desi Lohrenz

Dually Jackson
Dude Schwartz
Duncan Hindman
Ebony Bushong (†)
Flap Maly
Fonzie Schroth (†)
Frank Edlund
Geraldine Bushong (†)
Ginger Chase (†)
Grayton Friedlander
Gretchen Scharlach (†)
Guadalupe Tortilla Holmberg
Jemimah Bushong (†)
Kate Davidson (†)
Linus Black (†)
Lizzy Prominski
Loftus Meadows
Lucy Spaulding (†)
Maddie Bushong
Maxwell Haus (†) and my lenses

Midnight Lunsford (†)
Mini Hana (Indian Princess)
Molly Holmberg (†)
Muttly Chase (†)
Pancho Villa Holmberg (†)
Peanut Schroth
Pepper Miller
Petra Chase (†)
Powers Jackson
Sammie Chase
Sapphire Miller (†)
Sebastian Miller (†)
Susi Bueso
Teddy Schroth
Toby Schroth (†)
Toto Walker (†)
Travis Chase (†)
Tuffy Beman

(†) = R.I.P.

Preface

PURPOSE AND CONTENT

The purpose of *Radiologic Science for Technologists: Physics, Biology, and Protection* is threefold: to convey a working knowledge of radiologic physics, to prepare radiography students for the certification examination by the ARRT, and to provide a base of knowledge from which practicing radiographers can make informed decisions about technical factors, diagnostic image quality, and radiation management for both patients and personnel.

This textbook provides a solid presentation of radiologic science, including the fundamentals of radiologic physics, diagnostic imaging, radiobiology, and radiation management. Special topics include mammography, fluoroscopy, interventional procedures, multislice spiral computed tomography, and the various emerging modes of digital imaging.

The fundamentals of radiologic science cannot be removed from mathematics, but this textbook does not assume a mathematics background for the readers. The few mathematical equations presented are always followed by sample problems with direct clinical application. As a further aid to learning, all mathematical formulas are highlighted with their own icon.

Likewise, the most important ideas under discussion are presented with their own colorful penguin icon and box:

The use of the penguin icon is described early in Chapter 1.

This ninth edition improves this popular feature of information bullets by including even more key concepts and definitions in each chapter. This edition also presents learning objectives, chapter overviews, and chapter summaries that encourage students and make the text user friendly for all. Challenge Questions at the end of each chapter include definition exercises, short-answer questions, and a few calculations. These questions can be used for homework assignments, review sessions, or self-directed testing and practice. Answers to all questions are provided on the Evolve site at http://evolve.elsevier.com.

HISTORICAL PERSPECTIVE

For seven decades after Roentgen's discovery of x-rays in 1895, diagnostic radiology remained a relatively stable field of study and practice. Truly great changes during that time can be counted on one hand: the Crookes tube, the radiographic grid, radiographic intensifying screens, and image intensification.

Since the publication of the first edition of this textbook in 1975, however, newer systems for diagnostic imaging have come into routine use: multislice spiral computed tomography, computed radiography, digital radiography, and digital fluoroscopy. Truly spectacular advances in computer technology and x-ray tube and image receptor design have made these innovations possible, and they continue to transform the diagnostic imaging sciences.

NEW TO THIS EDITION

Currently we are accelerating to all-digital imaging. Digital radiography is replacing screen-film radiography rapidly and this requires that radiologic technologists acquire a new and different fund of knowledge in addition to what has been required previously—and in the same length of training time!

This ninth edition includes eight new chapters on digital imaging. Much of the material in the other 32 chapters has been reprocessed for brevity so that the size of this edition remains essentially the same as the previous edition. Another recent innovation described in this textbook is the imaging characteristics associated with the use of amorphous silicon and amorphous selenium. There is a new discussion of charge-coupled devices and the advantages for interventional radiology procedures.

Also presented are many updates in the areas of special imaging, in which the greatest advances in radiologic technology have occurred. There is a new chapter on multislice spiral computed tomography. Also discussed are advances in target composition, compression, and digital imaging for mammography. Pay particular attention to Chapter 30, Digital Display Quality

Control, a field that requires new skills on the part of the radiographic technologist. The AAPM TG-18 recommendations will become as standard as processor quality control.

The ninth edition also includes more in-text definitions and chapter cross-references. All boldface terms are defined when first introduced and are collected in an expanded glossary. New radiographs and line drawings keep this text fresh and fun.

ANCILLARIES
Student Workbook and Laboratory Manual

This three-part resource has been updated to reflect the changes in the text and the rapid advancements in the field of radiologic science. Part I offers a complete selection of worksheets organized by textbook chapter. Part II, the Math Tutor, provides an outstanding refresher for any student. Part III, Laboratory Experiments, collects experiments designed to demonstrate important concepts in radiologic science.

Evolve Resources

Instructor ancillaries, including an ExamView Test Bank of over 900 questions, an image collection of all of the images in the text, and a PowerPoint lecture presentation are all available at http://evolve.elsevier.com.

Mosby's Radiography Online

Instructional materials to support teaching and learning online, radiologic physics, radiographic imaging, radiobiology, and radiation protection have been developed by Elsevier and may be obtained by contacting the publisher directly.

A NOTE ON THE TEXT

Although the ARRT has not formally adopted the International System of Units (SI units), they are presented in this textbook. With this system come the corresponding units of radiation and radioactivity. The roentgen, the rad, and the rem are being replaced the gray (Gy), and the sievert (Sv), respectively. A summary of special quantities and units in radiologic science can be found on the inside front cover of the text.

Radiation exposure is measured in SI units of C/kg, or in terms of air kerma, measured in mGy. Because mGy is also a unit of dose, a measurement of air kerma is distinguished from tissue dose by applying a subscript a or t to mGy, according to the recommendations of Archer and Wagner (*Minimizing Risk From Fluoroscopic X-rays*, PRM, 2007). Therefore, when the SI is used, air kerma is measured in mGy_a and tissue dose in mGy_t.

ACKNOWLEDGMENTS

For the preparation of the ninth edition, I am indebted to the many readers of the eighth edition who submitted suggestions, criticisms, corrections, and compliments.

I am particularly indebted to the following radiologic science educators and students for their suggestions for change and clarification. Many supplied radiographic illustrations, and they are additionally acknowledged with the illustration.

Kimberley Adams, Mississippi State University; **Aldo Badano,** Center for Devices and Radiation Control; **Ed Barnes,** Medical Technology Management Institute; **Tammy Bauman,** Banner Thunderbird Medical Center; **Richard Bayless,** University of Montana; **Stephenie Belella,** CDRH; **Ronald Bresell,** University of Wisconsin; **Jeffrey Brown,** Kaiser Permanente; **Barry Burns,** UNC School of Medicine; **Quinn Carroll,** Midland Community College; **David Clayton,** MD Anderson Cancer Center; **Suzanne Crandall,** Mercy College of Health Sciences; **Mike Emory,** Sandhills Community College; **Michael Flynn,** Henry Ford Health System; **Eugene Frank,** Riverland Community College; **Brian Fraser,** Gateway Community College; **Roger Friemark,** Oregon Imaging Centers; **Camille Gaudet,** Hospital Regional Dumant; **Tim Gienapp,** Apollo College; **Ed Goldschmidt,** New Jersey Medical College; **Jeff Hamzeh,** Keiser College; **Phil Heintz,** University of New Mexico; **Linda Holden,** Laramie County Community College; **Cheryl Kates,** MGH Institute of Health Professions; **Diane Kawamura,** Weber State University; **Sonny La,** Sweden; **Kent Lambert,** Drexel University; **John Lampignano,** Gateway Community College; **Pam Lee,** Tacoma Community College; **Kurt Loveland,** Drexel University; **David Ludema,** Delaware Technical and Community College; **Robert Luke,** Boise State University; **Starla Mason,** Laramie County Community College; **John Mayes,** Military Continuing Education; **Rita McLaughlin,** British Columbia Institute of Technology; **Rene Michel,** VA San Diego Healthcare System; **Norman Miller,** CDRH; **Rex Miller,** Lansing Community College; **Ryan Minic,** Pima Medical Institute; **Glen Mitchell,** Laughlin Memorial Hospital; **Mary Jane Reynolds,** Citizens Medical Center; **Rita Robinson,** Memorial Hermann Hospital System; **Dorothy Saia,** Stamford Hospital; **Eshan Samei,** Duke University Medical Center; **Ralph Schaetzing,** Agfa; **David Schaver,** NCRP; **Deborah Schroth,** St. Anthony Hospitals; **Euclid Seeram,** British Columbia Institute of Technology; **Susan Sprinkle-Vincent,** Advanced Health Education Center; **Steve Strickland,** Aiken Technical College; **Don Summers,** Athens Technical College; **Rune Sylvarnes,** Norway; **Ian Thompson,** New Zealand; **Kyle Thornton,** City College of San Francisco; **Beth Veale,** Midwestern State University; **Nancy Wardlow,** Tyler Junior College; **Jo Ellen Watson,** Santa Barbara City College; **Judy Williams,** Grady Memorial Hospital; **Charles Willis,** MD Anderson Cancer Center; **Sherrill Wilson,** Brandon Community College; **Ian Yorkston,** Kodak; **Paula Young,** University of Mississippi; **Elvia Zuazo,** Keiser College.

My colleague, Ben Archer, is the author of the Penguin Tale (Chapter 1), which for me has become a particularly effective teaching tool. Special thanks to **Linda Rarey**, MA, CNMT, ARRT at St. Joseph Health System for her excellent and conscientious work on the accompanying Test Bank and PowerPoint presentation.

As you, student or educator, use this text and have questions or comments, I hope you will email me at *sbushong@bcm.edu* so that together we can strive to make this very difficult material easier to learn.

"Physics is fun" is the motto of my radiologic science courses, and I believe this text will help make physics enjoyable for the student radiologic technologist.

Stewart Carlyle Bushong

Contents

PART I

RADIOLOGIC PHYSICS

1   Concepts of Radiologic Science, 2
2   Fundamentals of Radiologic Science, 16
3   The Structure of Matter, 37
4   Electromagnetic Energy, 56
5   Electricity, Magnetism, and Electromagnetism, 72

PART II

THE X-RAY BEAM

6   The X-ray Imaging System, 100
7   The X-ray Tube, 119
8   X-ray Production, 138
9   X-ray Emission, 151
10   X-ray Interaction With Matter, 162

PART III

THE RADIOGRAPH

11   Radiographic Film, 180
12   Processing the Latent Image, 193
13   Radiographic Intensifying Screens, 207
14   Control of Scatter Radiation, 223
15   Radiographic Technique, 244
16   Image Quality, 272
17   Image Artifacts, 297
18   Quality Control, 304

PART IV

ADVANCED X-RAY IMAGING

19   Mammography, 318
20   Mammography Quality Control, 331
21   Fluoroscopy, 346
22   Interventional Radiology, 360
23   Multislice Spiral Computed Tomography, 367

PART V

DIGITAL IMAGING

24   Computer Science, 396
25   Computed Radiography, 412
26   Digital Radiography, 426
27   Digital Fluoroscopy, 436
28   The Digital Image, 449
29   Viewing the Digital Image, 466
30   Digital Display Quality Control, 478
31   Digital Image Artifacts, 486

PART VI

RADIOBIOLOGY

32   Human Biology, 500
33   Fundamental Principles of Radiobiology, 512
34   Molecular and Cellular Radiobiology, 520
35   Early Effects of Radiation, 534
36   Late Effects of Radiation, 549

PART VII

RADIATION PROTECTION

37   Health Physics, 570
38   Designing for Radiation Protection, 580
39   Patient Radiation Dose Management, 597
40   Occupational Radiation Dose Management, 613

GLOSSARY, 631

ILLUSTRATION CREDITS, 651

PART I

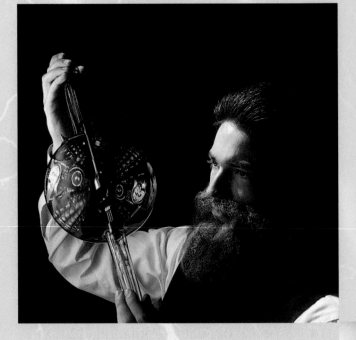

RADIOLOGIC PHYSICS

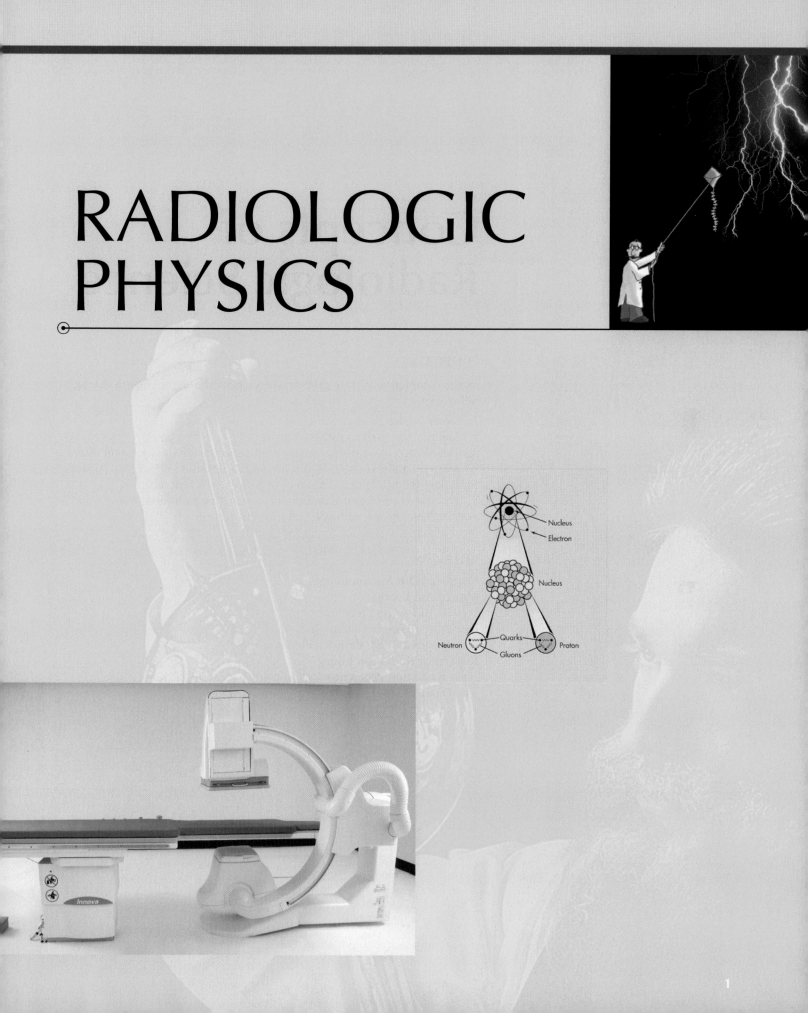

Nucleus
Electron
Nucleus
Neutron
Quarks
Gluons
Proton

Concepts of Radiologic Science

OBJECTIVES

At the completion of this chapter, the student should be able to do the following:

1. Describe the characteristics of matter and energy
2. Identify the various forms of energy
3. Define electromagnetic radiation and specifically ionizing radiation
4. State the relative intensity of ionizing radiation from various sources
5. Relate the accidental discovery of x-rays by Roentgen
6. Discuss examples of human injury caused by radiation
7. List the concepts of basic radiation protection

OUTLINE

Nature of Our Surroundings
Matter and Energy
Sources of Ionizing Radiation
Discovery of X-rays
Development of Modern Radiology
Reports of Radiation Injury
Basic Radiation Protection
The Diagnostic Imaging Team

THIS CHAPTER explores the basic concepts of the science and technology of x-ray imaging. These include the study of matter, energy, the electromagnetic spectrum, and ionizing radiation. The production and use of ionizing radiation as a diagnostic tool serve as the basis for radiography. Radiologic technologists who deal specifically with x-ray imaging are radiographers. Radiographers have a great responsibility in performing x-ray examinations in accordance with established radiation protection standards for the safety of patients and medical personnel. Radiography is a career choice with great, yet diverse, opportunities. Welcome to the field of medical imaging!

NATURE OF OUR SURROUNDINGS

In a physical analysis, all things can be classified as matter or energy. Matter is anything that occupies space and has mass. It is the material substance of which physical objects are composed. All matter is composed of fundamental building blocks called *atoms*, which are arranged in various complex ways. These atomic arrangements are considered at great length in Chapter 3.

A primary, distinguishing characteristic of matter is **mass,** the quantity of matter contained in any physical object. We generally use the term *weight* when describing the mass of an object, and for our purposes, we may consider mass and weight to be the same. Remember, however, that in the strictest sense they are not the same. Mass is actually described by its energy equivalence, whereas weight is the force exerted on a body under the influence of gravity.

> Mass is the quantity of matter as described by its energy equivalence.

Mass is measured in kilograms (kg). For example, on Earth, a 200-lb (91-kg) man weighs more than a 120-lb (55-kg) woman. This occurs because of the mutual attraction, called *gravity*, between the Earth's mass and the mass of the man or woman. On the moon, the man and the woman would weigh only about one-sixth what they weigh on Earth because the mass of the moon is much less than that of the Earth. However, the mass of the man and the woman remains unchanged at 91 kg and 55 kg, respectively.

MATTER AND ENERGY

Matter is anything that occupies space. It is the material substance with mass of which physical objects are composed. The fundamental, complex building blocks of matter are **atoms** and **molecules.** The kilogram, the scientific unit of mass, is unrelated to gravitational effects. The prefix **kilo** stands for 1000; a kilogram (kg) is equal to 1000 grams (g).

A Penguin Tale by Benjamin Archer

In the vast and beautiful expanse of the Antarctic region, there was once a great, isolated iceberg floating in the serene sea. Because of its location and accessibility, the great iceberg became a Mecca for penguins from the entire area. As more and more penguins flocked to their new home and began to cover the slopes of the ice field, the iceberg began to sink further and further into the sea. Penguins kept climbing on, forcing others off the iceberg and back into the ocean. Soon, the iceberg became nearly submerged owing to the sheer number of penguins that attempted to take up residence there.

Moral: The **PENGUIN** represents an important fact or bit of information that we must learn to understand a subject. The brain, similar to the iceberg, can retain only so much information before it becomes overloaded. When this happens, concepts begin to become dislodged, like penguins from the sinking iceberg. So, the key to learning is to reserve space for true "penguins" to fill the valuable and limited confines of our brains. Thus, key points in this book are highlighted and referred to as **"PENGUINS."**

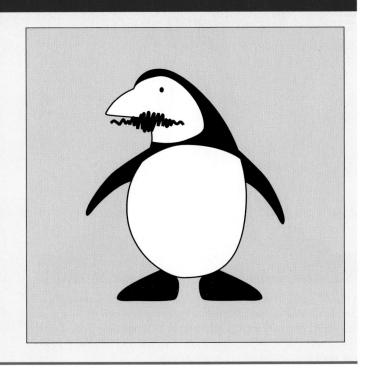

Although mass, the quantity of matter, remains unchanged regardless of its state, it can be transformed from one size, shape, and form to another. Consider a 1-kg block of ice, in which shape changes as the block of ice melts into a puddle of water. If the puddle is allowed to dry, the water apparently disappears entirely. We know, however, that the ice is transformed from a solid state to a liquid state, and that liquid water becomes water vapor suspended in air. If we could gather all the molecules that make up the ice, the water, and the water vapor and measure their masses, we would find that each form has the same mass.

Similar to matter, energy can exist in several forms. In the International System (SI), energy is measured in joules (J). In radiology, the unit electron volt (eV) is often used.

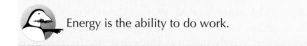

Energy is the ability to do work.

Potential energy is the ability to do work by virtue of position. A guillotine blade held aloft by a rope and pulley is an example of an object that possesses potential energy (Figure 1-1). If the rope is cut, the blade will descend and do its ghastly task. Work was required to get the blade to its high position, and because of this position, the blade is said to possess potential energy. Other examples of objects that possess potential energy

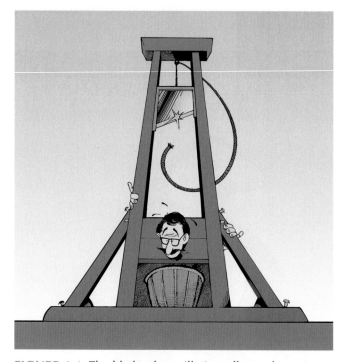

FIGURE 1-1 The blade of a guillotine offers a dramatic example of both potential and kinetic energy. When the blade is pulled to its maximum height and is locked into place, it has potential energy. When the blade is allowed to fall, the potential energy is released as kinetic energy.

include a roller coaster on top of the incline and the stretched spring of an open screen door.

Kinetic energy is the energy of motion. It is possessed by all matter in motion: a moving automobile, a turning windmill wheel, a falling guillotine blade. These systems can all do work because of their motion.

Chemical energy is the energy released by a chemical reaction. An important example of this type of energy is that which is provided to our bodies through chemical reactions involving the foods we eat. At the molecular level, this area of science is called **biochemistry.** The energy released when dynamite explodes is a more dramatic example of chemical energy.

Electrical energy represents the work that can be done when an electron moves through an electric potential difference (voltage). The most familiar form of electrical energy is normal household electricity, which involves the movement of electrons through a copper wire by an electric potential difference of 110 volts (V). All electric apparatus, such as motors, heaters, and blowers, function through the use of electrical energy.

Thermal energy (**heat**) is the energy of motion at the molecular level. It is the kinetic energy of molecules and is closely related to temperature. The faster the molecules of a substance are vibrating, the more thermal energy the substance has and the higher is its temperature.

Nuclear energy is the energy that is contained within the nucleus of an atom. We control the release and use of this type of energy in electric nuclear power plants. An example of the uncontrolled release of nuclear energy is the atomic bomb.

Electromagnetic energy is perhaps the least familiar form of energy. It is the most important for our purposes, however, because it is the type of energy that is used in an x-ray. In addition to x-rays, electromagnetic energy includes radio waves, microwaves, and ultraviolet, infrared, and visible light.

Just as matter can be transformed from one size, shape, and form to another, so energy can be transformed from one type to another. In radiology, for example, electrical energy in the x-ray imaging system is used to produce electromagnetic energy (the x-ray), which then is converted to chemical energy in the radiographic film.

Reconsider now the statement that all things can be classified as matter or energy. Look around you and think of absolutely anything, and you should be convinced of this statement. You should be able to classify anything as matter, energy, or both. Frequently, matter and energy exist side by side—a moving automobile has mass and kinetic energy; boiling water has mass and thermal energy; the Leaning Tower of Pisa has mass and potential energy.

Perhaps the strangest property associated with matter and energy is that they are interchangeable, a characteristic first described by Albert Einstein in his famous theory of relativity. Einstein's **mass-energy equivalence** equation is a cornerstone of that theory.

Mass-Energy

$E = mc^2$

where E is energy, m is mass, and c is the speed of light in a vacuum.

This mass-energy equivalence serves as the basis for the atomic bomb, nuclear power plants, and certain nuclear medicine imaging techniques.

Energy emitted and transferred through space is called **radiation.** When a piano string vibrates, it is said to radiate sound; the sound is a form of radiation. Ripples or waves radiate from the point where a pebble is dropped into a still pond. Visible light, a form of electromagnetic energy, is radiated by the sun and often is called **electromagnetic radiation.** In fact, electromagnetic energy that travels through space is usually referred to as electromagnetic radiation or, simply, **radiation.**

 Radiation is the transfer of energy.

Matter that intercepts radiation and absorbs part or all of it is said to be **exposed** or **irradiated.** Spending a day at the beach exposes you to ultraviolet light. Ultraviolet light is the type of radiation that causes sunburn. During a radiographic examination, the patient is exposed to x-rays. **The patient is said to be irradiated.**

Ionizing radiation is a special type of radiation that includes x-rays. Ionizing radiation is any type of radiation that is capable of removing an orbital electron from the atom with which it interacts (Figure 1-2). This type of interaction between radiation and matter is called **ionization.** Ionization occurs when an x-ray passes close to an orbital electron of an atom and transfers sufficient energy to the electron to remove it from the atom. The ionizing radiation may interact with and ionize additional atoms. The orbital electron and the atom from which it was separated are called an **ion pair.** The electron is a negative ion and the remaining atom is a positive ion.

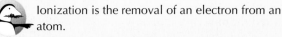 Ionization is the removal of an electron from an atom.

Thus any type of energy that is capable of ionizing matter is known as ionizing radiation. X-rays, gamma rays, and ultraviolet light are the only forms of electromagnetic radiation with sufficient energy to ionize. Some fast-moving particles (particles with high kinetic energy) are also capable of ionization. Examples of particle-type ionizing radiation are alpha and beta particles (see Chapter 3). Although alpha and beta particles are sometimes called *rays,* this designation is incorrect.

SOURCES OF IONIZING RADIATION

Many types of radiation are harmless, but ionizing radiation can injure humans. We are exposed to many sources of ionizing radiation (Figure 1-3). These sources can be divided into two main categories: **natural environmental radiation** and **man-made radiation.**

Natural environmental radiation results in an annual dose of approximately 300 millirem (mrem) (3 millisievert [mSv]). Man-made radiation results in approximately

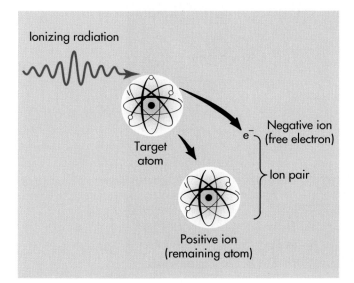

FIGURE 1-2 Ionization is the removal of an electron from an atom. The ejected electron and the resultant positively charged atom together are called an *ion pair.*

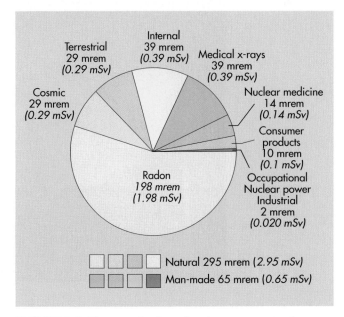

FIGURE 1-3 The contribution of various sources to the average U.S. population radiation dose, 1990.

60 mrem (0.6 mSv). An mrem is 1/1000 of a **rem.** The rem is the unit of radiation equivalent man. It is used to express radiation exposure of populations (see Chapter 2).

Natural environmental radiation consists of three components: **cosmic rays, terrestrial radiation,** and **internally deposited radionuclides.** Cosmic rays are particulate and electromagnetic radiation emitted by the sun and stars. On Earth, the intensity of cosmic radiation increases with altitude and latitude. Terrestrial radiation results from deposits of uranium, thorium, and other radionuclides in the Earth. The intensity is highly dependent on the geology of the local area. Internally deposited radionuclides, mainly potassium-40 (^{40}K), are natural metabolites. They have always been with us and contribute an equal dose to each of us.

The largest source of natural environmental radiation is **radon.** Radon is a radioactive gas that is produced by the natural radioactive decay of uranium, which is present in trace quantities in the Earth. All Earth-based materials, such as concrete, bricks, and gypsum wallboard, contain radon. Radon emits alpha particles, which are not penetrating, and therefore contributes a radiation dose only to the lung.

Collectively, these sources of natural environmental radiation result in approximately 2 to 10 microroentgens (μR)/hr at waist level in the United States (Figure 1-4). This equals an annual exposure of approximately 20 milliroentgen (mR)/yr (0.2 milligray [mGy]/yr) along the Gulf Coast and Florida to 90 mR/yr (0.9 mGy/yr) or higher in the Rocky Mountain region.

Remember, however, that humans have existed for several hundred thousand years in the presence of this natural environmental radiation level. Human evolution undoubtedly has been influenced by natural environmental radiation. Some geneticists contend that evolution is influenced primarily by ionizing radiation. If this is so, then we must indeed be concerned with control of unnecessary radiation exposure because over the past century, with increasing medical applications of radiation, the average annual exposure of our population to radiation has increased significantly.

Diagnostic x-rays constitute the largest man-made source of ionizing radiation (39 mrem/yr) (0.39 mSv/yr). This estimate was made in 1990 by the National Council on Radiation Protection and Measurements (NCRP). More recent estimates put this source at nearly 320 mrem/yr (3.2 mSv/yr), with increases due principally to the increasing use of multislice spiral computed tomography (MSCT) and high-level fluoroscopy.

The benefits derived from the application of x-rays in medicine are indisputable; however, such applications must be made with prudence and with care taken to reduce unnecessary exposure of patients and personnel. This responsibility falls primarily on the radiologic technologist because the technologist usually controls the operation of the x-ray imaging system during a radiologic examination.

The currently accepted approximate annual dose resulting from medical applications of ionizing radiation is 50 mrem (0.5 mSv). In contrast to the natural

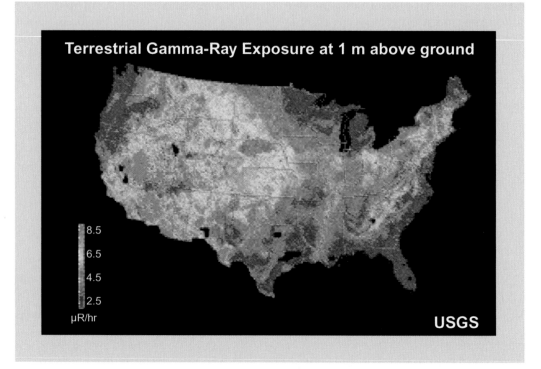

FIGURE 1-4 Radiation exposure at waist level throughout the United States. (Courtesy U.S. Geological Survey.)

environmental radiation dose, this level takes into account people who are not receiving a radiologic examination and those undergoing several within a year.

The medical radiation exposure for some in our population will be zero, but for others, it may be quite high. Although this average level is comparable with natural environmental radiation levels, it is actually a rather small amount of radiation. One could question, therefore, why it is necessary to be concerned about radiation control and radiation safety in radiology.

Question: What percentage of our annual average radiation dose is due to diagnostic x-rays? (see Figure 1-3)

Answer: $\dfrac{39 \text{ mrad}}{360 \text{ mrad}} = 0.108 \cong 11\%$

Other sources of man-made radiation include nuclear power generation, research applications, industrial sources, and consumer items. Nuclear power stations and other industrial applications contribute very little to our radiation dose. Consumer products such as watch dials, exit signs, smoke detectors, camping lantern mantles, and airport surveillance systems contribute a few millirems to our annual radiation dose.

DISCOVERY OF X-RAYS

X-rays were not developed; they were discovered, and quite by accident. During the 1870s and 1880s, many university physics laboratories were investigating the conduction of **cathode rays,** or electrons, through a large, partially evacuated glass tube known as a **Crookes tube.** Sir William Crookes was an Englishman from a rather humble background who was a self-taught genius.

The tube that bears his name was the forerunner of modern fluorescent lamps and x-ray tubes. There were many different types of Crookes tubes; most of them were capable of producing x-rays. Wilhelm Roentgen was experimenting with a type of Crookes tube when he discovered x-rays (Figure 1-5).

On November 8, 1895, Roentgen was working in his physics laboratory at Würzburg University in Germany. He had darkened his laboratory and completely enclosed his Crookes tube with black photographic paper so he could better visualize the effects of the cathode rays in the tube. A plate coated with **barium platinocyanide,** a fluorescent material, happened to be lying on a bench top several feet from the Crookes tube.

No visible light escaped from the Crookes tube because of the black paper that enclosed it, but Roentgen noted that the barium platinocyanide glowed. The intensity of the glow increased as the plate was brought closer to the tube; consequently, there was little doubt about the origin of the stimulus of the glow. This glow is called **fluorescence.**

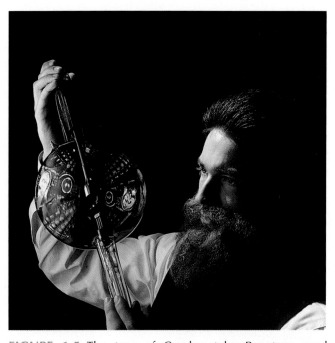

FIGURE 1-5 The type of Crookes tube Roentgen used when he discovered x-rays. Cathode rays (electrons) leaving the cathode are attracted by high voltage to the anode, where they produce x-rays and fluorescent light. (Courtesy Gary Leach, Memorial Hermann Hospital.)

Roentgen's immediate approach to investigating this "X-light," as he called it, was to interpose various materials—wood, aluminum, his hand!—between the Crookes tube and the fluorescing plate. The "X" was for unknown! He feverishly continued these investigations for several weeks.

Roentgen's initial investigations were extremely thorough, and he was able to report his experimental results to the scientific community before the end of 1895. For this work, in 1901 he received the first Nobel Prize in physics. Roentgen recognized the value of his discovery to medicine. He produced and published the first medical x-ray image in early 1896. It was an image of his wife's hand (Figure 1-6). Figure 1-7 is a photograph of what is reported to be the first x-ray examination in the United States, conducted in early February 1896, in the physics laboratory at Dartmouth College.

The discovery of x-rays is characterized by many amazing features, and this causes it to rank high among the events in human history. First, the discovery was accidental. Second, probably no fewer than a dozen contemporaries of Roentgen had previously observed x-radiation, but none of these other physicists had recognized its significance or investigated it. Third, Roentgen followed his discovery with such scientific vigor that within little more than a month, he had described x-radiation with nearly all the properties we recognize today.

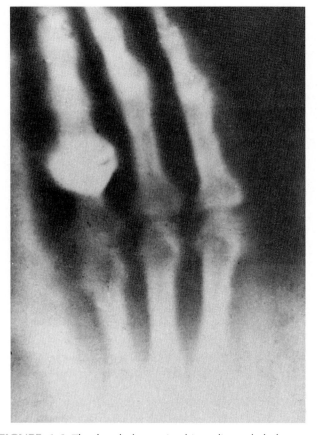

FIGURE 1-6 The hand shown in this radiograph belongs to Mrs. Roentgen. This first indication of the possible medical applications of x-rays was made within a few days of the discovery. (Courtesy Deutsches Roentgen Museum.)

DEVELOPMENT OF MODERN RADIOLOGY

There are two general types of x-ray examinations: **radiography** and **fluoroscopy.** Radiography uses x-ray film and usually an x-ray tube mounted from the ceiling on a track that allows the tube to be moved in any direction. Such examinations provide the radiologist with fixed images.

Fluoroscopy is usually conducted with an x-ray tube located under the examination table. The radiologist is provided with moving images on a television monitor or flat panel display. There are many variations of these two basic types of examinations, but in general, x-ray equipment is similar.

 To provide an x-ray beam that is satisfactory for imaging, you must supply the x-ray tube with a high voltage and a sufficient electric current.

X-ray voltages are measured in kilovolt peak (**kVp**). One kilovolt (**kV**) is equal to 1000 V of electric potential. X-ray currents are measured in milliampere (**mA**), where the ampere (A) is a measure of electric current. The prefix **milli** stands for 1/1000 or 0.001.

Question: The usual x-ray source-to-image receptor distance (SID) is 1 meter. How many millimeters is that?

Answer: 1 mm = 1/1000 m or 10^{-3}, therefore 1000 mm = 1 m.

Today, voltage and current are supplied to an x-ray tube through rather complicated electric circuits, but in Roentgen's time, only simple static generators were available. These units could provide currents of only a few milliamperes and voltages to 50 kVp. Today, 1000 mA and 150 kVp are commonly used.

Radiographic procedures that involve equipment with these limitations of electric current and potential often required exposure times of 30 minutes or longer for a satisfactory examination. Long exposure time results in image blur. One development that helped reduce this exposure time was the use of a fluorescent **intensifying screen** in conjunction with the glass photographic plates.

Michael Pupin is said to have demonstrated the use of a radiographic intensifying screen in 1896, but only many years later did it receive adequate recognition and use. Radiographs during Roentgen's time were made by exposing a glass plate with a layer of photographic emulsion coated on one side.

Charles L. Leonard found that by exposing two glass x-ray plates with the emulsion surfaces together, exposure time was halved and the image was considerably enhanced. This demonstration of double-emulsion radiography was conducted in 1904, but **double-emulsion film** did not become commercially available until 1918.

Much of the high-quality glass used in radiography came from Belgium and other European countries. This supply was interrupted during World War I; therefore radiologists began to make use of film rather than glass plates.

The demands of the army for increased radiologic services made necessary a substitute for the glass plate. The substitute was **cellulose nitrate,** and it quickly became apparent that the substitute was better than the original glass plate.

The **fluoroscope** was developed in 1898 by the American inventor Thomas A. Edison (Figure 1-8). Edison's original fluorescent material was barium platinocyanide, a widely used laboratory material. He investigated the fluorescent properties of more than 1800 other materials, including **zinc cadmium sulfide** and **calcium tungstate**—two materials in use today.

There is no telling what additional inventions Edison might have developed had he continued his x-ray research, but he abandoned it when his assistant and long-time friend, Clarence Dally, suffered a severe x-ray burn that eventually required amputation of both arms. Dally died in 1904 and is counted as the first x-ray fatality in the United States.

Two devices designed to reduce the exposure of patients to x-rays and thereby minimize the possibility of x-ray burn were introduced before the turn of the 20th

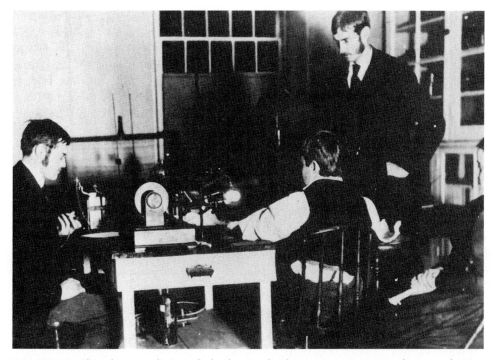

FIGURE 1-7 This photograph records the first medical x-ray examination in the United States. A young patient, Eddie McCarthy of Hanover, New Hampshire, broke his wrist while skating on the Connecticut River and submitted to having it photographed by the "X-light." With him are *(left to right)* Professor E.B. Frost, Dartmouth College, and his brother, Dr. G.D. Frost, Medical Director, Mary Hitchcock Hospital. The apparatus was assembled by Professor F.G. Austin in his physics laboratory at Reed Hall, Dartmouth College, on February 3, 1896. (Courtesy Mary Hitchcock Hospital.)

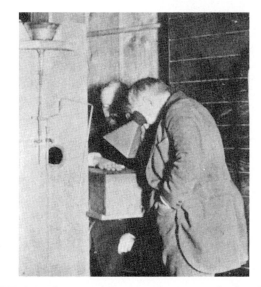

FIGURE 1-8 Thomas Edison is seen viewing the hand of his unfortunate assistant, Clarence Dally, through a fluoroscope of his own design. Dally's hand rests on the box that contains the x-ray tube.

century by a Boston dentist, William Rollins. Rollins used x-rays to image teeth and found that restricting the x-ray beam with a sheet of lead with a hole in the center, a **diaphragm,** and inserting a leather or aluminum filter improved the diagnostic quality of radiographs.

This first application of **collimation** and **filtration** was followed very slowly by general adoption of these techniques. It was later recognized that these devices reduce the hazard associated with x-rays.

Two developments that occurred at approximately the same time transformed the use of x-rays from a novelty in the hands of a few physicists into a valuable, large-scale medical specialty. In 1907, H.C. Snook introduced a substitute high-voltage power supply, an interrupterless **transformer,** for the static machines and induction coils then in use.

Although the Snook transformer was far superior to these other devices, its capability greatly exceeded the capability of the Crookes tube. It was not until the introduction of the Coolidge tube that the Snook transformer was widely adopted.

The type of Crookes tube that Roentgen used in 1895 had existed for a number of years. Although some modifications were made by x-ray workers, it remained essentially unchanged into the second decade of the 20th century.

After considerable clinical testing, William D. Coolidge unveiled his hot-cathode x-ray tube to the medical community in 1913. It was immediately recognized as far superior to the Crookes tube. It was a vacuum tube that allowed x-ray intensity and energy to be selected separately and with great accuracy. This had not been possible with gas-filled tubes, which made standards for techniques difficult to obtain. X-ray tubes in use today are refinements of the **Coolidge tube.**

 Radiology emerged as a medical specialty because of the Snook transformer and the Coolidge x-ray tube.

The era of modern radiography is dated from the matching of the Coolidge tube with the Snook transformer; only then did acceptable kVp and mA levels become possible. Few developments since that time have had such a major influence on diagnostic imaging.

In 1913, Gustav Bucky (German) invented the stationary grid ("Glitterblende"); 2 months later, he applied for a second patent for a moving grid. In 1915, H. Potter (American), probably unaware of Bucky's patent because of the First World War, also invented a moving grid. To his credit, Potter recognized Bucky's work, and the Potter-Bucky grid was introduced in 1921.

In 1946, the light amplifier tube was demonstrated at Bell Telephone Laboratories. This device was adapted for fluoroscopy by 1950. Today, image-intensified fluoroscopy is universal.

BOX 1-1 Important Dates in the Development of Modern Radiology

DATE	EVENT
1895	Roentgen discovers x-rays.
1896	First medical applications of x-rays in diagnosis and therapy are made.
1900	The American Roentgen Society, the first American radiology organization, is founded.
1901	Roentgen receives the first Nobel Prize in physics.
1905	Einstein introduces his theory of relativity and the famous equation $E=mc^2$.
1907	The Snook interrupterless transformer is introduced.
1913	Bohr theorizes his model of the atom, featuring a nucleus and planetary electrons.
1913	The Coolidge hot-filament x-ray tube is developed.
1917	The cellulose nitrate film base is widely adopted.
1920	Several investigators demonstrate the use of soluble iodine compounds as contrast media.
1920	The American Society of Radiologic Technologists (ASRT) is founded.
1921	The Potter-Bucky grid is introduced.
1922	Compton describes the scattering of x-rays.
1923	Cellulose acetate "safety" x-ray film is introduced (Eastman Kodak).
1925	The First International Congress of Radiology is convened in London.
1928	The roentgen is defined as the unit of x-ray intensity.
1929	Forssmann demonstrates cardiac catheterization...... on himself!
1929	The rotating anode x-ray tube is introduced.
1930	Tomographic devices are shown by several independent investigators.
1932	Blue tint is added to x-ray film (Dupont).
1932	The U.S. Committee on X-ray and Radium Protection (now the NCRP) issues first dose limits.
1942	Morgan exhibits an electronic phototiming device.
1942	First automatic film processor (Pako) is introduced.
1948	Coltman develops the first fluoroscopic image intensifier.
1951	Multidirectional tomography (polytomography) is introduced.
1953	The rad is officially adopted as the unit of absorbed dose.
1956	Xeroradiography is demonstrated.
1956	First automatic roller transport film processing (Eastman Kodak) is introduced.
1960	Polyester base film is introduced (Dupont).
1963	Kuhl and Edwards demonstrate single-photon emission computed tomography (SPECT).
1965	Ninety-second rapid processor is introduced (Eastman Kodak).
1966	Diagnostic ultrasound enters routine use.
1972	Single-emulsion film and one-screen mammography become available (Dupont).
1973	Hounsfield completes development of first computed tomography (CT) imaging system (EMI, Ltd.).
1973	Damadian and Lauterbur produce first magnetic resonance image (MRI).
1974	Rare Earth radiographic intensifying screens are introduced.
1977	Mistretta demonstrates digital subtraction fluoroscopy.
1979	The Nobel Prize in Physiology or Medicine is awarded to Allan Cormack and Godfrey Hounsfield for CT.
1980	First commercial superconducting MRI system is introduced.
1981	Slot scan chest radiography is demonstrated by Barnes.

BOX 1-1	Important Dates in the Development of Modern Radiology—cont'd

DATE	EVENT
1981	The International System of Units (SI) is adopted by the International Commission on Radiation Units and Measurements (ICRU).
1982	Picture archiving and communications system (PACS) becomes available.
1983	First tabular grain film emulsion (Eastman Kodak) is developed.
1984	Laser-stimulable phosphors for computed radiography appear (Fuji).
1988	A superconducting quantum interference device (SQUID) for magnetoencephalography (MEG) is first used.
1990	Last xeromammography system is produced.
1990	Spiral CT is introduced (Toshiba).
1991	Twin-slice CT is developed (Elscint).
1992	Mammography Quality Standard Acts (MQSA) is passed.
1996	Digital radiography that uses thin-film transistors (TFTs) is developed.
1997	Charge-coupled device (CCD) digital radiography is introduced by Swissray.
1997	Amorphous selenium flat panel image receptor is demonstrated by Rowlands.
1998	Multislice CT is introduced (General Electric).
1998	Amorphous silicon-CsI image receptor is demonstrated for digital radiography.
2000	The first direct digital mammographic imaging system is made available (General Electric).
2002	Sixteen-slice spiral CT is introduced.
2002	Positron emission tomography (PET) is placed into routine clinical service.
2003	The Nobel in Physiology or Medicine is awarded to Paul Lauterbur and Sir Peter Mansfield for MRI.
2004	Sixty-four–slice spiral CT is introduced.
2005	Dual-source CT is announced (Siemens).
2006	Two hundred fifty six–slice spiral CT is introduced (Toshiba).

Each recent decade has seen remarkable improvements in medical imaging. Diagnostic ultrasound appeared in the 1960s, as did the gamma camera; positron emission tomography (PET) and x-ray computed tomography (CT) were developed in the 1970s. Magnetic resonance imaging (MRI) became an accepted modality in the 1980s, and now, magnetoencephalography (MEG) is being investigated. Box 1-1 chronologically summarizes some of the more important developments.

REPORTS OF RADIATION INJURY

The first x-ray fatality in the United States occurred in 1904. Unfortunately, radiation injuries occurred rather frequently in the early years. These injuries usually took the form of skin damage (sometimes severe), loss of hair, and anemia. Physicians and, more commonly, patients were injured, primarily because the low energy of radiation then available resulted in the necessity for long exposure times to obtain an acceptable radiograph.

By about 1910, these acute injuries began to be controlled as the biologic effects of x-rays were scientifically investigated and reported. With the introduction of the Coolidge tube and the Snook transformer, the frequency of reports of injuries to superficial tissues decreased.

Years later, it was discovered that blood disorders such as aplastic anemia and leukemia were occurring in radiologists at a much higher rate than in others. Because of these observations, protective devices and apparel, such as lead gloves and aprons, were developed for use by radiologists. X-ray workers were routinely observed for any effects of their occupational exposure and were provided with personnel radiation monitoring devices. This attention to radiation safety in radiology has been effective.

Because of effective radiation protection practices, radiology is now considered a safe occupation.

BASIC RADIATION PROTECTION

Today, the emphasis on radiation control in diagnostic radiology has shifted back to protection of the patient. Current studies suggest that even the low doses of x-radiation used in routine diagnostic procedures may result in a small incidence of latent harmful effects. It is also well established that the human fetus is sensitive to x-radiation early in pregnancy.

It is hoped that this introduction has emphasized the importance of providing adequate protection for both radiologic technologist and patient. As you progress through your training in radiologic technology, you will quickly learn how to operate your x-ray imaging systems safely, with minimal radiation exposures, by following standard radiation protection procedures.

One caution is in order early in your training—After you have worked with x-ray imaging systems, you will become so familiar with your work environment that you may become complacent about radiation control. Do not allow yourself to develop this attitude because it can lead to unnecessary radiation exposure. Radiation

BOX 1-2   The Ten Commandments of Radiation Protection

1. Understand and apply the cardinal principles of radiation control: time, distance, and shielding.
2. Do not allow familiarity to result in false security.
3. Never stand in the primary beam.
4. Always wear protective apparel when not behind a protective barrier.
5. Always wear an occupational radiation monitor and position it outside the protective apron at the collar.
6. Never hold a patient during radiographic examination. Use mechanical restraining devices when possible. Otherwise, have parents or friends hold the patient.
7. The person who is holding the patient must always wear a protective apron and, if possible, protective gloves.
8. Use gonadal shields on all people of childbearing age when such use will not interfere with the examination.
9. Examination of the pelvis and lower abdomen of a pregnant patient should be avoided whenever possible, especially during the first trimester.
10. Always collimate to the smallest field size appropriate for the examination.

protection must be an important consideration during each x-ray procedure. Box 1-2 reports the Ten Commandments of Radiation Protection.

 Always practice ALARA: Keep radiation exposures As Low As Reasonably Achievable.

Minimizing radiation exposure to technologist and patient is easy if the radiographic and fluoroscopic imaging systems designed for this purpose are recognized and understood. A brief description of some of the primary radiation protection devices follows.

Filtration

Metal filters, usually aluminum or copper, are inserted into the x-ray tube housing so that low- energy x-rays are absorbed before they reach the patient. These x-rays have little diagnostic value.

Collimation

Collimation restricts the useful x-ray beam to that part of the body to be imaged and thereby spares adjacent tissue from unnecessary exposure. Collimators take many different forms. Adjustable light-locating collimators are the most frequently used collimating devices. Collimation also reduces scatter radiation and thus improves image contrast.

Intensifying Screens

Today, most x-ray films are exposed in a cassette, with radiographic intensifying screens on both sides of the film. Examinations conducted with radiographic intensifying screens reduce exposure of the patient to x-rays by more than 95% compared with examinations conducted without radiographic intensifying screens.

Protective Apparel

Lead-impregnated material is used to make aprons and gloves worn by radiologists and radiologic technologists during fluoroscopy and some radiographic procedures.

Gonadal Shielding

The same lead-impregnated material used in aprons and gloves is used to fabricate gonadal shields. Gonadal shields should be used with all persons of childbearing age when the gonads are in or near the useful x-ray beam and when use of such shielding will not interfere with the diagnostic value of the examination.

Protective Barriers

The radiographic control console is always located behind a protective barrier. Often, the barrier is lead-lined and is equipped with a leaded-glass window. Under normal circumstances, personnel remain behind the barrier during radiographic examination. Figure 1-9 is a rendering of a radiographic/fluoroscopic examination room. Many radiation safety features are illustrated.

Other procedures should be followed. Abdominal/pelvic x-ray examinations of expectant mothers should not be conducted during the first trimester unless absolutely necessary. Every effort should be made to ensure that an examination will not have to be repeated because of technical error. Repeat examinations subject the patient to twice the necessary radiation.

When shielding patients for x-ray examination, one should consider the medical management of the patient. Except for screening mammography, examination of asymptomatic patients is not indicated.

Patients who require assistance during examination should never be held by x-ray personnel. Mechanical immobilization devices should be used. When necessary, a member of the patient's family should provide the necessary assistance.

THE DIAGNOSTIC IMAGING TEAM

To become part of this exciting profession, a student must complete the prescribed academic courses, obtain clinical experience, and pass the national certification examination given by the American Registry of Radiologic Technologists (ARRT). Both academic expertise and clinical skills are required of radiographers (Box 1-3).

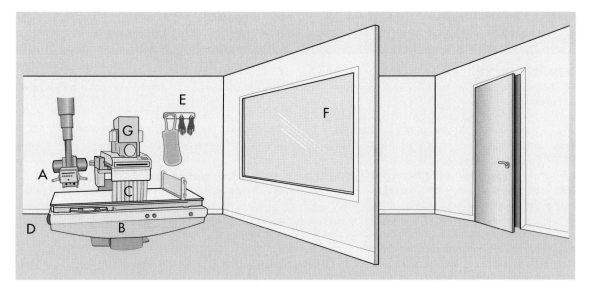

FIGURE 1-9 The general purpose radiographic/fluoroscopic (R&F) imaging system includes an overhead radiographic tube **(A)** and a fluoroscopic examining table **(B)** with an x-ray tube under the table. Some of the more common radiation protection devices are the lead curtain **(C)**, the Bucky slot cover **(D)**, leaded apron and gloves **(E)**, and the protective viewing window **(F)**. The location of the image intensifier **(G)** and of associated imaging equipment is shown.

BOX 1-3 Task Inventory for Radiography as Required for Examination by the American Registry of Radiologic Technologists

PATIENT CARE
1. Confirm patient's identity.
2. Evaluate patient's ability to understand and comply with requirements for the requested examination.
3. Explain and confirm patient's preparation (e.g., dietary restrictions, preparatory medications) before performing radio graphic/fluoroscopic examinations.
4. Examine radiographic requisition to verify accuracy and completeness of information (e.g., patient history, clinical diagnosis).
5. Sequence imaging procedures to avoid effects of residual contrast material on future exams.
6. Maintain responsibility for medical equipment attached to patients (e.g., IVs, oxygen) during radiographic procedures.
7. Provide for patient safety, comfort, and modesty.
8. Communicate scheduling delays to waiting patients.
9. Verify or obtain patient consent as necessary (e.g., with contrast studies).
10. Explain procedure instructions to patient or patient's family.
11. Practice standard precautions.
12. Follow appropriate procedures when in contact with patient in isolation.
13. Select immobilization devices, when indicated, to prevent patient movement.
14. Use proper body mechanics and/or mechanical transfer devices when assisting patient.
15. Before administration of a contrast agent, gather information to determine appropriate dosage, and to discern whether patient is at increased risk for an adverse reaction.
16. Confirm type of contrast media to be used and prepare for administration.
17. Use sterile or aseptic technique when indicated.
18. Perform venipuncture.
19. Administer IV contrast media.
20. Observe patient after administration of contrast media to detect adverse reactions.
21. Obtain vital signs.
22. Recognize need for prompt medical attention and administer emergency care.
23. Explain postprocedural instructions to patient or patient's family.
24. Maintain confidentiality of patient's information.
25. Document required information (e.g., radiographic requisitions, radiographs) on patient's medical record.

Continued

BOX 1-3   Task Inventory for Radiography as Required for Examination by the American Registry of Radiologic Technologists—cont'd

RADIATION PROTECTION

26. Clean, disinfect, or sterilize facilities and equipment, and dispose of contaminated items in preparation for next examination.
27. Evaluate the need for and use of protective shielding.
28. Take appropriate precautions to minimize radiation exposure to patient.
29. Question female patient of childbearing age about possible pregnancy, and take appropriate action (i.e., document response, contact physician).
30. Restrict beam to limit exposure area, improve image quality, and reduce radiation dose.
31. Set kVp, mA, and time or automatic exposure system to achieve optimum image quality, safe operating conditions, and minimum radiation dose.
32. Prevent all unnecessary persons from remaining in area during x-ray exposure.
33. Take appropriate precaution to minimize occupational radiation exposure.
34. Wear a personnel monitoring device while on duty.
35. Evaluate individual occupational exposure reports to determine whether values for the reporting period are within established limits.

EQUIPMENT OPERATION

36. Prepare and operate radiographic unit and accessories.
37. Prepare and operate fluoroscopy unit and accessories.
38. Prepare and operate specialized units.
39. Prepare and operate digital imaging devices.

IMAGE PRODUCTION

40. Remove from patient or table all radiopaque materials that could interfere with the radiographic image.
41. Select appropriate film-screen combination.
42. Select appropriate equipment and accessories (e.g., grid, compensating filters, shielding) for the examination requested.
43. Use radiopaque markers to indicate anatomical side, position, or other relevant information (e.g., time, upright, decubitus, postvoid).
44. Explain breathing instructions before beginning the exposure.
45. Position patient to demonstrate the desired anatomy with body landmarks.
46. Using calipers and technique charts, determine appropriate exposure factors.
47. Modify exposure factors for circumstances such as involuntary motion, casts and splints, pathologic conditions, or the patient's inability to cooperate.
48. Process exposed image.
49. Reload cassettes and magazines by selecting film of proper size and type.
50. Prepare digital/computed image receptor for exposure.
51. Verify accuracy of patient identification on radiograph.
52. Evaluate radiographs for diagnostic quality.
53. Determine corrective measures that should be used if radiograph is not of diagnostic quality, and take appropriate action.
54. Store and handle film/cassette in a manner that will reduce the possibility of artifact production.

EQUIPMENT MAINTENANCE

55. Recognize and report malfunctions in the radiographic or fluoroscopic unit and accessories.
56. Perform basic evaluations of radiographic equipment and accessories.
57. Recognize and report malfunctions in processing equipment.
58. Perform basic evaluations of processing equipment and accessories.

RADIOGRAPHIC PROCEDURES

59. Position patient, x-ray tube, and image receptor to produce diagnostic images of the following:
    - Thorax
    - Abdomen and GI studies
    - Urologic studies
    - Spine and pelvis
    - Cranium
    - Extremities
    - Other: arthrography, myelography, venography....

SUMMARY

Radiology offers a career in many areas of medical imaging, and it requires a modest knowledge of medicine, biology, and physics (radiologic science). This first chapter weaves the history and development of radiography with an introduction to medical physics.

Medical physics includes the study of matter, energy, and the electromagnetic spectrum of which x-radiation is a part. The production of x-radiation and its safe, diagnostic use serve as the basis of radiology. As well as emphasizing the importance of radiation safety, this chapter presents a detailed list of clinical and patient care skills required of the radiographer.

CHALLENGE QUESTIONS

1. Define or otherwise identify the following:
   a. Energy
   b. Einstein's mass–energy equivalence equation
   c. Ionizing radiation
   d. The mrad
   e. The average level of natural environmental radiation
   f. The Coolidge tube
   g. Fluoroscopy
   h. Collimation
   i. The term applied to the chemistry of the body
   j. Barium platinocyanide
2. Match the following dates with the appropriate event:

a. 1901	1. Roentgen discovers x-rays
b. 1907	2. Roentgen wins first Nobel Prize in physics
c. 1913	3. The Snook transformer is developed
d. 1895	4. The Coolidge hot-cathode x-ray tube is introduced

3. Describe how weight is different from mass.
4. Name four examples of electromagnetic radiation.
5. How is x-ray interaction different from that seen in other types of electromagnetic radiation?
6. What is the purpose of x-ray beam filtration?
7. Describe the process that results in the formation of a negative ion and a positive ion.
8. What percentage of average radiation exposure to a human is due to medical x-rays?
9. Why was the discovery of x-rays such an amazing event in human history?
10. Why is radiography now considered a radiation-safe occupation?
11. The acronym ALARA stands for what?
12. Name devices designed to minimize radiation exposure to the patient and the operator.
13. Briefly describe the history of x-ray film.
14. What are the three natural sources of whole-body radiation exposure?
15. What naturally occurring radiation source is responsible for dosing to lung?
16. How would you define the term "radiation"?
17. What are cathode rays?
18. Place the following in chronologic order of appearance:
    a. Digital fluoroscopy
    b. American Society of Radiologic Technologists (ASRT)
    c. Computed tomography (CT)
    d. Radiographic grids
    e. Automatic film processing
19. List five clinical skills required by the ARRT.
20. List five personal skills required by the ARRT.

The answers to the Challenge Questions can be found by logging on to our website at http://evolve.elsevier.com.

Fundamentals of Radiologic Science

OBJECTIVES

At the completion of this chapter, the student should be able to do the following:

1. Discuss the derivation of scientific systems of measurement
2. List the three systems of measurement
3. Identify nine categories of mechanics
4. Calculate problems using fractions, decimals, exponents, and algebraic equations
5. Identify scientific exponential notation and associated prefixes
6. List and define units of radiation and radioactivity

OUTLINE

Standard Units of Measurement
   Length
   Mass
   Time
   Units
Mechanics
   Velocity
   Acceleration
   Newton's Laws of Motion
   Weight
   Momentum
   Work
   Power
   Energy
   Heat

Mathematics for Radiologic Science
   Fractions
   Decimals
   Significant Figures
   Algebra
   Number Systems
   Rules for Exponents
   Graphing
Terminology for Radiologic Science
   Numeric Prefixes
   Radiologic Units

I N CHAPTER 1, matter and energy were defined. Mechanics, which involves matter in motion, is discussed in this chapter. However, when dealing with matter, energy, or mechanics, standards of measurement are required. This chapter also deals with such standards.

The instant an x-ray tube produces x-rays, all the laws of physics are evident. The projectile electron from the cathode hits the target of the anode, producing x-rays. Some x-rays interact with tissue and other x-rays interact with the image receptor, forming an image. The physics of radiography deals with the production and interaction of x-rays.

This chapter defines and illustrates the units of radiation and radioactivity used in medical imaging. To help the reader understand such units, a brief review of mathematics is offered. Emphasis is placed on basic mathematics as it applies to x-ray imaging: number systems, algebra, exponents, and graphing.

STANDARD UNITS OF MEASUREMENT

Physics is the study of interactions of matter and energy in all their diverse forms. Similar to all scientists, physicists strive for exactness or certainty in describing these interactions. They try to remove the uncertainties by eliminating subjective descriptions of events.

Consider, for example, the act of kicking a football. If several observers were asked to describe this event, each would give a description based on his or her perception. One might describe the stature of the kicker and the kicking stance. Another might simply conclude that "a football was kicked about 30 yards" or "the kick was wide left." There could be as many different descriptions as observers.

Physicists, however, try to remove uncertainty by eliminating subjective descriptions such as these. A physicist describing this event might determine quantities such as the mass of the football, the initial velocity of the ball, the wind velocity, and the exact distance the football travels.

Each of these requires a measurement and ultimately can be represented by a number. Assuming that all measurements are correctly made, all observers who use the methods of physics will obtain exactly the same results.

In addition to seeking certainty, physicists strive for simplicity; therefore, only three measurable quantities are considered basic. These base quantities are **mass, length,** and **time,** and they are the building blocks of all other quantities. Figure 2-1 indicates the role these base quantities play in supporting some of the other quantities used in radiologic science.

The secondary quantities are called derived quantities because they are derived from a combination of one or more of the three base quantities. For example, volume is length cubed (l^3), mass density is mass divided by volume (m/l^3), and velocity is length divided by time (l/t).

Additional quantities are designed to support measurement in specialized areas of science and technology. These additional quantities are called *special quantities;* in radiologic science, special quantities are those of exposure, dose, equivalent dose, and radioactivity.

Whether a physicist is studying something large, such as the universe, or something small, such as an atom, meaningful measurements must be reproducible. Therefore, once the fundamental quantities are established, it is essential that they be related to a well-defined and invariable standard. Standards are normally defined by international organizations and usually are redefined when the progress of science requires greater precision.

Length

For many years, the standard unit of length was accepted to be the distance between two lines engraved on a platinum-iridium bar kept at the International Bureau of Weights and Measures in Paris, France. This distance was defined to be exactly 1 meter (m).

The English-speaking countries also base their standards of length on the meter:

$$1 \text{ yd} = 0.9144 \text{ m}$$
$$1 \text{ in} = 2.54 \text{ cm} = 0.0254 \text{ m}$$

In 1960, the need for a more accurate standard of length led to redefinition of the meter in terms of the wavelength of orange light emitted from an isotope of krypton (krypton-86). One meter is now defined as the distance traveled by light in 1/299,792,468 second.

> The meter is based on the speed of light.

Mass

The kilogram was originally defined to be the mass of 1000 cm³ of water at 4° Celsius (° C). In the same vault in Paris where the standard meter was kept, a platinum-iridium cylinder represents the standard unit of mass—the **kilogram (kg),** which has the same mass as 1000 cm³ of water. The kilogram is a unit of mass, whereas the **newton** and the **pound,** a British unit, are units of weight.

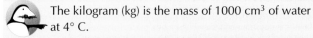

> The kilogram (kg) is the mass of 1000 cm³ of water at 4° C.

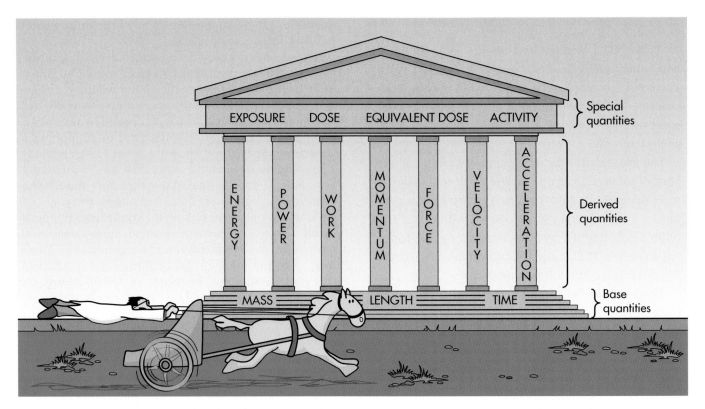

FIGURE 2-1   Base quantities support derived quantities, which in turn support the special quantities of radiologic science.

Time

The standard unit of time is the **second (s)**. Originally, the second was defined in terms of the rotation of the Earth on its axis—the mean solar day. In 1956, it was redefined as a certain fraction of the tropical year 1900. In 1964, the need for a better standard of time led to another redefinition.

Now, time is measured by an atomic clock and is based on the vibration of cesium atoms. The atomic clock is capable of keeping time correctly to about 1 second in 5000 years.

 The second (s) is based on the vibration of atoms of cesium.

Units

Every measurement has two parts: a **magnitude** and a **unit.** For example, the standard source-to-image receptor distance (SID) is 100 cm. The magnitude, 100, is not meaningful unless a unit is also designated. Here, the unit of measurement is the centimeter.

Table 2-1 shows four **systems of units** that represent base quantities. The MKS (meters, kilograms, seconds) and the CGS (centimeters, grams, and seconds) systems are more widely used in science and in most countries of the world than is the British system.

The International System (Le Système International d'Unités, SI), an extension of the MKS system, represents the current state of units. SI includes the three base units of the MKS system plus an additional four. Derived units and special units of the SI represent derived quantities and special quantities of radiologic science (Table 2-2).

Table 2-1	System of Units			
	SI*	**MKS**	**CGS**	**British**
Length	Meter (m)	Meter (m)	Centimeter (cm)	Foot (ft)
Mass	Kilogram (kg)	Kilogram (kg)	Gram (g)	Pound (lb)†
Time	Second (s)	Second (s)	Second (s)	Second (s)

CGS, System of centimeters, grams, and seconds; *MKS*, system of meters, kilograms, and seconds; *SI*, International System.
*The SI includes four additional base units.
†The pound is actually a unit of force that is related to mass.

Table 2-2	Special Quantities of Radiologic Science and Their Units	
Radiographic Quantities	Special Units	SI (International System) Units
Exposure	C/kg	Air kerma (Gy$_a$)
Dose	J/kg	Gray$_t$ (Gy$_t$)
Equivalent dose	J/kg	Sievert (Sv)
Radioactivity	s^{-1}	Becquerel (Bq)

 The same system of units must always be used when one is working on problems or reporting answers.

The following would be unacceptable because of inconsistent units: mass density = 8.1 g/ft^3 and pressure = 700 lb/cm^2.

Mass density should be reported with units of grams per cubic centimeter (g/cm^3) or kilograms per cubic meter (kg/m^3). Pressure should be given in Newtons per square meter (N/m^2).

Question: The dimensions of a box are 30 cm × 86 cm × 4.2 m. Find the volume.
Answer: Formula for the volume of an object:
$V = \text{length} \times \text{width} \times \text{height}$
or
$V = lwh$

Because the dimensions are given in different systems of units, however, we must choose only one system. Therefore,
$$V = (0.30 \text{ m})(0.86 \text{ m})(4.2 \text{ m})$$
$$= 1.1 \text{ m}^3$$

Note that the units are multiplied also: m × m × m = m^3.

Question: Find the mass density of a ball with a volume of 200 cm^3 and a mass of 0.4 kg.
Answer: D = mass/volume (change 0.4 kg to 400 g)
= 400 g/200 cm^3
= 2 g/cm^3
or (change 200 cm^3 to 2 × 10^{-4} m^{-3})
$$D = \frac{0.4 \ kg}{200 \ cm^3 \times \frac{1 \ m^3}{10^6 \ cm^3}}$$
$$= \frac{0.4 \ kg}{2 \times 19^{-4} \ m^3}$$
$$= \frac{0.4 \ kg}{2 \ m^3} \times 10^4$$
$$= 4000 \ kg/2 \ m^3$$
$$= 2000 \ kg/m^3$$

Question: A 9-inch-thick patient has a coin placed on the skin. The SID is 100 cm. What will be the magnification of the coin?
Answer: The formula for magnification is
$$M = \frac{SID}{SOD} = \frac{source\,to\,image \text{ receptor distance}}{source\,to\,object \text{ distance}}$$
$$M = \frac{SID}{SOD} = \frac{100 \ cm}{100 \ cm - 9 \ in}$$

The 9 inches must be converted to centimeters so that units are consistent.
$$M = \frac{SID}{SOD} = \frac{100 \ cm}{100 \ cm - (9 \ in \times 2.54 \ cm/in)}$$
$$= \frac{100 \ cm}{100 \ cm - (23 \ cm)}$$
$$= \frac{100 \ cm}{77 \ cm}$$
$$= 1.3 \ cm$$

The image of the coin will be 1.3 times the size of the coin.

MECHANICS

Mechanics is a segment of physics that deals with objects at rest (statics) and objects in motion (dynamics).

Velocity

The motion of an object can be described with the use of two terms: **velocity** and **acceleration.** Velocity, sometimes called **speed,** is a measure of how fast something is moving or, more precisely, the rate of change of its position with time.

The velocity of a car is measured in miles per hour (kilometers per hour). Units of velocity in SI are meters per second (m/s). The equation for velocity (v) is as follows:

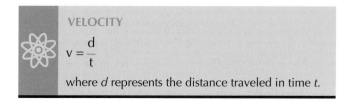

VELOCITY
$$v = \frac{d}{t}$$
where *d* represents the distance traveled in time *t*.

Question: What is the velocity of a ball that travels 60 m in 4 s?
Answer: $v = \frac{d}{t}$
= 60 m/4 s
= 15 m/s

Question: Light is capable of traveling 669 million miles in 1 hour. What is its velocity in SI units?

Answer:
$$v = \frac{d}{t}$$

$$= \frac{6.69 \times 10^8 \; mi}{hr} \times \frac{1609 \; m/mi}{3600 \; s/hr}$$

$$= 2.99 \times 10^8 \; m/s$$

> The velocity of light is constant and is symbolized by c: $c = 3 \times 10^8$ m/s.

Often, the velocity of an object changes as its position changes. For example, a dragster running a race starts from rest and finishes with a velocity of 80 m/s. The **initial velocity,** designated by v_o, is 0 (Figure 2-2). The **final velocity,** represented by v_f, is 80 m/s. The **average velocity** can be calculated from the following expression:

> ## AVERAGE VELOCITY
> $$\bar{v} = \frac{v_f - v_o}{t}$$
> where the bar over the "v" represents average velocity.

Question: What is the average velocity of the dragster?

Answer:
$$\bar{v} = \frac{0 \; m/s + 80 \; m/s}{2}$$

$$= 40 \; m/s$$

Question: A Corvette can reach a velocity of 88 mph in one quarter of a mile. What is its average velocity?

Answer:
$$\bar{v} = \frac{v_o + v_t}{2}$$

$$v = \frac{0 \; mph + 88 \; mph}{2}$$

$$v = 44 \; mph$$

Acceleration

The rate of change of velocity with time is **acceleration.** It is how "quickly or slowly" the velocity is changing. Because acceleration is velocity divided by time, the unit is meters per second squared (m/s²).

If velocity is constant, acceleration is zero. On the other hand, a constant acceleration of 2 m/s² means that the velocity of an object increased by 2 m/s each second. The defining equation for acceleration is given by the following:

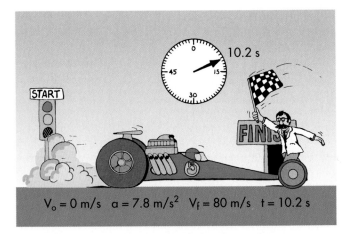

$$V_o = 0 \; m/s \quad a = 7.8 \; m/s^2 \quad V_f = 80 \; m/s \quad t = 10.2 \; s$$

FIGURE 2-2 Drag racing provides a familiar example of the relationships among initial velocity, final velocity, acceleration, and time.

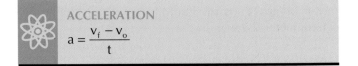

> ## ACCELERATION
> $$a = \frac{v_f - v_o}{t}$$

Question: What is the acceleration of the dragster?

Answer:
$$a = \frac{80 \; m/s - 0 \; m/s}{10.2 \; s}$$

$$= 7.8 \; m/s^2$$

Question: A 5L Mustang can accelerate to 60 mph in 5.9 s. What is the acceleration in SI units?

Answer:
$$a = \frac{v_f - v_o}{t}$$

$$v_f = (60 \; mph \times \frac{1609 \; m}{mi}) \div \frac{3600 \; s}{hr}$$

$$= 26.8 \; m/s$$

$$a = \frac{26.8 \; m/s - 0 \; m/s}{5.9 \; s}$$

$$= 4.5 \; m/s^2$$

Newton's Laws of Motion

In 1686, the English scientist Isaac Newton presented three principles that even today are recognized as **fundamental laws of motion.**

> Newton's First Law: Inertia—A body will remain at rest or will continue to move with constant velocity in a straight line unless acted on by an external force.

Newton's first law states that if no force acts on an object, there will be no acceleration. The property of matter that acts to resist a change in its state of motion is called **inertia**. Newton's first law is thus often referred to as the **Law of Inertia** (Figure 2-3). A mobile x-ray imaging system obviously will not move until forced by a push. Once in motion, however, it will continue to move forever, even when the pushing force is removed, unless an opposing force is present—friction.

 Newton's Second Law: Force—The force (F) that acts on an object is equal to the mass (m) of the object multiplied by the acceleration (a) produced.

Newton's second law is a definition of the concept of **force**. Force can be thought of as a push or pull on an object. If a body of mass *m* has an acceleration *a*, then **the force on it is given by the mass times the acceleration**. Newton's second law is illustrated in Figure 2-4. Mathematically, this law can be expressed as follows:

 FORCE
$F = ma$
The SI unit of force is the **newton (N)**.

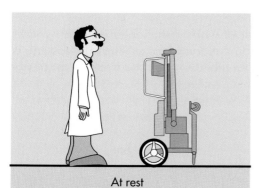

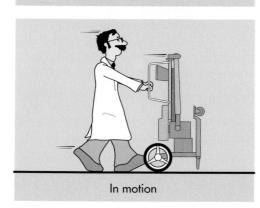

FIGURE 2-3 Newton's first law states that a body at rest will remain at rest and a body in motion will continue in motion until acted on by an outside force.

Question: Find the force on a 55-kg mass accelerated at 14 m/s².

Answer: $F = ma$
(55 kg) (14 m/s²)
770 N

Question: For a 3600-lb (1636-kg) Ford Explorer to accelerate at 15 m/s², what force is required?

Answer: $F = ma$
(1636 kg) (15 m/s²)
24,540 N

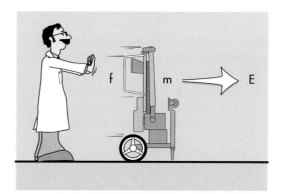 Newton's Third Law: Action/reaction—For every action, there is an equal and opposite reaction.

Newton's third law of motion states that **for every action, there is an equal and opposite reaction**. "Action" was Newton's word for "force." According to this law, if you push on a heavy block, the block will push back on you with the same force that you apply. On the other hand, if you were the physics professor illustrated in Figure 2-5, whose crazed students had tricked him into the clamp room, no matter how hard you pushed, the walls would continue to close.

FIGURE 2-4 Newton's second law states that the force applied to move an object is equal to the mass of the object multiplied by the acceleration.

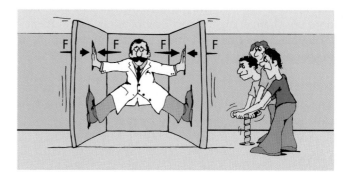

FIGURE 2-5 Crazed student technologists performing a routine physics experiment to prove Newton's third law.

Weight

Weight (Wt) is a **force** on a body caused by the pull of gravity on it. Experiments have shown that objects that fall to Earth accelerate at a constant rate. This rate, termed the **acceleration due to gravity** and represented by the symbol **g,** has the following values on Earth:

$$g = 9.8 \text{ m/s}^2 \text{ in SI units}$$

$$g = 32 \text{ ft/s}^2 \text{ in British units}$$

The value of acceleration due to gravity on the moon is only about one-sixth that on the Earth. "Weightlessness" observed in outer space is due to the absence of gravity. Thus, the value of gravity in outer space is zero. The weight of an object is equal to the product of its mass and the acceleration of gravity.

> **WEIGHT**
>
> Wt = mg
> Units of weight are the same as those for force: newtons and pounds.

> Weight is the product of mass and the acceleration of gravity on Earth: 1 lb = 4.5 N.

Question: A student technologist has a mass of 75 kg. What is her weight on the Earth? On the moon?

Answer: Earth: g = 9.8 m/s²
Wt = mg
= 75 kg (9.8 m/s²)
= 735 N
Moon: g = 1.6 m/s²
Wt = mg
= 75 kg (1.6 m/s²)
= 120 N

This example displays an important concept. The weight of an object can vary according to the value of gravity acting on it. Note, however, that the mass of an object does not change, regardless of its location. The student's 75 kg mass remains the same on Earth, on the moon, or in space.

Momentum

The product of the mass of an object and its velocity is called **momentum,** represented by **p.**

> **MOMENTUM**
>
> p = mv

The greater the velocity of an object, the more momentum the object possesses. A truck accelerating down a hill, for example, gains momentum as its velocity increases.

Momentum is the product of mass and velocity.

The total momentum before any interaction is equal to the total momentum after the interaction. Imagine a billiard ball colliding with two other balls at rest (Figure 2-6). The total momentum before the collision is the mass times the velocity of the cue ball. After the collision, this momentum is shared by the three balls. Thus, the original momentum of the cue ball is conserved after the interaction.

Work

Work, as used in physics, has specific meaning. The work done on an object is the force applied times the distance over which it is applied. In mathematical terms,

> **WORK**
>
> W = Fd

The unit of work is the joule (J). When you lift a cassette, you are doing work. When the cassette is merely held motionless, however, no work (in the physics sense)

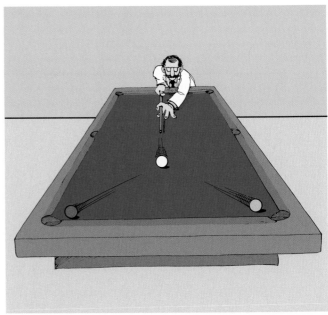

FIGURE 2-6 The conservation of momentum occurs with every billiard shot.

is being performed, even though considerable effort is being expended.

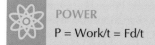 Work is the product of force and distance.

Question: Find the work done in lifting an infant patient weighing 90 N (20 lb) to a height of 1.5 m.

Answer:
$$\text{Work} = Fd$$
$$= (90 \text{ N}) (1.5 \text{ m})$$
$$= 135 \text{ J}$$

Power

Power is the rate of doing work. The same amount of work is required to lift a cassette to a given height, whether it takes 1 second or 1 minute to do so. Power gives us a way to include the time required to perform the work.

POWER
$P = \text{Work}/t = Fd/t$

The SI unit of power is the joule/second (J/s), which is a **watt (W)**. The British unit of power is the **horsepower (hp)**.

$$1 \text{ hp} = 746 \text{ W}$$
$$1000 \text{ W} = 1 \text{ kilowatt (kW)}$$

 Power is the quotient of work by time.

Question: A radiographer lifts a 0.8-kg cassette from the floor to the top of a 1.5-m table with an acceleration of 3 m/s². What is the power exerted if it takes 1.0 s?

Answer: This is a multistep problem. We know that P = work/t; however, the value of work is not given in the problem. Recall that work = Fd and F = ma. First, find F.
$$F = ma$$
$$= (0.8 \text{ kg}) (3 \text{ m/s}^2)$$
$$= 2.4 \text{ N}$$
Next, find work:
$$\text{Work} = Fd$$
$$= (2.4 \text{ N}) (1.5 \text{ m})$$
$$= 3.6 \text{ J}$$
Now, P can be determined:
$$P = \text{Work}/t$$
$$= 3.6 \text{ J}/1.0 \text{ s}$$
$$= 3.6 \text{ W}$$

Question: A hurried radiographer pushes a 35-kg mobile imaging system down a 25-m hall in 9 s with a final velocity of 3 m/s. How much power did this require?

Answer:
$$a = \frac{v_f - v_o}{t}$$
$$a = \frac{3 - 0}{9}$$
$$= 0.33 \text{ m/s}^2$$
$$F = ma$$
$$= 35 \text{ kg} \times 0.33 \text{ m/s}^2$$
$$= 11.6 \text{ N}$$
$$\text{Work} = Fd$$
$$= 11.6 \text{ N} \times 25 \text{ m}$$
$$= 290 \text{ J}$$
$$P = \frac{290 \text{ J}}{9 \text{ s}}$$
$$= 32 \text{ W}$$

Energy

There are many forms of energy, as discussed in Chapter 1. The law of conservation of energy states that **energy may be transformed from one form to another, but it cannot be created or destroyed;** the total amount of energy is constant. For example, electrical energy is converted into light energy and heat energy in an electric light bulb. The unit of energy and work is the same, the joule.

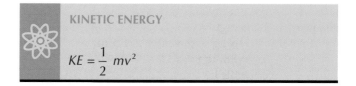 Energy is the ability to do work.

Two forms of **mechanical energy** often are used in radiologic science: kinetic energy and potential energy. **Kinetic energy (KE)** is the energy associated with the motion of an object as expressed by the following:

KINETIC ENERGY
$KE = \dfrac{1}{2} mv^2$

It is apparent that kinetic energy depends on the mass of the object and on the **square** of its velocity.

Question: Consider two rodeo chuck wagons, A and B, with the same mass. If B has twice the velocity of A, verify that the KE of chuck wagon B is four times that of chuck wagon A.

Answer:

$$KE_A = \frac{1}{2}mv_A^2$$ Chuck wagon A:

$$KE_B = \frac{1}{2}mv_B^2$$ Chuck wagon B:

However, $m_A = m_B, v_B = 2v_A$

therefore, $KE_B = \frac{1}{2}m_A(2v_A)^2$

$$= \frac{1}{2}m_A(4v_A^2)$$

$$KE_B = 2mv_A^2$$

$$= 4(\frac{1}{2}mv_A^2)$$

$$= 4\,KE_A$$

Potential energy (PE) is the stored energy of position or configuration. A textbook on a desk has PE because of its height above the floor … and the potential for a better job if it is read? It has the ability to do work by falling to the ground. Gravitational potential energy is given by the following:

POTENTIAL ENERGY

PE = mgh
where *h* is the distance above the Earth's surface.

A skier at the top of a jump, a coiled spring, and a stretched rubber band are examples of other systems that have PE because of their position or configuration.

If a scientist held a ball in the air atop the Leaning Tower of Pisa (Figure 2-7), the ball would have only PE, no KE. When it is released and begins to fall, the PE decreases as the height decreases. At the same time, the KE is increasing as the ball accelerates. Just before impact, the KE of the ball becomes maximum as its velocity reaches maximum. Because it now has no height, the PE becomes zero. All the initial PE of the ball has been converted into KE during the fall.

Question: A radiographer holds a 6-kg x-ray tube 1.5 m above the ground. What is its potential energy?

Answer: PE = mgh
= 6 kg × 9.8 m/s^2 × 1.5 m
= 88 kg m^2/s^2
= 88 J

Table 2-3 presents a summary of the quantities and units in mechanics.

Heat

Heat is a form of energy that is very important to the radiologic technologist. Excessive heat, a deadly enemy of an x-ray tube, can cause permanent damage.

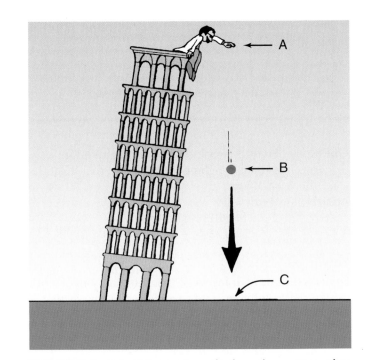

FIGURE 2-7 Potential energy results from the position of an object. Kinetic energy is the energy of motion. **A,** Maximum potential energy, no kinetic energy. **B,** Potential energy and kinetic energy. **C,** Maximum kinetic energy, no potential energy.

For this reason, the technologist should be aware of the properties of heat.

Heat is the kinetic energy of the random motion of molecules.

The more rapid and disordered the motion of molecules, the more heat an object contains. The unit of heat, the **calorie,** is defined as the heat necessary to raise the temperature of 1 g of water through 1° C. The same amount of heat will have different effects on different materials. For example, the heat required to change the temperature of 1 g of silver by 1° C is approximately 0.05 calorie, or only $\frac{1}{20}$ that required for a similar temperature change in water.

Heat is transferred by conduction, convection, and radiation.

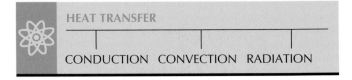

HEAT TRANSFER

CONDUCTION CONVECTION RADIATION

Conduction is the transfer of heat through a material or by touching. Molecular motion from a high-temperature object that touches a lower-temperature object equalizes the temperature of both.

Table 2-3	Summary of Quantities, Equations, and Units Used in Mechanics			
Quantity	**Symbol**	**Defining Equation**	**SI**	**British**
Velocity	v	$v = d/t$	m/s	ft/s
Average velocity	$\bar{v}$	$\bar{v} = \dfrac{v_0 - v_1}{2}$	m/s	ft/s
Acceleration	a	$a = \dfrac{v_1 - v_0}{t}$	m/s^2	ft/s^2
Force	F	$F = ma$	N	lb
Weight	Wt	$Wt = mg$	N	lb
Momentum	p	$p = mv$	kg-m/s	ft-lb/s
Work	W	$W = Fd$	J	ft-lb
Power	P	$P = W/t$	W	hp
Kinetic energy	KE	$KE = \frac{1}{2}\,mv^2$	J	ft-lb
Potential energy	PE	$PE = mgh$	J	ft-lb

Conduction is easily observed when a hot object and a cold object are placed in contact. After a short time, heat conducted to the cooler object results in equal temperatures of the two objects. Heat is conducted from an x-ray tube anode through the rotor to the insulating oil.

Convection is the mechanical transfer of "hot" molecules in a gas or liquid from one place to another. A steam radiator or forced-air furnace warms a room by convection. The air around the radiator is heated, causing it to rise, while cooler air circulates in and takes its place.

Thermal radiation is the transfer of heat by the emission of **infrared radiation**. The reddish glow emitted by hot objects is evidence of heat transfer by radiation. **An x-ray tube cools primarily by radiation.**

A forced-air furnace blows heated air into the room, providing forced circulation to complement the natural convection. Heat is convected from the housing of an x-ray tube to air.

Temperature normally is measured with a **thermometer.** A thermometer is usually calibrated at two reference points—the freezing and boiling points of water. The three scales that have been developed to measure temperature are Celsius (°C), Fahrenheit (°F), and Kelvin (K) (Figure 2-8).

These scales are interrelated as follows:

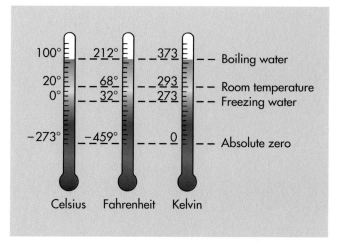

FIGURE 2-8 Three scales used to represent temperature. Celsius is the adopted scale for weather reporting everywhere except the United States. Kelvin is the scientific scale.

Question: Convert 77° F to degrees Celsius.

Answer:
$$T_c = \frac{5}{9}(T_f - 32)$$
$$= \frac{5}{9}(77 - 32) = \frac{5}{9}(45) = 25°\,C$$

One can use the following for easy, approximate conversion:

TEMPERATURE SCALES

$T_c = 5/9\ (T_f - 32)$

$T_f = 9/5\ T_c + 32$

$T_k = T_c + 273$

The subscripts *c, f,* and *k* refer to Celsius, Fahrenheit, and Kelvin, respectively.

APPROXIMATE TEMPERATURE CONVERSION

From °F to °C, subtract 30 and divide by 2.
From °C to °F, double, then add 30.

Magnetic resonance imaging (MRI) with a superconducting magnet requires extremely cold liquids called *cryogens.* Liquid nitrogen, which boils at 77 K, and liquid helium, which boils at 4 K, are the two cryogens that are used.

Question: Liquid helium is used to cool superconducting wire in MRI systems. What is its temperature in degrees Fahrenheit?

Answer:
$$T_k = T_c + 273$$
$$T_c = Tk - 273$$
$$T_c = 4 - 273$$
$$T_c = -269° \text{ C}$$
$$T_f = 9/5 \, T_c + 32$$
$$T_f = -484 + 32$$
$$T_f = -452° \text{ F}$$

The relationship between temperature and energy is often represented by an energy thermometer (Figure 2-9). We consider x-rays to be energetic, although on the cosmic scale they are rather ordinary.

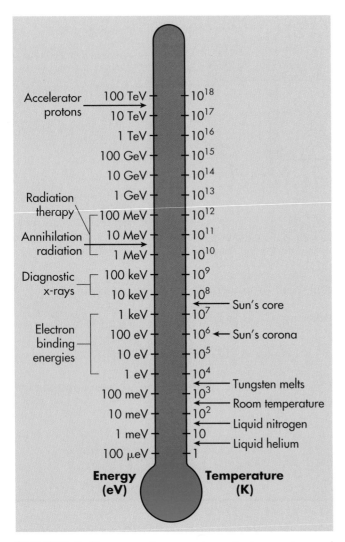

FIGURE 2-9 The energy thermometer scales temperature and energy together.

MATHEMATICS FOR RADIOLOGIC SCIENCE

Physics owes a great deal of its certainty to the use of mathematics, and accordingly, most of the concepts of physics can be expressed mathematically. It is therefore important in the study of radiologic science to have a solid foundation in the basic concept of mathematics. The following sections review fundamental mathematics. You should become proficient at working each type of problem presented in this review.

Fractions

A **fraction** is a numeric value expressed by dividing one number by another; it is also called the *quotient* of two numbers. A fraction has a numerator and a denominator.

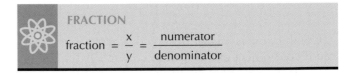

FRACTION

$$\text{fraction} = \frac{x}{y} = \frac{\text{numerator}}{\text{denominator}}$$

If the quotient of the numerator divided by the denominator is less than one, the value is a **proper fraction**. **Improper factions** have values greater than one.

Question: Give examples of a proper fraction.
Answer: $\dfrac{1}{2}, \dfrac{3}{5}, \dfrac{5}{7}, \dfrac{9}{10}$

Question: Give examples of an improper fraction.
Answer: $\dfrac{3}{2}, \dfrac{6}{5}, \dfrac{10}{7}, \dfrac{13}{10}$

Addition and Subtraction. First, find a common denominator, then add or subtract.

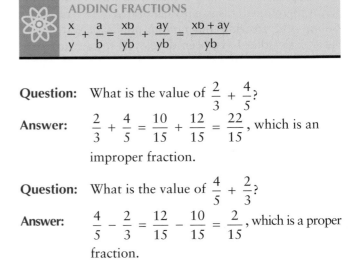

ADDING FRACTIONS

$$\frac{x}{y} + \frac{a}{b} = \frac{xb}{yb} + \frac{ay}{yb} = \frac{xb + ay}{yb}$$

Question: What is the value of $\dfrac{2}{3} + \dfrac{4}{5}$?

Answer: $\dfrac{2}{3} + \dfrac{4}{5} = \dfrac{10}{15} + \dfrac{12}{15} = \dfrac{22}{15}$, which is an improper fraction.

Question: What is the value of $\dfrac{4}{5} + \dfrac{2}{3}$?

Answer: $\dfrac{4}{5} - \dfrac{2}{3} = \dfrac{12}{15} - \dfrac{10}{15} = \dfrac{2}{15}$, which is a proper fraction.

Multiplication. To multiply fractions, simply multiply numerators and denominators.

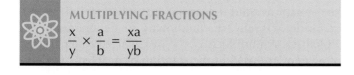

MULTIPLYING FRACTIONS

$$\frac{x}{y} \times \frac{a}{b} = \frac{xa}{yb}$$

Question: What is the value of $\frac{2}{5} \times \frac{7}{4}$?

Answer: $\frac{2}{5} \times \frac{7}{4} = \frac{14}{20} = \frac{7}{10}$, which is a proper fraction.

Question: What is the value of $\frac{9}{8} \times \frac{12}{7}$?

Answer: $\frac{9}{8} \times \frac{12}{7} = \frac{108}{56} = \frac{27}{14}$, which is an improper fraction.

Division. To divide fractions, invert the second fraction and multiply.

DIVIDING FRACTIONS

$$\frac{x}{y} \div \frac{a}{b} = \frac{x}{y} \times \frac{b}{a} = \frac{xb}{ya}$$

Question: What is the value of $\frac{5}{2} \div \frac{7}{4}$?

Answer: $\frac{5}{2} \div \frac{7}{4} = \frac{5}{2} \times \frac{4}{7} = \frac{20}{14} = \frac{10}{7}$, which is an improper fraction.

Question: What is the value of $\frac{3}{10} \div \frac{7}{2}$?

Answer: $\frac{3}{10} \div \frac{7}{2} = \frac{3}{10} \times \frac{2}{7} = \frac{6}{70} = \frac{3}{35}$, which is a proper fraction.

A special application of fractions to radiology is the **ratio**. Ratios express the mathematical relationship between similar quantities, such as feet to the mile or pounds to the kilogram.

Question: What is the ratio of feet to a mile?
Answer: There are 5280 feet in a mile; therefore, the ratio is 5280 ft/mi.

Question: What is the ratio of pound to the kilograms?
Answer: There are 2.2 pounds in a kilogram; therefore, the ratio is $\frac{2.2 \text{ lb}}{\text{kg}}$

Decimals

Fractions in which the denominator is a power of 10 may easily be converted to decimals.

CONVERTING FRACTIONS TO DECIMALS

$$\frac{3}{10} = 0.3 \qquad \frac{161}{10,000} = 0.0161$$

$$\frac{3}{1000} = 0.003 \qquad \frac{1527}{10,000} = 0.1527$$

If the denominator is not a power of 10, the decimal equivalent can be found by division or with a calculator.

$$\frac{5}{12} = \text{(long division equation)}$$

$$\begin{array}{r} 0.41\overline{6} \\ 12\overline{)5.000} \\ \underline{48} \\ 20 \\ \underline{12} \\ 80 \\ \underline{72} \\ 8 \end{array}$$

The bar above the 6 indicates that this digit is repeating. When one divides 5 by 12, the answer is 0.416666.............

Rarely do we convert fractions to decimals without a hand calculator or computer. Depending on the calculator, it is simply a matter of keying numbers in the proper sequence.

Question: What is the decimal equivalent of the proper fraction $\frac{3}{7}$?
Answer: $\frac{3}{7} = 0.429$

Question: What is the decimal equivalent of the improper fraction $\frac{123}{69}$?
Answer: $\frac{123}{69} = 1.78$

Significant Figures

Students often wonder how many decimal places to report in an answer. For example, suppose you were asked to find the area of a circle.

Question: What is the area of a circle with a radius of 1.25 cm?
Answer: $A = \pi r^2$
$= (3.14)(1.25 \text{ cm})^2$
$= (3.14)(1.5625 \text{ cm}^2)$
$= 4.90625 \text{ cm}^2$

This answer is unsuitable because it implies much greater precision in the measurement of the area than we actually have. This result must be rounded off according to specific rules.

In addition and subtraction, round to the same number of decimal places as the entry with the least number of digits to the right of the decimal point.

Question: Add 5.0631, 117.2, and 21.42 and round off the answer.

Answer:

$$
\begin{array}{r}
5.0631 \\
117.2 \\
+\,21.42 \\
\hline
143.6831
\end{array}
$$

Since 117.2 has one digit, 2, to the right of the decimal point, the answer is 143.7.

Question: Solve the following and round off the answer: 42.83 − 7.6147.

Answer:

$$
\begin{array}{r}
42.83 \\
-7.6147 \\
\hline
35.2153
\end{array}
$$

Because 42.83 has two digits, 83, to the right of the decimal point, the answer is 35.22.

In multiplication and division, round to the same number of digits as the entry with the least number of significant digits.

Question: What is the product of 17.24 and 0.382?

Answer:

$$
\begin{array}{r}
17.24 \\
\times\,0.382 \\
\hline
6.58568
\end{array}
$$

Since 0.382 has three significant digits (the zero is not significant) and 17.24 has four, the answer must have three digits. The answer is 6.59.

Question: How would you report the area of the circle discussed previously?

Answer: 4.91 cm^2

Question: What is the quotient of 3.1416 by 1.05?

Answer: $\dfrac{3.1416}{1.05} = 2.992$

Because 1.05 has three significant digits (in this case, the zero is significant because it is followed by a number greater than zero) and 3.1416 five significant digits, the answer must have three digits. The answer is 2.99.

Algebra

Rules of algebra provide definite ways to manipulate fractions and equations to solve for unknown quantities. Usually, the unknowns are designated by an alphabetic symbol such as x, y, or z. Three principal rules of algebra are used in the solution of problems in diagnostic imaging.

When an unknown, x, is multiplied by a number, divide both sides of the equation by that number.

$$ax = c$$
$$\frac{ax}{a} = \frac{c}{a}$$
$$x = \frac{c}{a}$$

Question: Solve the equation 5x = 10 for x.

Answer:
$$5x = 10$$
$$\frac{5x}{5} = \frac{10}{5}$$
$$x = 2$$

When numbers are added to an unknown, x, subtract that number from both sides of the equation.

$$x + a = b$$
$$x + a - a = b - a$$
$$x = b - a$$

Question: Solve the equation x + 7 = 10.

Answer:
$$x + 7 - 7 = 10 - 7$$
$$x = 3$$

When an equation is presented in the form of a proportion, cross-multiply and then solve for the unknown, x.

$$\frac{x}{a} = \frac{b}{c}$$
$$\frac{x}{a} \,\bowtie\, \frac{b}{c}$$
$$cx = ab$$
$$x = \frac{ab}{c}$$

The crossed arrows show the direction of cross-multiplication.

Question: Solve the equation $\dfrac{x}{5} = \dfrac{3}{8}$ for x.

Answer:
$$\frac{x}{5} = \frac{3}{8}$$
$$8x = 3 \times 5$$
$$8x = 15$$
$$\frac{8x}{8} = \frac{15}{8}$$
$$x = 1\frac{7}{8}$$

Often, all three rules may be necessary to solve a particular problem.

Question: Solve $6x + 3 = 15$ for the value of x.

Answer:
$$6x + 3 = 15$$
$$6x + 3 - 3 = 15 - 3$$
$$6x = 12$$
$$\frac{6x}{6} = \frac{12}{6}$$
$$x = 2$$

Question: Solve $\dfrac{4}{x} = \left(\dfrac{3}{4}\right)^2$ for the value of x.

Answer:
$$\frac{4}{x} = \left(\frac{3}{4}\right)^2$$
$$\frac{4}{x} = \frac{9}{16}$$
$$64 = 9x$$
$$9x = 64$$
$$\frac{9x}{9} = \frac{64}{9}$$
$$x = 7.1$$

Question: Solve $ABx + C = D$ for x.

Answer:
$$ABx + C = D$$
$$ABx + C - C = D - C$$
$$ABx = D - C$$
$$\frac{ABx}{AB} = \frac{D - C}{AB}$$
$$x = \frac{D - C}{AB}$$

Note that the first and third of the previous examples are nearly identical in form. Symbols are often used in physics equations instead of numbers.

A special application of fractions and rules of algebra to radiology is the **proportion**. A proportion expresses the equality of two ratios. The ratio of a radiographic grid is directly proportional to the quotient of the height to the interspace between grid lines.

Question: If the grid height is 800 µm and the interspace 80 µm, what is the grid ratio?

Answer: $\dfrac{800\ \mu m}{80\ \mu m} = \dfrac{10}{1}$ the grid ratio.

Sometimes this is written 10:1 and is expressed as "10 to 1 ratio."

The statement "gas mileage is inversely proportional to automobile weight" can be used as a numerical proportion to solve for an unknown quantity.

Question: A 1650-pound compact car gets 34 mpg. What is the expected mileage for a 3600-pound luxury car?

Answer: Set up the inverse proportion as follows:
$$\frac{x}{1650\ lb} = \frac{34\ mpg}{3600\ lb}$$

and use the rules of algebra to solve for x.

$$x = \frac{(34\ mpg)(1650\ lb)}{3600\ lb}$$
$$x = 15.6\ mpg$$

Radiation output is directly proportional to the mAs of a radiographic imaging system.

Question: At 50 mAs, the entrance skin exposure (ESE) is 240 mR (2.4 mGy$_a$). What will be the ESE if the technique is increased to 60 mAs?

Answer: $\dfrac{x}{60\ mAs} = \dfrac{240\ mR}{50\ mAs}$

$$x = \frac{(240\ mR)(60\ mAs)}{50\ mAs}$$
$$x = 288\ mR$$

Number Systems

We use a system of numbers that is based on multiples of 10, called the **decimal system**. The origin of this system is unknown, but theories have been proposed (Figure 2-10). Numbers in this system can be represented in various ways, four of which are shown in Table 2-4.

The superscript on "10" in the exponential form of Table 2-4 is called the exponent. The exponential form, also referred to as power-of-ten notation or scientific notation, is particularly useful in radiology.

Note that very large and very small numbers are difficult to write in decimal and fractional forms. In radiology, many numbers are very large or very small. Exponential form allows these numbers to be written and manipulated with relative ease.

To express a number in exponential form, first write the number in decimal form. If there are digits to the left of the decimal point, the exponent will be positive.

To determine the value of this positive exponent, position the decimal point after the first digit and count the number of digits the decimal point was moved. For example, the national debt of the United States was approximately $9 trillion on November 25, 2007. To express this in scientific notation, we must position the decimal point after the first 9 and count the number of digits that was moved. This indicates that the exponent will be + 12.

United States National Debt = $9,001,574,661,231 = $9.0 × 10^{12}

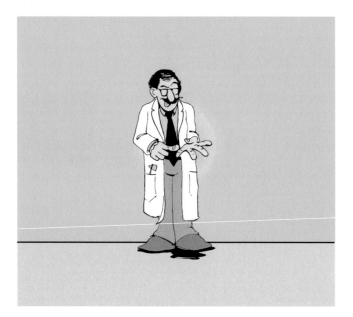

FIGURE 2-10   The probable origin of the decimal number system.

If there are no nonzero digits to the left of the decimal point, the exponent will be negative. The value of this negative exponent is found by positioning the decimal point to the right of the first nonzero digit and counting the number of digits the decimal point was moved.

A string on Robert Earle Keene's guitar has a diameter of 0.00075 m. What is its diameter in scientific notation? First, position the decimal point between the 7 and the 5. Next, count the number of digits the decimal point has moved and express this quantity as the negative exponent.

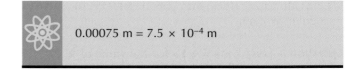

0.00075 m = 7.5 × 10^{-4} m

Another example from physics is a number called **Planck's constant,** symbolized by **h.** Planck's constant is related to the energy of an x-ray. Its decimal form is as follows:

h = 0.000000000000000000000000000000000663 J s

Obviously this form is too cumbersome to write each time. Thus, Planck's constant is always written in exponential form:

$$h = 6.63 \times 10^{-34} \text{ J s}$$

Question: Express 4050 in exponential form.
Answer: $4050 = 4.05 \times 10^3$

Question: Express in exponential form. $\dfrac{1}{2000}$

Answer: First, convert to decimal form.

$$\frac{1}{2000} = 0.0005$$
$$0.0005 = 5 \times 10^{-4}$$

Table 2-4	Various Ways to Represent Numbers in the Decimal System		
Fractional Form	**Decimal Form**	**Exponential Form**	**Logarithmic Form**
10,000	10,000	10^4	4.000
1000	1000	10^3	3.000
100	100	10^2	2.000
10	10	10^1	1.000
1	1	10^0	0.000
1/10	0.1	10^{-1}	−1.000
1/100	0.01	10^{-2}	−2.000
1/1000	0.001	10^{-3}	−3.000
1/10,000	0.0001	10^{-4}	−4.000

Question: X-rays have a velocity of 300,000,000 m/s. Express this in exponential form.

Answer: $300{,}000{,}000 = 3 \times 10^8$ m/s

Question: Dedicated chest x-ray imaging systems used to be installed with a 10-ft source-to-image receptor distance (SID). Express this in centimeters in exponential form.

Answer: $10 \text{ ft} \times \dfrac{12 \text{ in}}{\text{ft}} \times \dfrac{2.54 \text{ cm}}{\text{in}} = 304.8$ cm

$304.8 \text{ cm} = 3.048 \times 10^2$ cm

Actually, today's dedicated chest units are installed at a 3-m SID.

Rules for Exponents

Another advantage of handling numbers in exponential form is evident in operations other than addition and subtraction. The general rules for these types of numerical operations are shown in Table 2-5.

The following examples should sufficiently emphasize the principles involved.

Multiplication. Add the exponents.

Question: Simplify $10^6 \times 10^8$.

Answer: $10^6 \times 10^8 = 10^{(6+8)} = 10^{14}$

Question: Simplify $2^8 \times 2^{12}$.

Answer: $2^8 \times 2^{12} = 2^{(8+12)} = 2^{20}$

Division. Subtract the exponents.

Question: $10^{10} \div 10^2$

Answer: $10^{10} \div 10^2 = 10^{(10-2)} = 10^8$

Question: Simplify $\dfrac{2^3}{3^5}$

Answer: $\dfrac{2^3}{2^6} = 2^{(3-5)} = 2^{-2} = \dfrac{1}{2^2} = \dfrac{1}{4}$

Raising to a Power. Multiply the exponents.

Question: Simplify $(3 \times 10^{10})^2$

Answer: $(3 \times 10^{10})^2 = 3^2 \times (10^{10})^2$

$= 9 \times 10^{20}$

Question: Simplify $(2.718 \times 10^{-4})^3$

Answer: $(2.718 \times 10^{-4})^3 = (2.718)^3 \times (10^{-4})^3$

$= 20.08 \times 10^{-12}$

$= 2.008 \times 10^{-11}$

Note that the rules for exponents apply only when the numbers raised to a power are the same.

Question: Given $a = 6.62 \times 10^{-27}$, $b = 3.766 \times 10^{12}$, what is $a \times b$?

Answer: $a \times b = (6.62 \times 10^{-27}) \times (3.766 \times 10^{12})$

$= (6.62 \times 3.766) \times 10^{-27} \times 10^{12}$

$= 24.931 \times 10^{(-27+12)}$

$= 24.93 \times 10^{-15}$

$= 2.49 \times 10^{-14}$

Graphing

Knowledge of graphing is essential to the study of radiologic science. It is important not only to be able to read information from graphs but to graph data obtained from measurements or observations.

Most graphs are based on two **axes:** a horizontal or **x-axis** and a vertical or **y-axis.** The point where the two axes meet is called the **origin** (labeled 0 in Figure 2-11). Coordinates have the form of **ordered pairs** (x,y), where the first number of the pair represents a distance along the x-axis and the second number indicates a distance up the y-axis.

The ordered pair (3,2) represents a point 3 units over on the x-axis and 2 units up on the y-axis. This point is plotted in Figure 2-11. How does it differ from the point (2,3)? If the value of one additional ordered pair is known [e.g., (8,10)], a straight-line graph can be constructed.

In radiologic science, the axes of graphs are not usually labeled x and y. Usually, the relationship between two specific quantities is desired. Suppose, for example, that you were asked to graph the effect of mAs on optical density (OD), the darkening of a radiograph.

The first step is to draw the axes. In this example, the data are recorded in ordered pairs, where mAs represents the x-value and OD represents the y-value.

Next, note the range of each quantity and choose a convenient scale that allows the data adequately to fill the graph. Then, label the axes and carefully plot each point. Finally, draw the best smooth curve through

Table 2-5	**Rules for Handling Numbers in Exponential Form**	
Operation	**Rule**	**Example**
Multiplication	$10^x \times 10^y = 10^{(x+y)}$	$10^2 \times 10^3 = 10^{(2+3)} = 10^5$
Division	$10^x \div 10^y = 10^{(x-y)}$	$10^6 \div 10^4 = 10^{(6-4)} = 10^2$
Raising to a power	$(10^x)^y = 10^{xy}$	$(10^5)^3 = 10^{5\times3} = 10^{15}$
Inverse	$10^{-x} = 1/10^x$	$10^{-3} = 1/10^3 = 1/1000$
Unity	$10^0 = 1$	$3.7 \times 10^0 = 3.7$

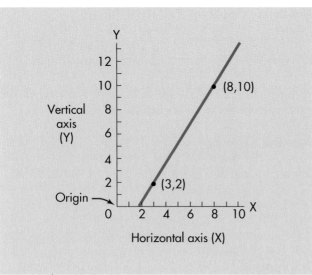

FIGURE 2-11 The principal features of any graph are x- and y-axes that intersect at the origin. Points of data are entered as ordered pairs.

MAS vs. OD	
mAs	**OD**
0	0.15
10	0.25
20	0.46
30	0.70
40	0.91
60	1.24
80	1.45
100	1.60

the points. The curve need not touch each of the plotted points. A completed graph of the preceding data is shown in Figure 2-12.

Question: The following data were obtained from an experiment conducted to determine how much x-radiation it takes to kill 50% of irradiated mice in 60 days ($LD_{50/60}$). Plot these data and estimate the ($LD_{50/60}$).

Radiation Dose (rad)	Number of Mice Irradiated	Number of Mice Dead Within 60 Days	Percentage Lethality
700	36	0	0
750	36	2	6
800	46	5	11
850	36	13	36
900	46	29	63
950	36	31	86
1000	40	37	93

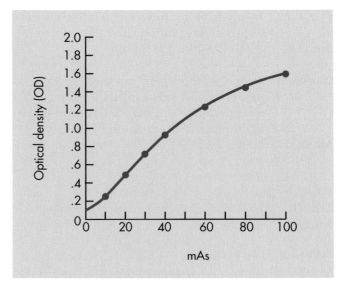

FIGURE 2-12 Relationship of optical density to milliampere seconds from the data presented in the text.

Answer: The columns of data to be plotted are the first and the last. Label the axes so that the range of data is covered. Now, plot the ordered pairs of data and connect them with a smooth curve.

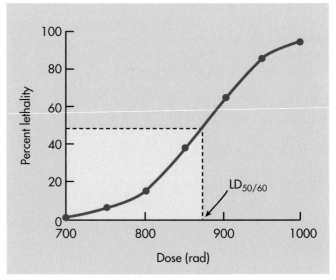

Finally, draw a horizontal line at the 50% lethality level and, when it intersects the smooth curve, drop to the dose axis.

This is the $LD_{50/60}$ for the mice in this experiment (approximately 880 rad). The $LD_{50/60}$ for humans is approximately 350 rad (3.5 Gy_t).

Often the data to be plotted are in scientific notation and therefore extend over a very large range of values. In these situations, a linear scale is not adequate, and a logarithmic scale must be used (Figure 2-13).

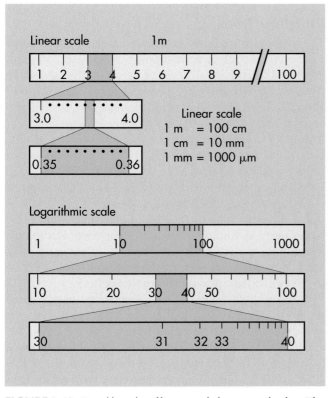

FIGURE 2-13 Equal lengths of linear scale have equal value. The logarithm scale allows a large range of values to be plotted.

Radiologic data frequently require a graph that uses a semilogarithmic scale (Figure 2-14). The y-axis on a semilog scale is logarithmic and is used to accommodate a wide range of values. The x-axis is a linear scale.

Question: The following data were obtained to determine how much lead would be required to reduce x-ray intensity from 330 mR to 10 mR.

Lead thickness (mm)	0	2	4	6	8
X-ray intensity (mR)	330	140	58	25	11

Plot these data on linear and semilog graph paper, and estimate the thickness of lead required.

Answer: From the semilog plot of Figure 2-14, it is easy to see that the answer is 8.2 mm Pb. The linear plot is not so easy to read.

TERMINOLOGY FOR RADIOLOGIC SCIENCE

Every profession has its own language. Radiologic science is no exception. Several words and phrases characteristic of radiologic science already have been identified;

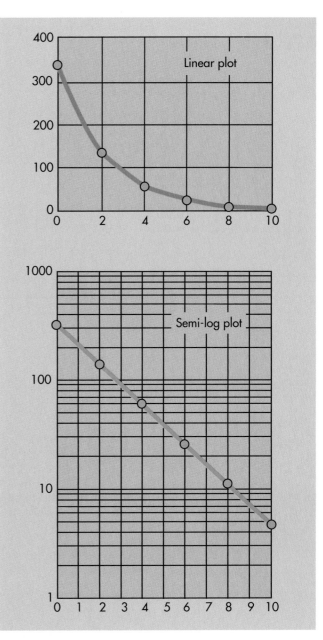

FIGURE 2-14 Semilogarithmic paper is often used for plotting radiologic data.

many more will be defined and used throughout this book. For now, an introduction to this terminology should be sufficient.

Numeric Prefixes

Often in radiologic science, we must describe very large or very small multiples of standard units. Two units, milliampere (mA) and kilovolt peak (kVp), already have been discussed. By writing 70 kVp instead of 70,000 volt peak, we can understandably express the same quantity with fewer characters. For such economy of expression, scientists have devised a system of prefixes and symbols (Table 2-6).

Table 2-6	Standard Scientific and Engineering Prefixes	
Multiple	Prefix	Symbol
10^{18}	exa-	E
10^{15}	peta-	P
10^{12}	**tera-**	**T**
10^9	**giga-**	**G**
10^6	**mega-**	**M**
10^3	**kilo-**	**k**
10^2	hecto-	h
10	deka-	da
10^{-1}	deci-	d
10^{-2}	**centi-**	**c**
10^{-3}	**milli-**	**m**
10^{-6}	**micro-**	μ
10^{-9}	**nano-**	**n**
10^{-12}	pico-	p
10^{-15}	femto-	f
10^{-18}	atto-	a

Boldfaced prefixes are those most frequently used in radiologic science.

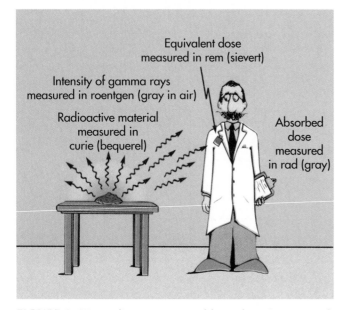

FIGURE 2-15 Radiation is emitted by radioactive material. The quantity of radioactive material is measured in curie. Radiation quantity is measured in roentgen, rad, or rem, depending on the precise use. In diagnostic imaging, we may consider 1 R = 1 rad = 1 rem.

Question: How many kilovolts equals 37,000 volts?
Answer: 37,000 V = 37 × 10^3 V
                = 37 kV
Question: The diameter of a blood cell is approximately 10 micrometers (μ). How many meters is that?
Answer: 10 μ = 10 × 10^{-6} m
                = 10^{-5} m
                = 0.00001 m

Radiologic Units

The four units used to measure radiation should become a familiar part of your vocabulary. Figure 2-15 relates them to a hypothetical situation in which they would be used. Table 2-7 shows the relationship of the customary radiologic units to their International System (SI) equivalents.

In 1981, the International Commission on Radiation Units and Measurements (ICRU) issued standard units based on SI that have since been adopted by all countries except the United States. Most U.S. scientific journals and societies have adopted Le Système International d'Unités (The International System, SI), but regulatory agencies and the American Registry of Radiologic Technologists (ARRT) have not. Consequently, this book uses the customary radiologic units followed by the SI equivalent in parentheses throughout.

Roentgen (R) (Gy_a). The roentgen is equal to the radiation intensity that will create $2.08 × 10^8$ ion pairs in a cubic centimeter of air; that is, 1 R = $2.08 × 10^8$ ip/cm^3. The official definition, however, is expressed in terms of electric charge per unit mass of air (1 R = $2.58 × 10^{-4}$ C/kg). The charge refers to the electrons liberated by ionization.

The roentgen was first defined as a unit of radiation quantity in 1928. Since then, the definition has been revised many times. Radiation monitors usually are calibrated in roentgens. The output of x-ray imaging systems is usually specified in milliroentgens (mR). The roentgen applies only to x-rays and gamma rays and their interactions with air. In keeping with the adoption of the Wagner/Archer method described in the preface, the SI unit of air kerma (mGy_a) is used.

> The roentgen (Gy_a) is the unit of radiation exposure or intensity.

Question: The output intensity of an x-ray imaging system is 100 mR. What is this value in SI units?
Answer: 100 R = 1 Gy_a
                100 mR = .001 Gy_a
                100 mR = 1 mGy_a

Rad (Gy_t). Biologic effects usually are related to the radiation absorbed dose; therefore, the rad is the unit most often used when one is describing the quantity of radiation received by a patient. The rad is used for any type of ionizing radiation and any exposed matter, not just air. One rad is equal to 100 erg/g (10^{-2} Gy_t), where the erg (joule) is a unit of energy and the gram (kilogram) is a unit of mass. The units Gy_a and Gy_t refer to radiation dose in air and tissue, respectively.

Table 2-7	Special Quantities of Radiologic Science and Their Associated Special Units				
	CUSTOMARY UNIT			**SI UNIT**	
Quantity	Name		Symbol	Name	Symbol
Exposure	roentgen		R	air kerma	Gy_a
Absorbed dose	rad		rad	gray	Gy_t
Equivalent dose	rem		rem	seivert	Sv
Radioactivity	curie		Ci	becquerel	Bq
Multiply	R	by	0.01	to obtain	Gy_a
Multiply	rad	by	0.01	to obtain	Gy_t
Multiply	rem	by	0.01	to obtain	Sv
Multiply	Ci	by	3.7×10^{10}	to obtain	Bq

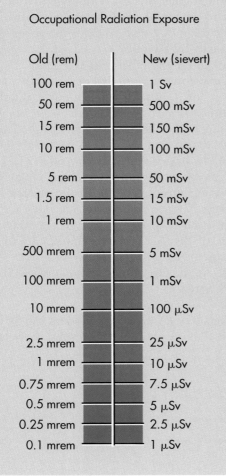

Occupational Radiation Exposure

Old (rem)	New (sievert)
100 rem	1 Sv
50 rem	500 mSv
15 rem	150 mSv
10 rem	100 mSv
5 rem	50 mSv
1.5 rem	15 mSv
1 rem	10 mSv
500 mrem	5 mSv
100 mrem	1 mSv
10 mrem	100 μSv
2.5 mrem	25 μSv
1 mrem	10 μSv
0.75 mrem	7.5 μSv
0.5 mrem	5 μSv
0.25 mrem	2.5 μSv
0.1 mrem	1 μSv

FIGURE 2-16 Scales for radiation equivalent dose.

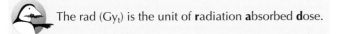 The rad (Gy_t) is the unit of **r**adiation **a**bsorbed **d**ose.

Rem (Sv). Occupational radiation monitoring devices are analyzed in terms of rem (radiation equivalent man). The rem is used to express the quantity of radiation received by radiation workers and populations.

Some types of radiation produce more damage than x-rays. The rem accounts for these differences in biologic effectiveness. This is particularly important for persons working near nuclear reactors or particle accelerators.

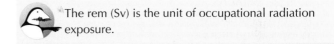 The rem (Sv) is the unit of occupational radiation exposure.

Figure 2-16 summarizes the conversion from conventional units of occupational radiation exposure to SI units.

Curie (Ci) (Bq). The curie is the unit of quantity of radioactive material, not the radiation emitted by that material. One curie is that quantity of radioactivity in which 3.7×10^{10} nuclei disintegrate every second (3.7×10^{10} becquerels [Bq]). The millicurie (mCi) and the microcurie (μCi) are common quantities of radioactive material. Radioactivity and the curie have nothing to do with x-rays.

Question: 0.05 μCi iodine-125 is used for radioimmunoassay. What is this radioactivity in becquerels?

Answer: $0.05 \, \mu Ci = 0.05 \times 10^{-6} \, Ci$
$= (0.05 \times 10^{-6} \, Ci) (3.7 \times 10^{10} \, Bq/Ci)$
$= 0.185 \times 10^4 \, Bq = 1850 \, Bq$

The curie (Bq) is a unit of radioactivity.

Diagnostic radiology is concerned primarily with x-rays. We may consider 1 R is equal to 1 rad is equal to 1 rem ($1 \, mGy_a = 1 \, mGy_t = 1 \, mSv$). With other types of ionizing radiation, this generalization is not true.

SUMMARY

This chapter introduces the various standards of measurement and applies them to concepts associated with mechanics and several areas that are associated with radiologic science. Table 2-3 summarizes the concepts addressed in this chapter. Practice the Challenge Questions using that table as a reference.

The technical aspects of radiologic science are complex. A basic knowledge of mathematics is required, as are identification and proper use of the units of radiation measurements.

As you review this chapter, consider again fraction/decimal conversion, algebraic relations, numeric prefixes/exponents, and graphing. All are important to understanding the principles of radiologic science related to x-ray imaging.

CHALLENGE QUESTIONS

1. Define or otherwise identify the following:
   a. Base quantity
   b. Derived quantity
   c. Special quantity
   d. Inertia
   e. Acceleration
   f. Convection
   g. Work
   h. Velocity
   i. Scalar versus vector quantity
   j. Newton's Second Law of Motion
2. The dimensions of a radiographic cassette are 27 cm × 36 cm × 3 cm. Find the volume.
3. What is the volume of a rectangular radiographic positioning sponge that measure 5 inches by 5 inches by 10 inches?
4. What is the velocity of a ball that travels 50 meters in 4 seconds?
5. What is the velocity of the mobile x-ray imaging system in the hospital elevator if the elevator travels 20 meters to the next floor in 30 seconds?
6. A Corvette can reach a velocity of 88 mph in ¼ mile. What is the average velocity?
7. Moving down a ramp, the C-arm fluoroscope reaches a velocity of 1 ft/s after 5 seconds. What is the average velocity?
8. A 5L Mustang can accelerate to 60 mph in 5.9 seconds. What is its acceleration in SI units?
9. Find the force on a 55-kg object accelerated at 14 m/s².
10. For a 2500-pound (1136-kg) car to accelerate at 12 m/s², what force is required?
11. A professor has a mass of 90 kg. What is his weight on the Earth? On the moon?
12. Find the work done lifting an infant patient weighing 60 N to a height of 2.0 meters.
13. A radiographer lifts a 1.0-kg cassette from the floor to the top of a 1.5-meter table with an acceleration of 2 m/s². What is the power exerted if it takes 1.2 seconds?
14. A rushed radiographer pushes a 25-kg portable down a 50-m hall in 10 s with a final velocity of 10 m/s. How much power did this require?
15. A radiographer holds a 3-kg x-ray tube 2.0 m above the ground. What is its potential energy?
16. Liquid hydrogen with a boiling point of 77 K is used to cool some superconducting magnets. What is its temperature in degrees Fahrenheit?
17. Convert 77° F to degrees Celsius.
18. Convert 80° F to degrees Celsius.
19. What are the four special quantities of radiation measurement?
20. What are the three units common to the SI and MKS systems?

The answers to the Challenge Questions can be found by logging on to our website at http://evolve.elsevier.com.

The Structure of Matter

OBJECTIVES

At the completion of this chapter, the student should be able to do the following:

1. Relate the history of the atom
2. Identify the structure of the atom
3. Describe electron shells and instability within atomic structure
4. Discuss radioactivity and the characteristics of alpha and beta particles
5. Explain the difference between two forms of ionizing radiation: particulate and electromagnetic

OUTLINE

Centuries of Discovery
   Greek Atom
   Dalton Atom
   Thomson Atom
   Bohr Atom
Fundamental Particles
Atomic Structure
   Electron Arrangement
   Electron Binding Energy
Atomic Nomenclature
Combinations of Atoms
Radioactivity
   Radioisotopes
   Radioactive Half-life
Types of Ionizing Radiation
   Particulate Radiation
   Electromagnetic Radiation

THIS CHAPTER diverges from the study of energy and force to return to the basis of matter itself. What composes matter? What is the magnitude of matter?

From the inner space of the atom to the outer space of the universe, there is an enormous range in the size of matter. More than 40 orders of magnitude are needed to identify objects as small as the atom and as large as the universe. Because matter spans such a large magnitude, exponential form is used to express the measurements of objects. Figure 3-1 shows the orders of magnitude and illustrates how matter in our surroundings varies in size.

The atom is the building block of the radiographer's understanding of the interaction between ionizing radiation and matter. This chapter explains what happens when energy in the form of an x-ray interacts with tissue. Although tissue has an extremely complex structure, it is made up of atoms and combinations of atoms. By examining the structure of atoms, we can learn what happens when the structure is changed.

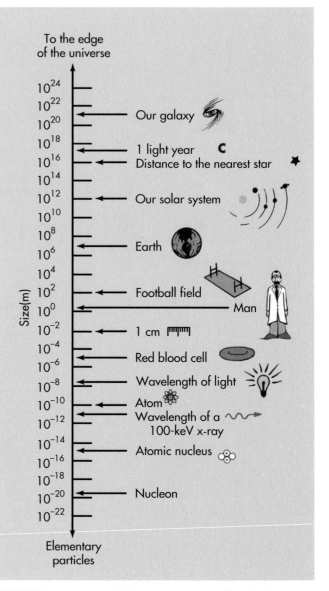

FIGURE 3-1 The size of objects varies enormously. The range of sizes in nature requires that scientific notation be used because more than 40 orders of magnitude are necessary.

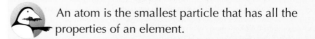

An atom is the smallest particle that has all the properties of an element.

CENTURIES OF DISCOVERY
Greek Atom

One of civilization's most pronounced continuing scientific investigations has sought to determine precisely the structure of matter. The earliest recorded reference to this investigation comes from the Greeks, several hundred years BC. Scientists at that time thought that all matter was composed of four **substances:** earth, water, air, and fire. According to them, all matter could be described as combinations of these four basic substances in various proportions, modified by four basic **essences:** wet, dry, hot, and cold. Figure 3-2 shows how this theory of matter was represented at that time.

The Greeks used the term *atom,* meaning "indivisible" [a (not) + temon (cut)] to describe the smallest part of the four substances of matter. Each type of atom was represented by a symbol (Figure 3-3, *A*). Today, 112 substances or **elements** have been identified; 92 are naturally occurring and the additional 20 have been artificially produced in high-energy particle accelerators. We now know that the atom is the smallest particle of matter that has the properties of an element. Many particles are much smaller than the atom; these are called subatomic particles.

Dalton Atom

The Greek description of the structure of matter persisted for hundreds of years. In fact, it formed the theoretical basis for the vain efforts by medieval alchemists to transform lead into gold. It was not until the 19th century that the foundation for modern atomic theory was laid. In 1808, John Dalton, an English schoolteacher, published a book summarizing his experiments, which showed that the elements could be classified according to integral values of atomic mass.

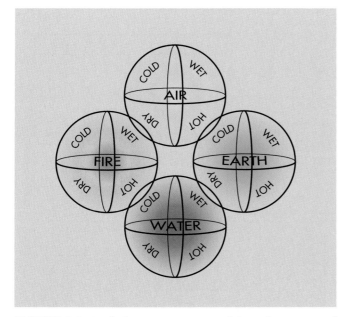

FIGURE 3-2 Symbolic representation of the substances and essences of matter as viewed by the ancient Greeks.

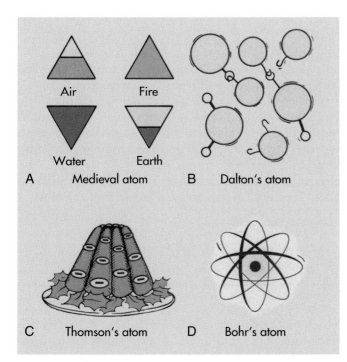

FIGURE 3-3 Through the years, the atom has been represented by many symbols. **A,** The Greeks envisioned four different atoms, representing air, fire, earth, and water. These triangular symbols were adopted by medieval alchemists. **B,** Dalton's atoms had hooks and eyes to account for chemical combination. **C,** Thomson's model of the atom has been described as a plum pudding, with the plums representing the electrons. **D,** The Bohr atom has a small, dense, positively charged nucleus surrounded by electrons at precise energy levels.

According to Dalton, an element was composed of identical atoms that reacted the same way chemically. For example, all oxygen atoms were alike. They looked alike, they were constructed alike, and they reacted alike. They were, however, very different from atoms of any other element. The physical combination of one type of atom with another was visualized as being an eye-and-hook affair (Figure 3-3, *B*). The size and number of the eyes and hooks were different for each element.

Some 50 years after Dalton's work, a Russian scholar, Dmitri Mendeleev, showed that if the elements were arranged in order of increasing atomic mass, a periodic repetition of similar chemical properties occurred. At that time, about 65 elements had been identified. Mendeleev's work resulted in the first **periodic table of the elements.** Although there were many holes in Mendeleev's table, it showed that all the then-known elements could be placed in one of eight groups.

Figure 3-4 is a rendering of the periodic table of elements. Each block represents an element. The superscript is the atomic number. The subscript is the elemental mass.

All elements in the same group (i.e., column) react chemically in a similar fashion and have similar physical properties. Except for hydrogen, the elements of group I, called the alkali metals, are all soft metals that combine readily with oxygen and react violently with water. The elements of group VII, called halogens, are easily vaporized and combine with metals to form water-soluble salts. Group VIII elements, called the noble gases, are highly resistant to reaction with other elements.

These elemental groupings are determined by the placement of electrons in each atom. This is considered more fully later.

Thomson Atom

After the publication of Mendeleev's periodic table, additional elements were separated and identified and the periodic table slowly became filled. Knowledge of the structure of the atom, however, remained scanty.

Before the turn of the 20th century, atoms were considered indivisible. The only difference between the atoms of one element and the atoms of another was their mass. Through the efforts of many scientists, it slowly became apparent that there was an electrical nature to the structure of an atom.

In the late 1890s, while investigating the physical properties of **cathode rays (electrons),** J.J. Thomson concluded that electrons were an integral part of all atoms. He described the atom as looking something like a plum pudding, where the plums represented negative electric charges (electrons) and the pudding was a shapeless mass of uniform positive electrification (Figure 3-3, *C*). The number of electrons was thought to equal the quantity of positive electrification because the atom was known to be electrically neutral.

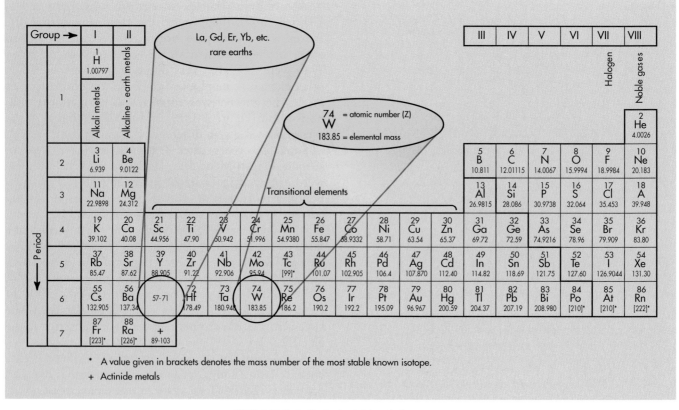

FIGURE 3-4 Periodic table of elements.

Through a series of ingenious experiments, Ernest Rutherford in 1911 disproved Thomson's model of the atom. Rutherford introduced the nuclear model, which described the atom as containing a small, dense, positively charged center surrounded by a negative cloud of electrons. He called the center of the atom the **nucleus.**

Bohr Atom

In 1913, Niels Bohr improved Rutherford's description of the atom. Bohr's model was a miniature solar system in which the electrons revolved about the nucleus in prescribed orbits or **energy levels.** For our purposes, the Bohr atom (Figure 3-3, *D*) represents the best way to picture the atom, although the details of atomic structure are more accurately described by a newer model, called **quantum chromodynamics (QCD).**

Simply put, the Bohr atom contains a small, dense, positively charged nucleus surrounded by negatively charged electrons that revolve in fixed, well-defined orbits about the nucleus. In the normal atom, the number of electrons is equal to the number of positive charges in the nucleus.

FUNDAMENTAL PARTICLES

Our understanding of the atom today is essentially that which Bohr presented nearly a century ago. With the development of high-energy **particle accelerators,** or "atom smashers," as some call them, the structure of the atomic nucleus is slowly being mapped and identified. More than

100 subatomic particles have been detected and described by physicists working with particle accelerators.

Nuclear structure is now well defined (Figure 3-5). Nucleons—protons and neutrons—are composed of quarks that are held together by gluons. These particles, however, are of little consequence to radiologic science. Only the three primary constituents of an atom, the **electron,** the **proton,** and the **neutron,** are considered here. They are the **fundamental particles** (Table 3-1).

> The fundamental particles of an atom are the electron, the proton, and the neutron.

The atom can be viewed as a miniature solar system whose sun is the nucleus and whose planets are the electrons. The arrangement of electrons around the nucleus determines the manner in which atoms interact.

Electrons are very small particles that carry one unit of negative electric charge. Their mass is only 9.1×10^{-31} kg. They can be pictured as revolving about the nucleus in precisely fixed orbits, just as the planets in our solar system revolve around the sun.

Because an atomic particle is extremely small, its mass is expressed in **atomic mass units (amu)** for convenience. One atomic mass unit is equal to one half the mass of a carbon-12 atom. The electron mass is 0.000549 amu. When precision is not necessary, a system of whole numbers called **atomic mass numbers** is used. The atomic mass number of an electron is zero.

The nucleus contains particles called **nucleons,** of which there are two types: protons and neutrons. Both have nearly 2000 times the mass of an electron. The mass of a proton is 1.673×10^{-27} kg; the neutron is just slightly heavier, at 1.675×10^{-27} kg. The atomic mass number of each is one. The primary difference between a proton and a neutron is electric charge. The proton carries one unit of positive electric charge. The neutron carries no charge; it is electrically neutral.

ATOMIC STRUCTURE

You might be tempted to visualize the atom as a beehive of subatomic activity because classical representations of it usually appear like that shown in Figure 3-3, *D.*

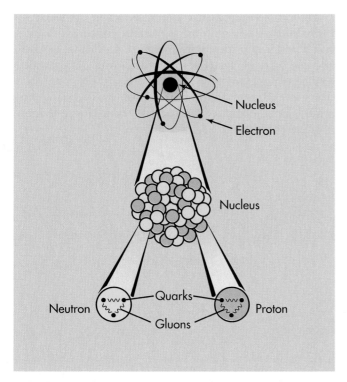

FIGURE 3-5 The nucleus consists of protons and neutrons, which are made of quarks bound together by gluons.

Because of the space limitations of the printed page, Figure 3-3, *D* is greatly oversimplified. In fact, the atom is mostly empty space, similar to our solar system. The nucleus of an atom is very small but contains nearly all the mass of the atom.

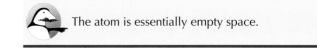

The atom is essentially empty space.

If a basketball, whose diameter is 9.6 in (0.23 m), represented the size of the uranium nucleus, the largest naturally occurring atom, the path of the orbital electrons would take them more than 8 miles (12.8 km) away. Because it contains all the neutrons and protons, the nucleus of the atom contains most of its mass. For example, the nucleus of a uranium atom contains 99.998% of the entire mass of the atom.

Possible electron orbits are grouped into different "shells." The arrangement of these shells helps reveal how an atom reacts chemically, that is, how it combines with other atoms to form molecules. Because a neutral atom has the same number of electrons in orbit as protons in the nucleus, the number of protons ultimately determines the chemical behavior of an atom.

The number of protons determines the **chemical element.** Atoms that have the same number of protons but differ in the number of neutrons are **isotopes;** they behave in the same way during chemical reactions.

The periodic table of the elements (see Figure 3-4) lists matter in order of increasing complexity, beginning with hydrogen (H). An atom of hydrogen contains one proton in its nucleus and one electron outside the nucleus. Helium (He), the second atom in the table, contains two protons, two neutrons, and two electrons.

The third atom, lithium (Li), contains three protons, four neutrons, and three electrons. Two of these electrons are in the same orbital shell, the K shell, as are the electrons of hydrogen and helium. The third electron is in the next farther orbital shell from the nucleus, the L shell.

Electrons can exist only in certain **shells,** which represent different **electron binding energies** or **energy levels.** For identification purposes, electron orbital shells

Table 3-1	**Important Characteristics of the Fundamental Particles**						
			MASS				
Particle	**Location**	**Relative**	**Kilograms**	**amu**	**Number**	**Charge**	**Symbol**
Electron	Shells	1	9.109×10^{-31}	0.000549	0	−1	−
Proton	Nucleus	1836	1.673×10^{-27}	1.00728	1	+1	+
Neutron	Nucleus	1838	1.675×10^{-27}	1.00867	1	0	O

amu, Atomic mass units.

are given the codes K, L, M, N, and so forth, to represent the relative binding energies of electrons from closest to the nucleus to farthest from the nucleus. The closer an electron is to the nucleus, the greater is its binding energy.

The next atom on the periodic table, beryllium (Be), has four protons and five neutrons in the nucleus. Two electrons are in the K shell and two are in the L shell.

The complexity of the electron configuration of atoms increases as one progresses through the periodic table to the most complex naturally occurring element, uranium (U). Uranium has 92 protons and 146 neutrons. The electron distribution is as follows: 2 in the K shell, 8 in the L shell, 18 in the M shell, 32 in the N shell, 21 in the O shell, 9 in the P shell, and 2 in the Q shell.

Figure 3-6 is a schematic representation of four atoms. Although these atoms are mostly empty space, they have been diagrammed on one page. If the actual size of the helium nucleus were that in Figure 3-6, the K-shell electrons would be several city blocks away.

In their normal state, *atoms are electrically neutral;* the electric charge on the atom is zero.

The total number of electrons in the orbital shells is exactly equal to the number of protons in the nucleus. If an atom has an extra electron or has had an electron removed, it is said to be **ionized.** An ionized atom is not electrically neutral but carries a charge equal in magnitude to the difference between the numbers of electrons and protons.

You might assume that atoms can be ionized by changing the number of positive charges as well as the number of negative charges. Atoms, however, cannot be ionized by the addition or subtraction of protons because they are bound very strongly together, and that action would change the type of atom. An alteration in the number of neutrons does not ionize an atom because the neutron is electrically neutral.

Figure 3-7 represents the interaction between an x-ray and a carbon atom, a primary constituent of tissue. The x-ray transfers its energy to an orbital electron and ejects that electron from the atom. This process requires approximately 34 eV of energy. The x-ray may cease to exist and an ion pair is formed. The remaining atom is now a positive ion because it contains one more positive charge than negative charge.

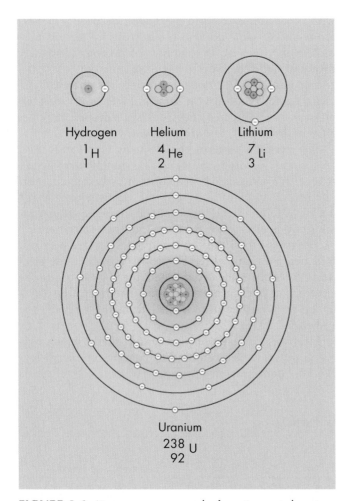

FIGURE 3-6 Atoms are composed of neutrons and protons in the nucleus and electrons in specific orbits surrounding the nucleus. Shown here are the three smaller atoms and the largest naturally occurring atom, uranium.

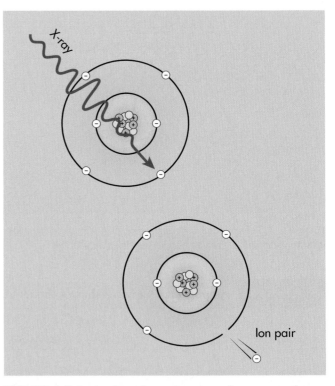

FIGURE 3-7 Ionization of a carbon atom by an x-ray leaves the atom with a net electric charge of +1. The ionized atom and the released electron are called an *ion pair.*

Ionization is the removal of an orbital electron from an atom.

In all except the lightest atoms, the number of neutrons is always greater than the number of protons. The larger the atom, the greater the abundance of neutrons over protons.

Electron Arrangement

The maximum number of electrons that can exist in each shell (Table 3-2) increases with the distance of the shell from the nucleus. These numbers need not be memorized because the electron limit per shell can be calculated from the expression:

MAXIMUM ELECTRONS PER SHELL

$2n^2$

where n is the shell number.

Question: What is the maximum number of electrons that can exist in the O shell?

Answer: The O shell is the fifth shell from the nucleus; therefore:

$$n = 5$$
$$2n^2 = 2(5)^2$$
$$= 2(25)$$
$$= 50 \text{ electrons}$$

This answer, 50 electrons, is a theoretical value. Even the largest atom does not completely fill shell O or higher.

Physicists call the shell number n the **principal quantum number.** Every electron in every atom can be precisely identified by four quantum numbers, the most important of which is the principal quantum number. The other three quantum numbers represent the existence of subshells, which are not important to radiologic science.

Table 3-2	Maximum Number of Electrons That Can Occupy Each Electron Shell	
Shell Number	Shell Symbol	Number of Electrons
1	K	2
2	L	8
3	M	18
4	N	32
5	O	50
6	P	72
7	Q	98

The observant reader may have noticed a relationship between the number of shells in an atom and its position in the periodic table of the elements. Oxygen has eight electrons; two occupy the K shell and six occupy the L shell. Oxygen is in the second period and the sixth group of the periodic table (see Figure 3-4).

Aluminum has the following electron configuration: K shell, two electrons; L shell, eight electrons; M shell, three electrons. Therefore, aluminum is in the third period (M shell) and third group (three electrons) of the periodic table.

ELECTRON ARRANGEMENT

The number of electrons in the outermost shell of an atom is equal to its group in the periodic table. The number of electrons in the outermost shell determines the valence of an atom. The number of the outermost electron shell of an atom is equal to its period in the periodic table.

Question: What are the period and group for the gastrointestinal contrast agent, barium (refer to Figure 3-4)?

Answer: Period 6 and group II.

 No outer shell can contain more than eight electrons.

Why does the periodic table show elements repeating similar chemical properties in groups of eight? In addition to the limitation on the maximum number of electrons allowed in any shell, the outer shell is always limited to eight electrons.

All atoms that have one electron in the outer shell lie in group I of the periodic table; atoms with two electrons in the outer shell fall in group II, and so forth. When eight electrons are in the outer shell, the shell is filled. Atoms with filled outer shells lie in group VIII, the noble gases, and are very stable.

The orderly scheme of atomic progression from smallest to largest atom is interrupted in the fourth period. Instead of simply adding electrons to the next outer shell, electrons are added to an inner shell.

The atoms associated with this phenomenon are called the **transitional elements.** Even in these elements, no outer shell ever contains more than eight electrons. The chemical properties of the transitional elements depend on the number of electrons in the two outermost shells.

The shell notation of the electron arrangement of an atom not only identifies the relative distance of an electron from the nucleus but indicates the relative energy by which the electron is attached to the nucleus. You might expect that an electron would spontaneously fly off from the nucleus, just as a ball twirling on the end of a string would do if the string were cut. The type of force that prevents this from happening is called **centripetal force** or "center-seeking" force, which results from a basic law of electricity that states that opposite charges attract one another and like charges repel.

 The force that keeps an electron in orbit is the centripetal force.

You might therefore expect that the electrons would drop into the nucleus because of the strong electrostatic attraction. In the normal atom, the centripetal force just balances the force created by the electron velocity, the **centrifugal force** or flying-out-from-the-center force, so that electrons maintain their distance from the nucleus while traveling in a circular or elliptical path.

Figure 3-8 is a representation of this state of affairs for a small atom. In more complex atoms, the same balance of force exists and each electron can be considered separately.

Electron Binding Energy

The strength of attachment of an electron to the nucleus is called the **electron binding energy**, designated E_b. The closer an electron is to the nucleus, the more tightly it is bound. K-shell electrons have higher binding energies than L-shell electrons, L-shell electrons are more tightly bound to the nucleus than M-shell electrons, and so forth.

Not all K-shell electrons of all atoms are bound with the same binding energy. The greater the total number of electrons in an atom, the more tightly each is bound.

To put it differently, the larger and more complex the atom, the higher is the E_b for electrons in any given shell. Because electrons of atoms with many protons are more tightly bound to the nucleus than those of small atoms, it generally takes more energy to ionize a large atom than a small atom.

Figure 3-9 represents the binding energy of electrons of several atoms of radiologic importance. The metals tungsten (W) and molybdenum (Mo) are the primary constituents of the target of an x-ray tube. Barium (Ba) and iodine (I) are used extensively as radiographic and fluoroscopic contrast agents.

Question: How much energy is required to ionize tungsten through removal of a K-shell electron?

Answer: The minimum energy must equal E_b or 69 keV—with less than that, the atom cannot be ionized.

Carbon (C) is an important component of human tissue. As with other tissue atoms, E_b for the outer shell electrons is only approximately 10 eV. Yet approximately 34 eV is necessary to ionize tissue atoms.

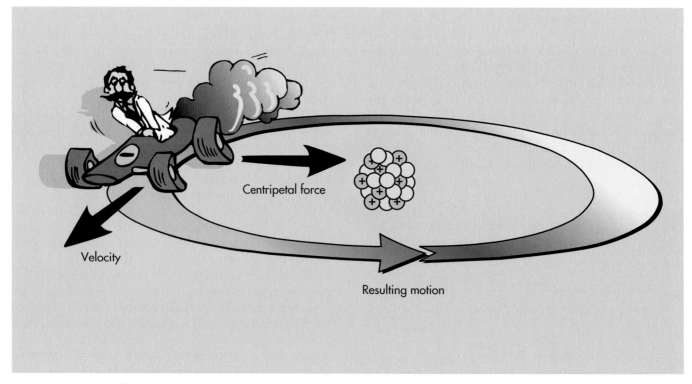

FIGURE 3-8 Electrons revolve about the nucleus in fixed orbits or shells. Electrostatic attraction results in a specific electron path about the nucleus.

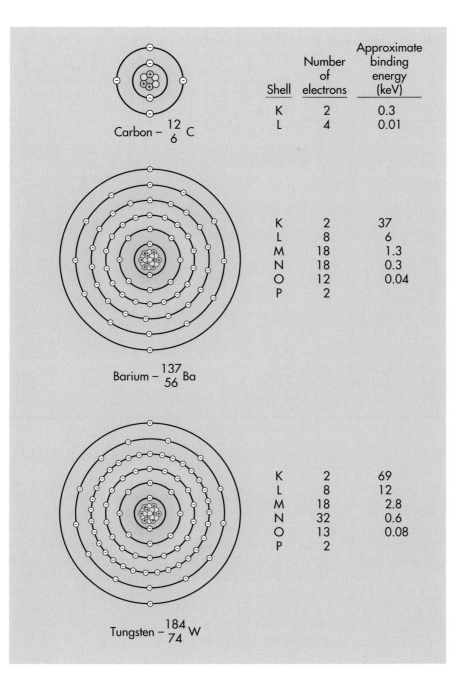

Shell	Number of electrons	Approximate binding energy (keV)
K	2	0.3
L	4	0.01

Carbon – $^{12}_{6}$C

Shell	Number of electrons	Approximate binding energy (keV)
K	2	37
L	8	6
M	18	1.3
N	18	0.3
O	12	0.04
P	2	

Barium – $^{137}_{56}$Ba

Shell	Number of electrons	Approximate binding energy (keV)
K	2	69
L	8	12
M	18	2.8
N	32	0.6
O	13	0.08
P	2	

Tungsten – $^{184}_{74}$W

FIGURE 3-9 Atomic configurations and approximate electron binding energies for three radiologically important atoms. As atoms get bigger, electrons in a given shell become more tightly bound.

The value, 34 eV, is called the **ionization potential.** The difference, 24 eV, causes multiple electron excitations, which ultimately result in heat. The concept of ionization potential is important to the description of linear energy transfer (LET), which is discussed in Chapter 33.

Question: How much more energy is necessary to ionize barium than to ionize carbon by removal of K-shell electrons?

Answer:
E_b (Ba) = 37,400 eV
E_b (C) = 300 eV
Difference = 37,100 eV
= 37.1 keV

ATOMIC NOMENCLATURE

Often an element is indicated by an alphabetic abbreviation. Such abbreviations are called **chemical symbols.** Table 3-3 lists some of the important elements and their chemical symbols.

The chemical properties of an element are determined by the number and arrangement of electrons. In the neutral atom, the number of electrons equals the number of protons. The number of protons is called the atomic number, represented by Z. Table 3-3 shows that the atomic number of barium is 56, thus indicating that 56 protons are in the barium nucleus.

TABLE 3-3	Characteristics of Some Elements Important to Radiologic Science					
Element	Chemical Symbol	Atomic Number (Z)	Atomic Mass Number (A)*	Number of Naturally Occurring Isotopes	Elemental Mass (amu)†	K-Shell Electron Binding Energy (keV)
Beryllium	Be	4	9	1	9.012	0.11
Carbon	C	6	12	3	12.01	0.28
Oxygen	O	8	16	3	15	0.53
Aluminum	Al	13	27	1	26.98	1.56
Calcium	Ca	20	40	6	40.08	4.04
Iron	Fe	26	56	4	55.84	7.11
Copper	Cu	29	63	2	63.54	8.98
Molybdenum	Mo	42	98	7	95.94	20
Rhodium	Rh	45	103	5	102.9	23.2
Ruthenium	Ru	44	102	7	101	22.1
Silver	Ag	47	107	2	107.9	25.7
Tin	Sn	50	120	10	118.6	29.2
Iodine	I	53	127	1	126.9	33.2
Barium	Ba	56	138	7	137.3	37.4
Tungsten	W	74	184	5	183.8	69.5
Rhenium	Re	75	186	2	185.9	71.7
Gold	Au	79	197	1	196.9	80.7
Lead	Pb	82	208	4	207.1	88
Uranium	U	92	238	3	238	116

amu, Atomic mass units; *keV*, electron kilovolt.
*Most abundant isotope.
†Average of naturally occurring isotopes.

The number of protons plus the number of neutrons in the nucleus of an atom is called the atomic mass number, symbolized by A. The atomic mass number is always a whole number. The use of atomic mass numbers is helpful in many areas of radiologic science.

> The atomic mass number and the precise mass of an atom are not equal.

An atom's atomic mass number is a whole number that is equal to the number of nucleons in the atom. The actual **atomic mass** of an atom is determined by measurement and rarely is a whole number. ^{135}Ba has A = 135 because its nucleus contains 56 protons and 79 neutrons. The atomic mass of ^{135}Ba is 134.91 amu.

Only one atom, ^{12}C, has an atomic mass equal to its atomic mass number. This occurs because the ^{12}C atom is the arbitrary standard for atomic measure.

Many elements in their natural state are composed of atoms with different atomic mass numbers and different atomic masses but identical atomic numbers. The characteristic mass of an element, the **elemental mass**, is determined by the relative abundance of isotopes and their respective atomic masses.

Barium, for example, has an atomic number of 56. The atomic mass number of its most abundant isotope is 138. Natural barium, however, consists of seven different isotopes with atomic mass numbers of 130, 132, 134, 135, 136, 137, and 138; the elemental mass is determined by calculating the average weight of all these isotopes.

With the protocol described in Figure 3-10, the atoms of Figure 3-6 would have the following symbolic representation:

$$^{1}_{1}\text{H}, \,^{4}_{2}\text{He}, \,^{7}_{3}\text{Li}, \,^{238}_{92}\text{U}$$

Because the chemical symbol also indicates the atomic number, the subscript is often omitted.

$$^{1}\text{H}, \,^{4}\text{He}, \,^{7}\text{Li}, \,^{238}\text{U}$$

> **Isotopes**
> Atoms that have the same atomic number but different atomic mass numbers are isotopes.

Isotopes of a given element contain the same number of protons but varying numbers of neutrons. Most

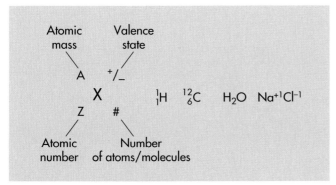

FIGURE 3-10 Protocol for representing elements in a molecule.

elements have more than one stable isotope. The seven natural isotopes of barium are as follows:

$$^{130}Ba, \, ^{132}Ba, \, ^{134}Ba, \, ^{135}Ba, \, ^{136}Ba, \, ^{137}Ba, \, ^{138}Ba$$

The term *isotope* describes all atoms of a given element. Such atoms have different nuclear configurations but nevertheless react the same way chemically.

Question: How many protons and neutrons are in each of the seven naturally occurring isotopes of barium?

Answer: The number of protons in each isotope is 56. The number of neutrons is equal to A-Z. Therefore,
^{130}Ba: $130 - 56 = 74$ neutrons
^{132}Ba: $132 - 56 = 76$ neutrons
^{134}Ba: $134 - 56 = 78$ neutrons
and so forth.

Isobar
Atomic nuclei that have the same atomic mass number but different atomic numbers are isobars.

Isobars are atoms that have different numbers of protons and different numbers of neutrons but the same total number of nucleons. Isobaric radioactive transitions from parent atom to daughter atom result from the release of a beta particle or a positron. The parent and the daughter are atoms of different elements.

Isotone
Atoms that have the same number of neutrons but different numbers of protons are isotones.

Isotones are atoms with different atomic numbers and different mass numbers but a constant value for the

quantity A-Z. Consequently, isotones are atoms with the same number of neutrons in the nucleus.

The final category of atomic configuration is the **isomer.**

Isomer
Isomers have the same atomic number and the same atomic mass number.

In fact, isomers are identical atoms, except that they exist at different energy states because of differences in nucleon arrangement. Technetium-99m decays to technetium-99 with the emission of a 140-keV gamma ray, which is very useful in nuclear medicine. Table 3-4 presents a summary of the characteristics of these nuclear arrangements.

Question: From the following list of atoms, pick out those that are isotopes, isobars, and isotones.

$$^{131}_{54}Xe, \, ^{130}_{53}I, \, ^{132}_{55}Cs, \, ^{131}_{53}I$$

Answer: ^{130}I and ^{131}I are isotopes. ^{131}I and ^{131}Xe are isobars. ^{130}I, ^{131}Xe, and ^{132}Cs are isotones.

COMBINATIONS OF ATOMS

Molecule
Atoms of various elements may combine to form structures called *molecules.*

Four atoms of hydrogen (H_2) and two atoms of oxygen (O_2) can combine to form two molecules of water ($2 H_2O$). The following equation represents this atomic combination:

$$2H_2 + O_2 \rightarrow 2H_2O$$

Table 3-4	Characteristics of Various Nuclear Arrangements		
Arrangement	Atomic Number	Atomic Mass Number	Neutron Number
Isotope	Same	Different	Different
Isobar	Different	Same	Different
Isotone	Different	Different	Same
Isomer	Same	Same	Same

An atom of sodium (Na) can combine with an atom of chlorine (Cl) to form a molecule of sodium chloride (NaCl), which is common table salt:

$$Na + Cl \rightarrow NaCl$$

Both of these molecules are common in the human body. Molecules, in turn, may combine to form even larger structures: cells and tissues.

Compound

A *chemical compound* is any quantity of one type of molecule.

Although more than 100 different elements are known, most elements are rare. Approximately 95% of the Earth and its atmosphere consists of only a dozen elements. Similarly, hydrogen, oxygen, carbon, and nitrogen compose over 95% of the human body. Water molecules make up approximately 80% of the human body.

There is an organized scheme for representing elements in a molecule (see Figure 3-10). The shorthand notation that incorporates the chemical symbol with subscripts and superscripts is used to identify atoms.

The chemical symbol (X) is positioned between two subscripts and two superscripts. The subscript and superscript to the left of the chemical symbol represent atomic number and atomic mass number, respectively. The subscript and superscript to the right are values for the number of atoms per molecule and the valence state of the atom, respectively.

The formula NaCl represents one molecule of the compound sodium chloride. Sodium chloride has properties that are different from those of sodium or chlorine. Atoms combine with each other to form compounds (chemical bonding) in two main ways. The examples of H_2O and NaCl can be used to describe these two types of chemical bonds.

Oxygen and hydrogen combine into water through **covalent bonds.** Oxygen has six electrons in its outermost shell. It has room for two more electrons, so in a water molecule, two hydrogen atoms share their single electrons with the oxygen. The hydrogen electrons orbit the H and the O, thus binding the atoms together. This covalent bonding is characterized by the sharing of electrons.

Sodium and chlorine combine into salt through **ionic bonds.** Sodium has one electron in its outermost shell. Chlorine has space for one more electron in its outermost shell. The sodium atom will give up its electron to the chlorine. When it does, it becomes ionized because it has lost an electron and now has an imbalance of electric charges.

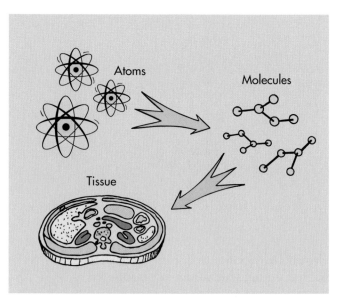

FIGURE 3-11 Matter has many levels of organization. Atoms combine to make molecules and molecules combine to make tissues.

The chlorine atom also becomes ionized because it has gained an electron and now has more electrons than protons. The two atoms are attracted to each other, resulting in an ionic bond because they have opposite electrostatic charges.

Sodium, hydrogen, carbon, and oxygen atoms can combine to form a molecule of sodium bicarbonate ($NaHCO_3$). A measurable quantity of sodium bicarbonate constitutes a chemical compound commonly called **baking soda.**

The smallest particle of an element is an atom; the smallest particle of a compound is a molecule.

The interrelations between atoms, elements, molecules, and compounds are orderly. This organizational scheme is what the ancient Greeks were trying to describe by their substances and essences. Figure 3-11 is a diagram of this current scheme of matter.

RADIOACTIVITY

Some atoms exist in an abnormally excited state characterized by an unstable nucleus. To reach stability, the nucleus spontaneously emits particles and energy and transforms itself into another atom. This process is called **radioactive disintegration** or **radioactive decay.** The atoms involved are **radionuclides.** Any nuclear arrangement is called a **nuclide;** only nuclei that undergo radioactive decay are radionuclides.

Radioactivity
Radioactivity is the emission of particles and energy in order to become stable.

Radioisotopes

Many factors affect nuclear stability. Perhaps the most important is the number of neutrons. When a nucleus contains too few or too many neutrons, the atom can disintegrate radioactively, bringing the number of neutrons and protons into a stable and proper ratio.

In addition to stable isotopes, many elements have radioactive isotopes or **radioisotopes.** These may be artificially produced in machines such as particle accelerators or nuclear reactors. Seven radioisotopes of barium have been discovered, all of which are artificially produced. In the following list of barium isotopes, the radioisotopes are boldface:

$$^{127}\textbf{Ba}, \; ^{128}\textbf{Ba}, \; ^{129}\textbf{Ba}, \; ^{130}\textbf{Ba}, \; ^{131}\textbf{Ba}, \; ^{132}\textbf{Ba}, \; ^{133}\textbf{Ba},$$
$$^{134}\textbf{Ba}, \; ^{135}\textbf{Ba}, \; ^{136}\text{Ba}, \; ^{137}\text{Ba}, \; ^{138}\text{Ba}, \; ^{139}\textbf{Ba}, \; ^{140}\textbf{Ba}$$

Artificially produced radioisotopes have been identified for nearly all elements. A few elements have naturally occurring radioisotopes as well.

There are two primary sources of naturally occurring radioisotopes. Some originated at the time of the Earth's formation and are still decaying very slowly. An example is uranium, which ultimately decays to radium, which in turn, decays to radon. These and other decay products of uranium are radioactive. Others, such as ^{14}C, are continuously produced in the upper atmosphere through the action of cosmic radiation.

Radioisotopes can decay to stability in many ways, but only two, **beta emission** and **alpha emission,** are of particular importance here.

During beta emission, an electron created in the nucleus is ejected from the nucleus with considerable kinetic energy and escapes from the atom. The result is the loss of a small quantity of mass and one unit of negative electric charge from the nucleus of the atom. Simultaneously, a neutron undergoes conversion to a proton.

The result of beta emission therefore is to increase the atomic number by one ($Z \rightarrow Z+1$), while the atomic mass number remains the same ($A = $ constant). This nuclear transformation results in the changing of an atom from one type of element to another (Figure 3-12).

Radioactivity decay by alpha emission is a much more violent process. The alpha particle consists of two protons and two neutrons bound together; its atomic mass number is 4. A nucleus must be extremely unstable to emit an alpha particle, but when it does, it loses two units of positive charge and four units of mass. The transformation is significant because the resulting atom is not only chemically different but is also lighter by 4 amu (Figure 3-13).

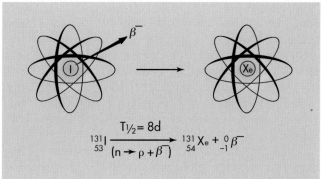

FIGURE 3-12 ^{131}I decays to ^{131}Xe with the emission of a beta particle.

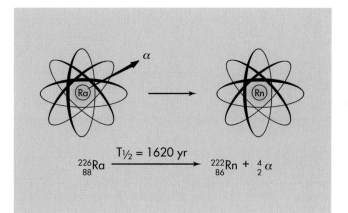

FIGURE 3-13 The decay of ^{226}Ra to ^{222}Rn is accompanied by alpha emission.

Radioactive decay results in emission of alpha particles, beta particles, and usually gamma rays.

Beta emission occurs much more frequently than alpha emission. Virtually all radioisotopes are capable of transformation by beta emission, but only heavy radioisotopes are capable of alpha emission. Some radioisotopes are pure beta emitters or pure alpha emitters, but most emit gamma rays simultaneously with the particle emission.

Question: ^{139}Ba is a radioisotope that decays by beta emission. What will be the values of A and Z for the atom that results from this emission?

Answer: In beta emission a neutron is converted to a proton and a beta particle: $n \rightarrow p + \beta$, therefore $^{139}_{56}\text{Ba} \rightarrow {}^{139}_{57}?$ Lanthanum is the element with Z = 57; thus, $^{139}_{57}\text{La}$ is the result of the beta decay of $^{139}_{56}\text{Ba}$.

Radioactive Half-life

Radioactive matter is not here one day and gone the next. Rather, radioisotopes disintegrate into stable isotopes of different elements at a decreasing rate, so that the quantity of radioactive material never quite reaches zero. Remember from Chapter 2 that radioactive material is measured in curies (Ci) and that 1 Ci is equal to disintegration of 3.7×10^{10} atoms each second (3.7×10^{10} Bq).

The rate of radioactive decay and the quantity of material present at any given time are described mathematically by a formula known as the **radioactive decay law.** From this formula we obtain a quantity known as **half-life ($T\frac{1}{2}$).** Half-lives of radioisotopes vary from less than a second to many years. Each radioisotope has a unique, characteristic half-life.

Half-life

The half-life of a radioisotope is the time required for a quantity of radioactivity to be reduced to one-half its original value.

The half-life of ^{131}I is 8 days (Figure 3-14). If 100 mCi (3.7×10^9 Bq) of ^{131}I was present on January 1 at noon, then at noon on January 9, only 50 mCi (1.85×10^9 Bq) would remain. On January 17, 25 mCi (9.25×10^8 Bq) would remain, and on January 25, 12.5 mCi (4.63×10^8 Bq) would remain. A plot of the radioactive decay of ^{131}I allows one to determine the amount of radioactivity remaining after any given length of time (see Figure 3-14).

After approximately 24 days, or three half-lives, the linear-linear plot of the decay of ^{131}I becomes very difficult to read and interpret. Consequently, such graphs are usually presented in semilogarithmic form (Figure 3-15). With a presentation such as this, one can estimate radioactivity after a very long time.

Question: On Monday at 8 AM, 100 μCi (3.7 MBq) of ^{131}I is present. How much will remain on Friday at 5 PM?

Answer: The time of decay is $4\frac{1}{3}$ days. According to Figure 3-15, at $4\frac{1}{3}$ days, approximately 63% of the original activity will remain. Therefore, 63 μCI (2.33 MBq) will be present on Friday at 5 PM.

Theoretically, all the radioactivity of a radioisotope never disappears. After each period of time equivalent to one half-life, one-half the activity present at the beginning of that time will remain. Therefore, although the quantity of a radioisotope progressively decreases, it never quite reaches zero.

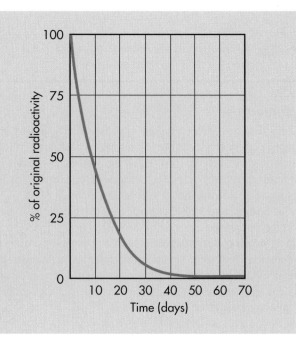

FIGURE 3-14 ^{131}I decays with a half-life of 8 days. This linear graph allows estimation of radioactivity only for a short time.

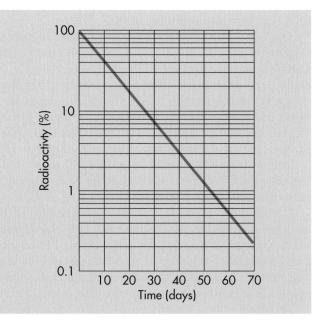

FIGURE 3-15 This semilog graph is useful for estimating the radioactivity of ^{131}I at any given time.

Figure 3-16 shows two similar graphs used to estimate the quantity of any radioisotope remaining after any length of time. In these graphs, the percentage of original radioactivity remaining is plotted against time, measured in units of half-life. To use these graphs, one must express the initial radioactivity as 100% and convert the time of interest into units of half-life. For decay times exceeding three half-lives, the semilog form is easier to use.

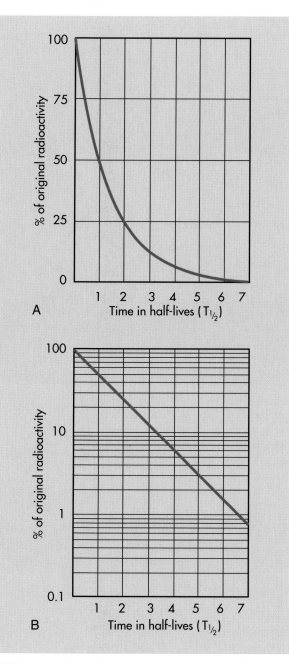

FIGURE 3-16 The radioactivity after any period can be estimated from the linear **(A)** or the semilog **(B)** graph. The original quantity is assigned a value of 100%, and the time of decay is expressed in units of half-life.

Question: 65 mCi (2.4×10^9 Bq) of ^{131}I is present at noon on Wednesday. How much will remain 1 week later?

Answer: 7 days = $\frac{7}{8}$ T$\frac{1}{2}$ = 0.875 T$\frac{1}{2}$. Figure 3-16 shows that at 0.875 T$\frac{1}{2}$, approximately 55% of the initial radioactivity will remain; 55% × 65 mCi (2.4×10^9 Bq) = 0.55×65 = 35.8 mCi (1.32×10^9 Bq).

^{14}C is a naturally occurring radioisotope with T$\frac{1}{2}$ = 5730 years. The concentration of ^{14}C in the environment is constant, and ^{14}C is incorporated into living material at a constant rate. Trees of the Petrified Forest contain less ^{14}C than living trees because the ^{14}C of living trees is in equilibrium with the atmosphere; the carbon in a petrified tree was fixed many thousands of years ago, and the fixed ^{14}C is reduced over time by radioactive decay (Figure 3-17).

Question: If a piece of petrified wood contains 25% of the ^{14}C that a tree living today contains, how old is the petrified wood?

Answer: The ^{14}C in living matter remains constant as long as the matter is alive because it is constantly exchanged with the environment. In this case, the petrified wood has been dead long enough for the ^{14}C to decay to 25% of its original value. That time period represents two half-lives. Consequently, we can estimate that the petrified wood sample is approximately 2 × 5730 = 11,460 years old.

Question: How many half-lives are required before a quantity of radioactive material has decayed to less than 1% of its original value?

Answer: A simple approach to this type of problem is to count half-lives.

Half-life number	Radioactivity remaining
1	50%
2	25%
3	12.5%
4	6.25%
5	3.12%
6	1.56%
7	0.78%

A simpler approach finds the answer more precisely on Figure 3-16: 6.5 half-lives. Another approach is to use the following relationship:

RADIOACTIVE DECAY
Activity Remaining = Original Activity $(0.5)^n$
where n = number of half-lives.

The concept of half-life is essential to radiologic science. It is used daily in nuclear medicine and has an exact parallel in x-ray terminology, the **half-value layer.** The better you understand half-life now, the better you will understand the meaning of half-value layer later.

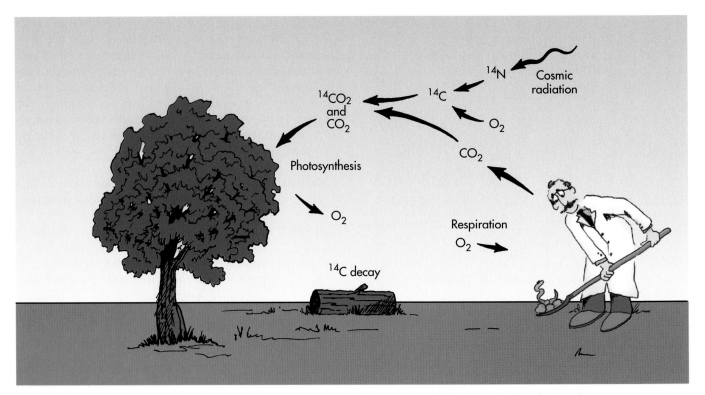

FIGURE 3-17 Carbon is a biologically active element. A small fraction of all carbon is the radioisotope ^{14}C. As a tree grows, ^{14}C is incorporated into the wood in proportion to the amount of ^{14}C in the atmosphere. When the tree dies, further exchange of ^{14}C with the atmosphere does not take place. If the dead wood is preserved by petrification, the ^{14}C content diminishes as it radioactively decays. This phenomenon serves as the basis for radiocarbon dating.

Table 3-5	General Classification of Ionizing Radiation			
Type of Radiation	**Symbol**	**Atomic Mass Number**	**Charge**	**Origin**
PARTICULATE				
Alpha radiation	α	4	+2	Nucleus
Beta radiation	β^-	0	−1	Nucleus
	β^+	0	+1	Nucleus
ELECTROMAGNETIC				
Gamma rays	γ	0	0	Nucleus
X-rays	X	0	0	Electron cloud

TYPES OF IONIZING RADIATION

All ionizing radiation can be conveniently classified into two categories: **particulate radiation** and **electromagnetic radiation** (Table 3-5). The types of radiation used in diagnostic ultrasound and in magnetic resonance imaging are **nonionizing radiation.**

Although all ionizing radiation acts on biologic tissue in the same manner, there are fundamental differences between various types of radiation. These differences can be analyzed according to five physical characteristics: mass, energy, velocity, charge, and origin.

Particulate Radiation

Many subatomic particles are capable of causing ionization. Consequently, electrons, protons, and even rare nuclear fragments all can be classified as particulate ionizing radiation if they are in motion and possess sufficient kinetic energy. At rest, they cannot cause ionization.

There are two main types of particulate radiation: **alpha particles** and **beta particles**. Both are associated with radioactive decay.

The alpha particle is equivalent to a helium nucleus. It contains two protons and two neutrons. Its mass is approximately 4 amu, and it carries two units of positive electric charge. Compared with an electron, the alpha particle is large and exerts great electrostatic force. Alpha particles are emitted only from the nuclei of heavy elements. Light elements cannot emit alpha particles because they do not have enough excess mass (excess energy).

ALPHA PARTICLE

An alpha particle is a helium nucleus that contains two protons and two neutrons.

Once emitted from a radioactive atom, the alpha particle travels with high velocity through matter. Because of its great mass and charge, however, it easily transfers this kinetic energy to orbital electrons of other atoms.

Ionization accompanies alpha radiation. The average alpha particle possesses 4 to 7 MeV of kinetic energy and ionizes approximately 40,000 atoms for every centimeter of travel through air.

Because of this amount of ionization, the energy of an alpha particle is quickly lost. It has a very short range in matter. In air, alpha particles can travel approximately 5 cm, whereas in soft tissue, the range may be less than 100 μm. Consequently, alpha radiation from an external source is nearly harmless because the radiation energy is deposited in the superficial layers of the skin.

With an internal source of radiation, just the opposite is true. If an alpha-emitting radioisotope is deposited in the body, it can intensely irradiate the local tissue.

Beta particles differ from alpha particles in terms of mass and charge. They are light particles with an atomic mass number of 0 and carry one unit of negative or positive charge. The only difference between electrons and negative beta particles is their origin. Beta particles originate in the nuclei of radioactive atoms and electrons exist in shells outside the nuclei of all atoms. Positive beta particles are positrons. They have the same mass as electrons and are considered to be antimatter. We will see positrons again when we discuss pair production.

BETA PARTICLE

A beta particle is an electron emitted from the nucleus of a radioactive atom.

Once emitted from a radioisotope, beta particles traverse air, ionizing several hundred atoms per centimeter. The beta particle range is longer than that for the alpha particle. Depending on its energy, a beta particle may traverse 10 to 100 cm of air and approximately 1 to 2 cm of soft tissue.

Electromagnetic Radiation

X-rays and gamma rays are forms of electromagnetic ionizing radiation. This type of radiation is covered more completely in the next chapter; the discussion here is necessarily brief.

X-rays and gamma rays are often called **photons.** Photons have no mass and no charge. They travel at the speed of light ($c = 3 \times 10^8$ m/s) and are considered energy disturbances in space.

X-rays and gamma rays are the only forms of ionizing electromagnetic radiation of radiologic interest.

Just as the only difference between beta particles and electrons is their origin, so the only difference between x-rays and gamma rays is their origin. Gamma rays are emitted from the nucleus of a radioisotope and are usually associated with alpha or beta emission. X-rays are produced outside the nucleus in the electron shells.

X-rays and gamma rays exist at the speed of light or not at all. Once emitted, they have an ionization rate in air of approximately 100 ion pairs/cm, about equal to that for beta particles. In contrast to beta particles, however, x-rays and gamma rays have an unlimited range in matter.

Photon radiation loses intensity with distance but theoretically never reaches zero. Particulate radiation, on the other hand, has a finite range in matter, and that range depends on the particle's energy.

Table 3-6 summarizes the more important characteristics of each of these types of ionizing radiation. In nuclear medicine, beta and gamma radiation are most important. In radiography, only x-rays are important. The penetrability and low ionization rate of x-rays make them particularly useful for medical imaging (Figure 3-18).

SUMMARY

As a miniature solar system, the Bohr atom set the stage for the modern interpretation of the structure of matter. An atom is the smallest part of an element, and a molecule is the smallest part of a compound.

The three fundamental particles of the atom are the electron, proton, and neutron. Electrons are negatively charged particles that orbit the nucleus in configurations or shells held in place by electrostatic forces. Chemical reactions occur when outermost orbital electrons are shared or given up to other atoms. Nucleons, neutrons, and protons each have nearly 2000 times the mass of electrons. Protons are positively charged and neutrons have no charge.

Elements are grouped in a periodic table in order of increasing complexity. The groups on the table indicate the number of electrons in the outermost shell. The

Table 3-6	Characteristics of Several Types of Ionizing Radiation				
			APPROXIMATE RANGE		
Type of Radiation	Approximate Energy	In Air	In Soft Tissue	Origin	
PARTICULATE					
Alpha particles	4-7 MeV	1-10 cm	Up to 0.1 mm	Heavy radioactive nuclei	
Beta particles	0-7 MeV	0-10 m	0-2 cm	Radioactive nuclei	
ELECTROMAGNETIC					
X-rays	0-25 MeV	0-100 m	0-30 cm	Electron cloud	
Gamma rays	0-5 MeV	0-100 m	0-30 cm	Radioactive nuclei	

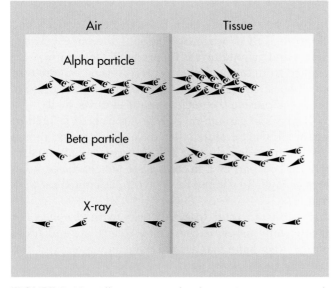

FIGURE 3-18 Different types of radiation ionize matter with different degrees of efficiency. Alpha particles represent highly ionizing radiation with a very short range in matter. Beta particles do not ionize so readily and have a longer range. X-rays have a low ionization rate and a very long range.

elements in the periods on the periodic table have the same number of orbital shells.

Some atoms have the same number of protons and electrons as other elements but a different number of neutrons, giving the element a different atomic mass. These are isotopes.

Some atoms, which contain too many or too few neutrons in the nucleus, can disintegrate. This is called *radioactivity*. Two types of particulate emission that occur after radioactive disintegration are alpha and beta particles. The half-life of a radioactive element or a radioisotope is the time required for the quantity of radioactivity to be reduced to one-half its original value.

Ionizing radiation consists of particulate and electromagnetic radiation. Alpha and beta particles produce particulate radiation. Alpha particles have four atomic mass units, are positive in charge, and originate from

the nucleus of heavy elements. Beta particles have an atomic mass number of zero and have one unit of negative charge. Beta particles originate in the nucleus of radioactive atoms.

X-rays and gamma rays are forms of electromagnetic radiation called *photons*. These rays have no mass and no charge. X-rays are produced in the electron shells, and gamma rays are emitted from the nucleus of a radioisotope.

CHALLENGE QUESTIONS

1. Define or otherwise identify the following:
   a. Photon
   b. The Rutherford atom
   c. Positron
   d. Nucleons
   e. The arrangement of the periodic table of the elements
   f. Radioactive half-life
   g. W (chemical symbol for what element?)
   h. Alpha particle
   i. K shell
   j. Chemical compound
2. Figure 3-1 shows the following approximate sizes: an atom, 10^{-10} m; the Earth, 10^7 m. By how many orders of magnitude do these objects differ?
3. How many protons, neutrons, electrons, and nucleons are found in the following?

$$^{17}_{8}\text{O}, \, ^{27}_{13}\text{Al}, \, ^{60}_{27}\text{Co}, \, ^{226}_{88}\text{Ra}$$

4. Using the data in Table 3-1, determine the mass of ^{99}Tc in atomic mass units and in grams.
5. Diagram the expected electron configuration of ^{40}Ca.
6. If atoms large enough to have electrons in the T-shell existed, what would be the maximum number allowed in that shell?
7. How much more tightly bound are K-shell electrons in tungsten than (a) L-shell electrons, (b) M-shell electrons, (c) free electrons? (Refer to Figure 3-9.)

8. From the following list of nuclides, identify sets of isotopes, isobars, and isotones.

$$^{60}_{28}\text{Ni} \quad ^{61}_{28}\text{Ni} \quad ^{62}_{28}\text{Ni}$$

$$^{59}_{27}\text{Co} \quad ^{60}_{27}\text{Co} \quad ^{61}_{27}\text{Co}$$

$$^{58}_{28}\text{Fe} \quad ^{59}_{28}\text{Fe} \quad ^{60}_{28}\text{Fe}$$

9. $^{90}_{38}\text{Sr}$ has a half-life of 29 years. If 10 Ci (3.7×10^{11} Bq) were present in 1950, approximately how much would remain in 2010?

10. Complete the following table with relative values.

Type of radiation	Mass	Energy	Charge	Origin
α				
β				
β+				
γ				
X				

11. For what is Mendeleev remembered?

12. Who developed the concept of the atom as a miniature solar system?

13. List the fundamental particles within an atom.

14. What property of an atom does binding energy describe?

15. Can atoms be ionized by changing the number of positive charges?

16. Describe how ion pairs are formed.

17. What determines the chemical properties of an element?

18. Why doesn't an electron spontaneously fly away from the nucleus of an atom?

19. Describe the difference between alpha and beta emission.

20. How does carbon-14 dating determine the age of petrified wood?

The answers to the Challenge Questions can be found by logging onto our website at http://evolve.elsevier.com.

Electromagnetic Energy

OBJECTIVES

At the completion of this chapter, the student should be able to do the following:

1. Identify the properties of photons
2. Explain the inverse square law
3. Define wave theory and quantum theory
4. Discuss the electromagnetic spectrum

OUTLINE

Photons
    Velocity and Amplitude
    Frequency and Wavelength
Electromagnetic Spectrum
    Measurement of the Electromagnetic Spectrum
    Visible Light
    Radiofrequency
    Ionizing Radiation
Wave-Particle Duality
    Wave Model: Visible Light
    Inverse Square Law
    Particle Model: Quantum Theory
Matter and Energy

PHOTONS WERE first described by the ancient Greeks. Today, photons are known as electromagnetic energy; however, these words are commonly used interchangeably. Electromagnetic energy is present everywhere and exists over a wide energy range. X-rays, visible light, and radiofrequencies are examples of electromagnetic energy.

The properties of electromagnetic energy include frequency, wavelength, velocity, and amplitude. In this chapter, discussions of visible light, radiofrequency, and ionizing radiation highlight these properties and the importance of electromagnetic energy in medical imaging. The wave equation and the inverse square law are mathematical formulas that further describe how electromagnetic energy behaves.

The wave-particle duality of electromagnetic energy is introduced as wave theory and quantum theory. Matter and energy, as well as their importance to medical imaging, are summarized.

PHOTONS

Ever present all around us is a field or state of energy called **electromagnetic energy.** This energy exists over a wide range called an energy **continuum.** A continuum is an uninterrupted (continuous) ordered sequence. Examples of continuums are free-flowing rivers and sidewalks. If the river is dammed or the sidewalk curbed, then the continuum is interrupted. Only an extremely small segment of the electromagnetic energy continuum—the visible light segment—is naturally apparent to us.

The ancient Greeks recognized the unique nature of light. It was not one of their four basic essences, but light was given entirely separate status. They called an atom of light a **photon.** Today, many types of electromagnetic energy in addition to visible light are recognized, but the term *photon* is still used.

A photon is the smallest quantity of any type of electromagnetic energy, just as an atom is the smallest quantity of an element. A photon may be pictured as a small bundle of energy, sometimes called a **quantum,** that travels through space at the speed of light. We speak of x-ray photons, light photons, and other types of electromagnetic energy as photon radiation.

An x-ray photon is a quantum of electromagnetic energy.

The physics of visible light has always been a subject of investigation apart from other areas of science. Nearly all the classical laws of optics were described hundreds of years ago. Late in the 19th century, James Clerk Maxwell showed that visible light has both electric and magnetic properties, hence the term **electromagnetic energy.**

By the beginning of the 20th century, other types of electromagnetic energy had been described and a uniform theory evolved. Electromagnetic energy is best explained by reference to a model, in much the same way that the atom is best described by the Bohr model.

Velocity and Amplitude

Photons are energy disturbances that move through space at the speed of light *(c)*. Some sources give the speed of light as 186,000 miles per second, but in the SI system of units, it is 3×10^8 m/s.

Question: What is the value of c in miles per second, given $c = 3 \times 10^8$ m/s?

Answer:

$$C = \frac{3 \times 10^8 \ m}{s} \times \frac{mi}{5280 \ ft} \times \frac{3.2808 \ ft}{m}$$
$$= \frac{3 \times 10^8 \ m \times 10^8 \ m-mi-ft}{5.280 \times 10^3 \ s-ft-m}$$
$$= 1.854 \times 10^5 \ mi/s$$
$$= 186,400 \ mi/s$$

The velocity of all electromagnetic radiation is 3×10^8 m/s.

Although photons have no mass and therefore no identifiable form, they do have electric and magnetic fields that are continuously changing in a **sinusoidal** fashion. Physicists use the term *field* to describe interactions among different energies, forces, or masses that can otherwise be described only mathematically. For instance, we can understand the gravitational field even though we cannot see it. We know the gravitational field exists because we are held to the Earth by it.

The gravitational field governs the interaction of different masses. Similarly, the electric field governs the interaction of electrostatic charges, and the magnetic field, the interaction of magnetic poles.

Figure 4-1 shows three examples of a sinusoidal variation. This type of variation is usually called a **sine wave.** Sine waves can be described by a mathematical formula and therefore have many applications in physics.

Sine waves exist in nature and are associated with many familiar objects (Figure 4-2). Simplistically, sine waves are variations of amplitude over time.

Alternating electric current consists of electrons moving back and forth sinusoidally through a conductor. A long rope fastened at one end vibrates as a sine wave if the free end is moved up and down in whiplike fashion.

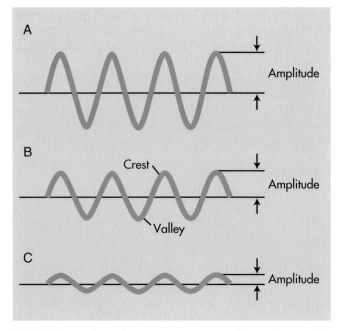

FIGURE 4-1 These three sine waves are identical except for their amplitudes.

The arms of a tuning fork vibrate sinusoidally after being struck with a hard object. The weight on the end of a coil spring varies sinusoidally up and down after the spring has been stretched.

The sine waves in Figure 4-1 are identical except for their amplitude; sine wave A has the largest amplitude and sine wave C has the smallest. Sine wave amplitude is discussed later in connection with high-voltage generation and rectification in an x-ray imaging system.

> *Amplitude* is one-half the range from crest to valley over which the sine wave varies.

Frequency and Wavelength

The sine wave model of electromagnetic energy describes variations in the electric and magnetic fields as the photon travels with velocity c. The important properties of this model are **frequency**, represented by f, and **wavelength**, represented by the Greek letter *lambda* (λ).

Another interpretation of the vibrating rope in Figure 4-2 is the Texas roadside critter observing the motion of the rope from a point midway between the fastened end and the scientist (Figure 4-3).

What does the critter see? If he moves his field of view along the rope, he will observe the crest of the sine wave traveling along the rope to the end. If he fixes his attention on one segment of the rope such as point A, he will see the rope rise and fall harmonically as the waves pass. The more rapidly the scientist holding the loose end moves the rope up and down, the faster the sequence of the rise and fall.

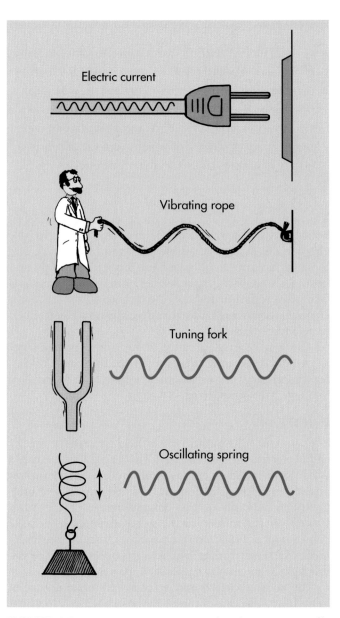

FIGURE 4-2 Sine waves are associated with many naturally occurring phenomena in addition to electromagnetic energy.

The rate of rise and fall is frequency. It is usually identified as cycles per second. The unit of measurement is the hertz (Hz). One hertz is equal to 1 cycle per second. The frequency is equal to the number of crests or the number of valleys that pass the point of an observer per unit of time. If the critter used a stopwatch and counted 20 crests passing in 10 s, then the frequency would be 20 cycles in 10 s, or 2 Hz. If the scientist doubles the rate at which he moves the rope up and down, the critter would count 40 crests passing in 10 s and the frequency would be 4 Hz.

> *Frequency* is the number of wavelengths that pass a point of observation per second.

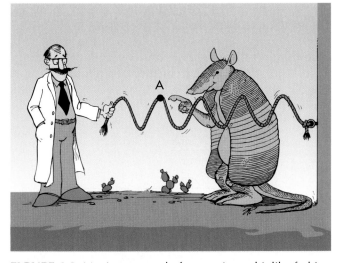

FIGURE 4-3 Moving one end of a rope in a whiplike fashion will set into motion sine waves that travel down the rope to the fastened end. An observer, midway, can determine the frequency of oscillation by counting the crests or valleys that pass a point (**A**) per unit time.

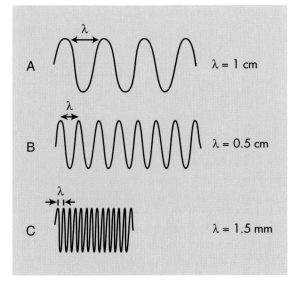

FIGURE 4-4 These three sine waves have different wavelengths. The shorter the wavelength (λ), the higher is the frequency.

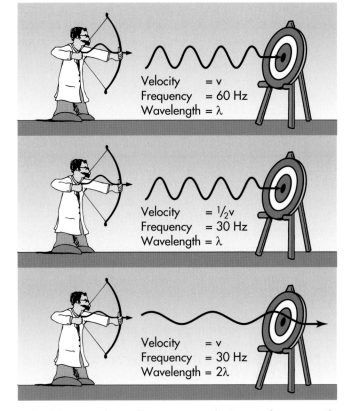

FIGURE 4-5 Relationships among velocity (v), frequency (f), and wavelength for any sine wave.

The **wavelength** is the distance from one crest to another, from one valley to another, or from any point on the sine wave to the next corresponding point. Figure 4-4 shows sine waves of three different wavelengths. With a meter rule, you can verify that wave *A* repeats every 1 cm and therefore has a wavelength of 1 cm. Similarly, wave *B* has a wavelength of 0.5 cm, and wave *C* has a wavelength of 1.5 mm. Clearly, then, as the frequency is increased, the wavelength is reduced. The wave amplitude is not related to wavelength or frequency.

Three wave parameters—velocity, frequency, and wavelength—are needed to describe electromagnetic energy. The relationship among these parameters is important. A change in one affects the value of the other. Velocity is constant.

Suppose a radiologic technologist is positioned to observe the flight of the sine wave arrows to determine their frequency (Figure 4-5). The first sine wave is measured and is found to have a frequency of 60 Hz, which signifies 60 oscillations (wavelengths) of the sine wave every second.

The unknown archer now puts an identical sine wave arrow into his bow and shoots it with less force so that this second arrow has only half the velocity of the first arrow. The observer correctly measures the frequency at 30 Hz, even though the wavelength of the second arrow was the same as that of the first arrow. In other words, as the velocity decreases, the frequency decreases proportionately.

Now the archer shoots a third sine wave arrow with precisely the same velocity as the first but with a wavelength twice as long as that of the first. What should be the observed frequency? The correct answer is 30 Hz.

At a given velocity, wavelength and frequency are inversely proportional.

This brief analogy demonstrates how the three parameters associated with a sine wave are interrelated. A simple mathematical formula, called the **wave equation,** expresses this interrelationship:

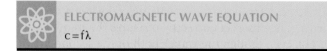

THE WAVE EQUATION

$$Wavelength = Velocity/Frequency$$
or
$$v = f\lambda$$

The wave equation is used for both sound and electromagnetic energy. However, keep in mind that sound waves are very different from electromagnetic photons. The sources of sound are different, they are propagated in different ways, and their velocities vary greatly. The velocity of sound depends on the density of the material through which it passes. Sound cannot travel through a vacuum.

Question: The speed of sound in air is approximately 340 m/s. The highest treble tone that a person can hear is about 20 kHz. What is the wavelength of this sound?

Answer: $v = f\lambda$

$$\lambda = \frac{v}{f}$$

$$= \frac{340 \text{ m/s}}{20 \text{ kHz}}$$

$$= \frac{3.40 \times 10^2 \text{ m}}{s} \times \frac{s}{2 \times 10^4 \text{ cycle}}$$

$$= 1.7 \times 10^{-2} \text{ m}$$

$$= 1.7 \text{ cm}$$

When dealing with electromagnetic energy, we can simplify the wave equation because all such energy travels with the same velocity.

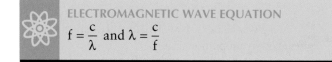

ELECTROMAGNETIC WAVE EQUATION

$$c = f\lambda$$

The product of frequency and wavelength always equals the velocity of light for electromagnetic energy. Stated differently, **for electromagnetic energy, frequency and wavelength are inversely proportional.** The following are alternative forms of the electromagnetic wave equation.

ELECTROMAGNETIC WAVE EQUATION

$$f = \frac{c}{\lambda} \text{ and } \lambda = \frac{c}{f}$$

As the frequency of electromagnetic energy increases, the wavelength decreases, and vice versa.

Question: Yellow light has a wavelength of 580 nm. What is the frequency of a photon of yellow light?

Answer: $f = \dfrac{c}{\lambda}$

$$= \frac{3 \times 10^8 \text{ m/s}}{580 \text{ nm}}$$

$$= \frac{3 \times 10^8 \text{ m}}{s} \times \frac{1}{580 \times 10^{-9} \text{ m}}$$

$$= \frac{3 \times 10^8 \text{ m}}{s} \times \frac{1}{5.8 \times 10^{-7} \text{ m}}$$

$$= 0.517 \times 10^{15} \text{ cycles/s}$$

$$= 5.17 \times 10^{14} \text{ Hz}$$

Question: The highest energy x-ray produced at 100 kVp (100 keV) has a frequency of 2.42 10^{19} Hz. What is its wavelength?

Answer: $x = \dfrac{c}{f}$

$$= \frac{3 \times 10^8 \text{ m}}{s} \times \frac{s}{2.42 \times 10^{19} \text{ cycle}}$$

$$= 1.24 \times 10^{-11} \text{ m}$$

$$= 12.4 \text{ pm}$$

ELECTROMAGNETIC SPECTRUM

The frequency range of electromagnetic energy extends from approximately 10^2 to 10^{24} Hz. The photon wavelengths associated with these radiations are approximately 10^7 to 10^{-16} m, respectively. This wide range of values covers many types of electromagnetic energy, most of which are familiar to us. Grouped together, these types of energy make up the **electromagnetic spectrum.**

The electromagnetic spectrum includes the entire range of electromagnetic energy.

The known electromagnetic spectrum has three regions most important to radiologic science: visible light, x-radiation, and radiofrequency. Other portions of the spectrum include ultraviolet light, infrared light, and microwave radiation.

With all of these various types of energy, photons are essentially the same. Each can be represented as a bundle of energy consisting of varying electric and magnetic fields that travel at the speed of light. The photons of these various portions of the electromagnetic spectrum differ only in frequency and wavelength.

Ultrasound is not produced in photon form and does not have a constant velocity. Ultrasound is a wave of moving molecules. Ultrasound requires matter; electromagnetic energy can exist in a vacuum.

> Diagnostic ultrasound is not a part of the electromagnetic spectrum.

Measurement of the Electromagnetic Spectrum

The electromagnetic spectrum shown in Figure 4-6 contains three different scales, one each for energy, frequency, and wavelength. Because the velocity of all electromagnetic energy is constant, the wavelength and frequency are inversely related.

Although segments of the electromagnetic spectrum are often given precise ranges, these ranges actually overlap because of production methods and detection techniques. For example, by definition, ultraviolet light has a shorter wavelength than violet light and cannot be sensed by the eye. What is visible violet light to one observer, however, may be ultraviolet light to another. Similarly, microwaves and infrared light are indistinguishable in their common region of the spectrum.

The earliest investigations focused on visible light. Studies of reflection, refraction, and diffraction showed

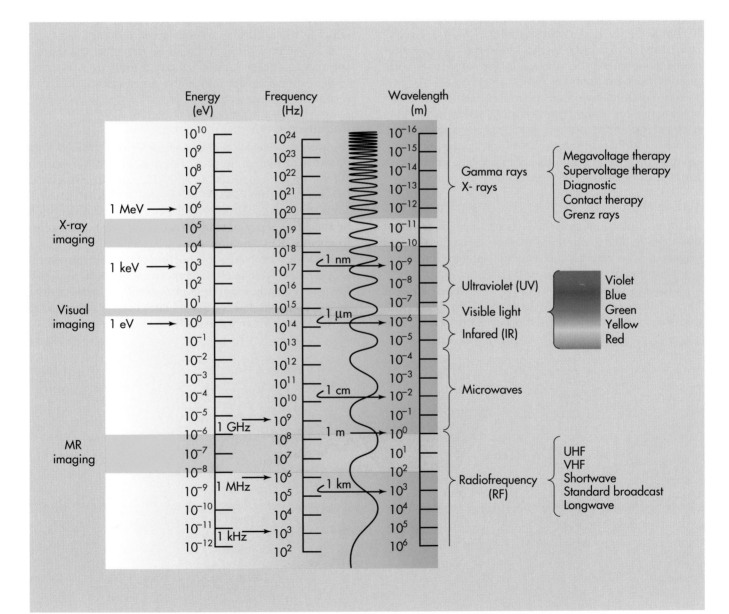

FIGURE 4-6 The electromagnetic spectrum extends over more than 25 orders of magnitude. This chart shows the values of energy, frequency, and wavelength and identifies the three imaging windows.

light to be wavelike. Consequently, visible light is described by wavelength, measured in meters.

In the 1880s, some scientists began to experiment with the radio, which required the oscillation of electrons in a conductor. Consequently, the unit of frequency, the hertz, is used to describe radio waves.

Finally, in 1895, Roentgen discovered x-rays by applying an electric potential (kilovolts) across a Crookes tube. Consequently, x-rays are described in terms of a unit of energy, the electron volt (eV).

 The energy of a photon is directly proportional to its frequency.

It should be clear that these three scales are directly related mathematically. If you know the value of electromagnetic energy on one scale, you can easily compute its value on the other two.

The electromagnetic spectrum has been scientifically investigated for longer than a century. Scientists working with energy in one portion of the spectrum were often unaware of others investigating another portion. Consequently, there is no generally accepted, single dimension for measuring electromagnetic energy.

Visible Light

An optical physicist describes visible light in terms of wavelength. When sunlight passes through a prism (Figure 4-7), it emerges not as white sunlight but as the colors of the rainbow.

Although photons of visible light travel in straight lines, their course can be deviated when they pass from one transparent medium to another. This deviation in line of travel, called *refraction*, is the cause of many peculiar but familiar phenomena, such as a rainbow or the apparent bending of a straw in a glass of water.

White light is composed of photons of a range of wavelengths, and the prism acts to separate and group the emerging light into colors because different wavelengths are refracted through different angles. The component colors of white light have wavelength values ranging from approximately 400 nm for violet to 700 nm for red.

Visible light occupies the smallest segment of the electromagnetic spectrum, and yet it is the only portion that we can sense directly. Sunlight also contains two types of invisible light: infrared and ultraviolet.

Infrared light consists of photons with wavelengths longer than those of visible light but shorter than those of microwaves. Infrared light heats any substance on which it shines. It may be considered radiant heat.

Ultraviolet light is located in the electromagnetic spectrum between visible light and ionizing radiation. It is responsible for molecular interactions that can result in sunburn.

Radiofrequency

A radio or television engineer describes radio waves in terms of their frequency. For example, radio station WIMP might broadcast at 960 kHz, and its associated television station WIMP-TV might broadcast at 63.7 MHz. Communication broadcasts are usually identified by their frequency of transmission and are called **radiofrequency (RF)** emissions.

RF covers a considerable portion of the electromagnetic spectrum. RF has relatively low energy and relatively long wavelength. Ham operators speak of broadcasting on the 10-m band or the 30-m band; these numbers refer to the approximate wavelength of emission.

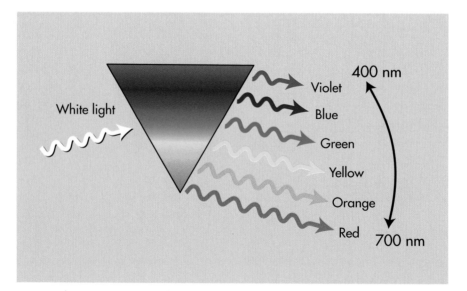

FIGURE 4-7 When it passes through a prism, white light is refracted into its component colors. These colors have wavelengths that extend from approximately 400 to 700 nm.

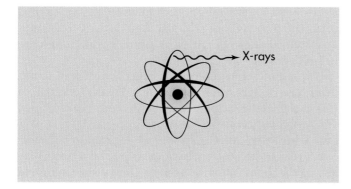

FIGURE 4-8 X-rays are produced outside the nucleus of excited atoms.

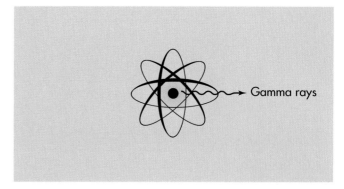

FIGURE 4-9 Gamma rays are produced inside the nucleus of radioactive atoms.

Standard AM radio broadcasts have a wavelength of about 100 m. Television and FM broadcasting occur at much shorter wavelengths. Because microwaves are also used for communication, RF and microwave emissions overlap considerably.

Very-short-wavelength RF is **microwave** radiation. Microwave frequencies vary according to use but are always higher than broadcast RF and lower than infrared. Microwaves have many uses, such as cellular telephone communication, highway speed monitoring, medical diathermy, and hot dog preparation.

Ionizing Radiation

Different from RF or visible light, ionizing electromagnetic energy usually is characterized by the energy contained in a photon. When an x-ray imaging system is operated at 80 kVp, the x-rays it produces contain energies ranging from 0 to 80 keV.

An x-ray photon contains considerably more energy than a visible light photon or an RF photon. The frequency of x-radiation is much higher and the wavelength much shorter than for other types of electromagnetic energy.

It is sometimes said that gamma rays have higher energy than x-rays. In the early days of radiology, this was true because of the limited capacity of available x-ray imaging systems. Today, linear accelerators make it possible to produce x-rays of considerably higher energies than gamma ray emissions. Consequently, the distinction by energy is not appropriate.

 The only difference between x-rays and gamma rays is their origin.

X-rays are emitted from the electron cloud of an atom that has been stimulated artificially (Figure 4-8). Gamma rays, on the other hand, come from inside the nucleus of a radioactive atom (Figure 4-9).

X-rays are produced in diagnostic imaging systems, whereas gamma rays are emitted spontaneously from radioactive material. Nevertheless, given an x-ray and a gamma ray of equal energy, one could not tell them apart.

This situation is analogous to the difference between beta particles and electrons. These particles are the same except that beta particles come from the nucleus and electrons come from outside the nucleus.

 Visible light is identified by wavelength, RF is identified by frequency, and x-rays are identified by energy.

Once again, three regions of the electromagnetic spectrum are particularly important to radiologic science. Naturally, the x-ray region is fundamental to producing a high-quality radiograph. The visible light region is also important because the viewing conditions of a radiographic or fluoroscopic image are critical to diagnosis. With the introduction of magnetic resonance imaging (MRI), the radiofrequency region has become more important in medical imaging.

The electromagnetic relationship triangle (Figure 4-10) can be helpful in relating each scale to the other two.

WAVE-PARTICLE DUALITY

A photon of x-radiation and a photon of visible light are fundamentally the same, except that x-radiation has much higher frequency, and hence a shorter wavelength, than visible light. These differences result in differences in the way these photons interact with matter.

Visible-light photons tend to behave more like waves than particles. The opposite is true of x-ray photons, which behave more like particles than waves. In fact, both types of photons exhibit both types of behavior—a phenomenon known as the **wave-particle duality** of electromagnetic energy.

Photons interact with matter most easily when the matter is approximately the same size as the photon wavelength.

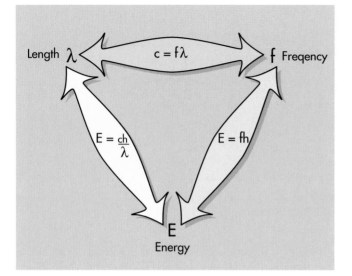

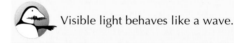

FIGURE 4-10 The electromagnetic relationship triangle.

Another general way to consider the interaction of electromagnetic radiation with matter is as a function of wavelength. Radio and TV waves, whose wavelengths are measured in meters, interact with metal rods or wires called *antennas.*

Microwaves, whose wavelengths are measured in centimeters, interact most easily with objects of the same size, such as hot dogs and hamburgers.

The wavelength of visible light is measured in nanometers (nm); visible light interacts with living cells, such as the rods and cones of the eye. Ultraviolet light interacts with molecules, and x-rays interact with electrons and atoms. All radiation with wavelength longer than those of x-radiation interacts primarily as a wave phenomenon.

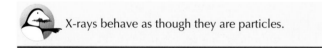 X-rays behave as though they are particles.

Wave Model: Visible Light

One of the unique features of animal life is the sense of vision. It is interesting that we have developed organs that sense only a very narrow portion of the enormous spread of the electromagnetic spectrum. This narrow portion is called **visible light.**

The visible-light spectrum extends from short-wavelength violet radiation through green and yellow to long-wavelength red radiation. On either side of the visible-light spectrum are ultraviolet light and infrared light. Neither can be detected by the human eye, but they can be detected by other means, such as a photographic emulsion.

Visible light interacts with matter very differently from x-rays. When a photon of light strikes an object, it sets the object's molecules into vibration. The orbital electrons of some atoms of certain molecules are excited to an energy level that is higher than normal. This energy is immediately re-emitted as another photon of light; it is reflected.

The atomic and molecular structures of any object determine which wavelengths of light are reflected. A leaf in the sunlight appears green because nearly all the visible-light photons are absorbed by the leaf. Only photons with wavelengths in the green region are reflected. Similarly, a balloon may appear red by absorbing all visible light photons except long-wavelength red photons, which are reflected.

Many familiar phenomena of light, such as reflection, absorption, and transmission, are most easily explained by using the wave model of electromagnetic energy. When a pebble is dropped into a still pond, ripples radiate from the center of the disturbance like miniature waves.

This situation is similar to the wave nature of visible light. Figure 4-11 shows the difference in the water waves between an initial disturbance caused by a small object and one caused by a large object. The distance between the crests of waves is much greater with the large object than with the small object.

 Visible light behaves like a wave.

With these water waves, the difference in wavelength is proportional to the energy introduced into the system. With light, the opposite is true: The shorter the photon wavelength, the higher is the photon energy.

If the analogy of the pebble in the pond is extended to a continuous succession of pebbles dropped into a smooth ocean, then at the edge of the ocean, the waves will appear straight rather than circular. Light waves behave as though they were straight rather than circular because the distance from the source is so great. The manner in which light is reflected from or transmitted through a surface is a consequence of this straight wavelike motion.

When the waves of the ocean crash into a vertical bulkhead (Figure 4-12), the reflected waves scatter from the bulkhead at the same angle at which the incident waves struck it. When the bulkhead is removed and replaced with a beach, the water waves simply crash onto the beach, dissipate their energy, and are absorbed. When an intermediate condition exists in which the bulkhead has been replaced by a line of pilings, the energy of the waves is scattered and absorbed.

Electromagnetic energy attenuation is the reduction in intensity that results from scattering and absorption.

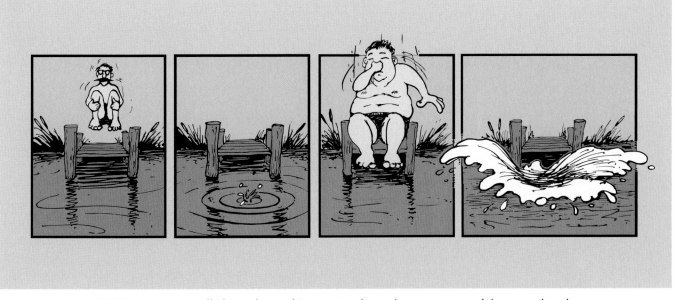

FIGURE 4-11 A small object dropped into a smooth pond creates waves of short wavelength. A large object creates waves of much longer wavelength.

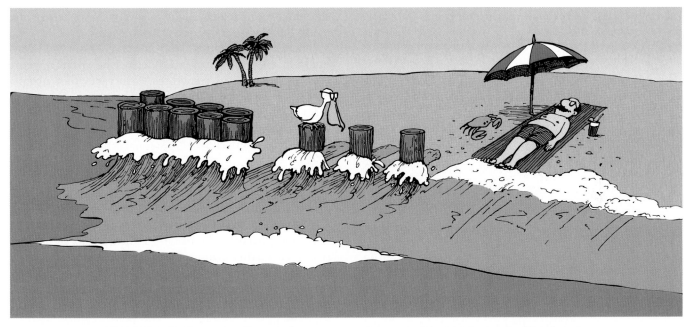

FIGURE 4-12 Energy is reflected when waves crash into a bulkhead. It is absorbed by a beach. It is partially absorbed or attenuated by a line of pilings. Light is also reflected, absorbed, or attenuated, depending on the composition of the surface on which it is incident.

Visible light can similarly interact with matter. **Reflection** from the silvered surface of a mirror is common. Examples of **transmission, absorption,** and **attenuation** of light are equally easy to identify. When light waves are absorbed, the energy deposited in the absorber reappears as heat. A black asphalt road reflects very little visible light but absorbs a considerable amount. In so doing, the road surface can become quite hot.

Just a slight modification can change how some materials transmit or absorb light. There are three degrees of interaction between light and an absorbing material: transparency, translucency, and opacity (Figure 4-13).

Window glass is transparent; it allows light to be transmitted almost unaltered. One can see through glass because the surface is smooth and the molecular structure is tight and orderly. Incident light waves cause molecular and electronic vibrations within the glass. These vibrations are transmitted through the glass and are re-irradiated almost without change.

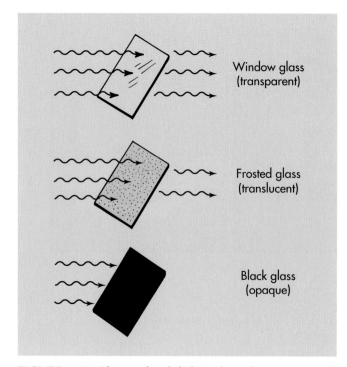

FIGURE 4-13 Objects absorb light in three degrees: not at all (transmission), partially (attenuation), and completely (absorption). The objects associated with these degrees of absorption are called transparent, translucent, and opaque, respectively.

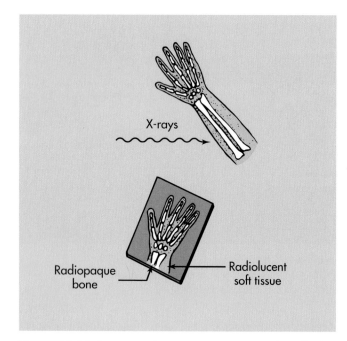

FIGURE 4-14 Structures that attenuate x-rays are described as radiolucent or radiopaque, depending on the relative degree of x-ray transmission or absorption, respectively.

When the surface of the glass is roughened with sandpaper, light is still transmitted through the glass but is greatly scattered and reduced in intensity. Instead of seeing clearly, one sees only blurred forms. Such glass is translucent.

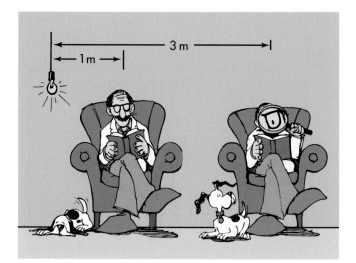

FIGURE 4-15 The inverse square law describes the relationship between radiation intensity and distance from the radiation source.

When the glass is painted black, the characteristics of the pigment in the paint are such that no light can pass through. Any incident light is totally absorbed in the paint. Such glass is opaque to visible light.

The terms *radiopaque* and *radiolucent* are used routinely in x-ray diagnosis to describe the visual appearance of anatomical structures. Structures that absorb x-rays are called radiopaque. Structures that transmit x-rays are called radiolucent (Figure 4-14). Bone is radiopaque, whereas lung tissue and to some extent soft tissue are radiolucent.

Inverse Square Law

When light is emitted from a source such as the sun or a light bulb, the intensity decreases rapidly with the distance from the source. X-rays exhibit precisely the same property. Figure 4-15 shows that as a book is moved farther from a light source, the intensity of light falls.

This decrease in intensity is inversely proportional to the square of the distance of the object from the source. Mathematically, this is called the **inverse square law** and is expressed as follows:

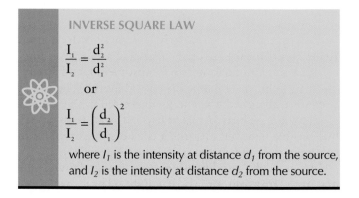

INVERSE SQUARE LAW

$$\frac{I_1}{I_2} = \frac{d_2^2}{d_1^2}$$

or

$$\frac{I_1}{I_2} = \left(\frac{d_2}{d_1}\right)^2$$

where I_1 is the intensity at distance d_1 from the source, and I_2 is the intensity at distance d_2 from the source.

The reason for the rapid decrease in intensity with increasing distance is that the total light emitted is spread out over an increasingly larger area. The equivalent of this phenomenon in the water wave analogy is the reduction of wave amplitude with distance from the source. The wavelength remains fixed.

 Electromagnetic energy (radiation) intensity is inversely related to the square of the distance from the source.

If the source of electromagnetic energy is not a point but rather a line, such as a fluorescent lamp, the inverse square law does not hold at distances close to the source. At great distances from the source, the inverse square law can be applied.

 The inverse square law can be applied to distances greater than seven times the longest dimension of the source.

To apply the inverse square law, you must know three of the four parameters, which consist of *two distances* and *two intensities*. The usual situation involves a known intensity at a fixed distance from the source and an unknown intensity at a greater distance.

Question: The intensity of light from a reading lamp is 100 millilumens (mlm), I_2, at a distance of 1 m, d_2. (The lumen is a unit of light intensity.) What is the intensity, I_1, of this light at 3 m, d_1?

Answer:
$$\frac{I_1}{I_2} = \frac{d_2^2}{d_1^2}$$

$$\frac{I_1}{100\ mlm} = \frac{1\ m^2}{3\ m^2}$$

$$I = (100\ mlm)\left(\frac{1\ m}{3\ m}\right)^2$$

$$= (100\ mlm)(1/9)$$

$$= 11\ mlm$$

This relationship between electromagnetic energy (radiation) intensity and distance from the source applies equally well to x-ray intensity.

Question: The exposure from an x-ray tube operated at 70 kVp, 200 mAs is 400 mR (4 mGy$_a$) at 90 cm. What will the exposure be at 180 cm?

Answer:
$$\frac{I_1}{I_2} = \left(\frac{d_2}{d_1}\right)^2$$

$$I_1 = I_2\left(\frac{d_1}{d_2}\right)^2$$

$$= (400\ mR)\ \frac{90\ cm^2}{180\ cm}$$

$$= (400\ mR)\left(\frac{1}{2}\right)^2$$

$$= (400\ mR)\left(\frac{1}{4}\right)$$

$$= 100\ mR$$

This example illustrates that when the distance from the source is doubled, the intensity of radiation is reduced by one fourth; conversely, when the distance is halved, the intensity is increased by a factor of four.

Question: For a given technique, the x-ray intensity at 1 m is 450 mR (4.5 mGy$_a$). What is the intensity at the edge of the control booth, a distance of 3 m, if the useful beam is directed at the booth? (This, of course, should never be done!)

Answer:
$$\frac{I_1}{I_2} = \left(\frac{d_2}{d_1}\right)^2$$

$$I_1 = I_2\left(\frac{d_1}{d_2}\right)^2$$

$$= (450\ mR)$$

$$\frac{1\ cm^2}{3\ cm} = 450\ mR\left(\frac{1}{3}\right)^2$$

$$= 450\ mR\left(\frac{1}{9}\right)$$

$$= 50\ mR$$

Often it is necessary to determine the distance from the source at which the radiation has a given intensity. This type of problem is commonly encountered in designing radiologic facilities.

Question: A temporary chest radiographic imaging system is to be set up in a large hall. The technique used results in an exposure of 25 mR (0.25 mGy$_a$) at 180 cm. The area behind the chest stand in which the exposure intensity exceeds 1 mR is to be cordoned off. How far from the x-ray tube will this area extend?

Answer:

$$\frac{I_1}{I_2} = \frac{d_2^2}{d_1^1}$$

$$\frac{25\ mR}{1\ mR} = \frac{(d_2)^2}{(180\ cm)^2}$$

$$(d_2)^2 = (180\ cm)^2 \left(\frac{25\ mR}{1\ mR}\right)$$

$$d_2 = \left[(180\ cm)^2 \left(\frac{25}{1}\right)\right]^{1/2}$$

$$= (180)(25)^{1/2}$$

$$= (180)(5)$$

$$= 900\ cm$$

$$= 9\ m$$

In the previous exercises, the intensity of the x-ray beam is calculated at a distance that assumes that the source is constant. In practical radiography, it is usual to work the other way around. One must calculate what the intensity of the beam should be at the source (i.e., the x-ray focal spot), so that exposure at the distance to the image receptor will remain constant. Thus, later, we will use the above formula but with one side inverted and will call it The Square Law.

Particle Model: Quantum Theory

In contrast to other portions of the electromagnetic spectrum, x-rays are usually identified by their energy, measured in electron volts (eV). X-ray energy ranges from approximately 10 keV to 50 MeV. The associated wavelength for this range of x-radiation is approximately 10^{-10} to 10^{-14} m. The frequency of these photons ranges from approximately 10^{18} to 10^{22} Hz.

Table 4-1 describes the various types of x-rays produced and the general use that is made of each. We are interested primarily in the diagnostic range of x-radiation, although what is said for that range holds equally well for other types of x-radiation.

An x-ray photon can be thought of as containing an electric field and a magnetic field that vary sinusoidally at right angles to each other with a beginning and an end that have diminishing amplitude (Figure 4-16). The wavelength of an x-ray photon is measured similarly to that of any electromagnetic energy: It is the distance from any position on the sine wave to the corresponding position of the next wave. The frequency of an x-ray photon is calculated similarly to the frequency of any electromagnetic photon, with use of the wave equation.

 The x-ray photon is a discrete bundle of energy.

X-rays are created with the speed of light (c), and they exist with velocity (**c**) or they do not exist at all. That is one of the substantive statements of **Planck's quantum theory.** Max Planck was a German physicist whose mathematical and physical theories synthesized our understanding of electromagnetic radiation into a uniform model; for this work, he received the Nobel Prize in 1918.

Another important consequence of this theory is the relationship between energy and frequency: Photon energy is directly proportional to photon frequency. The constant of proportionality, known as **Planck's constant** and symbolized by h, has a numeric value of 4.15×10^{-15} eVs or 6.63×10^{-34} Js. Mathematically, the relationship between energy and frequency is expressed as follows:

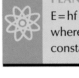

PLANCK'S QUANTUM EQUATION

$E = hf$

where E is the photon energy, h is Planck's constant, and f is the photon frequency in hertz.

The energy of a photon is directly proportional to its frequency.

Question: What is the frequency of a 70 keV x-ray?

Answer:

$$E = hf$$

$$f = \frac{E}{h}$$

$$= \frac{7 \times 10^4\ eV}{4.15 \times 10^{-15}\ eVs}$$

$$= 1.69 \times 10^{19}\ /s$$

$$= 1.69 \times 10^{19}\ Hz$$

Question: What is the energy in one photon of radiation from radio station WIMP-AM, which has a broadcast frequency of 960 kHz?

Answer:

$$E = hf$$

$$= (4.15 \times 10^{-15}\ eVs)(9.6 \times 10^5/s)$$

$$= 3.98 \times 10^{-9}\ eV$$

An extension of Planck's equation is the relationship between photon energy and photon wavelength; this relationship is useful in computing equivalent wavelengths of x-rays and other types of radiation.

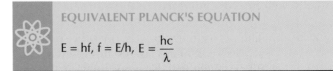

EQUIVALENT PLANCK'S EQUATION

$E = hf,\ f = E/h,\ E = \dfrac{hc}{\lambda}$

Table 4-1	Examples of the Wide Range of X-rays Produced by Application in Medicine, Research, and Industry	
Type of X-ray	Approximate Energy	Application
Diffraction	<10 kVp	Research: structural and molecular analysis
Grenz rays*	10-20 kVp	Medicine: dermatology
Superficial	50-100 kVp	Medicine: therapy of superficial tissues
Diagnostic	30-150 kVp	Medicine: imaging anatomical structures and tissues
Orthovoltage*	200-300 kVp	Medicine: therapy of deep-lying tissues
Supervoltage*	300-1000 kVp	Medicine: therapy of deep-lying tissues
Megavoltage	>1 MV	Medicine: therapy of deep-lying tissues
		Industry: checking integrity of welded metals

*These radiation therapy modalities are no longer in use.

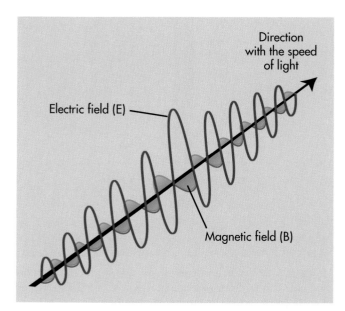

FIGURE 4-16 All electromagnetic radiation, including x-rays, can be visualized as two perpendicular sine waves that travel in a straight line at the speed of light. One of the sine waves represents an electric field and the other a magnetic field.

In other words, photon energy is inversely proportional to photon wavelength. In this relationship, the constant of proportionality is a combination of two constants, Planck's constant and the speed of light. The longer the wavelength of electromagnetic energy, the lower is the energy of each photon.

Question: What is the energy in one photon of green light whose wavelength is 550 nm?

Answer:

$$E = \frac{hc}{\lambda}$$

$$= \frac{\left(4.15 \times 10^{-15} \text{ eVs}\right)\left(3 \times 10^8 \text{ m/s}\right)}{550 \times 10^{-9} \text{ m}}$$

$$= \frac{12.45 \times 10^{-7} \text{ eVm}}{5.5 \times 10^{-7} \text{ m}}$$

$$= 2.26 \text{ eV}$$

MATTER AND ENERGY

We began Chapter 1 with the statement that everything in existence can be classified as matter or energy. We further stated that matter and energy are really manifestations of each other. According to classical physics, matter can be neither created nor destroyed, a law known as the **law of conservation of matter.** A similar law, the **law of conservation of energy,** states that energy can be neither created nor destroyed.

Einstein and Planck greatly extended these theories. According to quantum physics and the physics of relativity, matter can be transformed into energy and vice versa. Nuclear fission, the basis for generating electricity, is an example of converting matter into energy. In radiology, a process known as *pair production* (see Chapter 10) is an example of the conversion of energy into mass.

A simple relationship introduced in Chapter 1 allows the calculation of energy equivalence of mass and mass equivalence of energy. This equation is a consequence of Einstein's theory of relativity and is familiar to all.

Like the electron volt, the joule (J) is a unit of energy. One joule is equal to 6.24×10^{18} eV.

> **RELATIVITY**
> $E = mc^2$
> *E* in the equation is the energy measured in joules, *m* is the mass measured in kilograms, and *c* is the velocity of light measured in meters per second.

Question: What is the energy equivalence of an electron (mass = 9.109×10^{-31} kg), as measured in joules and in electron volts?

Answer:

$$E = mc^2$$

$$= \left(9.109 \times 10^{-31} \text{ kg}\right)\left(3 \times 10^8 \text{ m/s}\right)^2$$

$$= 81.972 \times 10^{-15} \text{ J}$$

$$= \left(8.1972 \times 10^{-14} \text{ J}\right)\left(\frac{6.24 \times 10^{18} \text{ eV}}{\text{J}}\right)$$

$$= 51.15 \times 10^4 \text{ eV}$$

$$= 511.5 \text{ keV}$$

The problem might be stated in the opposite direction as follows.

Question: What is the mass equivalent of a 70 keV x-ray?

Answer: $E = mc^2$

$$m = \frac{E}{c^2}$$

$$= \frac{(70 \times 10^3 \text{ eV}) \left(\dfrac{J}{6.24 \times 10^{18} \text{ eV}} \right)}{(3.8 \times 10^8 \text{ m/s})^2}$$

$$= \frac{11.2 \times 10^{-15} \text{ J}}{9 \times 10^{-16} \text{ m}^2/\text{s}^2}$$

$$= 1.25 \times 10^{-31} \text{ kg}$$

By using the relationships reported earlier, one can calculate the mass equivalence of a photon when only the photon wavelength or photon frequency is known.

Question: What is the mass equivalence of one photon of 1000 MHz microwave radiation?

Answer: $E = hf = mc^2$

$$m = \frac{hf}{c^2}$$

$$= \frac{(6.626 \times 10^{-34} \text{ Js})(1000 \times 10^6 \times Hz)}{(3 \times 10^8 \text{ m/s})^2}$$

$$= 0.736 \times 10^{-41} \text{ kg}$$

$$= 7.36 \times 10^{-42} \text{ kg}$$

Question: What is the mass equivalence of a 330-nm photon of ultraviolet light?

Answer: $E = \dfrac{hc}{\lambda} = mc^2$

$$m = \left(\frac{hc}{\lambda} \right) \left(\frac{1}{c^2} \right) = \frac{h}{\lambda c}$$

$$= \frac{6.626 \times 10^{-34} \text{ Js}}{(330 \times 10^{-9} \text{ m})(3 \times 10^8 \text{ m/s})}$$

$$= 0.00669 \times 10^{-33} \text{ kg}$$

$$= 6.69 \times 10^{-36} \text{ kg}$$

Calculations of this type can be used to set up a scale of mass equivalence for the electromagnetic spectrum (Figure 4-17). This scale can be used to check the answers to the above examples and to some of the problems in the companion *Workbook and Laboratory Manual.*

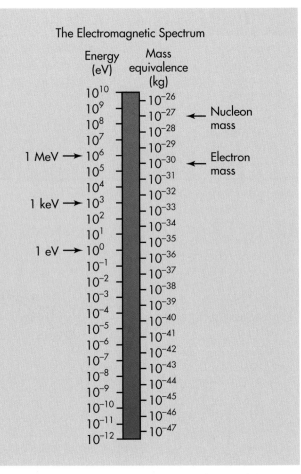

FIGURE 4-17 Mass and energy are two forms of the same medium. This scale shows the equivalence of mass measured in kilograms to energy measured in electron volts.

SUMMARY

Although matter and energy are interchangeable, x-ray imaging is based on energy in the form of x-ray photons that interact with tissue and an image receptor.

X-rays are one type of photon of electromagnetic energy. Frequency, wavelength, velocity, and amplitude are used to describe the various imaging regions of the electromagnetic spectrum. These characteristics of electromagnetic energy determine how such radiation interacts with matter.

CHALLENGE QUESTIONS

1. Define or otherwise identify the following:
   a. Photon
   b. Radiolucency
   c. The inverse square law
   d. Frequency
   e. The law of conservation of energy
   f. Gamma ray
   g. Electromagnetic spectrum

h. Sinusoidal (sine) variation
i. Quantum
j. Visible light

2. Accurately diagram one photon of orange light ($\lambda = 620$ nm) and identify its velocity, electric field, magnetic field, and wavelength.

3. A thunder clap associated with lightning has a frequency of 800 Hz. If its wavelength is 50 cm, what is its velocity? How far away is the thunder if the time interval between seeing the lightning and hearing the thunder is 6 s?

4. What is the frequency associated with a photon of microwave radiation that has a wavelength of 10^{-4} m?

5. Radio station WIMP-FM broadcasts at 104 MHz. What is the wavelength of this radiation?

6. In mammography, 28 keV x-rays are used. What is the frequency of this radiation?

7. Radiography of a barium-filled colon calls for high-kVp technique. These x-rays can have energy of 110 keV. What is the frequency and wavelength of this radiation?

8. What is the energy of the 110 keV x-ray in question 7 when expressed in joules? What is its mass equivalence?

9. The output intensity of a normal radiographic imaging system is 5 mR/mAs at 100 cm. What is the output intensity of such a system at 200 cm?

10. A mobile x-ray imaging system has an output intensity of 4 mR/mAs at 100 cm. Conditions require that a particular examination be conducted at 75 cm SID. What will be the output intensity at this distance?

11. Write the wave equation.

12. How are frequency and wavelength related?

13. Write the inverse square law and describe its meaning.

14. The intensity of light from a reading lamp is 200 millilumens (mlm) at a distance of 2 meters (m). What is the intensity of light at 3 m?

15. What are the three imaging windows of the electromagnetic spectrum and what unit of measure is applied to each?

16. What is the energy range of diagnostic x-rays?

17. What is the difference between x-rays and gamma rays?

18. Some regions of the electromagnetic spectrum behave like waves and some regions behave like particles in their interaction with matter. What is this phenomenon called?

19. Define attenuation.

20. What is the frequency of a 70-keV x-ray photon?

The answers to the Challenge Questions can be found by logging on to our website at http://evolve.elsevier.com.

Electricity, Magnetism, and Electromagnetism

OBJECTIVES

At the completion of this chapter, the student should be able to do the following:

1. Define electrification and provide examples
2. List the laws of electrostatics
3. Identify units of electric current, electric potential, and electric power
4. Identify the interactions between matter and magnetic fields
5. Discuss the four laws of magnetism
6. Relate the experiments of Oersted, Lenz, and Faraday in defining the relationships between electricity and magnetism
7. Identify the laws of electromagnetic induction

OUTLINE

Electrostatics
    Electrostatic Laws
    Electric Potential
Electrodynamics
    Electric Circuits
    Electric Power
Magnetism
    Magnetic Laws
    Magnetic Induction
Electromagnetism
    Electromagnetic Induction
    Electromagnetic Devices

THIS CHAPTER on electricity, magnetism, and electromagnetism briefly introduces the basic concepts needed for further study of the x-ray imaging system and its various components.

Because the primary function of the x-ray imaging system is to convert electric energy into electromagnetic energy—x-rays—the study of electricity, magnetism, and electromagnetism is particularly important.

This chapter begins by introducing some examples of familiar devices that convert electricity into other forms of energy. Electrostatics is the science of stationary electric charges. Electrodynamics is the science of electric charges in motion. Electromagnetism describes how electrons are given electric potential energy (voltage) and how electrons in motion create magnetism.

Magnetism has become increasingly important in diagnostic imaging with the application of magnetic resonance imaging (MRI) as a medical diagnostic tool. This chapter describes the nature of magnetism by discussing the laws that govern magnetic fields. These laws are similar to those that govern electric fields; knowing them is essential to understanding the function of several components of the x-ray imaging system. Electromagnetic induction is a means of transferring electric potential energy from one position to another, as in a transformer.

The primary function of an x-ray imaging system (Figure 5-1) is to convert electric energy into electromagnetic energy. Electric energy is supplied to the x-ray imaging system in the form of well-controlled electric current. A conversion takes place in the x-ray tube, where most of this electric energy is transformed into heat, some of it into x-rays.

Figure 5-2 shows other, more familiar examples of electric energy conversion. When an automobile battery runs down, an electric charge restores the chemical energy of the battery. Electric energy is converted into mechanical energy with a device known as an electric motor, which can be used to drive a circular saw. A kitchen toaster or electric range converts electric energy into thermal energy. There are, of course, many other examples of converting electric energy into other forms of energy.

ELECTROSTATICS

> Matter has mass and energy equivalence. Matter also may have electric charge.

Electric charge comes in discrete units that are **positive** or **negative**. Electrons and protons are the smallest units of electric charge. The electron has one unit of negative charge; the proton has one unit of positive charge. Thus, **the electric charges associated with an electron and a proton have the same magnitude but opposite signs.**

> *Electrostatics* is the study of stationary electric charges.

Because of the way atoms are constructed, electrons often are free to travel from the outermost shell of one atom to another atom. Protons, on the other hand, are fixed inside the nucleus of an atom and are not free to move. Consequently, nearly all discussions of electric charge deal with negative electric charges—those associated with the electron.

On touching a metal doorknob after having walked across a deep-pile carpet in winter, you get a shock (by contact). Such a shock occurs because electrons are rubbed off the carpet onto your shoes (by friction), causing you to become electrified. An object is said to be **electrified** if it has too few or too many electrons.

> Electrification can be created by contact, friction, or induction.

However, the outer shell electrons of some types of atoms are loosely bound and can be removed easily. Removal of these electrons electrifies the substances from which they were removed and results in static electricity.

If you run a comb through your hair, electrons are removed from the hair and deposited on the comb. The comb becomes electrified with too many negative charges. An electrified comb can pick up tiny pieces of paper as though the comb were a magnet (Figure 5-3). Because of its excess electrons, the comb repels some electrons in the paper, causing the closest end of the paper to become slightly positively charged. This results in a small electrostatic attractive force. Similarly, hair is electrified because it has an

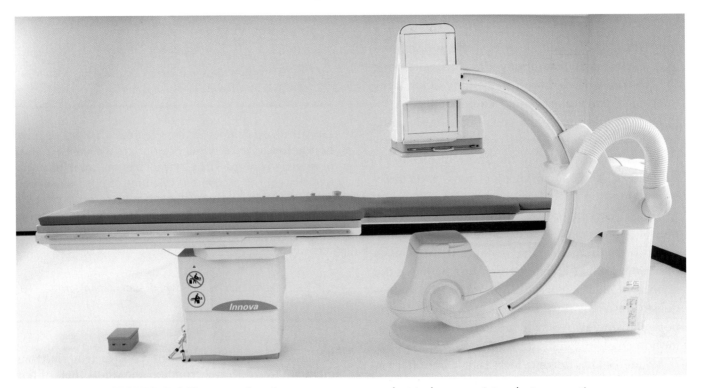

FIGURE 5-1 The x-ray imaging system converts electrical energy into electromagnetic energy. (Courtesy General Electric Medical Systems.)

abnormally low number of electrons and may stand on end because of mutual repulsion.

One object that is always available to accept electric charges from an electrified object is the Earth. The Earth behaves as a huge reservoir for stray electric charges. In this capacity, it is called an *electric ground*.

During a thunderstorm, wind and cloud movement can remove electrons from one cloud and deposit them on another (by induction). Both such clouds become electrified, one negatively and one positively.

If the electrification becomes sufficiently intense, a discharge can occur between the clouds; in this case, electrons are rapidly transported back to the cloud that is deficient. This phenomenon is called *lightning*. Although lightning can occur between clouds, it most frequently occurs between an electrified cloud and the Earth (Figure 5-4).

Another familiar example of electrification is seen in every Frankenstein movie. Usually, Dr. Frankenstein's laboratory is filled with electric gadgets, wire, and large steel balls with sparks flying in every direction (Figure 5-5). These sparks are created because the various objects—wires, steel balls, and so forth—are highly electrified.

The smallest unit of electric charge is the electron. This charge is much too small to be useful, so the fundamental unit of electric charge is the coulomb (C): $1 \text{ C} = 6 \times 10^{18}$ electron charges.

Question: What is the electrostatic charge of one electron?

Answer: One coulomb (C) is equivalent to 6.3×10^{18} electron charges; therefore,

$$\frac{1 \text{C}}{6.3 \times 10^{18} \text{ electron charges}}$$

$$= 1.6 \times 10^{-19} \text{ C/electron charge}$$

Question: The electrostatic charge transferred between two people after one has scuffed his feet across a nylon rug is one microcoulomb. How many electrons are transferred?

Answer: $1 \text{ C} = 6 \times 10^{18}$ electrons
$1 \text{ μC} = 6 \times 10^{12}$ electrons transferred

Question: One ampere is the flow of one coulomb per second; therefore "mAs" is a measure of what quantity?

Answer: $mAs = m \dfrac{C}{s} s = mC$, which is electrostatic charge

Electrostatic Laws

Four general laws of electrostatics describe how electric charges interact with each other and with neutral objects.

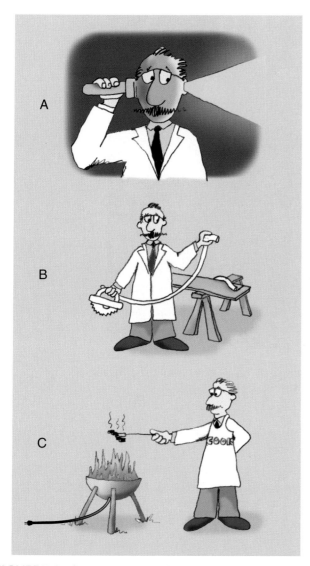

FIGURE 5-2 Electric energy can be converted from or to other forms by various devices, such as the battery **(A)** from chemical energy, the motor **(B)** to mechanical energy, and the barbecue **(C)** to thermal energy.

 Unlike charges attract; like charges repel.

Associated with each electric charge is an **electric field.** The electric field points outward from a positive charge and toward a negative charge. Uncharged particles do not have an electric field. In Figure 5-6, lines associated with each charged particle illustrate the intensity of the electric field.

When two similar electric charges—negative and negative or positive and positive—are brought close together, their electric fields are in opposite directions, which causes the electric charges to repel each other.

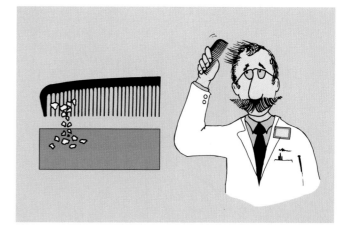

FIGURE 5-3 Running a comb briskly through your hair may cause both hair and comb to become electrified through the transfer of electrons from hair to comb. The electrified condition may make it possible to pick up small pieces of paper with the comb and may cause one's hair to stand on end.

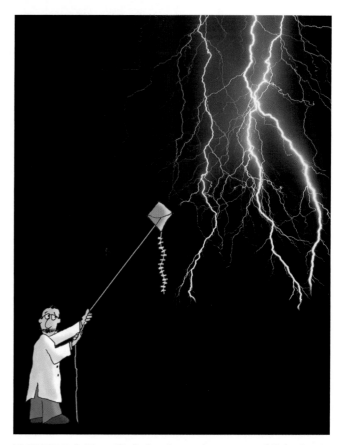

FIGURE 5-4 Electrified clouds are the source of lightning in a storm.

When unlike charges—one negative and one positive—are close to each other, the electric fields radiate in the same direction and cause the two charges to attract each other. The force of attraction between unlike charges or repulsion between like charges is due to the electric field. It is called an *electrostatic force.*

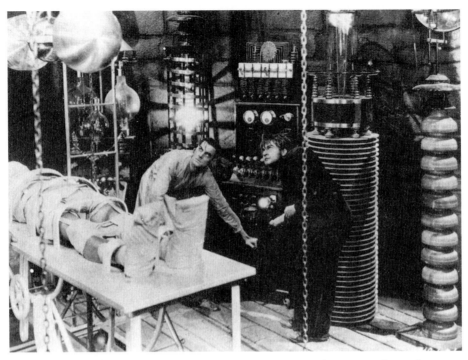

FIGURE 5-5 Early radiologic technologists are shown in this scene from the original *Frankenstein* movie (1931). (Courtesy Bettmann/Corbis.)

Coulomb's Law. The magnitude of the electrostatic force is given by Coulomb's law as follows:

COULOMB'S LAW

$$F = k \frac{Q_A Q_B}{d^2}$$

where F is the electrostatic force (newton), Q_A and Q_B are electrostatic charges (coulomb), d is the distance between the charges (meter), and k is a constant of proportionality.

 Coulomb's law: The electrostatic force is directly proportional to the product of the electrostatic charges and inversely proportional to the square of the distance between them.

The electrostatic force is very strong when objects are close but decreases rapidly as objects separate. This **inverse square** relationship for electrostatic force is the same as that for x-ray intensity (see Chapter 4).

 Electric charge distribution is uniform throughout or on the surface.

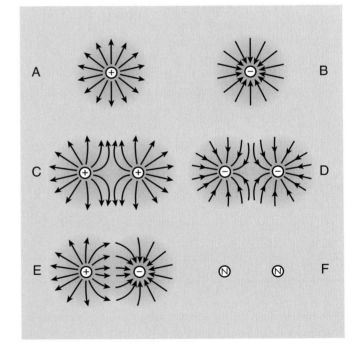

FIGURE 5-6 Electric fields radiate out from a positive charge **(A)** and toward a negative charge **(B).** Like charges repel one another **(C** and **D).** Unlike charges attract one another **(E).** Uncharged particles do not have an electric field **(F).**

When a diffuse nonconductor such as a thunder cloud becomes electrified, the electric charges are distributed rather uniformly throughout. With electrified copper wire, excess electrons are distributed on the outer surface (Figure 5-7).

 Electric charge of a conductor is concentrated along the sharpest curvature of the surface.

With an electrified cattle prod (Figure 5-8), electric charges are equally distributed on the surface of the two electrodes, except at each tip, where electric charge is concentrated. "Our business is shocking" is the motto of the manufacturer of the cattle prod shown.

Electric Potential

The discussion of potential energy in Chapter 1 emphasized the relationship of such energy to work. A system that possesses potential energy is a system with stored energy. Such a system has the ability to do work when this energy is released.

Electric charges have potential energy. When positioned close to each other, like electric charges have electric potential energy because they can do work when they fly apart. Electrons bunched up at one end of a wire create an electric potential because the electrostatic repulsive force causes some electrons to move along the wire so that work can be done.

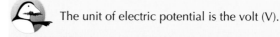 The unit of electric potential is the volt (V).

Electric potential is sometimes called *voltage;* the higher the voltage, the greater is the potential to do work. In the United States, the electric potential in homes and offices is 110 V. X-ray imaging systems usually require 220 V or higher. The volt is potential energy/unit charge, or *joule/coulomb* (1 V = 1 J/C).

ELECTRODYNAMICS

We recognized electrodynamic phenomena as electricity. If an electric potential is applied to objects such as copper wire, then electrons move along the wire. This is called an **electric current,** or **electricity.**

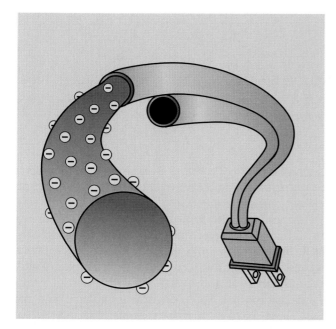

FIGURE 5-7 Cross section of an electrified copper wire, showing that the surface of the wire has excessive electrostatic charges.

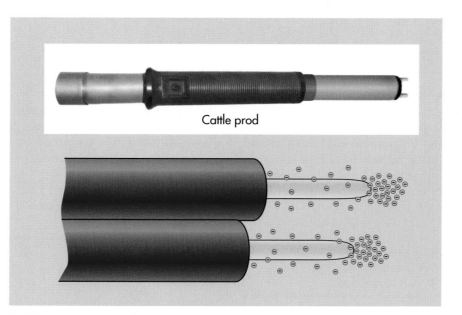

Cattle prod

FIGURE 5-8 Electrostatic charges are concentrated on surfaces of sharpest curvature. The cattle prod is a device that takes advantage of this electrostatic law.

Electric currents occur in many types of objects and range from the very small currents of the human body (such as those measured by electrocardiograms) to the very large currents of 440,000-V cross-country electric transmission lines.

 Electrodynamics is the study of electric charges in motion.

The direction of electric current is important. In his early classic experiments, Benjamin Franklin assumed that positive electric charges were conducted on his kite string. The unfortunate result is the convention that the direction of electric current is always opposite that of electron flow. Electrical engineers work with electric current, whereas physicists are usually concerned with electron flow.

A section of conventional household electric wire consists of a metal conducting wire, usually copper, coated with a rubber or plastic insulating material. The insulator confines the electron flow to the conductor. Touching the insulator does not result in a shock; touching the conductor does.

 A conductor is any substance through which electrons flow easily.

Most metals are good electric conductors; copper is one of the best. Water is also a good electric conductor because of the salts and other impurities it contains. That is why everyone should avoid water when operating power tools. Glass, clay, and other earthlike materials are usually good electric insulators.

 An insulator is any material that does not allow electron flow.

Other materials exhibit two entirely different electric characteristics. In 1946, William Shockley demonstrated *semiconduction.* The principal semiconductor materials are silicon (Si) and germanium (Ge). This development led to microchips and hence the explosive rise of computer technology.

A semiconductor is a material that under some conditions behaves as an insulator and in other conditions behaves as a conductor.

At room temperature, all material resists the flow of electricity. Resistance decreases as the temperature of

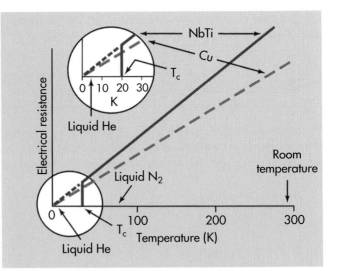

FIGURE 5-9 The electrical resistance of a conductor (Cu) and a superconductor (NbTi) as a function of temperature.

material is reduced (Figure 5-9). **Superconductivity** is the property of some materials to exhibit no resistance below a *critical temperature (Tc).*

Superconductivity was discovered in 1911 but was not developed commercially until the early 1960s. Scientific investigation into superconductivity has grown in recent years and now focuses on high-temperature superconductivity (Figure 5-10).

Superconducting materials such as niobium and titanium allow electrons to flow without resistance. Ohm's law, described in the next section, does not hold true for superconductors. A superconducting circuit can be viewed as one in perpetual motion because electric current exists without voltage. For material to behave as a superconductor, however, it must be made very cold, which requires energy.

Table 5-1 summarizes the four electric states of matter.

Electric Circuits

Modifying a conducting wire by reducing its diameter (wire gauge) or inserting different material (circuit elements) can increase its resistance. When this resistance is controlled and the conductor is made into a closed path, the result is an **electric circuit.**

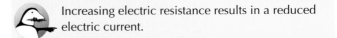 Increasing electric resistance results in a reduced electric current.

Electric current is measured in amperes (A). The ampere is proportional to the number of electrons flowing in the electric circuit. One ampere is equal to an electric charge of 1 C flowing through a conductor each second.

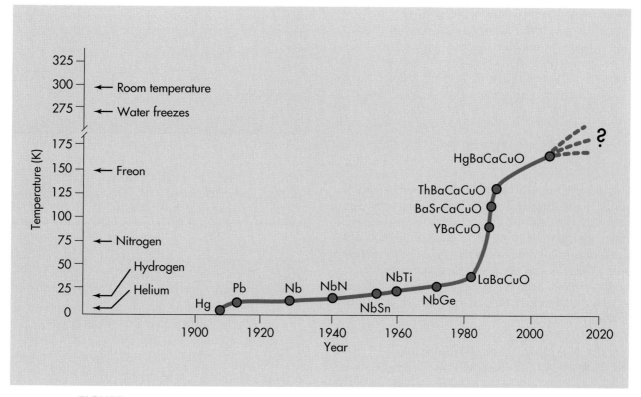

FIGURE 5-10 Recent years have seen a dramatic rise in the critical temperature for super-conducting materials.

Electric potential is measured in volts (V), and electric resistance is measured in ohms (Ω). Electrons at high voltage have high potential energy and high capacity to do work. If electron flow is inhibited, the circuit resistance is high.

The manner in which electric currents behave in an electric circuit is described by a relationship known as Ohm's law.

 Ohm's law: The voltage across the total circuit or any portion of the circuit is equal to the current times the resistance.

OHM'S LAW

$V = IR$

where V is the electric potential in volts, I is the electric current in amperes, and R is the electric resistance in ohms. Variations of this relationship are expressed as follows:

$$R = \frac{V}{I}$$

and

$$I = \frac{V}{R}$$

Table 5-1	**Four Electric States of Matter**	
State	**Material**	**Characteristics**
Superconductor	Niobium	No resistance to electron flow
	Titanium	No electric potential required
		Must be very cold
Conductor	Copper	Variable resistance
	Aluminum	Obeys Ohm's law
		Requires a voltage
Semiconductor	Silicon	Can be conductive
	Germanium	Can be resistive
		Basis for computers
Insulator	Rubber	Does not permit electron flow
	Glass	Extremely high resistance
		Necessary with high voltage

Question: If a current of 0.5 A passes through a conductor that has a resistance of 6 Ω, what is the voltage across the conductor?

Answer: V = IR
= (0.5 A) (6 Ω)
= 3 V

Question: A kitchen toaster draws a current of 2.5 A. If the household voltage is 110 V, what is the electric resistance of the toaster?

Answer:

$$R = \frac{V}{I}$$

$$= \frac{110\,\text{V}}{2.5\,\text{A}}$$

$$= 44\,\Omega$$

Most electric circuits, such as those used in radios, televisions, and other electronic devices, are very complicated. X-ray circuits are also complicated and contain a number of different types of circuit elements. Table 5-2 identifies some of the important types of circuit elements, the functions of each, and their symbols.

Usually, electric circuits can be reduced to one of two basic types: a series circuit (Figure 5-11) or a parallel circuit (Figure 5-12).

 In a *series circuit,* all circuit elements are connected in a line along the same conductor.

> **Rules for series circuits:**
> The total resistance is equal to the sum of the individual resistances.
>   The current through each circuit element is the same and is equal to the total circuit current.
>   The sum of the voltages across each circuit element is equal to the total circuit voltage.

 A *parallel circuit* contains elements that are connected at their ends rather than lying in a line along a conductor.

> **Rules for a parallel circuit:**
> The sum of the currents through each circuit element is equal to the total circuit current.
>   The voltage across each circuit element is the same and is equal to the total circuit voltage.
>   The total resistance is the inverse of the sum of the reciprocals of each individual resistance.

TABLE 5-2	Symbol and Function of Electric Circuit Elements	
Circuit Element	**Symbol**	**Function**
Resistor		Inhibits flow of electrons
Battery		Provides electric potential
Capacitor		Momentarily stores electric charge
Ammeter	(A)	Measures electric current
Voltmeter	(V)	Measures electric potential
Switch		Turns circuit on or off by providing infinite resistance
Transformer		Increases or decreases voltage by fixed amount (AC only)
Rheostat		Variable resistor
Diode		Allows electrons to flow in only one direction

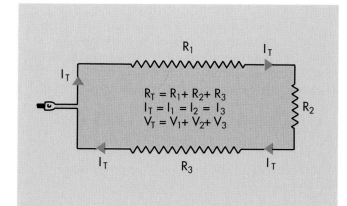

FIGURE 5-11 Series circuit and its basic rules.

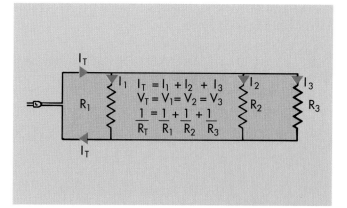

FIGURE 5-12 Parallel circuit and its basic rules.

Question: **A series circuit contains three resistive elements that have values of 8, 12, and 15 Ω. If the voltage is 110 V, what is the total resistance and current, the current through each resistor, and the voltage across each resistor?**

Answer: Refer to Figure 5-11:

let $R_1 = 8\ \Omega$, $R_2 = 12\ \Omega$, and $R_3 = 15\ \Omega$

$R_T = 8\ \Omega + 12\ \Omega + 15\ \Omega = 35\ \Omega$

$I_T = I_1 = I_2 = I_3 = V/R = 110/35 = 3.14\ A$

$V_1 = (3.14\ A)\ (8\ \Omega) = 25.12\ V$

$V_2 = (3.14\ A)\ (12\ \Omega) = 37.68\ V$

$V_3 = (3.14\ A)\ (15\ \Omega) = 47.10\ V$

Question: Suppose the previous example involved a parallel circuit rather than a series circuit. What would be the correct values for total resistance and current, the current through each resistor, and the voltage across each resistor?

Answer: Refer to Figure 5-12:

$$\frac{1}{R_T} = \frac{1}{8\ \Omega} + \frac{1}{12\ \Omega} + \frac{1}{15\ \Omega} = \frac{15}{120} + \frac{12}{120} + \frac{8}{120} = \frac{35}{120}$$

$$R_T = \frac{120}{35} = 3.4\ \Omega$$

$I_T = 110\ V/3.6\ \Omega = 30.2\ A$

$I_1 = 110\ V/8\ \Omega = 13.6\ A$

$I_2 = 110\ V/12\ \Omega = 9.2\ A$

$I_3 = 110\ V/15\ \Omega = 7.3\ A$

$V_1 = V_2 = V_3 = V_T = 110\ V$

Christmas lights are a good example of the difference between series and parallel circuits. Christmas lights wired in series have only one wire that connects each lamp; when one lamp burns out, the entire string of lights goes out. Christmas lights wired in parallel, on the other hand, have two wires that connect each lamp; when one lamp burns out, the rest remain lit.

Electric current, or electricity, is the flow of electrons through a conductor. These electrons can be made to flow in one direction along the conductor, in which case the electric current is called **direct current (DC)**.

Most applications of electricity require that the electrons be controlled so that they flow first in one direction and then in the opposite direction. Current in which electrons oscillate back and forth is called **alternating current (AC)**.

 Electrons that flow in only one direction constitute DC; electrons that flow alternately in opposite directions constitute AC.

Figure 5-13 diagrams the phenomenon of DC and shows how it can be described by a graph called a **waveform**. The horizontal axis, or x-axis, of the current waveform represents time; the vertical axis, or y-axis, represents the amplitude of the electric current. For DC, the electrons always flow in the same direction; therefore, DC is represented by a horizontal line. The vertical separation between this line and the time axis represents the magnitude of the current or the voltage.

The waveform for AC is a sine curve (Figure 5-14). Electrons flow first in a positive direction, then in a negative direction. At one instant in time (point 0 in Figure 5-14), all electrons are at rest. Then they move, first in the positive direction with increasing potential (segment A).

Once they reach maximum flow number, represented by the vertical distance from the time axis (point 1), the electric potential is reduced (segment B). They come to zero again momentarily (point 2) and then reverse motion and flow in the negative direction (segment C), increasing in negative electric potential to maximum (point 3). Next, the electric potential is reduced to zero (segment D).

This oscillation in electron direction occurs sinusoidally, with each requiring $\frac{1}{60}$ s. Consequently, AC is identified as a 60-Hz current (50 Hz in Europe and in much of the rest of the world).

Electric Power

Electric power is measured in **watts (W)**. Common household electric appliances, such as toasters, blenders, mixers, and radios, generally require 500 to 1500 W of electric power. Light bulbs require 30 to 150 W of electric power. An x-ray imaging system requires 20 to 150 kW of electric power.

> One watt is equal to 1 A of current flowing through an electric potential of 1 V. Power (W) = voltage (V) × current (A).

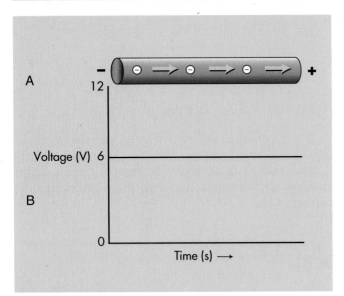

FIGURE 5-13 Representation of direct current. **A,** Electrons flow in one direction only. **B,** The graph of the associated electric waveform is a straight line.

Question: If the cost of electric power is 10 cents per kilowatt-hour (kW-hr), how much does it cost to operate a 100-W light bulb an average of 5 hours per day for 1 month?

Answer: Total on time = (30 days/mo) (5 hr/day)
= 150 hr/mo
Total power consumed = (150 hr/mo) (100 W)
= 15,000 W-hr/mo
= 15 kW-hr/mo
Total cost = (15 kW-hr/mo) (10 cents/kW-hr)
= $1.50/mo

> **ELECTRIC POWER**
>
> P = IV
> where *P* is the power in watts, *I* is the current in amperes, and *V* is the electric potential in volts; alternatively,
> P = IV = IIR
> therefore,
> P = I²R
> where *R* is resistance in ohms.

Question: An x-ray imaging system that draws a current of 80 A is supplied with 220 V. What is the power consumed?

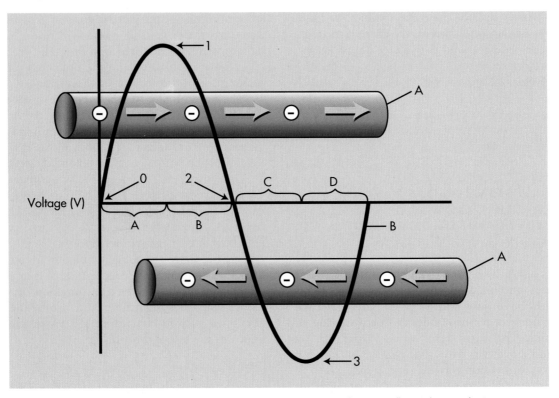

FIGURE 5-14 Representation of alternating current. **A,** Electrons flow alternately in one direction and then the other. **B,** Alternating current is represented graphically by a sinusoidal electric waveform.

Answer: P = IV
= (80 A) (220 V)
= 17,600 W
= 17.6 kW

Question: The overall resistance of a mobile x-ray imaging system is 10Ω. When plugged into a 110-V receptacle, how much current does it draw and how much power is consumed?

Answer: $I = \dfrac{V}{R} = \dfrac{110}{10} = 11A$

$P = IV$
$= (11A)(110V)$
$= 1210W$

$or\ P = I^2R$
$= (11A)^2 10$
$= 1210W$

MAGNETISM

Around 1000 BC, shepherds and dairy farmers near the village of Magnesia (what is now Western Turkey) discovered magnetite, an oxide of iron (Fe_3O_4). This rodlike stone, when suspended by a string, would rotate back and forth; when it came to rest, it pointed the way to water. It was called a **lodestone** or leading stone.

Of course, if you walk toward the North Pole from any spot on Earth, you will find water. So, the word **magnetism** comes from the name of that ancient village where the cows too were very curious. When milked, they produced Milk of Magnesia!

Magnetism is a fundamental property of some forms of matter. Ancient observers knew that lodestones would attract iron filings. They also knew that rubbing an amber rod with fur caused it to attract small, lightweight objects such as paper. They considered these phenomena to be different. We know them as magnetism and electrostatics, respectively; both are manifestations of the electromagnetic force.

Magnetism is perhaps more difficult to understand than other characteristic properties of matter, such as mass, energy, and electric charge, because magnetism is difficult to detect and measure. We can feel mass, visualize energy, and be shocked by electricity, but we cannot sense magnetism.

 Any charged particle in motion creates a magnetic field.

The magnetic field of a charged particle such as an electron in motion is perpendicular to the motion of that particle. The intensity of the magnetic field is represented by imaginary lines (Figure 5-15).

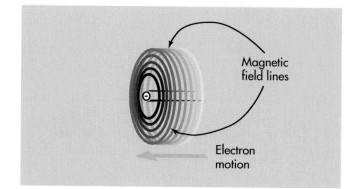

FIGURE 5-15 A moving charged particle induces a magnetic field in a plane perpendicular to its motion.

If the electron's motion is a closed loop, as with an electron circling a nucleus, magnetic field lines will be perpendicular to the plane of motion (Figure 5-16).

Electrons behave as if they rotate on an axis clockwise or counterclockwise. This rotation creates a property called *electron spin*. The electron spin creates a magnetic field, which is neutralized in electron pairs. Therefore, atoms that have an odd number of electrons in any shell exhibit a very small magnetic field.

Spinning electric charges also induce a magnetic field (Figure 5-17). The proton in a hydrogen nucleus spins on its axis and creates a nuclear magnetic dipole called a *magnetic moment*. This forms the basis of MRI.

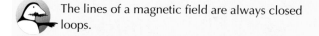 The lines of a magnetic field are always closed loops.

The lines of a magnetic field do not start or end as the lines of an electric field do. Such a field is called **bipolar** or **dipolar;** it always has a north and a south pole. The small magnet created by the electron orbit is called a **magnetic dipole.**

An accumulation of many atomic magnets with their dipoles aligned creates a **magnetic domain.** If all the magnetic domains in an object are aligned, it acts like a magnet. Under normal circumstances, magnetic domains are randomly distributed (Figure 5-18, *A*).

When acted on by an external magnetic field, however, such as the Earth in the case of naturally occurring ores or an electromagnet in the case of artificially induced magnetism, randomly oriented dipoles align with the magnetic field (Figure 5-18, *B*). This is what happens when ferromagnetic material is made into a permanent magnet.

The magnetic dipoles in a bar magnet can be thought of as generating imaginary lines of the magnetic field (Figure 5-19). If a nonmagnetic material is brought near such a magnet, these field lines are not disturbed. However, if ferromagnetic material such as soft iron is brought

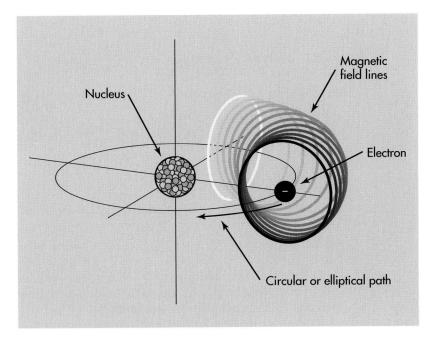

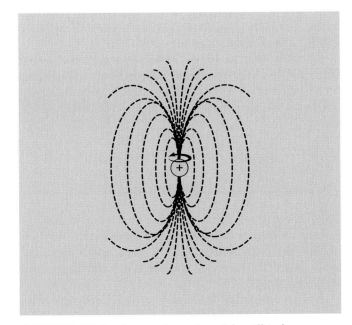

FIGURE 5-16 When a charged particle moves in a circular or elliptical path, the perpendicular magnetic field moves with the charged particle.

FIGURE 5-17 A spinning charged particle will induce a magnetic field along the axis of spin.

near the bar magnet, the magnetic field lines deviate and are concentrated into the ferromagnetic material.

 Magnetic permeability is the ability of a material to attract the lines of magnetic field intensity.

There are three principal types of magnets: naturally occurring magnets, artificially induced permanent magnets, and electromagnets.

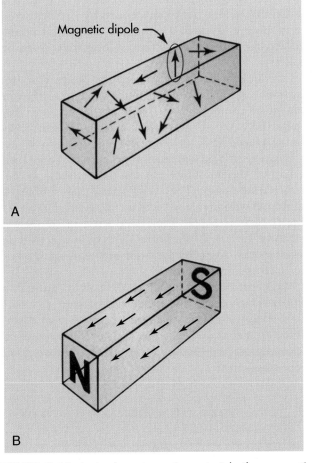

FIGURE 5-18 **A,** In ferromagnetic material, the magnetic dipoles are randomly oriented. **B,** This changes when the dipoles are brought under the influence of an external magnetic field.

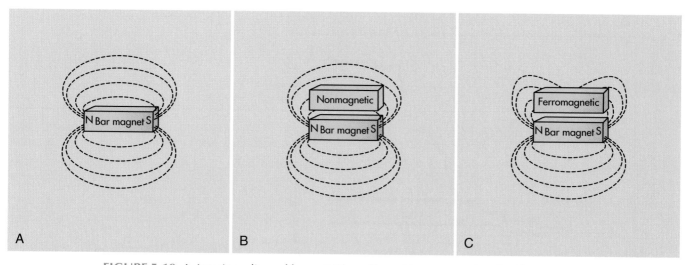

FIGURE 5-19 **A,** Imaginary lines of force. **B,** These lines of force are undisturbed by nonmagnetic material. **C,** They are deviated by ferromagnetic material.

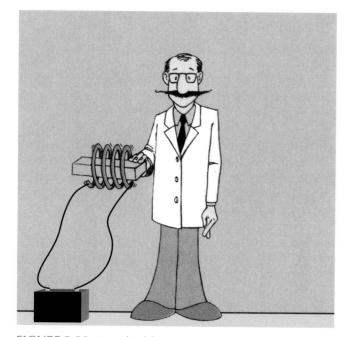

FIGURE 5-20 A method for using an electromagnet to render ceramic bricks magnetic.

 Magnets are classified according to the *origin* of the magnetic property.

The best example of a **natural magnet** is the Earth itself. The Earth has a magnetic field because it spins on an axis. Lodestones in the Earth exhibit strong magnetism presumably because they have remained undisturbed for a long time within the Earth's magnetic field.

Artificially produced **permanent magnets** are available in many sizes and shapes but principally as bar or horseshoe-shaped magnets, usually made of iron. A compass is a prime example of an artificial permanent magnet.

Permanent magnets are typically produced by aligning their domains in the field of an electromagnet (Figure 5-20).

Such permanent magnets do not necessarily stay permanent. One can destroy the magnetic property of a magnet by heating it or even by hitting it with a hammer. Either act causes individual magnetic domains to be jarred from their alignment. They thus again become randomly aligned, and magnetism is lost.

Electromagnets consist of wire wrapped around an iron core. When an electric current is conducted through the wire, a magnetic field is created. The intensity of the magnetic field is proportional to the electric current. The iron core greatly increases the intensity of the magnetic field.

 All matter can be classified according to the manner in which it interacts with an external magnetic field.

Many materials are unaffected when brought into a magnetic field. Such materials are nonmagnetic and include substances like wood and glass.

Diamagnetic materials are weakly repelled by either magnetic pole. They cannot be artificially magnetized and they are not attracted to a magnet. Examples of such diamagnetic materials are water and plastic.

Ferromagnetic materials include iron, cobalt, and nickel. These are strongly attracted by a magnet and usually can be permanently magnetized by exposure to a magnetic field. An alloy of aluminum, nickel, and cobalt called **alnico** is one of the more useful magnets produced from ferromagnetic material. Rare Earth ceramics have been developed recently and are considerably stronger magnets (Figure 5-21).

Paramagnetic materials lie somewhere between ferromagnetic and nonmagnetic. They are very slightly attracted to a magnet and are loosely influenced by an

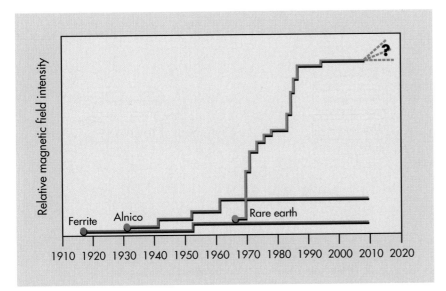

FIGURE 5-21 Developments in permanent magnet design have resulted in a great increase in magnetic field intensity.

TABLE 5-3	Four Magnetic States of Matter	
State	**Material**	**Characteristics**
Nonmagnetic	Wood, glass	Unaffected by a magnetic field
Diamagnetic	Water, plastic	Weakly repelled from both poles of a magnetic field
Paramagnetic	Gadolinium	Weakly attracted to both poles of a magnetic field
Ferromagnetic	Iron, nickel, cobalt	Can be strongly magnetized

external magnetic field. Contrast agents employed in MRI are paramagnetic.

 The degree to which a material can be magnetized is its *magnetic susceptibility*.

When wood is placed in a strong magnetic field, it does not increase the strength of the field: Wood has low magnetic susceptibility. On the other hand, when iron is placed in a magnetic field, it greatly increases the strength of the field: Iron has high magnetic susceptibility.

This phenomenon is used in transformers when the core of the transformer greatly enhances its efficiency. Unfortunately, some materials that are very susceptible are also reluctant to lose their magnetism. This condition is known as *hysteresis*.

Magnetic Laws

The physical laws of magnetism are similar to those of electrostatics and gravity. The forces associated with these three fields are fundamental (Table 5-3).

Note that the equations of force and the fields through which they act have the same form. Much work in theoretical physics involves the attempt to combine these fundamental forces with two others—the strong nuclear force and the weak interaction—to formulate a grand unified field theory.

In contrast to the case with electricity, there is no smallest unit of magnetism. Dividing a magnet simply creates two smaller magnets, which when divided again and again make baby magnets (Figure 5-22).

How do we know that these imaginary lines of the magnetic field exist? They can be demonstrated by the action of iron filings near a magnet (Figure 5-23).

If a magnet is placed on a surface with small iron filings, the filings attach most strongly and with greater concentration to the ends of the magnet. These ends are called *poles*, and every magnet has two poles, a north pole and a south pole, analogous to positive and negative electrostatic charges.

As with electric charges, like magnetic poles repel, and unlike magnetic poles attract. Also by convention, the imaginary lines of the magnetic field leave the north pole of a magnet and return to the south pole (Figure 5-24).

Magnetic Induction

Just as an electrostatic charge can be induced from one material to another, so some materials can be made magnetic by **induction**. The imaginary magnetic field lines just described are called *magnetic lines of induction*, and

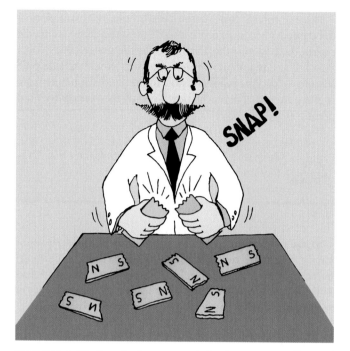

FIGURE 5-22 If a single magnet is broken into smaller and smaller pieces, baby magnets result.

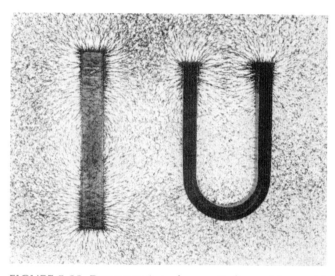

FIGURE 5-23 Demonstration of magnetic lines of force with iron filings.

the density of these lines is proportional to the intensity of the magnetic field.

> Ferromagnetic objects can be made into magnets by induction.

When ferromagnetic material, such as a piece of soft iron, is brought into the vicinity of an intense magnetic field, the lines of induction are altered by attraction to

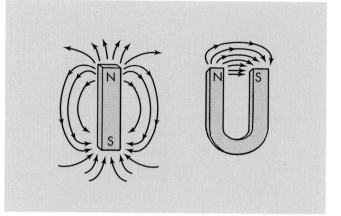

FIGURE 5-24 The imaginary lines of the magnetic field leave the north pole and enter the south pole.

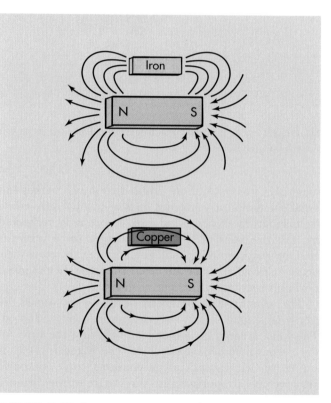

FIGURE 5-25 Ferromagnetic material such as iron attracts magnetic lines of induction, whereas nonmagnetic material such as copper does not.

the soft iron and the iron is made temporarily magnetic (Figure 5-25). If copper, a diamagnetic material, were to replace the soft iron, there would be no such effect.

This principle is employed with many MRI systems that use an iron magnetic shield to reduce the level of the fringe magnetic field. Ferromagnetic material acts as a magnetic sink by drawing the lines of the magnetic field into it.

When ferromagnetic material is removed from the magnetic field, it usually does not retain its strong

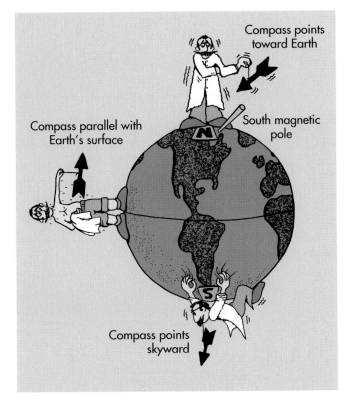

FIGURE 5-26 A compass reacts with the Earth as though it were a bar magnet seeking the north pole.

magnetic property. Soft iron, therefore, makes an excellent temporary magnet. It is a magnet only while its magnetism is being induced. If properly tempered by heat or exposed to an external field for a long period, however, some ferromagnetic materials retain their magnetism when removed from the external magnetic field and become permanent magnets.

The electric and magnetic forces were joined by Maxwell's field theory of electromagnetic radiation. The force created by a magnetic field and the force of the electric field behave similarly. This magnetic force is similar to electrostatic and gravitational forces that also are inversely proportional to the square of the distance between the objects under consideration. If the distance between two bar magnets is halved, the magnetic force increases by four times.

 The magnetic force is proportional to the product of the magnetic pole strengths divided by the square of the distance between them.

The Earth behaves as though it has a large bar magnet embedded in it. The polar convention of magnetism actually has its origin in the compass. At the equator, the north pole of a compass seeks the Earth's North Pole (which is actually the Earth's south magnetic pole).

As one travels toward the North Pole, the attraction of the compass becomes more intense until the compass needle points directly into the Earth, not at the geographic North Pole but at a region in northern Canada—the magnetic pole (Figure 5-26). The magnetic pole in the southern hemisphere is in Antarctica. There, the north end of the compass would point toward the sky.

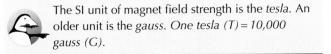 The SI unit of magnet field strength is the *tesla*. An older unit is the *gauss*. One tesla (T) = 10,000 *gauss (G)*.

The use of a compass might suggest that the Earth has a strong magnetic field, but it does not. The Earth's magnetic field is approximately 50 μT at the equator and 100 μT at the poles. This is far less than the magnet on a cabinet door latch, which is approximately 100 mT.

ELECTROMAGNETISM

Until the 19th century, electricity and magnetism were viewed as separate effects. Although many scientists suspected that the two were connected, research was hampered by the lack of any convenient way of producing and controlling electricity.

Thus the early study of electricity was limited to the investigation of static electricity, which could be produced by friction (e.g., the effect produced by rubbing fur on a rubber rod). Charges could be induced to move but only in a sudden discharge, as with a spark jumping a gap.

The development of methods for producing a steady flow of charges (i.e., an electric current) during the 19th century stimulated investigations of both electricity and magnetism. These investigations led to an enhanced understanding of electromagnetic phenomena and ultimately led to the electronic revolution on which today's technology is largely based.

In the late 1700s, an Italian anatomist, Luigi Galvani, made an accidental discovery. He observed that a dissected frog leg twitched when touched by two different metals, just as if it had been touched by an electrostatic charge. This prompted Alessandro Volta, an Italian physicist of the same era, to question whether an electric current might be produced when two different metals are brought into contact.

Using zinc and copper plates, Volta succeeded in producing a feeble electric current. To increase the current, he stacked the copper-zinc plates like a Dagwood sandwich to form what was called the **Voltaic pile,** a precursor of the modern battery. Each zinc-copper sandwich is called a **cell** of the battery.

Modern dry cells use a carbon rod as the positive electrode surrounded by an electrolytic paste housed in a negative zinc cylindrical can. Figure 5-27 shows

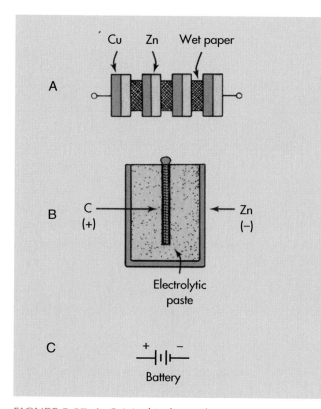

FIGURE 5-27 **A,** Original Voltaic pile. **B,** A modern dry cell. **C,** Symbol for a battery.

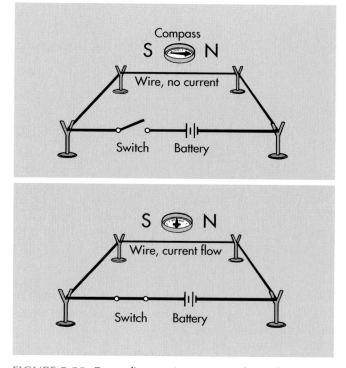

FIGURE 5-28 Oersted's experiment. **A,** With no electric current in the wire, the compass points north. **B,** With electric current, the compass points toward the wire.

the Voltaic pile, the modern battery, and the electronic symbol for the battery.

These devices are examples of sources of electromotive force. Any device that converts some form of energy directly into electric energy is said to be a source of electromotive force. Although still commonly used, this somewhat archaic term is a little misleading. Electromotive force is not really a force such as gravity; rather, the term refers to electric potential.

> Electric potential is measured in units of joule per coulomb, or volt.

Now that they finally had a source of constant electric current, scientists began extensive investigations into the possibility of a link between electric and magnetic forces. Hans Oersted, a Danish physicist, discovered the first such link in 1820.

Oersted fashioned a long straight wire, supported near a free-rotating magnetic compass (Figure 5-28). With no current in the wire, the magnetic compass pointed north as expected. When a current was passed through the wire, however, the compass needle swung to point straight at the wire. Here we have evidence of a direct link between electric and magnetic phenomena. The electric current evidently produced a magnetic

field strong enough to overpower the Earth's magnetic field and cause the magnetic compass to point toward the wire.

> Any charge in motion induces a magnetic field.

A charge at rest produces no magnetic field. Electrons that flow through a wire produce a magnetic field about that wire. The magnetic field is represented by imaginary lines that form concentric circles centered on the wire (Figure 5-29).

The direction of the magnetic field lines can be determined by using the right-hand rule. Imagine gripping the wire with the right hand. If the thumb is pointed in the direction of the electric current, the fingers of your hand will then curl in the direction of the magnetic field lines (Figure 5-30). Similarly, the left hand is used if the thumb is pointed in the direction of electron flow, which is opposite to current.

These same rules apply if the current is in a loop. Magnetic field lines form concentric circles around each tiny section of the wire. Because the wire is curved, however, these magnetic field lines overlap inside the loop. In particular, at the very center of the loop, all the field lines come together, making the magnetic field strong (Figure 5-31).

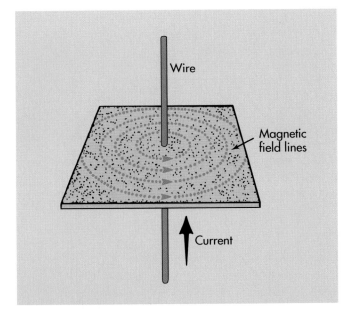

FIGURE 5-29 Magnetic field lines form concentric circles around the current-carrying wire.

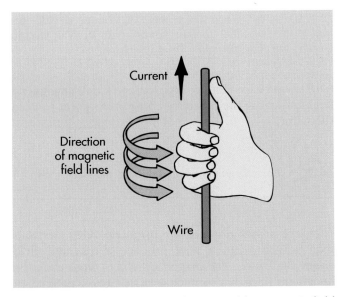

FIGURE 5-30 Determining the direction of the magnetic field around the wire using the right-hand rule.

Stacking more loops on top of each other increases the intensity of the magnetic field running through the center or axis of the stack of loops. The magnetic field of a solenoid is concentrated through the center of the coil (Figure 5-32).

A coil of wire is called a *solenoid*.

The magnetic field can be intensified further by wrapping the coil of wire around ferromagnetic material, such as iron. The iron core intensifies the magnetic field.

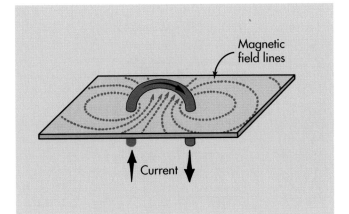

FIGURE 5-31 Magnetic field lines are concentrated on the inside of the loop.

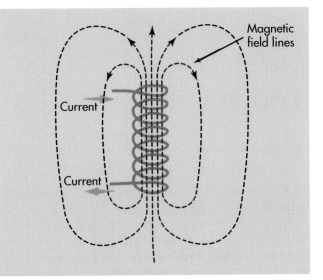

FIGURE 5-32 Magnetic field lines of a solenoid.

In this case, almost all of the magnetic field lines are concentrated inside the iron core, escaping only near the ends of the coil. This type of device is called an **electromagnet** (Figure 5-33).

 An electromagnet is a current-carrying coil of wire wrapped around an iron core, which intensifies the induced magnetic field.

The magnetic field produced by an electromagnet is the same as that produced by a bar magnet. That is, if both were hidden from view behind a piece of paper, the pattern of magnetic field lines revealed by iron filings sprinkled on the paper surface would be the same. Of course, the advantage of the electromagnet is that its magnetic field can be adjusted or turned on and off simply by varying the current through its coil of wire.

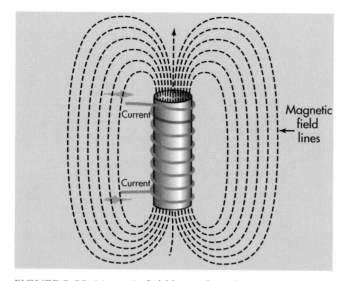

FIGURE 5-33 Magnetic field lines of an electromagnet.

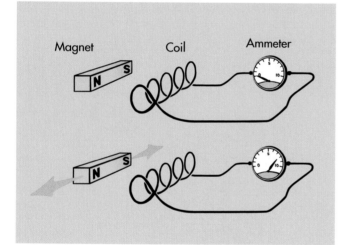

FIGURE 5-34 Schematic description of Faraday's experiment shows how a moving magnetic field induces an electric current.

Electromagnetic Induction

Oersted's experiment demonstrated that electricity can be used to generate magnetic fields. It is obvious, then, to wonder whether the reverse is true: Can magnetic fields somehow be used to generate electricity? Michael Faraday, a self-educated British experimenter, found the answer to that question.

From a series of experiments, Faraday concluded that an electric current cannot be induced in a circuit merely by the presence of a magnetic field. For example, consider the situation illustrated in Figure 5-34. A coil of wire is connected to a current-measuring device called an **ammeter.** If a bar magnet were set next to the coil, the meter would indicate no current in the coil.

However, Faraday discovered that when the magnet is moved, the coiled wire does have a current, as indicated

by the ammeter. Therefore, to induce a current with the use of a magnetic field, the magnetic field cannot be constant but must be changing.

Electromagnetic induction: An electric current is induced in a circuit if some part of that circuit is in a changing magnetic field.

This observation is summarized in what is called **Faraday's law,** or the first law of electromagnetics.

FARADAY'S LAW
The magnitude of the induced current depends on four factors:
1. The strength of the magnetic field
2. The velocity of the magnetic field as it moves past the conductor
3. The angle of the conductor to the magnetic field
4. The number of turns in the conductor

Actually, no physical motion is needed. An electromagnet can be fixed near a coil of wire. If the current in the electromagnet is then increased or decreased, its magnetic field will likewise change and induce a current in the coil.

A prime example of electromagnetic induction is radio reception (Figure 5-35). Radio emission consists of waves of electromagnetic radiation. Each wave has an oscillating electric field and an oscillating magnetic field. The oscillating magnetic field induces motion in electrons in the radio antennae, resulting in a radio signal. This signal is detected and decoded to produce sound.

The essential point in all these examples is that the intensity of the magnetic field at the wire must be changing to induce a current. If the magnetic field intensity is constant, there will be no induced current.

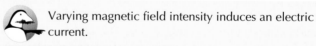
Varying magnetic field intensity induces an electric current.

Electromechanical Devices

Electric motors and generators are practical applications of Oersted's and Faraday's experiments. In one experiment, an electric current produces a mechanical motion (the motion of the compass needle). This is the basis of the electric motor. In the other experiment, mechanical motion (the motion of a magnet near a coil of wire) induces electricity in a coil of wire. This is the principle on which the electric generator operates.

Figure 5-36 shows the diagram of a simple electric generator. A coil of wire is placed in a strong magnetic

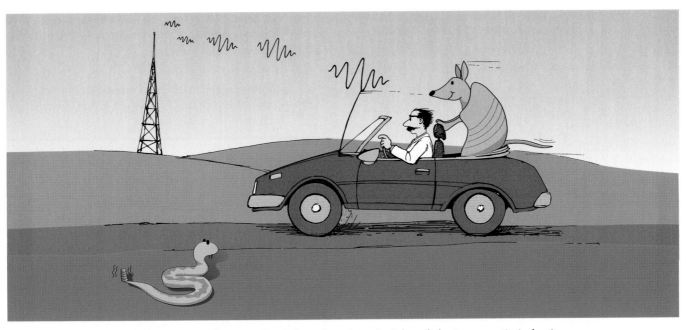

FIGURE 5-35 Radio reception is based on the principles of electromagnetic induction.

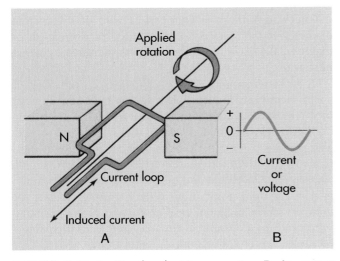

FIGURE 5-36 **A,** Simple electric generator. **B,** Its output waveform.

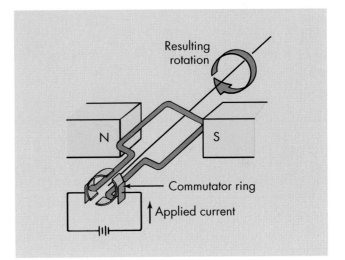

FIGURE 5-37 Simple direct current electric motor.

field between two magnetic poles. The coil is rotated by mechanical energy. The mechanical energy can be supplied by hand, by water flowing over a water wheel, or by steam flowing past the vanes of a turbine blade in a nuclear power plant. Because the coil of wire is moving in the magnetic field, a current is induced in the coil of wire.

The induced current is not constant, however. It varies according to the orientation of the coil's wire in the magnetic field. The induced current flows first in one direction and then the other, following a sinusoidal pattern. Thus, this type of simple electric generator produces an alternating current (AC).

The net effect of an electric generator is to convert mechanical energy into electrical energy. The

conversion process is, of course, not 100% efficient because of frictional losses in the mechanical moving parts and heat losses caused by resistance in the electrical components.

A simple electric motor has basically the same components as an electric generator (Figure 5-37). In this case, however, electric energy is supplied to the current loop to produce a mechanical motion—that is, a rotation of the loop in the magnetic field.

When a current is passed through the wire loop, a magnetic field is produced, making the loop behave like a tiny electromagnet. Being free to turn, the electromagnet current loop rotates as it attempts to align itself with the stronger magnetic field produced by the external bar magnet.

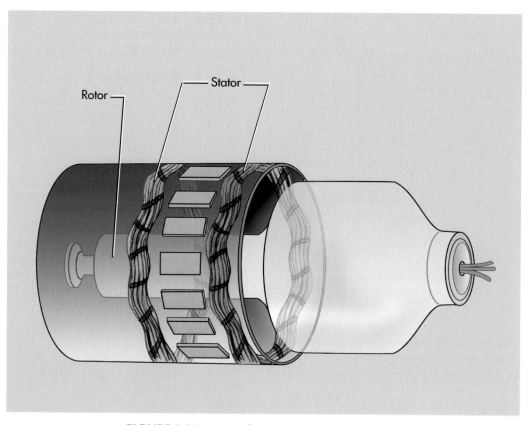

FIGURE 5-38 Principal parts of an induction motor.

Just as the current loop becomes aligned with the external magnetic field, the commutator ring switches the direction of current through the loop and therefore reverses the coil's required alignment.

Because of the reversal in current direction, the electromagnet is no longer aligned with the magnetic field of the bar magnet; it is now opposed to it. The electromagnet current loop rotates 180 degrees in an attempt to realign itself once again with the bar magnet field. As the electromagnet again nears alignment, the commutator ring switches the direction of current and forces the loop to rotate again.

The electromagnet current loop is never quite able to align itself with the magnetic field of the bar magnet. The net result is that the current loop rotates continuously.

A practical electric motor uses many turns of wire for the current loop and many bar magnets to create the external magnetic field. The principle of operation, however, is the same.

The type of motor used with x-ray tubes is an induction motor (Figure 5-38). In this type of motor, the rotating rotor is a shaft made of bars of copper and soft iron fabricated into one mass; however, the external magnetic field is supplied by several fixed electromagnets called *stators*.

An induction motor powers the rotating anode of an x-ray tube.

No electric current is passed to the rotor. Instead, current is produced in the rotor windings by induction. The electromagnets surrounding the rotor are energized in sequence, producing a changing magnetic field. The induced current produced in the rotor windings generates a magnetic field.

Just as in a conventional electric motor, this magnetic field attempts to align itself with the magnetic field of the external electromagnets. Because these electromagnets are being energized in sequence, the rotor begins to rotate, trying to bring its magnetic field into alignment.

The result is the same as in a conventional electric motor, that is, the rotor rotates continuously. The difference, however, is that the electrical energy is supplied to the external magnets rather than the rotor.

Another device that uses the interacting magnetic fields produced by changing electric currents is the **transformer**. However, the transformer does not convert one form of energy to another but rather transforms electric potential and current into higher or lower intensity.

A transformer changes the intensity of alternating voltage and current.

Consider an electromagnet with a ferromagnetic core bent around so that it forms a continuous loop

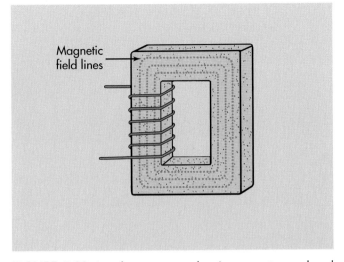

FIGURE 5-39 An electromagnet that incorporates a closed iron core produces a closed magnetic field that is primarily confined to the core.

(Figure 5-39). There are no end surfaces from which ferromagnetic field lines can escape. Therefore, the magnetic field tends to be confined to the loop of magnetic core material.

If a secondary coil is then wound around the other side of this loop of core material, almost all the magnetic field produced by the primary coil also passes through the center of the secondary coil. Thus, there is a good coupling between the magnetic field produced by the primary coil and the secondary coil. A changing current in the primary coil induces a changing current in the secondary coil. This type of device is a transformer.

A transformer will operate only with a changing electric current (AC). A direct current applied to the primary coil will induce no current in the secondary coil.

The transformer is used to change the magnitude of voltage and current in an AC circuit. The change in voltage is directly proportional to the ratio of the number of turns (windings) of the secondary coil (N_s) to the number of turns in the primary coil (N_p). If there are 10 turns on the secondary coil for every turn on the primary coil, then the voltage generated in the secondary circuit (V_s) will be 10 times the voltage supplied to the primary circuit (V_p). Mathematically, the transformer law is represented as follows:

TRANSFORMER LAW

$$\frac{V_S}{V_P} = \frac{N_S}{N_P}$$

The quantity N_s/N_p is known as the *turns ratio* of the transformer.

Question: The secondary side of a transformer has 300,000 turns; the primary side has 600 turns. What is the turns ratio?

Answer:
$$\text{Turns ratio} = \frac{N_S}{N_P}$$

$$N_s = 300{,}000$$
$$N_p = 600$$
$$= 300{,}000/600$$
$$= 500{:}1$$

The voltage change across the transformer is proportional to the turns ratio. A transformer with a turns ratio greater than 1 is a **step-up transformer** because the voltage is increased or stepped up from the primary side to the secondary side. When the turns ratio is less than 1, the transformer is a **step-down transformer**.

As the voltage changes across a transformer, the current *(I)* changes also; the transformer law may also be written as follows:

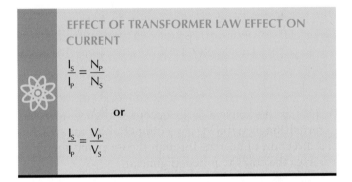

EFFECT OF TRANSFORMER LAW EFFECT ON CURRENT

$$\frac{I_S}{I_P} = \frac{N_P}{N_S}$$

or

$$\frac{I_S}{I_P} = \frac{V_P}{V_S}$$

Question: The turns ratio of a filament transformer is 0.125. What is the filament current if the current through the primary winding is 0.8 A?

Answer:
$$\frac{I_S}{I_P} = \frac{N_P}{N_S}$$

$$I_S = I_P \left(\frac{N_P}{N_S} \right)$$

$$= (0.8\,\text{A}) \left(\frac{1}{0.125} \right)$$

$$= 6.4\,\text{A}$$

The change in current across a transformer is in the opposite direction from the voltage change but in the same proportion: an inverse relationship. For example, if the voltage is doubled, the current is halved.

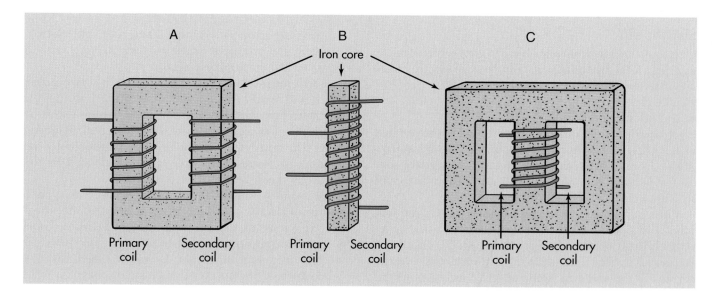

FIGURE 5-40 Type of transformers. **A,** Closed-core transformer. **B,** Autotransformer. **C,** Shell-type transformer.

In a step-up transformer, the current on the secondary side (I_s) is smaller than the current on the primary side (I_p). In a step-down transformer, the secondary current is larger than the primary current.

Question: There are 125 turns on the primary side of a transformer and 90,000 turns on the secondary side. If 110 V AC is supplied to the primary winding, what is the voltage induced in the secondary winding?

Answer:

$$\frac{V_s}{V_P} = \frac{N_S}{N_P}$$

$$V_s = V_p = \left[\frac{N_S}{N_P}\right]$$

$$= (110\,V)\left(\frac{90,000}{125}\right)$$

$$= (110)\,(720)\,V$$

$$= 79,200\,V$$

$$= 79.2\,kV$$

There are many ways to construct a transformer (Figure 5-40). The type of transformer discussed thus far, built about a square core of ferromagnetic material, is called a **closed-core transformer** (Figure 5-40, *A*).

The ferromagnetic core is not a single piece but rather is built up of laminated layers of iron. This layering helps reduce energy losses, resulting in greater efficiency.

Another type of transformer is the autotransformer (Figure 5-40, *B*). It consists of an iron core with only one winding of wire about it. This single winding acts as both the primary and the secondary winding. Connections are made at different points on the coil for both the primary and the secondary sides.

> The autotransformer has one winding and varies both voltage and current.

An autotransformer is generally smaller, and because the primary and the secondary sides are connected to the same wire, its use is generally restricted to cases in which only a small step up or step down in voltage is required. Thus, an autotransformer would not be suitable for use as the high-voltage transformer in an x-ray imaging system.

The third type of transformer is the **shell-type transformer** (Figure 5-40, *C*). This type of transformer confines even more of the magnet field lines of the primary winding because the secondary is wrapped around it and there are essentially two closed cores. This type is more efficient than the closed-core transformer. Most currently used transformers are shell-type.

The practical applications of the laws of electromagnetism appear in the electric motor (electric current produces mechanical motion), the electric generator (mechanical motion produces electric current), and the transformer (alternating electric current and electric potential are transformed in intensity). The transformer law describes how electric current and voltage change from the primary coil to the secondary coil.

SUMMARY

Electrons can flow from one object to another by contact, by friction, or by induction. The laws of electrostatics are as follows:

- Like charges repel
- Unlike charges attract

Electrostatic force is directly proportional to the product of the charges and inversely proportional to the square of the distance between them. Electric charges are concentrated along the sharpest curvature of the surface of the conductor.

Electrodynamics is the study of electrons in motion, otherwise known as *electricity*. Conductors are materials through which electrons flow easily. Insulators are materials that inhibit the flow of electrons. Electric current is measured in amperes (A), electric potential is measured in volts (V), and electric resistance is measured in ohms (Ω).

Electric power is energy produced or consumed per unit time. One watt of power is equal to 1 A of electricity flowing through an electric potential of 1 V.

Matter has magnetic properties because some atoms and molecules have an odd number of electrons in the outer shells. The unpaired spin of these electrons produces a magnetic field within the object. Natural magnets get their magnetism from the Earth, permanent magnets are artificially induced magnets, and electromagnets are produced when current-carrying wire is wrapped around an iron core.

Every magnet, no matter how small, has two poles: north and south. Like magnetic poles repel and unlike magnetic poles attract. Ferromagnetic material can be made magnetic when placed in an external magnetic field. The force between poles is proportional to the product of the magnetic pole strengths divided by the square of the distance between them.

Alessandro Volta's development of the battery as a source of electric potential energy prompted additional investigations of electric and magnetic fields. Hans Oersted demonstrated that electricity can be used to generate magnetic fields. It was Michael Faraday who observed the current in a changing magnetic field and described the first law of electromagnetism (Faraday's law).

Practical applications of the laws of electromagnetism appear in the electric motor (electric current produces mechanical motion), the electric generator (mechanical motion produces electric current), and the transformer (alternating electric current and electric potential are transformed in intensity). The transformer law describes how electric current and voltage change from the primary coil to the secondary coil.

CHALLENGE QUESTIONS

1. Define or otherwise identify the following:
   a. Electric charge and its unit
   b. Electrodynamics
   c. Electric power
   d. Electrostatics
   e. Dipole
   f. Induction
   g. Magnetic domain
   h. Autotransformer
   i. Gauss; Tesla
   j. Electric potential
2. What is the total circuit resistance when resistive elements of 5, 10, 15, and 20 Ω are connected in (a) series and (b) parallel?
3. If the total current in the circuit in question 2 is 7 A, what is the voltage across the 10 Ω resistor for (a) series and (b) parallel operation?
4. A radiographic exposure requires 100 mAs. How many electrons is this?
5. Describe three types of transformers.
6. What are the three ways to electrify an object?
7. List the four laws of electrostatics.
8. Why is electrification easier in dry Phoenix than in humid Houston?
9. A mobile x-ray imaging system operates on 110 V AC power. Its maximum capacity is 110 kVp and 100 mA. What is the turns ratio of the high-voltage transformer?
10. What should be the primary current in the previous question to produce a secondary current of 100 mA?
11. Magnetic fields in excess of 5 G can interfere with cardiac pacemakers. How many mT is this?
12. What is the role of magnetism in the study of x-ray imaging?
13. List the three principal types of magnets.
14. Describe an electromagnet.
15. Explain how a magnetic domain can cause an object to behave like a magnet.
16. State Ohm's how and describe its effect on electric circuits.
17. What happens when a bar magnet is heated to a very high temperature?
18. List three diamagnetic materials.
19. Where in everyday life might one find an electromagnet?
20. What is the range in intensity of the Earth's magnetic field?

The answers to the Challenge Questions can be found by logging on to our website at http://evolve.elsevier.com.

PART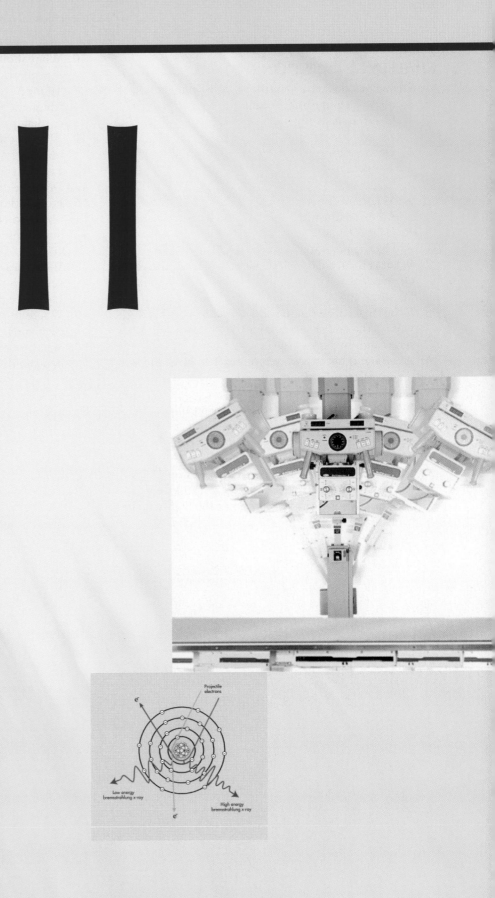

II

THE
X-RAY BEAM

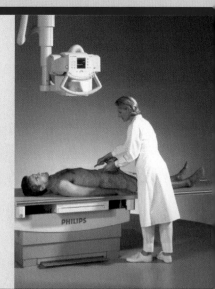

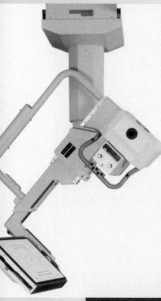

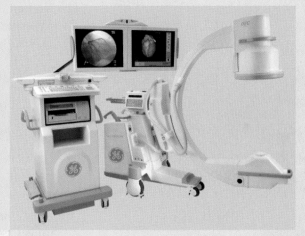

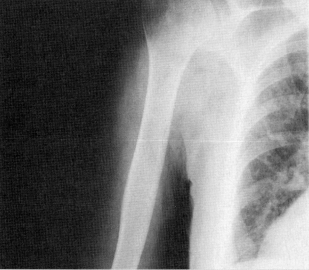

The X-ray Imaging System

OBJECTIVES

At the completion of this chapter, the student should be able
to do the following:

1. Identify the components of the operating console positioned outside
   the x-ray examination room
2. Explain the operation of the high-voltage generator, including the
   filament transformer and the rectifiers
3. Relate the important differences among single-phase, three-phase,
   and high-frequency power
4. Identify the voltage ripple associated with various high-voltage
   generators
5. Discuss the importance of voltage ripple to x-ray quantity and
   quality
6. Define the power rating of an x-ray imaging system

OUTLINE

Operating Console
Autotransformer
    Adjustment of Kilovolt Peak (kVp)
    Control of Milliamperage (mA)
    Filament Transformer
Exposure Timers
High-Voltage Generator
    High-Voltage Transformer
    Voltage Rectification
    Single-Phase Power
    Three-Phase Power
    High-Frequency Generator
    Capacitor Discharge Generator
    Voltage Ripple
    Power Rating
    X-Ray Circuit

WHEN FAST-MOVING electrons slam into a metal object, x-rays are produced. The kinetic energy of the electrons is transformed into electromagnetic energy. The function of the x-ray imaging system is to provide a controlled flow of electrons intense enough to produce an x-ray beam appropriate for imaging.

The three main components of an x-ray imaging system are (1) the x-ray tube, (2) the operating console, and (3) the high-voltage generator. The x-ray tube is discussed in Chapter 7. This chapter describes the components of the operating console. The operating console is used to control the voltage applied to the x-ray tube, the current through the x-ray tube, and the exposure time.

This chapter also discusses the high-voltage generator in its many forms. The high-voltage generator contains the high-voltage step-up transformer and the rectification circuit. The final section of this chapter combines all components into a single complete circuit diagram.

The many different types of x-ray imaging systems are usually identified according to the energy of the x-rays they produce or the purpose for which those x-rays are intended. Diagnostic x-ray imaging systems come in many different shapes and sizes, some of which are shown in Figure 6-1. These systems are usually operated at voltages of 25 to 150 kVp and at tube currents of 100 to 1200 mA.

The general purpose x-ray examination room contains a radiographic imaging system and a fluoroscopic imaging system. The fluoroscopic x-ray tube is usually located under the examining table; the radiographic x-ray tube is attached to an overhead movable crane assembly that permits easy positioning of the tube and aiming of the x-ray beam. Refer back to Chapter 1, Figure 1-9.

This type of equipment can be used for nearly all radiographic and fluoroscopic examinations. Rooms with a fluoroscope and two or more overhead radiographic tubes are used for special angiointerventional applications.

Regardless of the type of x-ray imaging system used, a patient-supporting examination table is required (Figure 6-2). This examination table may be flat or curved but must be uniform in thickness and as transparent to x-rays as possible. Carbon fiber tabletops are strong and absorb little x-radiation. This contributes to reduced patient radiation dose.

Most tabletops are floating—easily unlocked and moved by the radiologic technologist—or motor-driven. Just under the tabletop is an opening to hold a thin tray for a cassette and grid. If the table is used for fluoroscopy, the tray must move to the foot of the table and the opening must be automatically shielded for radiation protection with a Bucky slot cover (see Chapter 38). Fluoroscopic tables tilt and are identified by their degree of tilt. For example, a 90/30 table would tilt 90 degrees to the foot side and 30 degrees to the head side (Figure 6-3).

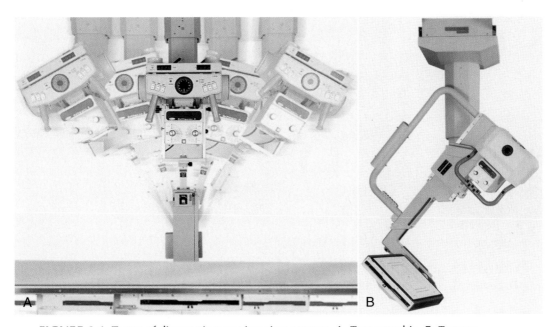

FIGURE 6-1 Types of diagnostic x-ray imaging systems. **A,** Tomographic. **B,** Trauma. (**A-B,** Courtesy Fischer Imaging.)

Continued

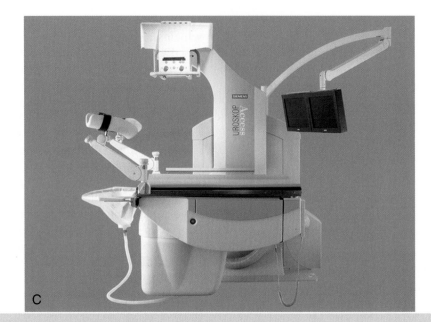

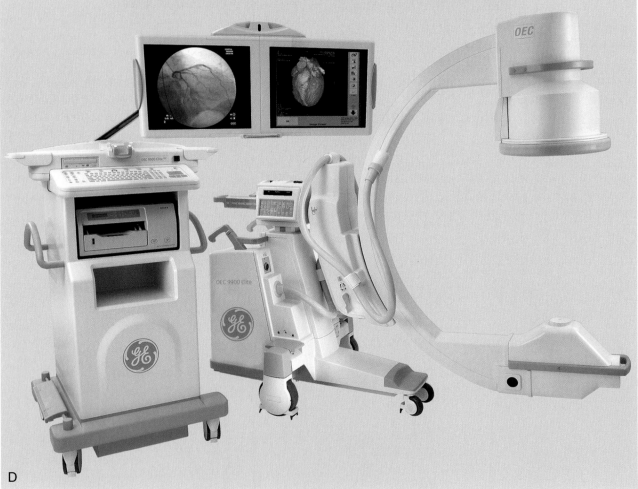

FIGURE 6-1—Cont'd **C,** Urologic. **D,** Mobile. (**C,** Courtesy Siemens Medical Systems; **D,** courtesy General Electric Medical Systems.)

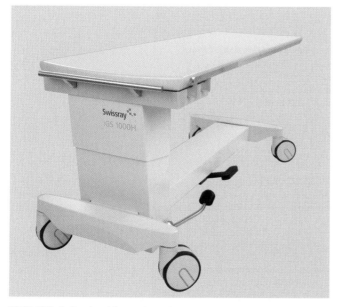

FIGURE 6-2 Flexible and mobile patient examination table. (Courtesy Swissray.)

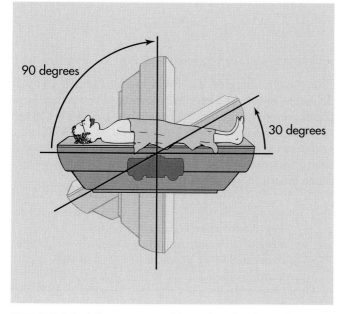

FIGURE 6-3 A fluoroscopic table is identified by its head and foot tilt.

Question: How far below horizontal will a patient's head go on a 90/15 fluoroscopic table?

Answer: 15 degrees below horizontal

Regardless of its design, every x-ray imaging system has three principal parts: the **x-ray tube** (see Chapter 7), the **operating console,** and the **high-voltage generator.** In some types of x-ray imaging systems, such as dental and portable machines, these three components are housed compactly. With most systems, however, the x-ray tube is located in the examination room and

the operating console is located in an adjoining room, with a protective barrier separating the two.

The protective barrier must have a window for viewing the patient during the examination. Ideally, the room should be designed so that it is possible to reach the operating console without having to enter the "radiation area" of the examination room.

The high-voltage generator may be housed in an equipment cabinet positioned against a wall. The high-voltage generator is always close to the x-ray tube, usually in the examination room. A few installations take advantage of false ceilings and place these generators out of sight above the examination room.

Newer generator designs that use high-frequency circuits require even less space. Figure 6-4 is a plan drawing of a conventional, general-purpose x-ray examination room.

OPERATING CONSOLE

The part of the x-ray imaging system most familiar to the radiologic technologist is the operating console. The operating console allows the radiologic technologist to control the x-ray tube current and voltage so that the useful x-ray beam is of proper quantity and quality (Figure 6-5).

Radiation quantity refers to the number of x-rays or the intensity of the x-ray beam. Radiation quantity is usually expressed in milliroentgens (mR) or milliroentgens/milliampere-second (mR/mAs). Radiation quality refers to the penetrability of the x-ray beam and is expressed in kilovolt peak (kVp) or, more precisely, half-value layer (HVL) (see Chapter 9).

The operating console usually provides for control of line compensation, kVp, mA, and exposure time. Meters are provided for monitoring kVp, mA, and exposure time. Some consoles also provide a meter for mAs. Imaging systems that incorporate automatic exposure control (AEC) may have separate controls for mAs.

All the electric circuits that connect the meters and controls on the operating console are at low voltage to minimize the possibility of hazardous shock. Figure 6-6 is a simplified schematic diagram for a typical operating console. A look inside an operating console will indicate how simplified this schematic drawing is!

Most operating consoles are based on computer technology. Controls and meters are digital, and techniques are selected with a touch screen. Numeric technique selection is sometimes replaced by icons indicating body part, size, and shape. Many of the features are automatic, but the radiologic technologist must know their purpose and proper use.

Most x-ray imaging systems are designed to operate on 220 V power, although some can operate on 110 V or 440 V. Unfortunately, electric power companies are not capable of providing 220 V accurately and continuously.

Because of variations in power distribution to the hospital and in power consumption by various sections

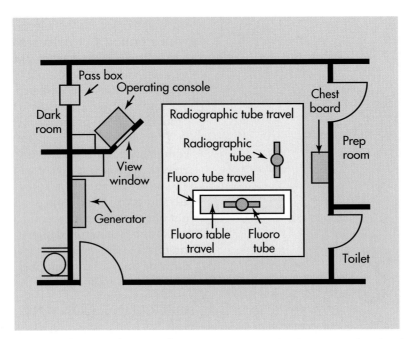

FIGURE 6-4 Plan drawing of a general purpose x-ray examination room, showing locations of the various x-ray apparatus items. Chapter 38 considers the layout of such rooms in greater detail.

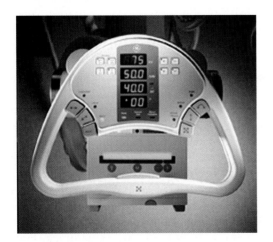

FIGURE 6-5 Typical operating console to control an overhead radiographic imaging system. Numbers of meters and controls depend on the complexity of the console. (Courtesy General Electric Medical Systems.)

of the hospital, the voltage provided to an x-ray unit easily may vary by as much as 5%. Such variation in supply voltage results in a large variation in the x-ray beam, which is inconsistent with production of high-quality images.

The **line compensator** measures the voltage provided to the x-ray imaging system and adjusts that voltage to precisely 220 V. Older units required technologists to adjust the supply voltage while observing a line voltage meter. Today's x-ray imaging systems have automatic line compensation and hence have no meter.

AUTOTRANSFORMER

The power supplied to the x-ray imaging system is delivered first to the autotransformer. The voltage supplied from the autotransformer to the high-voltage transformer is controlled but variable. It is much safer and easier to control a low voltage and then increase it than to increase a low voltage to the kilovolt level and then control its magnitude.

> The autotransformer has a single winding and is designed to supply a precise voltage to the filament circuit and to the high-voltage circuit of the x-ray imaging system.

The autotransformer works on the principle of electromagnetic induction but is very different from the conventional transformer. It has only one winding and one core. This single winding has a number of connections along its length (Figure 6-7). Two of the connections, A and A' as shown in the figure, conduct the input power to the autotransformer and are called *primary connections*.

Some of the secondary connections, such as C in the figure, are located closer to one end of the winding than are the primary connections. This allows the autotransformer to increase voltage. Other connections, such as E in the figure, allow a decrease in voltage. The autotransformer can be designed to step up voltage to approximately twice the input voltage value.

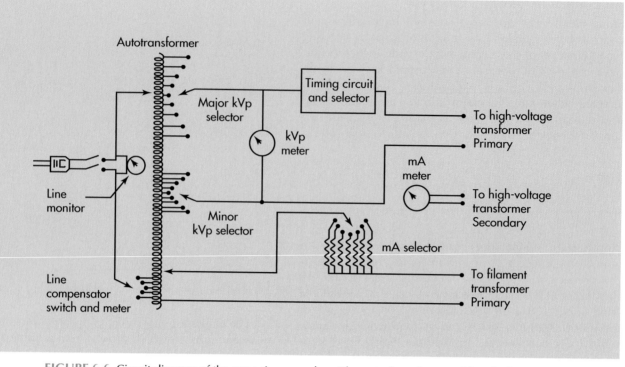

FIGURE 6-6 Circuit diagram of the operating console, with controls and meters identified.

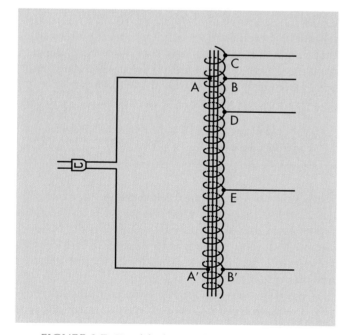

FIGURE 6-7 Simplified view of an autotransformer.

AUTOTRANSFORMER LAW

$$\frac{V_S}{V_P} = \frac{N_S}{N_P}$$

where

V_p = the primary voltage

V_s = the secondary voltage

N_p = the number of windings enclosed by primary connections

N_s = the number of windings enclosed by secondary connections

Question: If the autotransformer in Figure 6-7 is supplied with 220 V to the primary connections AA', which enclose 500 windings, what is the secondary voltage across BB' (500 windings), CB' (700 windings), and DE (200 windings)?

Answer:

$$BB : V_S = V_P \left(\frac{N_S}{N_P} \right)$$

$$= (220\,V) \left(\frac{500}{500} \right) = 220\,V$$

$$CB : V_S = (220\,V) \left(\frac{700}{500} \right)$$

$$= (220\,V)(1.4) = 308\,V$$

$$DE : V_S = (220\,V) \left(\frac{200}{500} \right)$$

$$= (220\,V)(0.4) = 88\,V$$

Because the autotransformer operates as an induction device, the voltage it receives (the primary voltage) and the voltage it provides (the secondary voltage) are related directly to the number of turns of the transformer enclosed by the respective connections. The autotransformer law is the same as the transformer law.

Adjustment of Kilovolt Peak (kVp)

Some older x-ray operating consoles have adjustment controls labeled **major kVp** and **minor kVp;** by selecting a combination of these controls, the radiologic technologist can provide precisely the required kilovolt peak. The minor kilovolt peak adjustment "fine tunes" the selected technique. The major kilovolt peak adjustment and the minor kilovolt peak adjustment represent two separate series of connections on the autotransformer.

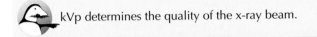

kVp determines the quality of the x-ray beam.

Appropriate connections can be selected with an adjustment knob, a push button, or a touch screen. If the primary voltage to the autotransformer is 220 V, the output of the autotransformer is usually controllable from about 100 to 400 V, depending on the design of the autotransformer. This low voltage from the autotransformer becomes the input to the high-voltage step-up transformer that increases the voltage to the chosen kilovolt peak.

Question: An autotransformer connected to a 440-V supply contains 4000 turns, all of which are enclosed by the primary connections. If 2300 turns are enclosed by secondary connections, what voltage is supplied to the high-voltage generator?

Answer:
$$V_S = V_P \left(\frac{N_S}{N_P} \right)$$
$$= (440 \text{ V}) \left(\frac{2300}{4000} \right)$$
$$= (440 \text{ V})(0.575)$$
$$= 253 \text{ V}$$

The kVp meter is placed across the output terminals of the autotransformer and therefore actually reads voltage, not kVp. The scale of the kVp meter, however, registers kilovolts because of the known multiplication factor of the turns ratio.

On most operating consoles, the kVp meter registers, even though no exposure is being made and the circuit has no current. This type of meter is known as a **prereading kVp meter.** It allows the voltage to be monitored before an exposure.

Control of Milliamperage (mA)

The x-ray tube current, crossing from cathode to anode, is measured in milliamperes (mA). The number of electrons emitted by the filament is determined by the temperature of the filament.

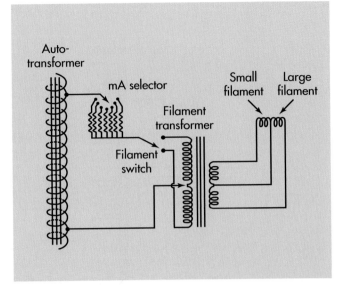

FIGURE 6-8 Filament circuit for dual-filament x-ray tube.

The filament temperature is in turn controlled by the filament current, which is measured in amperes (A). As filament current increases, the filament becomes hotter and more electrons are released by thermionic emission. Filaments normally operate at currents of 3 to 6 A.

A correction circuit has to be incorporated to counteract the *space charge effect*. As the kVp is raised, the anode becomes more attractive to those electrons that would not have enough energy to leave the filament area. These electrons also join the electron stream, which effectively increases the mA with kVp.

Thermionic emission is the release of electrons from a heated filament.

X-ray tube current is controlled through a separate circuit called the *filament circuit* (Figure 6-8). Connections on the autotransformer provide voltage for the filament circuit. Precision resistors are used to reduce this voltage to a value that corresponds to the selected milliamperage.

X-ray tube current normally is not continuously variable. Precision resistors result in fixed stations that provide tube currents of 100, 200, or 300 mA, and higher.

The falling load generator constitutes an exception (see Chapter 16). In a falling load generator, the exposure begins at maximum mA, and the mA drops as the anode heats. The result is minimum exposure time.

The product of x-ray tube current (mA) and exposure (s) is mAs, which is also electrostatic charge (C).

Question: An image is made at 400 mA and an exposure time of 100 ms. Express this in mAs
and as the total number of electrons.

Answer: 100 ms = 0.1 s
(400 mA) (0.1 s) = 40 mAs
40 mAs   = (40 mC/s) (s)
            [remember, 1 A = 1 C/s]
            = 40 mC
            = $(40 \times 10^{-3}$ C$)$ $(6.3 \times 10^{18}$ e^{-}/C$)$
            = 252×10^{15} e^{-}
            = 2.52×10^{17} electrons

The voltage from the mA selector switch is then
delivered to the filament transformer. The filament
transformer is a step-down transformer; therefore, the
voltage supplied to the filament is lower (by a factor
equal to the turns ratio) than the voltage supplied to the
filament transformer. Similarly, the current is increased
across the filament transformer in proportion to the
turns ratio.

Question: A filament transformer with a turns
ratio of 1/10 provides 6.2 A to the
filament. What is the current through
the primary coil of the filament
transformer?

Answer: $\dfrac{I_P}{I_S} = \dfrac{N_S}{N_P}$ where I_P = Primary current,

I_S = secondary current and $\dfrac{N_S}{N_P}$ = turns ratio

$I_P = I_S \left(\dfrac{N_S}{N_P} \right)$

$= (6.2) \left(\dfrac{1}{10} \right)$

$= 0.62\ A$

X-ray tube current is monitored with an mA meter that
is placed in the tube circuit. The mA meter is connected
at the center of the secondary winding of the high-voltage step-up transformer. The secondary voltage is alternating at 60 Hz such that the center of this winding is
always at zero volts (Figure 6-9).

In this way, no part of the meter is in contact with
the high voltage, and the meter may be safely put on
the operating console. Sometimes this meter allows that
mAs can be monitored in addition to mA.

Filament Transformer

The full title for this transformer is the Filament Heating
Isolation Step-down Transformer. It steps down the voltage
to approximately 12 V and provides the current to heat the
filament. Because the secondary windings are connected to
the high voltage supply for the x-ray tube, the secondary
windings are heavily insulated from the primary.

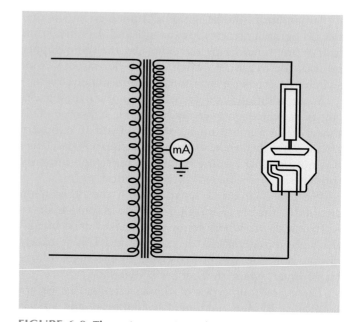

FIGURE 6-9 The mA meter is in the x-ray tube circuit at a
center tap of the output of the high-voltage step-up transformer.
This ensures electrical safety.

In the filament transformer, the primary windings are
of thin copper and carry a current of 0.5 to 1 A and
approximately 150 V. The secondary windings are thick
and at approximately 12 V electric potential and carry a
current of 5 to 8 A (not mA!).

EXPOSURE TIMERS

For any given radiographic examination, the number of
x-rays that reach the image receptor is directly related
to both the x-ray tube current and the time that the tube
is energized. X-ray operating consoles provide a wide
selection of x-ray beam-on times and, when used in conjunction with the appropriate mA station, provide an
even wider selection of values for mAs.

Question: A KUB examination (radiography of the
*k*idneys, *u*reters, and *b*ladder) calls for
70 kVp, 40 mAs. If the radiologic
technologist selects the 200 mA station,
what exposure time should be used?

Answer: $\dfrac{40\ \text{mAs}}{200\ \text{mA}} = 0.25\text{s} = 200\ \text{ms}$

Question: A lateral cerebral angiogram calls for
74 kVp, 20 mAs. If the generator has a
1000-mA capacity, what is the shortest
exposure time possible?

Answer: $\dfrac{20\ \text{mAs}}{1000\ \text{mA}} = 0.02\text{s} = 20\ \text{ms}$

Paramount in the design of all timing circuits is that the radiographer starts the exposure and the timer stops it. If at any time during the exposure, the radiographer releases the exposure switch or the fluoroscopic foot switch, the exposure is terminated immediately.

As an additional safety feature, another timing circuit is activated on every radiographic exposure. This timer, called a guard timer, will terminate an exposure after a prescribed time, usually approximately 6 s. Thus, it is not possible for any timing circuit to continuously irradiate a patient for an extensive period.

The timer circuit is separate from the other main circuits of the x-ray imaging system. It consists of an electronic device whose action is to "make" and "break" the high voltage across the x-ray tube. This is nearly always done on the **primary side** of the high-voltage transformer, where the voltage is lower.

There are four types of timing circuits. Three are controlled by the radiologic technologist and one is automatic. After studying this section, try to identify the types of timers on the equipment you use.

Synchronous Timers. In the United States, electric current is supplied at a frequency of 60 Hz. In Europe, Latin America, and other parts of the world, the frequency is 50 Hz. A special type of electric motor, known as a synchronous motor, is a precision device designed to drive a shaft at precisely 60 revolutions per second (rps). In some x-ray imaging systems, synchronous motors are used as timing mechanisms.

X-ray imaging systems with synchronous timers are recognizable because the minimum exposure time possible is 1/60 s (17 ms) and timing intervals increase by multiples thereof, such as 1/30, 1/20, and so on. Synchronous timers cannot be used for serial exposures because they must be reset after each exposure.

Electronic Timers. Electronic timers are the most sophisticated, most complicated, and most accurate of the x-ray exposure timers. Electronic timers consist of rather complex circuitry based on the time required to charge a capacitor through a variable resistance.

Electronic timers allow a wide range of time intervals to be selected and are accurate to intervals as small as 1 ms. Because they can be used for rapid serial exposures, they are particularly suitable for angiointerventional procedures.

> Most exposure timers are electronic and are controlled by a microprocessor.

mAs Timers. Most x-ray apparatus is designed for accurate control of tube current and exposure time. However, the product of mA and time—mAs—determines the number of x-rays emitted and, therefore, the exposure of the image receptor. A special kind of

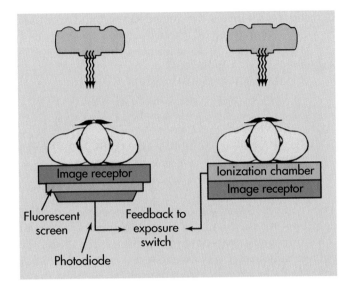

FIGURE 6-10 Automatic exposure control (AEC) terminates the x-ray exposure at the desired film optical density. This is done with an ionization chamber or a photodiode detector assembly.

electronic timer, called an *mAs timer*, monitors the product of mA and exposure time and terminates exposure when the desired mAs value is attained.

The mAs timer is usually designed to provide the highest safe tube current for the shortest exposure for any mAs selected. Because the mAs timer must monitor the actual tube current, it is located on the secondary side of the high-voltage transformer.

> mAs timers are used on falling-load and capacitor discharge imaging systems.

Automatic Exposure Control. The automatic exposure control (AEC) requires a special understanding on the part of the radiologic technologist. The AEC is a device that measures the quantity of radiation that reaches the image receptor. It automatically terminates the exposure when the image receptor has received the required radiation intensity. Figure 6-10 shows two types of AEC design.

The type of AEC used by most manufacturers incorporates a flat, parallel plate ionization chamber positioned between the patient and the image receptor. This chamber is made radiolucent so that it will not interfere with the radiographic image. Ionization within the chamber creates a charge. When the appropriate charge has been reached, the exposure is terminated.

When an AEC x-ray imaging system is installed, it must be calibrated. This calls for making exposures of a phantom and adjusting the AEC for the range of x-ray intensities required for quality images. The service engineer usually takes care of this calibration.

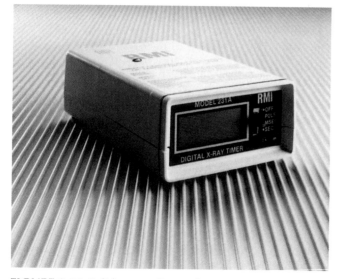

FIGURE 6-11 Solid-state radiation detectors are used to check timer accuracy. (Courtesy Gammex RMI.)

Once the AEC is in clinical operation, the radiologic technologist selects the type of examination, which then sets the appropriate mA and kVp. At the same time, the exposure timer is set to the backup time. When the electric charge from the ionization chamber reaches a preset level, a signal is returned to the operating console, where the exposure is terminated.

The AEC is now widely used and often is provided in addition to an electronic timer. The AEC mode requires particular care, especially in examinations that use low kVp such as mammography. Because of varying tissue thickness and composition, the AEC may not respond properly at low kVp.

When radiographs are taken in the AEC mode, the electronic timer should be set to 1.5 times the expected exposure time as a backup timer in case the AEC fails to terminate. This precaution should be followed for the protection of the patient and the x-ray tube. Many units automatically set this precaution.

Solid-state radiation detectors are now used for exposure-timer checks (Figure 6-11). These devices operate with a very accurate internal clock based on a quartz-crystal oscillator. They can measure exposure times as short as 1 ms and, when used with an oscilloscope, can display the radiation waveform.

HIGH-VOLTAGE GENERATOR

The high-voltage generator of an x-ray imaging system is responsible for increasing the output voltage from the autotransformer to the kVp necessary for x-ray production. A cutaway view of a typical high-voltage generator is shown in Figure 6-12. Although some heat is generated in the high-voltage section and is conducted to oil, the oil is used primarily for electrical insulation.

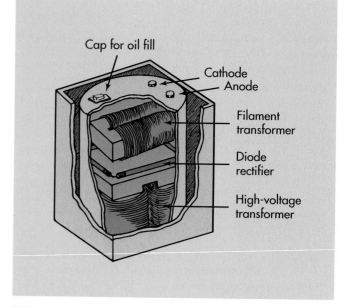

FIGURE 6-12 Cutaway view of a typical high-voltage generator, showing oil-immersed diodes and transformers.

The high-voltage generator contains three primary parts: the *high-voltage transformer*, the *filament transformer* (discussed previously), and *rectifiers*.

High-Voltage Transformer

The high voltage transformer is a step-up transformer, that is, the secondary voltage is higher than the primary voltage because the number of secondary windings is greater than the number of primary windings. The ratio of the number of secondary windings to the number of primary windings is called the **turns ratio** (see Chapter 5). The voltage increase is proportional to the turns ratio, according to the transformer law (also discussed in Chapter 5). Also, the current is reduced proportionately.

The turns ratio of a high-voltage transformer is usually between 500:1 and 1000:1. Because **transformers operate only on alternating current,** the voltage waveform on both sides of a high-voltage transformer is sinusoidal (Figure 6-13). The only difference between the primary and secondary waveforms is their **amplitude.** The primary voltage is measured in volts (V), and the secondary voltage is measured in kilovolt peak (kVp). The primary current is measured in amperes (A), and the secondary current is measured in milliamperes (mA).

Question: The turns ratio of a high-voltage transformer is 700:1 and the supply voltage is peaked at 120 V. What is the secondary voltage supplied to the x-ray tube?

Answer: (120 Vp) (700:1) = 84,000 Vp
= 84 kVp

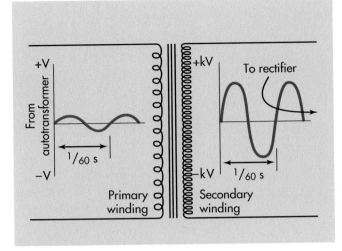

FIGURE 6-13 Voltage induced in the secondary winding of a high-voltage step-up transformer is alternating like the primary voltage but has a higher value.

Voltage Rectification

The current from a common wall plug is 60 Hz AC (alternating current). The current changes direction 120 times each second. However, an x-ray tube requires a direct current (DC), that is, electron flow in only one direction. Therefore, some means must be provided for converting AC to DC.

 Radiographers outside the United States and Japan may use a frequency of 50 Hz.

In the case of 50 Hz power, there are 100 half-cycles per second, each lasting 10 ms. In all other respects, the rectification process is the same.

Rectification is the process of converting AC to DC.

The electronic device that allows current flow in only one direction is a **rectifier.** Although transformers operate with alternating current, x-ray tubes must be provided with direct current. X-rays are produced by the acceleration of electrons from the cathode to the anode and cannot be produced by electrons flowing in the reverse direction, from anode to cathode.

Reversal of electron flow would be disastrous for the x-ray tube. The construction of the cathode assembly is such that it could not withstand the tremendous heat generated by such an operation, even if the anode could emit electrons thermionically. If the electron flow is to be only in the cathode-to-anode direction, the

secondary voltage of the high-voltage transformer must be **rectified.**

Voltage rectification is required to ensure that electrons flow from cathode to anode only.

Rectification is accomplished with diodes. A diode is an electronic device that contains two electrodes. Originally, all diode rectifiers were vacuum tubes called **valve tubes;** these have been replaced by solid-state rectifiers made of silicon (Figure 6-14).

It has long been known that metals are good conductors of electricity and that some other materials, such as glass and plastic, are poor conductors of electricity or insulators.

A third class of materials, called *semiconductors,* lie between the range of insulators and conductors in their ability to conduct electricity. Tiny crystals of these semiconductors have some useful electrical properties and allow semiconductors to serve as the basis for today's solid-state microchip marvels.

Semiconductors are classed into two types: n-type and p-type. N-type semiconductors have loosely bound electrons that are relatively free to move. P-type semiconductors have spaces, called *holes,* where there are no electrons. These holes are like the space between cars in heavy traffic. Holes are as mobile as electrons.

Consider a tiny crystal of n-type material placed in contact with a p-type crystal to form what is called a p-n junction (Figure 6-15). If a higher potential is placed on the p side of the junction, then the electrons and holes will both migrate toward the junction and wander across it. This flow of electrons and holes constitutes an electric current.

If, however, a positive potential is placed on the n side of the junction, both the electrons and the holes will be swept away from the junction, and no electrons will be available at the junction surface to form a current. Thus, in this case, no electric current passes through the p-n junction.

Therefore, a solid-state p-n junction tends to conduct electricity in only one direction. This type of p-n junction is called a solid-state diode. Solid-state diodes are rectifiers because they conduct electric current in only one direction. The arrowhead in the symbol for a diode indicates the direction of conventional electric current, which is opposite to the flow of electrons (Figure 6-16).

Electron flow is used when medical imaging systems are described.

Rectification is essential for the safe and efficient operation of the x-ray tube. Rectifiers are located in the high-voltage section.

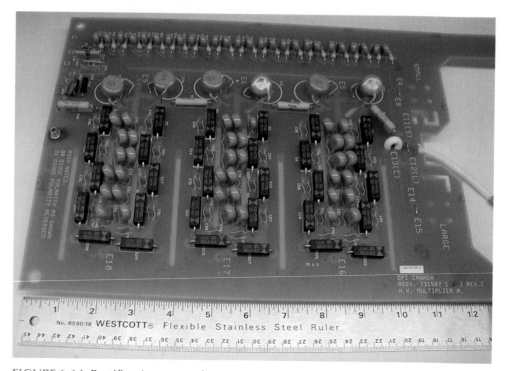

FIGURE 6-14 Rectifiers in most modern x-ray generators are the silicon, semiconductor type. The multiple black components on this 75-kVp high-voltage multiplier board are rectifiers. (Courtesy of CMP/CPII, Inc.)

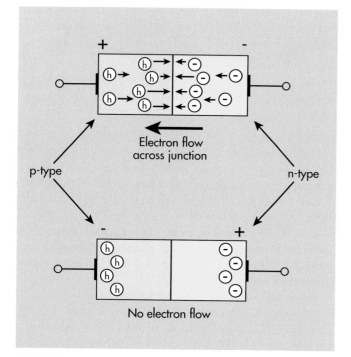

FIGURE 6-15 A p-n junction semiconductor shown as a solid-state diode.

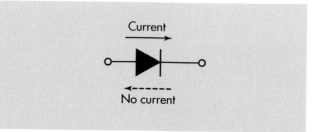

FIGURE 6-16 The electronic symbol for a solid-state diode.

The current that passes through the x-ray tube, however, exists only during the positive half of the cycle, when the anode is positive and the cathode is negative. During the negative half of the cycle, current can flow only from anode to cathode, but this does not occur because the anode is not constructed to emit electrons.

Half-Wave Rectification. The inverse voltage is removed from the supply to the x-ray tube by rectification. Half-wave rectification (Figure 6-18) is a condition in which the voltage is not allowed to swing negatively during the negative half of its cycle.

Rectifiers are assembled into electronic circuits to convert alternating current into the direct current necessary for the operation of an x-ray tube (Figure 6-19). During the positive portion of the AC waveform, the rectifier allows electric current to pass through the x-ray tube.

During the negative portion of the AC waveform, however, the rectifier does not conduct, and thus no

Unrectified Voltage. Figure 6-17 shows the unrectified voltage at the secondary side of the high-voltage step-up transformer. This voltage waveform appears as the voltage waveform supplied to the primary side of the high-voltage transformer, except its amplitude is much greater.

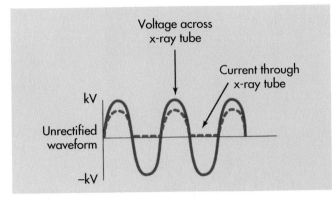

FIGURE 6-17 Unrectified voltage and current waveforms on the secondary side.

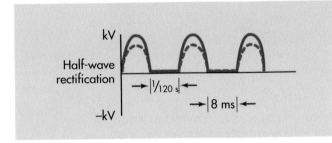

FIGURE 6-18 Half-wave rectification.

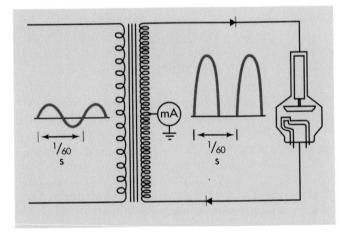

FIGURE 6-19 A half-wave–rectified circuit contains one or more diodes.

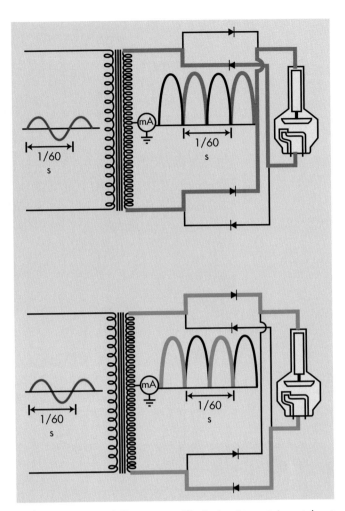

FIGURE 6-20 A full-wave–rectified circuit contains at least four diodes. Current is passed through the tube at 120 pulses per second.

electric current is allowed. The resultant electric current is a series of positive pulses separated by gaps when the negative current is not conducted.

This resultant electric current is a rectified current because electrons flow in only one direction. This form of rectification is called half-wave rectification because only one half of the AC waveform appears in the output.

In some portable and dental x-ray imaging systems, the x-ray tube serves as the vacuum tube rectifier. Such a system is said to be self-rectified, and the resulting waveform is the same as that of half-wave rectification.

Half-wave–rectified circuits contain zero, one, or two diodes. The x-ray output from a half-wave high-voltage generator pulsates, producing 60 x-ray pulses each second.

Full-Wave Rectification. One shortcoming of half-wave rectification is that it wastes half the supply of power. It also requires twice the exposure time. It is possible, however, to devise a circuit that rectifies the entire AC waveform. This form of voltage rectification is called *full-wave rectification*.

Full-wave–rectified x-ray imaging systems contain at least four diodes in the high-voltage circuit, usually arranged as in Figure 6-20. In a full-wave–rectified circuit, the negative half-cycle corresponding to the inverse voltage is reversed so that the anode is always positive (Figure 6-21).

The current through the circuit is shown during both the positive and the negative phases of the input waveform. Note that in both cases, the output voltage across the x-ray tube is positive. Also, there are no gaps in the output waveform. All of the input waveform is rectified into usable output.

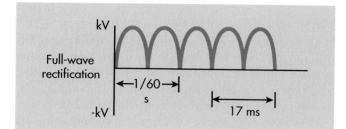

FIGURE 6-21 Voltage across a full-wave–rectified circuit is always positive.

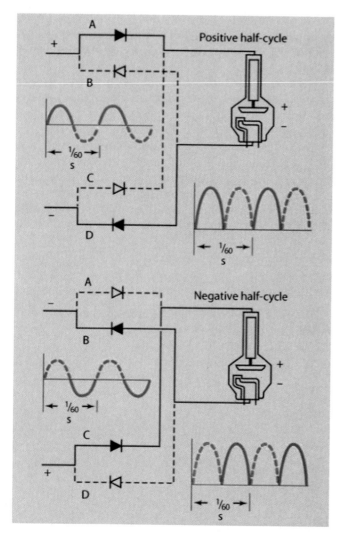

FIGURE 6-22 In a full-wave–rectified circuit, two diodes (*A* and *D*) conduct during the positive half-cycle and two (*B* and *C*) conduct during the negative half-cycle.

Figure 6-22 helps explain full-wave rectification. During the positive half-cycle of the secondary voltage waveform, electrons flow from the negative side to diodes C and D. Diode C is unable to conduct electrons in that direction, but diode D can. The electrons flow through diode D and the x-ray tube.

The electrons then butt into diodes A and B. Only diode A is positioned to conduct them, and they flow to the positive side of the transformer, thus completing the circuit.

During the negative half-cycle, diodes B and C are pressed into service while diodes A and D block electron flow. Note that the polarity of the x-ray tube remains unchanged. The cathode is always negative and the anode always positive, even though the induced secondary voltage alternates between positive and negative.

The main advantage of full-wave rectification is that the exposure time for any given technique is cut in half. The half-wave–rectified x-ray tube emits x-rays only half of the time. The pulsed x-ray output of a full-wave–rectified machine occurs 120 times each second instead of 60 times per second as with half-wave rectification.

Single-Phase Power

All of the voltage waveforms discussed so far are produced by single-phase electric power. Single-phase power results in a pulsating x-ray beam. This is caused by the alternate swing in voltage from zero to maximum potential 120 times each second under full-wave rectification.

The x-rays produced when the single-phase voltage waveform has a value near zero are of little diagnostic value because of their low energy; such x-rays have low penetrability. One method of overcoming this deficiency is to use some sophisticated electrical engineering principles to generate three simultaneous voltage waveforms that are out of step with one another. Such a manipulation results in **three-phase electric power.**

Three-Phase Power

The engineering required to produce three-phase power involves the manner in which the high-voltage step-up transformer is wired into the circuit, the details of which are beyond the scope of this discussion. Figure 6-23 shows the voltage waveforms for single-phase power, for three-phase power, and for full-wave–rectified three-phase power.

With three-phase power, multiple voltage waveforms are superimposed on one another, resulting in a waveform that maintains a nearly constant high voltage. There are six pulses per 1/60 s, compared with the two pulses characteristic of single-phase power.

 With three-phase power, the voltage impressed across the x-ray tube is nearly constant, never dropping to zero during exposure.

There are limitations to the speed of starting an exposure—**initiation time**—and ending an exposure—**extinction time.** Additional electronic circuits are necessary to correct this deficiency; this adds to the additional size and cost of the three-phase generator.

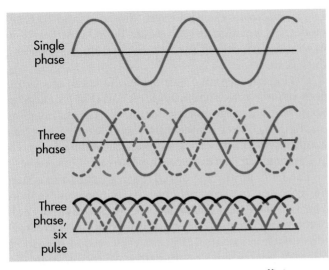

FIGURE 6-23 Three-phase power is a more efficient way to produce x-rays than is single-phase power. Shown are the voltage waveforms for unrectified single-phase power, unrectified three-phase power, and rectified three-phase power.

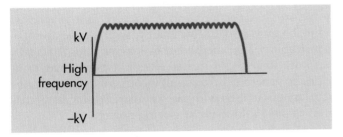

FIGURE 6-24 High-frequency voltage waveform.

High-Frequency Generator

High-frequency circuits are finding increasing application in generating high voltage for many x-ray imaging systems. Full-wave–rectified power at 60 Hz is converted to a higher frequency, usually 500 to 25,000 Hz, and then is transferred to high voltage (Figure 6-24).

One advantage of the high-frequency generator is its size. They are very much smaller than 60-Hz high-voltage generators. High-frequency generators produce a nearly constant potential voltage waveform, improving image quality at lower patient radiation dose.

This technology was first used with portable x-ray imaging systems. Now, nearly all mammography and spiral computed tomography systems use high-frequency circuits.

High-frequency voltage generation uses inverter circuits (Figure 6-25). Inverter circuits are high-speed switches, or choppers, that convert DC into a series of square pulses.

Many portable x-ray high-voltage generators use storage batteries and silicon-controlled rectifiers (SCRs) to generate square waves at 500 Hz; this becomes the input to the high-voltage step-up transformer. The high-voltage step-up transformer operating at 500 Hz is about 1/10 the size of a 60-Hz transformer, which is rather large and heavy. At 500 Hz, one can sometimes hear the transformer "sing" during exposure.

High-frequency x-ray generators are sometimes grouped by frequency (Table 6-1). The principal differences are found in the electric components designed as the inverter module. The real advantage of such circuits is that they are much smaller, less costly, and more efficient than 60-Hz high-voltage generators.

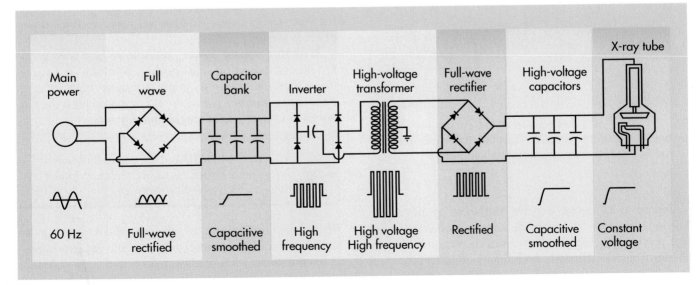

FIGURE 6-25 Inverter circuit of a high-voltage generator.

Full-wave rectification or high-frequency voltage generation is used in almost all stationary x-ray imaging systems.

Capacitor Discharge Generator

Some portable x-ray imaging systems still use a high-voltage generator, which operates by charging a series of SCRs from the DC voltage of a nickel-cadmium (NiCd) battery. By stacking (in an electric sense) the SCRs, the charge is stored at very high voltage. During exposure, the charge is released (discharged) to form the x-ray tube current needed to produce x-rays (Figure 6-26).

 During capacitor discharge, the voltage falls approximately 1 kV/mAs.

This falling voltage limits the available x-ray tube current and causes kVp to fall during exposure. The result is the need for precise radiographic technique charts.

After a given exposure time, the capacitor bank continues to discharge, which could cause continued x-ray emission. Such x-ray emission is stopped by a grid-controlled x-ray tube, an automatic lead beam stopper, or both. A grid-controlled x-ray tube has a specially designed cathode to control x-ray tube current.

Voltage Ripple

Another way to characterize these voltage waveforms is by **voltage ripple**. Single-phase power has **100% voltage ripple:** The voltage varies from zero to its maximum value. Three-phase, six-pulse power produces voltage with only approximately **14% ripple;** consequently, the voltage supplied to the x-ray tube never falls to below 86% of the maximum value.

A further improvement in three-phase power results in twelve pulses per cycle rather than six. Three-phase, twelve-pulse power results in only **4% ripple;** therefore, the voltage supplied to the x-ray tube does not fall to below 96% of the maximum value. High-frequency generators have approximately **1% ripple** and therefore greater x-ray quantity and quality.

Figure 6-27 shows these various power sources and the resultant voltage waveforms they provide to the x-ray tube, as well as the approximate voltage ripple. The most efficient method of x-ray production also involves the waveform with the lowest voltage ripple.

 Less voltage ripple results in greater radiation quantity and quality.

An x-ray tube voltage with less ripple offers many advantages. The principal advantage is the greater radiation quantity and quality that result from the more constant voltage supplied to the x-ray tube (Figure 6-28).

Table 6-1	Characteristics of High-Frequency X-ray Generators	
Frequency Range	**Inverter Features**	
<1 kHz	Thyristors	
1-10 kHz	Large silicon-controlled rectifier	
10-100 kHz	Power field effect transistors	

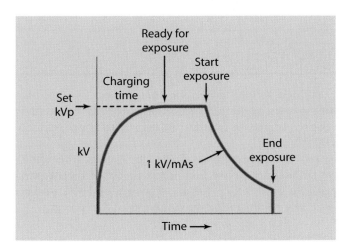

FIGURE 6-26 Tube voltage falls during exposure with a capacitor discharge generator.

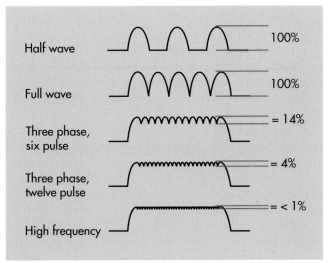

FIGURE 6-27 Voltage waveforms resulting from various power supplies. The ripple of the kilovoltage is indicated as a percentage for each waveform.

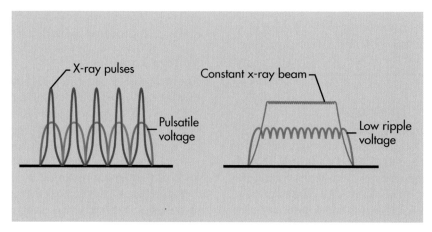

FIGURE 6-28 Both the number of x-rays and the x-ray energy increase as the voltage waveform increases.

The radiation quantity is greater because the efficiency of x-ray production is higher when x-ray tube voltage is high. Stated differently, for any projectile electron emitted by the x-ray tube filament, a greater number of x-rays are produced when the electron energy is high than when it is low.

Low-voltage ripple increases radiation quality because fewer low-energy projectile electrons pass from cathode to anode to produce low-energy x-rays. Consequently, the average x-ray energy is greater than that resulting from high-voltage ripple modes.

Because the x-ray beam intensity and penetrability are greater for less voltage ripple than for single-phase power, technique charts developed for one cannot be used on the other. New technique charts with three-phase or high-frequency x-ray imaging systems are needed.

Three-phase operation may require as much as a 10-kVp reduction to produce the same image receptor exposure when operated at the same mAs as single phase. A high-frequency generator may require a 12-kVp reduction.

Three-phase radiographic equipment is manufactured with tube currents as high as 1200 mA; therefore, exceedingly short, high-intensity exposures are possible. This capacity is particularly helpful in angiointerventional procedures.

When three-phase power is provided for a radiographic/fluoroscopic room, all radiographic exposures are performed with three-phase power. The fluoroscopic mode, however, usually remains single-phase and takes advantage of the electric capacitance of the x-ray tube cables.

Fluoroscopic mA is very low compared with radiographic mA. Because the x-ray cables are long, they have considerable capacitance, which results in a smoother voltage waveform (Figure 6-29).

The principal disadvantage of a three-phase x-ray apparatus is its initial cost. The costs of installation and

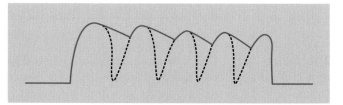

FIGURE 6-29 Voltage waveform is smoothed by the capacitance of long high-voltage cables.

operation, however, can be lower than those associated with single-phase equipment. The cost of high-frequency generators is moderate. Low-ripple generators have greater overall capacity and flexibility compared with single-phase equipment.

Power Rating

Transformers and high-voltage generators usually are identified by their power rating in kilowatts (kW). Electric power for any device is specified in watts, as was shown in the following equation from Chapter 5:

> Power = Current × Potential
> Watts = Amperes × Volts

A high-voltage generator for a basic radiographic unit is rated at 30 to 50 kW. Generators for angiointerventional suites have power ratings up to approximately 150 kW.

For specifying high-voltage generators, the industry standard is to use the maximum tube current (mA) possible at 100 kVp for an exposure of 100 ms. This generally results in the maximum available power.

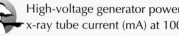 High-voltage generator power (kW) = maximum x-ray tube current (mA) at 100 kVp and 100 ms.

Power is the product of amperes and volts. This assumes constant current and voltage, which does not exist in single-phase x-ray imaging systems. However, the actual power is close enough to the low-ripple power of three-phase and high-frequency generators that the equation holds.

Question: When a system with low voltage ripple is energized at 100 kVp, 100 ms, the maximum possible tube current is 800 mA. What is the power rating?

Answer: Power rating = Current (A) × Potential (V)
= 800 mA × 100 kVp
= 80,000 mA × kVp
= 80,000 W
= 80 kW

Because the product of amperes volts = watts, the product of milliamperes kilovolts = watts. However, power rating is expressed in kilowatts, and so the defining equation for three-phase and high-frequency power is as follows:

$$\text{Power rating (kW)} = \frac{mA \times kVp}{1000}$$

Question: An angiointerventional system is capable of 1200 mA when operated in 100 kVp, 100 ms. What is the power rating?

Answer:
$$\text{Power rating (kW)} = \frac{1200\,mA \times 100\,kVp}{1000}$$
$$= 120\,kW$$

Single-phase generators have 100% voltage ripple and are less efficient x-ray generators. Consequently, the single-phase expression of power rating is as follows:

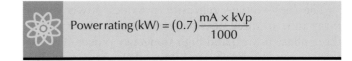

$$\text{Power rating (kW)} = (0.7)\frac{mA \times kVp}{1000}$$

Question: A single-phase radiographic unit installed in a private office reaches maximum capacity at 100 ms of 120 kVp and 500 mA. What is its power rating?

Answer:
$$\text{Power rating (kW)} = (0.7)\frac{(500\,mA)(120\,kVp)}{1000}$$
$$= 42\ kW$$

X-ray Circuit

Figure 6-30 is a simplified schematic diagram of the three main sections of the x-ray imaging system: the x-ray tube, the operating console, and the high-voltage

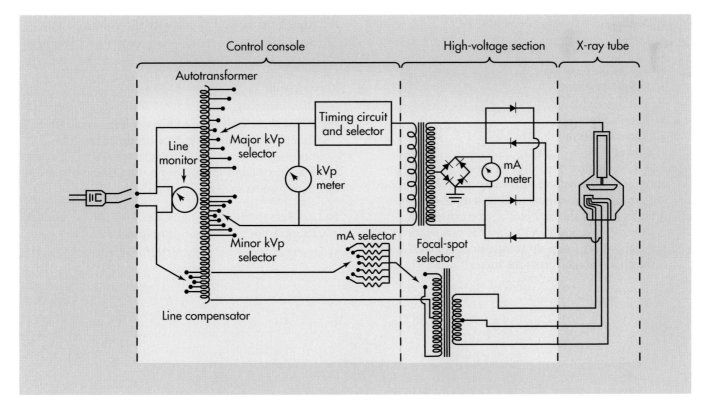

FIGURE 6-30 The schematic circuit of an x-ray imaging system.

generator. This figure also shows the locations of all meters, controls, and important components.

SUMMARY

The x-ray imaging system has three principal sections: (1) the x-ray tube, (2) the operating console, and (3) the high-voltage generator. The design and operation of the x-ray tube are discussed in Chapter 7.

The operating console consists of an on/off control and controls to select kVp, mA, and time or mAs. The AECs are also located on the operating console.

The high-voltage generator provides power to the x-ray tube in three possible ways: single-phase power, three-phase power, and high-frequency power. The difference between single- and three-phase power involves the manner in which the high-voltage step-up transformer is electrically positioned. With three-phase power, the voltage across the x-ray tube is nearly constant during exposure and never drops to zero, as does the voltage for single-phase power.

The components of an x-ray imaging system are sometimes identified by their power rating in kilowatts (kW). Maximum available power for high-voltage generators equals the maximum tube current (mA) at 100 kVp for an exposure of 100 ms.

CHALLENGE QUESTIONS

1. Define or otherwise identify the following:
   a. Semiconductor
   b. Automatic exposure control (AEC)
   c. Line compensation
   d. Capacitor
   e. mA meter location
   f. Diode
   g. Voltage ripple
   h. Rectification
   i. Autotransformer
   j. Power
2. 220 V is supplied across 1200 windings of the primary coil of the autotransformer. If 1650 windings are tapped, what voltage will be supplied to the primary coil of the high-voltage transformer?
3. A kVp meter reads 86 kVp and the turns ratio of the high-voltage step-up transformer is 1200. What is the true voltage across the meter?

4. The supply voltage from the autotransformer to the filament transformer is 60 V. If the turns ratio of the filament transformer is $1/12$, what is the filament voltage?
5. If the current in the primary of the filament transformer in question 4 were 0.5 A, what would be the filament current?
6. The supply to a high-voltage step-up transformer with a turns ratio of 550 is 190 V. What is the voltage across the x-ray tube?
7. Locate the various meters and controls shown in Figure 6-30 on an x-ray imaging system you operate.
8. The radiographic table must be radiolucent. Define *radiolucent*.
9. Describe the movements of a $90/20$ table.
10. List the five major controls on the operator's console.
11. What is the purpose of the autotransformer?
12. How does primary voltage relate to secondary voltage in an autotransformer?
13. What does the prereading kVp meter allow?
14. Operating console controls are set at 200 mA with an exposure time of $1/60$ s. What is the milliampere-seconds (mAs)?
15. In an examination of a pediatric patient, the operating console controls are set at 600 mA/30 ms. What is the mAs?
16. What is the difference between a high-voltage generator and a high-voltage transformer?
17. Why does the x-ray circuit require rectification?
18. Match the power source with the voltage ripple.

POWER	% VOLTAGE RIPPLE
Single-phase	4%
Three-phase, twelve-pulse	100%
Three-phase, six-pulse	14%
High-frequency	1%

19. What is the only type of high-voltage generator that can be positioned in or on the x-ray tube housing?
20. State the equations for computing single-phase and high-frequency power rating.

The answers to the Challenge Questions can be found by logging on to our website at http://evolve.elsevier.com.

The X-ray Tube

OBJECTIVES

At the completion of this chapter, the student should be able to do the following:

1. Describe the general design of an x-ray tube
2. List the external components that house and protect the x-ray tube
3. Identify the purpose of the glass or metal enclosure
4. Discuss the cathode and filament currents
5. Describe the parts of the anode and the induction motor
6. Define the line-focus principle and the heel effect
7. Identify the three causes of x-ray tube failure
8. Explain and interpret x-ray tube rating charts

OUTLINE

External Components
Ceiling Support System
Floor-to-Ceiling Support System
C-Arm Support System
Protective Housing
Glass or Metal Enclosure
Internal Components
Cathode
Anode
X-ray Tube Failure
Rating Charts
Radiographic Rating Chart
Anode Cooling Chart
Housing Cooling Chart

THE X-RAY tube is a component of the x-ray imaging system rarely seen by the radiologic technologist. It is contained in a protective housing and therefore is inaccessible. Figure 7-1 is a schematic diagram of a rotating anode diagnostic x-ray tube. Its components are considered separately, but it should be clear that there are two primary parts: the cathode and the anode. Each of these is an electrode, and any tube with two electrodes is a diode. An x-ray tube is a special type of diode.

The external structure of the x-ray tube consists of three parts: the support structure, the protective housing, and the glass or metal enclosure. The internal structures of the x-ray tube are the anode and the cathode.

An explanation of the external components of the x-ray tube and the internal structure of the x-ray tube follows. The causes and prevention of x-ray tube failure are discussed.

With proper use, an x-ray tube used in general radiography should last many years. X-ray tubes used in computed tomography (CT) and interventional radiology generally have a much shorter life.

EXTERNAL COMPONENTS

The x-ray tube and housing assembly are quite heavy; therefore, they require a support mechanism so the radiologic technologist can position them. Figure 7-2 illustrates the three main methods of x-ray tube support.

Ceiling Support System

The **ceiling support** system is probably the most frequently used. It consists of two perpendicular sets of ceiling-mounted rails. This allows for both longitudinal and transverse travel of the x-ray tube.

A telescoping column attaches the x-ray tube housing to the rails, allowing for variable source-to-image receptor distance (SID). When the x-ray tube is centered above the examination table at the standard SID, the x-ray tube is in a **preferred detent** position.

Other positions can be chosen and locked by the radiologic technologist. Some ceiling-supported x-ray tubes have a single control that removes all locks, allowing the tube to "float." This lock should be used only for minor adjustments and should not be used to move the tube farther than about a meter, because arm and shoulder strain can occur.

Floor-to-Ceiling Support System

The **floor-to-ceiling** support system has a single column with rollers at each end, one attached to a ceiling-mounted rail and the other attached to a floor-mounted

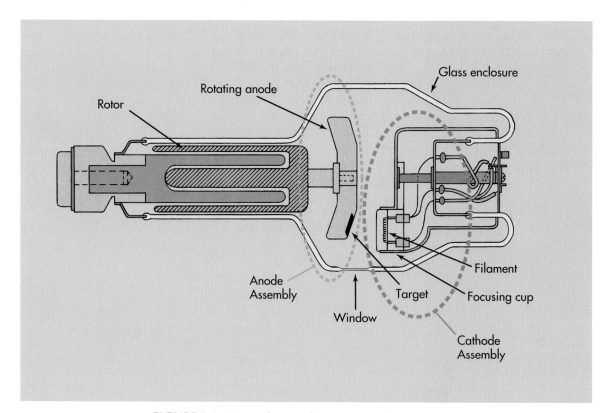

FIGURE 7-1 Principal parts of a rotating anode x-ray tube.

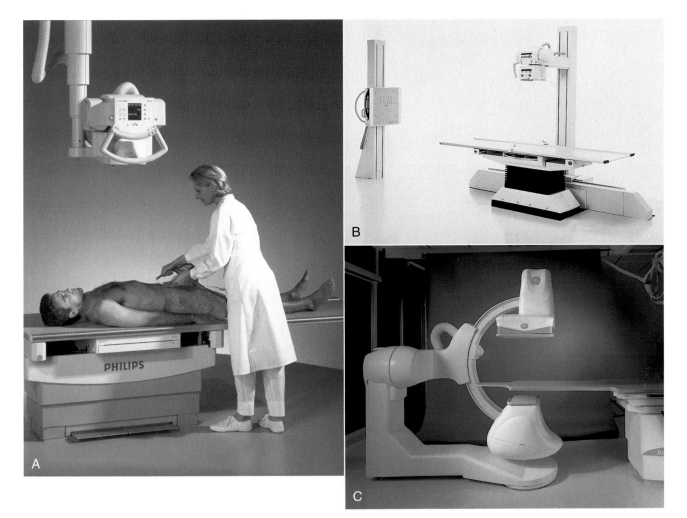

FIGURE 7-2 Three methods of supporting an x-ray tube. **A,** Ceiling support. **B,** Floor support. **C,** C-arm support. (**A,** Courtesy Philips Medical Systems. **B,** Courtesy Toshiba Corp. **C,** Courtesy General Electric Medical Systems.)

rail. The x-ray tube slides up and down the column as the column rotates. A variation of this type of support system has the column positioned on a single **floor support system** with one or two floor-mounted rails.

C-Arm Support System

Angiointerventional radiology suites often are equipped with C-arm support systems, so called because the system is shaped like a "C." These systems are ceiling mounted and provide for very flexible x-ray tube positioning. The image receptor is attached to the other end of the C-arm from the x-ray tube. Variations called *L-arm* or *U-arm support* are also common.

Protective Housing

When x-rays are produced, they are emitted **isotropically,** that is, with equal intensity in all directions. We use only those emitted through the special section of the x-ray tube called the **window** (Figure 7-3). Those x-rays emitted through the window are called the **useful beam.**

X-rays that escape through the protective housing are leakage radiation; they contribute nothing in the way of diagnostic information and result in unnecessary exposure of the patient and the radiologic technologist. Properly designed protective housing reduces the level of leakage radiation to less than 100 mR/hr at 1 m, when operated at maximum conditions.

Protective housing guards against excessive radiation exposure and electric shock.

The protective housing incorporates specially designed high-voltage receptacles to protect against accidental electric shock. Death by electrocution was a very real hazard for early radiologic technologists. The protective housing also provides **mechanical support** for the x-ray tube and protects the tube from damage caused by rough handling.

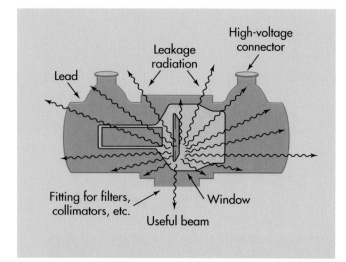

FIGURE 7-3 Protective housing reduces the intensity of leakage radiation to less than 100 mR/hr at 1 m.

The protective housing around some x-ray tubes contains oil that serves as both an **insulator** against electric shock and as a **thermal cushion** to dissipate heat. Some protective housings have a cooling fan to air-cool the tube or the oil in which the x-ray tube is immersed. A bellows-like device allows the oil to expand when heated. If the expansion is too great, a microswitch is activated, so the tube cannot be used until it cools.

Glass or Metal Enclosure

An x-ray tube is an electronic vacuum tube with components contained within a **glass** or **metal enclosure.** The x-ray tube, however, is a special type of vacuum tube that contains two electrodes: the cathode and the anode. It is relatively large, perhaps 30 to 50 cm long and 20 cm in diameter. The glass enclosure is made of Pyrex glass to enable it to withstand the tremendous heat generated.

The enclosure maintains a vacuum inside the tube. This vacuum allows for more efficient x-ray production and longer tube life. When just a little gas is in the enclosure, the electron flow from cathode to anode is reduced, fewer x-rays are produced, and more heat is generated.

Early x-ray tubes, modifications of the Crookes tube, were not vacuum tubes but rather contained controlled quantities of gas within the enclosure. The modern x-ray tube, the Coolidge tube, is a vacuum tube. If it becomes gassy, x-ray production falls and the tube can fail.

An improvement in tube design incorporates metal rather than glass as part or all of the enclosure. As a glass enclosure tube ages, some tungsten vaporizes and coats the inside of the glass enclosure. This alters the electrical properties of the tube, allowing tube current to stray and interact with the glass enclosure; the result is arcing and tube failure.

Metal enclosure tubes maintain a constant electric potential between the electrons of the tube current and the enclosure. Therefore, they have longer life and are less likely to fail. Virtually all high-capacity x-ray tubes now use metal enclosures.

> X-ray tubes are designed with a glass or a metal enclosure.

The x-ray tube window is an area of the glass or metal enclosure, approximately 5 cm², that is thin and through which the useful beam of x-rays is emitted. Such a window allows maximum emission of x-rays with minimum absorption.

INTERNAL COMPONENTS
Cathode

Figure 7-4 shows a photograph of a dual-filament cathode and a schematic drawing of its electric supply. The two filaments supply separate electron beams to produce two focal spots.

> The cathode is the negative side of the x-ray tube; it has two primary parts: a filament and a focusing cup.

Filament. The filament is a coil of wire similar to that in a kitchen toaster, except much smaller. The filament is approximately 2 mm in diameter and 1 or 2 cm long. In the kitchen toaster, an electric current is conducted through the coil, causing it to glow and emit a large quantity of heat.

An x-ray tube filament emits electrons when it is heated. When the current through the filament is sufficiently high, the outer-shell electrons of the filament atoms are "boiled off" and ejected from the filament. This phenomenon is known as **thermionic emission.**

Filaments are usually made of **thoriated tungsten.** Tungsten provides for higher thermionic emission than other metals. Its melting point is 3410° C; therefore, it is not likely to burn out like the filament of a light bulb. Also, tungsten does not vaporize easily. If it did, the tube would become gassy quickly and its internal parts would be coated with tungsten. The addition of 1% to 2% thorium to the tungsten filament enhances the efficiency of thermionic emission and prolongs tube life.

> Tungsten vaporization with deposition on the inside of the glass enclosure is the most common cause of tube failure.

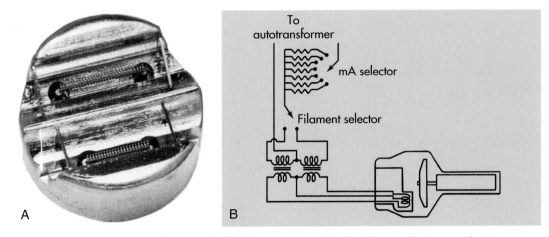

FIGURE 7-4 A, Dual-filament cathode designed to provide focal spots of 0.5 mm and 1.5 mm. **B,** Schematic for dual-filament cathode. (**A** courtesy The Machlett Laboratories, Inc.)

Ultimately, however, tungsten metal does vaporize and is deposited on internal components. This upsets some of the electric characteristics of the tube and can cause arcing and lead to tube failure. Such malfunction is usually abrupt.

Focusing Cup. The filament is embedded in a metal cup called the **focusing cup** (Figure 7-5). Because all the electrons accelerated from cathode to anode are electrically negative, the electron beam tends to spread out owing to electrostatic repulsion. Some electrons can even miss the anode completely.

The focusing cup is negatively charged so that it electrostatically confines the electron beam to a small area of the anode (Figure 7-6). The effectiveness of the focusing cup is determined by its size and shape, its charge, the filament size and shape, and the position of the filament in the focusing cup.

Most rotating anode x-ray tubes have two filaments mounted in the cathode assemble "side by side," creating large and small focal spot sizes. Filaments in biangle x-ray tubes have to be placed "end to end," with the small focus filament above the large filament.

Certain types of x-ray tubes called *grid-controlled tubes* are designed to be turned on and off very rapidly. Grid-controlled tubes are used in portable capacitor discharge imaging systems and in digital subtraction angiography, digital radiography, and cineradiography, each of which requires multiple exposures for precise exposure time.

The term *grid* is borrowed from vacuum tube electronics and refers to an element in the tube that acts as the switch. In a grid-controlled x-ray tube, the focusing cup is the grid and, therefore, the exposure switch.

Filament Current. When the x-ray imaging system is first turned on, a low current passes through the filament to warm it and prepare it for the thermal jolt necessary for x-ray production. At low filament current, there is no tube current because the filament does not get

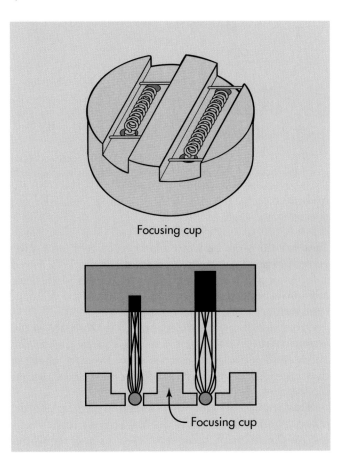

FIGURE 7-5 The focusing cup is a metal shroud that surrounds the filament.

hot enough for thermionic emission. Once the filament current is high enough for thermionic emission, a small rise in filament current results in a large rise in tube current.

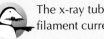 The x-ray tube current is adjusted by controlling the filament current.

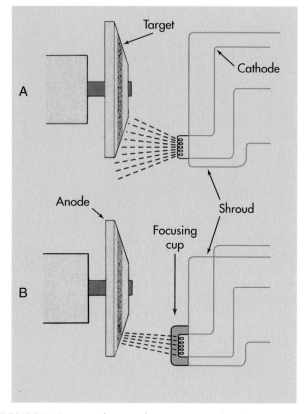

FIGURE 7-6 A, Without a focusing cup, the electron beam is spread beyond the anode because of mutual electrostatic repulsion among the electrons. **B,** With a focusing cup that is negatively charged, the electron beam is condensed and directed to the target.

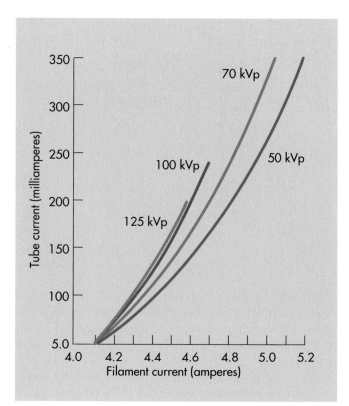

FIGURE 7-7 The x-ray tube current is actually controlled by changing the filament current. Because of thermionic emission, a small change in filament current results in a large change in tube current.

This relationship between filament current and tube current depends on the tube voltage (Figure 7-7). Fixed stations of 100, 200, and 300 mA, and so forth, usually correspond to discrete connections on the filament transformer or to precision resistors.

When emitted from the filament, electrons are in the vicinity of the filament before they are accelerated to the anode. Because these electrons carry negative charges, they repel one another and tend to form a cloud around the filament.

This cloud of electrons, called a *space charge*, makes it difficult for subsequent electrons to be emitted by the filament because of electrostatic repulsion. This phenomenon is called the *space charge effect*. A major obstacle in producing x-ray tubes with currents that exceed 1000 mA is the design of adequate space charge–compensating devices.

> Thermionic emission at low kVp and high mA can be space charge limited.

At any given filament current, say, 5.2 A (Figure 7-8), the x-ray tube current rises with increasing voltage to a maximum value. A further increase in kVp does

not result in a higher mA because all of the available electrons have been used. This is the **saturation current.**

Saturation current is not reached at a lower kVp because of space charge limitation. When an x-ray tube is operated at the saturation current, it is said to be emission limited.

Most diagnostic x-ray tubes have two focal spots—one large and the other small. The small focal spot is used when better spatial resolution is required. The large focal spot is used when large body parts are imaged, and when other techniques that produce high heat are required.

Selection of one or the other focal spot is usually made with the mA station selector on the operating console. Normally, either filament can be used with the lower mA station—approximately 300 mA or less. At approximately 400 mA and up, only the larger focal spot is allowed because the heat capacity of the anode could be exceeded if the small focal spot were used.

Small focal spots range from 0.1 to 1 mm; large focal spots range from 0.3 to 2 mm. Each filament of a dual-filament cathode assembly is embedded in the focusing cup (Figure 7-9). The small focal spot size is associated with the small filament and the large focal spot size with the large filament. An electric current is directed through the appropriate filament.

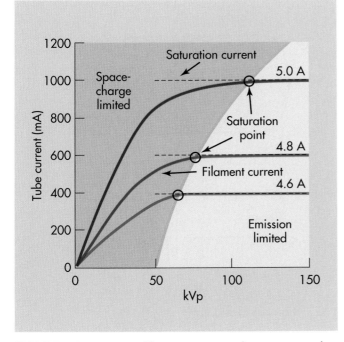

FIGURE 7-8 At a given filament current, tube current reaches a maximum level called *saturation current*.

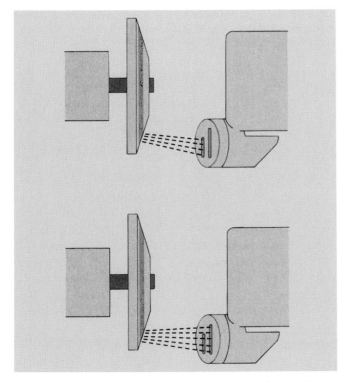

FIGURE 7-9 In a dual-focus x-ray tube, focal spot size is controlled by heating one of the two filaments.

Anode

The anode is the positive side of the x-ray tube. There are two types of anodes—**stationary** and **rotating** (Figure 7-10). Stationary anode x-ray tubes are used in dental x-ray imaging systems, some portable imaging systems, and other special purpose units in which high tube current

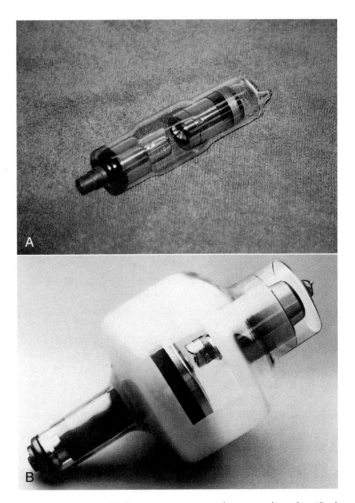

FIGURE 7-10 All diagnostic x-ray tubes can be classified according to type of anode. **A,** Stationary anode. **B,** Rotating anode. (Courtesy Philips Medical Systems.)

and power are not required. General purpose x-ray tubes use the rotating anode because they must be capable of producing high-intensity x-ray beams in a short time.

 The anode is the positive side of the x-ray tube; it conducts electricity and radiates heat and contains the target.

The anode serves three functions in an x-ray tube. The anode is an **electrical conductor.** It receives electrons emitted by the cathode and conducts them through the tube to the connecting cables and back to the high-voltage generator. The anode also provides **mechanical support** for the target.

The anode also must be a good **thermal dissipator.** When the projectile electrons from the cathode interact with the anode, more than 99% of their kinetic energy is converted into heat. This heat must be dissipated quickly. Copper, molybdenum, and graphite are the most common anode materials. Adequate heat dissipation is the major engineering hurdle in designing higher-capacity x-ray tubes.

Target. The **target** is the area of the anode struck by the electrons from the cathode. In stationary anode tubes, the target consists of a tungsten alloy embedded in the copper anode (Figure 7-11, A). In rotating anode tubes, the entire rotating disc is the target (Figure 7-11, B).

Alloying the tungsten (usually with rhenium) gives it added mechanical strength to withstand the stresses of high-speed rotation and the effects of repetitive expansion and contraction. High-capacity x-ray tubes have molybdenum or graphite layered under the tungsten target (Figure 7-12). Both molybdenum and graphite have lower mass density than tungsten, making the anode lighter and easier to rotate.

Tungsten is the material of choice for the target for general radiography for three main reasons:
1. **Atomic number**—Tungsten's high atomic number, 74, results in high-efficiency x-ray production and in high-energy x-rays. The reason for this is discussed more fully in Chapter 9.
2. **Thermal conductivity**—Tungsten has a thermal conductivity nearly equal to that of copper. It is therefore an efficient metal for dissipating the heat produced.
3. **High melting point**—Any material, if heated sufficiently, will melt and become liquid. Tungsten has a high melting point (3400°C, compared with 1100°C for copper) and therefore can stand up under high tube current without pitting or bubbling.

Specialty x-ray tubes for mammography have molybdenum or rhodium targets principally because of their low atomic number and low K-characteristic x-ray energy. This concept is discussed fully in Chapter 8. Table 7-1 summarizes the properties of these target materials.

Rotating Anode. The rotating anode x-ray tube allows the electron beam to interact with a much larger target area; therefore, the heating of the anode is not confined to one small spot, as in a stationary anode tube. Figure 7-13 compares the target areas of typical stationary anode and rotating anode x-ray tubes with 1-mm focal spots.

The actual target for the stationary tube is 1 mm × 4 mm = 4 mm². If the rotating anode diameter is 15 cm, then the radius of the target area is approximately 7 cm (70 mm). The total target area of the rotating anode is $2\pi(70) \times 4$ mm = 1760 mm². Thus, the rotating anode tube provides nearly 500 times more area to interact with the electron beam than is provided by a stationary anode tube.

 Higher tube currents and shorter exposure times are possible with the rotating anode.

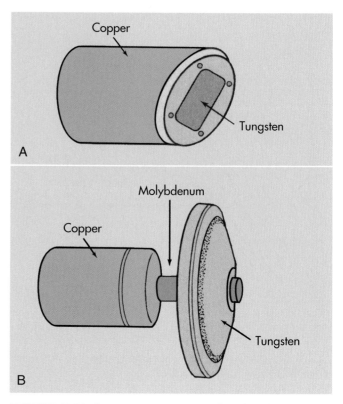

FIGURE 7-11 A, In a stationary anode tube, the target is embedded in the anode. **B,** In a rotating anode tube, the target is the rotating disc.

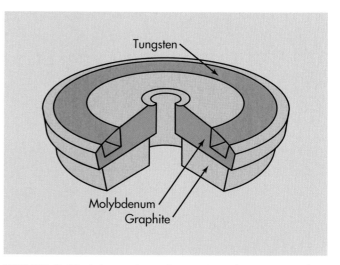

FIGURE 7-12 A layered anode consists of a target surface backed by one or more layers to increase heat capacity.

Heat capacity can be further improved by increasing the speed of anode rotation. Most rotating anodes revolve at 3600 rpm (revolutions per minute). The anodes of high-capacity tubes rotate at up to 10,000 rpm.

The stem of the anode is the shaft between the anode and the rotor. It is narrow so as to reduce its thermal conductivity. The stem usually is made of molybdenum because it is a poor heat conductor.

Table 7-1	Characteristics of X-ray Targets			
Element	**Chemical Symbol**	**Atomic Number**	**K X-ray Energy***	**Melting Temperature**
Tungsten	W	74	69 keV	3400° C
Molybdenum	Mo	42	19 keV	2600° C
Rhodium	Rh	45	23 keV	3200° C

*X-rays resulting from electron transitions into the K shell.

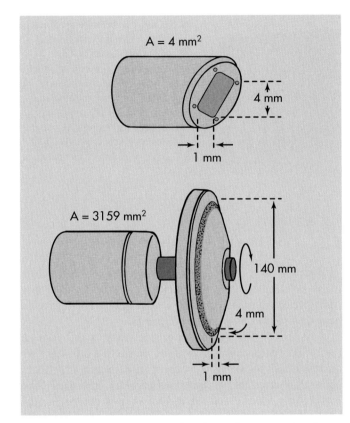

FIGURE 7-13 Stationary anode tube with a 1-mm focal spot may have a target area of 4 mm². A comparable 15 cm–diameter rotating anode tube can have a target area of approximately 1800 mm², which increases the heating capacity of the tube by a factor of nearly 500.

Occasionally, the rotor mechanism of a rotating anode tube fails. When this happens, the anode becomes overheated and pits or cracks, causing tube failure (Figure 7-14).

Induction Motor. How does the anode rotate inside an enclosure with no mechanical connection to the outside? Most things that revolve are powered by chains or axles or gears of some sort.

An electromagnetic induction motor is used to turn the anode. An induction motor consists of two principal parts separated from each other by the glass or metal enclosure (Figure 7-15). The part outside the enclosure, called the *stator,* consists of a series of electromagnets

equally spaced around the neck of the tube. Inside the enclosure is a shaft made of bars of copper and soft iron fabricated into one mass. This part is called the *rotor.*

> The rotating anode is powered by an electromagnetic *induction motor.*

The induction motor works through electromagnetic induction, similar to a transformer. Current in each stator winding induces a magnetic field that surrounds the rotor. The stator windings are energized sequentially so that the induced magnetic field rotates on the axis of the stator. This magnetic field interacts with the ferromagnetic rotor, causing it to rotate synchronously with the activated stator windings.

When the radiologic technologist pushes the exposure button of a radiographic imaging system, there is a short delay before an exposure is made. This allows the rotor to accelerate to its designated rpm while the filament is heated. Only then is the kVp applied to the x-ray tube.

During this time, filament current is increased to provide the correct x-ray tube current. When a two-position exposure switch is used, the switch should be pushed to its final position in one motion. This minimizes the time that the filament is heated and prolongs tube life.

When the exposure is completed on imaging systems equipped with high-speed rotors, one can hear the rotor slow down and stop within approximately 1 min. The high-speed rotor slows down as quickly as it does because the induction motor is put into reverse. The rotor is a precisely balanced, low-friction device that, if left alone, might take many minutes to coast to rest after use.

In a new x-ray tube, the **coast time** is approximately 60 s. With age, the coast time is reduced because of wear of the rotor bearings.

One design that allows for massive anodes uses a shaft fixed at each end (Figure 7-16). In this x-ray tube, the anode is attached to the enclosure, and the whole insert rotates. The cathode is positioned on the axis and the electron beam is deflected electromagnetically onto the anode.

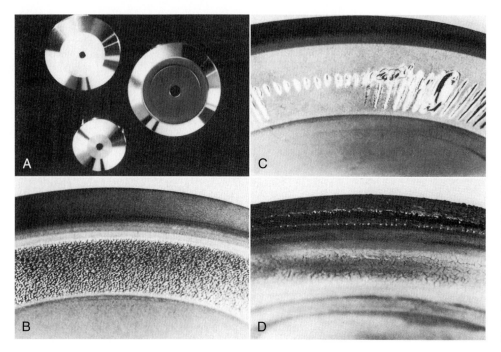

FIGURE 7-14 Comparison of smooth, shiny appearances of rotating anodes when new **(A)** versus their appearance alter failure **(B-D)**. Examples of anode separation and surface melting shown were caused by slow rotation due to bearing damage **(B)**, repeated overload **(C)**, and exceeding of maximum heat storage capacity **(D)**. (Courtesy Philips Medical Systems.)

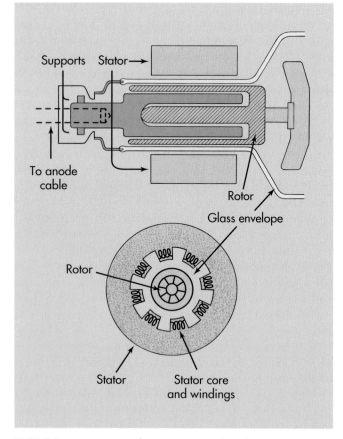

FIGURE 7-15 Target of a rotating anode tube is powered by an induction motor, the principal components of which are the stator and the rotor.

Because the disc is part of the enclosure, the cooling oil is in contact with the back of the anode, allowing optimum cooling. The principal advantages are improved heat dissipation and greater capacity.

Line-Focus Principle. The focal spot is the area of the target from which x-rays are emitted. Radiology requires small focal spots because the smaller the focal spot, the better the spatial resolution of the image. Unfortunately, as the size of the focal spot decreases, the heating of the target is concentrated onto a smaller area. This is the limiting factor to focal spot size.

> The focal spot is the actual x-ray source.

Before the rotating anode was developed, another design was incorporated into x-ray tube targets to allow a large area for heating while maintaining a small focal spot. This design is known as the **line-focus principle.** By angling the target (Figure 7-17), one makes the effective area of the target much smaller than the actual area of electron interaction.

The effective target area, or effective focal spot size, is the area projected onto the patient and the image receptor. This is the value given when large or small focal spots are identified. When the target angle is made smaller, the effective focal spot size also is made smaller. Diagnostic x-ray tubes have target angles that vary from approximately 5 to 20 degrees.

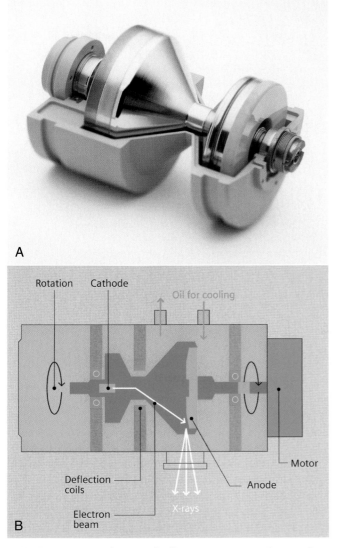

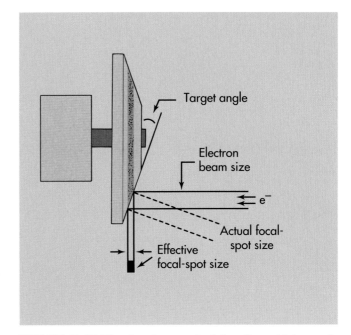

FIGURE 7-17 The line-focus principle allows high anode heating with small effective focal spots. As the target angle decreases, so does the effective focal spot size.

FIGURE 7-16 A, This very high capacity x-ray tube revolves in a bath of oil for complete heat dissipation. **B,** The cooling capacity is greater than any heat load. (Courtesy Siemens Medical Systems.)

The limiting factor in target angle is the ability of the cone of x-rays produced to adequately cover the largest field size used. In general radiography, this is usually taken as the diagonal of a 17 × 14-in (35 × 43-cm) image receptor, which is approximately 22 in or 55 cm.

When a smaller image receptor is used, the anode angle can be steeper. The advantage of the line-focus principle is that it simultaneously improves spatial resolution and heat capacity.

 The line-focus principle results in an effective focal spot size much less than the actual focal spot size.

Biangular targets are available that produce two focal spot sizes because of two different target angles on the anode (Figure 7-18). Combining biangular targets with different-length filaments results in a very flexible combination.

A circular effective focal spot is preferred. Usually, however, it has a shape characterized as a double banana (Figure 7-19). These differences in x-ray intensity across the focal spot are controlled principally by the design of the filament and focusing cup and by the voltage on the focusing cup. Round focal spots are particularly important for high-resolution magnification radiography and mammography.

The National Electrical Manufacturers Association (NEMA) has established standards and variances for focal spot sizes. When a manufacturer states a focal spot size, that is its nominal size. Table 7-2 shows the maximum measured size permitted that is still within the standard.

Heel Effect. One unfortunate consequence of the line-focus principle is that the radiation intensity on the cathode side of the x-ray field is greater than that on the anode side. Electrons interact with target atoms at various depths into the target.

The x-rays that constitute the useful beam emitted toward the anode side must traverse a greater thickness of target material than the x-rays emitted toward the cathode direction (Figure 7-20). The intensity of x-rays that are emitted through the "heel" of the target is reduced because they have a longer path through the target, and therefore increased absorption. This is the **heel effect.**

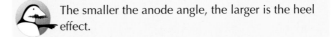 The smaller the anode angle, the larger is the heel effect.

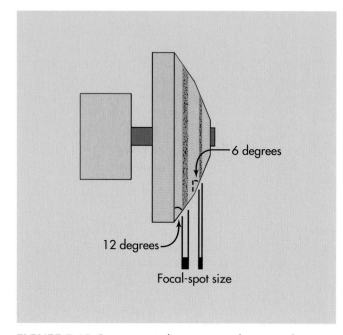

FIGURE 7-18 Some targets have two angles to produce two focal spots. To achieve this, the filaments must be placed one above the other.

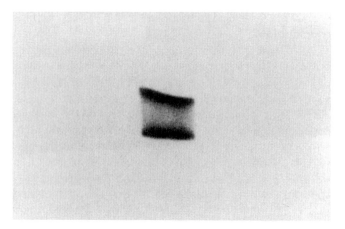

FIGURE 7-19 The usual shape of a focal spot is the double banana. (Courtesy Donald Jacobson, Medical College of Wisconsin.)

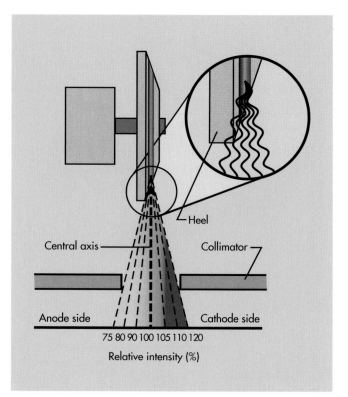

FIGURE 7-20 The heel effect results in reduced x-ray intensity on the anode side of the useful beam caused by absorption in the "heel" of the target.

The difference in radiation intensity across the useful beam of an x-ray field can vary by as much as 45%. The **central ray** of the useful beam is the imaginary line generated by the centermost x-ray in the beam. If the radiation intensity along the central ray is designated as 100%, then the intensity on the cathode side may be as high as 120%, and that on the anode side may be as low as 75%.

The heel effect is important when one is imaging anatomical structures that differ greatly in thickness or mass density. In general, positioning the cathode side of the x-ray tube over the thicker part of the anatomy provides more uniform radiation exposure of the image receptor. The cathode and anode directions are usually indicated on the protective housing, sometimes near the cable connectors.

Table 7-2	Nominal Focal Spot Size Compared With Maximum Acceptable Dimensions				
NOMINAL FOCAL SPOT SIZE (mm)			**ACCEPTABLE MEASURED FOCAL SPOT SIZE (mm)**		
Width	**×**	**Length**	**Width**	**×**	**Length**
0.1	×	0.1	0.15	×	0.15
0.3	×	0.3	0.45	×	0.65
0.4	×	0.4	0.6	×	0.85
0.5	×	0.5	0.75	×	1.1
1.0	×	1.0	1.4	×	2.0
2.0	×	2.0	2.6	×	3.7

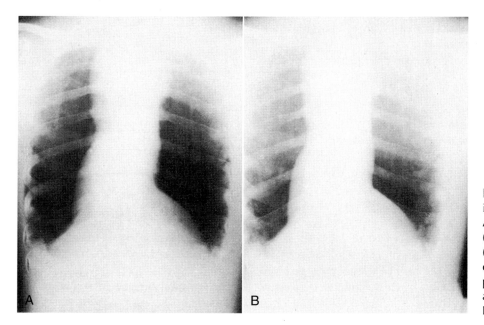

FIGURE 7-21 Posteroanterior chest images demonstrate the heel effect. **A,** Images taken with the cathode up (superior). **B,** Image with cathode down (inferior). More uniform radiographic density is obtained with the cathode positioned to the thicker side of the anatomy, as in **B.** (Courtesy Pat Duffy, Roxbury Community College.)

In chest radiography, for example, the cathode should be inferior. The lower thorax in the region of the diaphragm is considerably thicker than the upper thorax, and therefore requires higher radiation intensity if x-ray exposure of the image receptor is to be uniform.

In abdominal imaging, on the other hand, the cathode should be superior. The upper abdomen is thicker than the lower abdomen and pelvis and requires greater x-ray intensity for uniform x-ray exposure.

Figure 7-21 shows two posteroanterior chest images—one taken with the cathode down, the other with the cathode up. Can you tell the difference? Which do you think represents better radiographic quality? Resolve the difference before looking at the figure legend.

In mammography, the x-ray tube is designed so that the more intense side of the x-ray beam, the cathode side, is positioned toward the chest wall. With angling of the x-ray tube, advantage can be taken of the foreshortening that occurs to the focal spot size, resulting in an even smaller effective focal spot size.

Another important consequence of the heel effect is changing focal spot size. The effective focal spot is smaller on the anode side of the x-ray field than on the cathode side (Figure 7-22). Some manufacturers of mammography equipment take advantage of this property by angling the x-ray tube to produce the smaller focal spot along the chest wall.

> The heel effect results in smaller effective focal spot and less radiation intensity on the anode side of the x-ray beam.

Off Focus Radiation. X-ray tubes are designed so that projectile electrons from the cathode interact with the target only at the focal spot. However, some of the electrons bounce off the focal spot and then land on other areas of the target, causing x-rays to be produced from outside of the focal spot (Figure 7-23).

These x-rays are called *off-focus radiation.* This is not unlike squirting a water pistol at a concrete pavement: Some of the water splashes off the pavement and lands in a larger area.

Off focus radiation is undesirable because it extends the size of the focal spot. The additional x-ray beam area increases skin dose modestly but unnecessarily. Off focus radiation can significantly reduce image contrast.

Finally, off focus radiation can image patient tissue that was intended to be excluded by the variable-aperture collimators. Examples of such undesirable images are the ears in a skull examination, the soft tissue beyond the cervical spine, and the lung beyond the borders of the thoracic spine.

Off focus radiation is reduced by designing a fixed diaphragm in the tube housing near the window of the x-ray tube (Figure 7-24). This is a geometric solution.

Another effective solution is the metal enclosure x-ray tube. Electrons reflected from the focal spot are extracted by the metal enclosure and conducted away. Therefore, they are not available to be attracted to the target outside of the focal spot. The use of a grid does not reduce off focus radiation.

X-RAY TUBE FAILURE

With careful use, x-ray tubes can provide many years of service. With inconsiderate use, x-ray tube life may be shortened substantially.

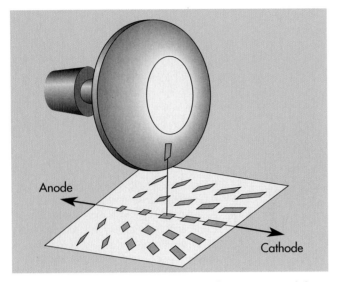

FIGURE 7-22 The effective focal spot changes size and shape across the projected x-ray field.

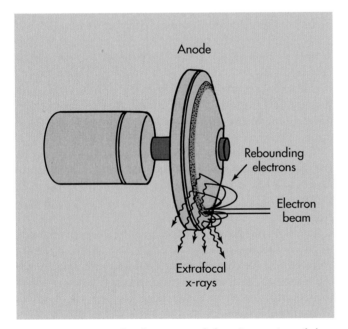

FIGURE 7-23 Extrafocal x-rays result from interaction of electrons with the anode off of the focal spot.

The length of x-ray tube life is primarily under the control of the radiologic technologist. Basically, x-ray tube life is extended by using the minimum radiographic factors of mA, kVp, and exposure time that are appropriate for each examination. The use of faster image receptors results in longer tube life.

X-ray tube failure has several causes, most of which are related to the thermal characteristics of the x-ray tube. Enormous heat is generated in the anode of the x-ray tube during x-ray exposure. This heat must be dissipated for the x-ray tube to continue to function.

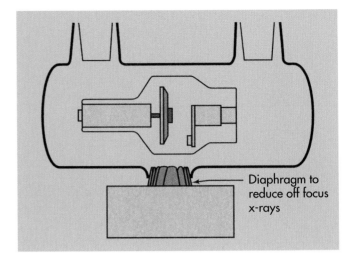

FIGURE 7-24 An additional diaphragm is positioned close to the focal spot to reduce extrafocal radiation.

This heat can be dissipated in one of three ways: radiation, conduction, or convection (Figure 7-25). **Radiation** is the transfer of heat by the emission of infrared radiation. Heat lamps emit not only visible light but infrared energy.

Conduction is the transfer of energy from one area of an object to another. The handle of a heated iron skillet becomes hot because of conduction. **Convection** is the transfer of heat by the movement of a heated substance from one place to another. Many homes and offices are heated by the convection of hot air.

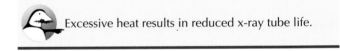

Excessive heat results in reduced x-ray tube life.

All three modes of heat transfer occur in an x-ray tube. Most of the heat is dissipated by radiation during exposure. The anode may glow red hot. It always emits infrared energy.

Unfortunately, some heat is conducted through the neck of the anode to the rotor and glass enclosure. The heated glass enclosure raises the temperature of the oil bath; this convects the heat to the tube housing and then to room air.

When the temperature of the anode is excessive during a single exposure, localized surface melting and pitting of the anode can occur. These surface irregularities result in variable and reduced radiation output. If surface melting is sufficiently severe, the tungsten can be vaporized and can plate the inside of the glass enclosure. This can cause filtering of the x-ray beam and interference with electron flow from cathode to anode.

If the temperature of the anode increases too rapidly, the anode may crack, becoming unstable in rotation and

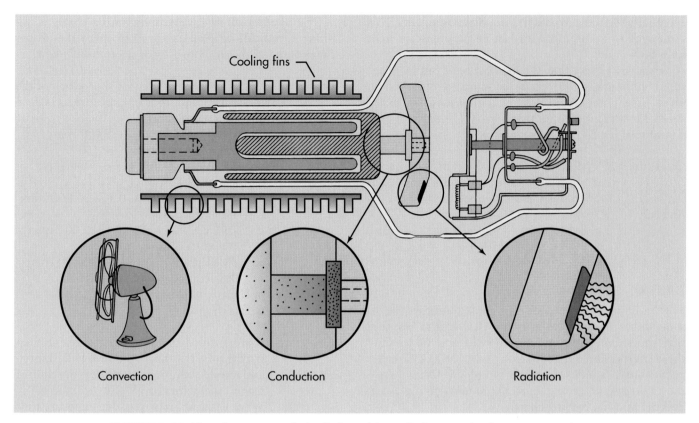

Cooling fins

Convection   Conduction   Radiation

FIGURE 7-25 Heat from an anode is dissipated by radiation, conduction, or convection, most often radiation.

rendering the tube useless. If maximum techniques are required for a particular examination, the anode should first be warmed by low-technique operation.

 Maximum radiographic techniques should never be applied to a cold anode.

A second type of x-ray tube failure results from maintaining the anode at elevated temperatures for prolonged periods. During exposures lasting 1 to 3 s, the temperature of the anode may be sufficient to cause it to glow like an incandescent light bulb. During exposure, heat is dissipated by radiation.

Between exposures, heat is dissipated, primarily through conduction, to the oil bath in which the tube is immersed. Some heat is conducted through the narrow molybdenum neck to the rotor assembly; this can cause subsequent heating of the rotor bearings. Excessive heating of the bearings results in increased rotational friction and an imbalance of the rotor anode assembly. Bearing damage is another cause of tube failure.

If thermal stress on the x-ray tube anode is maintained for prolonged periods, such as during fluoroscopy, the thermal capacity of the total anode system and of the x-ray tube housing is the limitation to operation. During

fluoroscopy, the x-ray tube current is usually less than 5 mA, rather than hundreds of mA as in radiography.

Under such fluoroscopic conditions, the rate of heat dissipation from the rotating target attains equilibrium with the rate of heat input, and this rate rarely is sufficient to cause surface defects in the target. However, the x-ray tube can fail because of the continuous heat delivered to the rotor assembly, the oil bath, and the x-ray tube housing. Bearings can fail, the glass enclosure can crack, and the tube housing can fail.

A final cause of tube failure involves the filament. Because of the high temperature of the filament, tungsten atoms are vaporized slowly and plate the inside of the glass or metal enclosure, even with normal use. This tungsten, along with that vaporized from the anode, can disturb the electric balance of the x-ray tube, causing abrupt, intermittent changes in tube current, which often lead to arcing and tube failure.

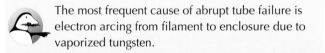 The most frequent cause of abrupt tube failure is electron arcing from filament to enclosure due to vaporized tungsten.

With excessive heating of the filament caused by high mA operation for prolonged periods, more tungsten is vaporized. The filament wire becomes thinner and eventually breaks, producing an **open filament**. This same type of failure occurs when an incandescent light bulb burns out.

In the same way that the life of a light bulb is measured in hours—2000 hours is standard—that of an x-ray tube is measured in tens of thousands of exposures. Most computed tomography (CT) tubes are now guaranteed for 50,000 exposures.

Question: A 7-MHU spiral CT x-ray tube is guaranteed for 50,000 scans, each scan limited to 5 s. What is the x-ray tube life in hours?

Answer:
$$\text{Guaranteed tube life} = (50{,}000 \text{ scans}) (5 \text{ s/scan})$$
$$= 250{,}000 \text{ s}$$
$$= 69 \text{ hr}$$

RATING CHARTS

The radiologic technologist is guided in the use of x-ray tubes by **x-ray tube rating charts.** It is essential that the technologist be able to read and understand these charts. Three types of x-ray tube rating charts are particularly significant to the radiologic technologist: the radiographic rating chart, the anode cooling chart, and the housing cooling chart.

Radiographic Rating Chart

Of the three rating charts, the radiographic rating chart is the most important because it conveys which radiographic techniques are safe and which techniques are unsafe for x-ray tube operation. Each chart shown in Figure 7-26 contains a family of curves that represent the various tube currents in mA. The x-axis and the y-axis show scales of the two other radiographic parameters, time and kVp.

For a given mA, any combination of kVp and time that lies below the mA curve is safe. Any combination of kVp and time that lies above the curve representing the desired mA is unsafe. If an unsafe exposure was made, the tube might fail abruptly. Most x-ray imaging systems have a microprocessor control that does not allow an exposure to be made when the technique selected would cause the tube to exceed the safe conditions of the radiographic rating chart.

A series of radiographic rating charts accompanies every x-ray tube. These charts cover the various modes of operation possible with that tube. There are different charts for the filament in use (large or small focal spot), the speed of anode rotation (3600 rpm or 10,000 rpm), the target angle, and the voltage rectification (half-wave, full-wave, three-phase, high-frequency).

Be sure to use the proper radiographic rating chart with each tube. This is particularly important after x-ray tubes have been replaced. An appropriate radiographic rating chart is supplied with each replacement x-ray tube and can be different from that of the original tube.

The application of radiographic rating charts is not difficult and can be used as a tool to check the proper functioning of the microprocessor protection circuit.

Question: With reference to Figure 7-26, which of the following conditions of exposure are safe and which are unsafe?
a. 95 kVp, 150 mA, 1 s; 3400 rpm; 0.6-mm focal spot
b. 85 kVp, 400 mA, 0.5 s; 3400 rpm; 1-mm focal spot
c. 125 kVp, 500 mA, 0.1 s; 10,000 rpm; 1-mm focal spot
d. 75 kVp, 700 mA, 0.3 s; 10,000 rpm; 1-mm focal spot
e. 88 kVp, 400 mA, 0.1 s; 10,000 rpm; 0.6-mm focal spot

Answer: a. Unsafe; b. Unsafe; c. Safe; d. Safe; e. Unsafe.

Question: Radiographic examination of the abdomen with a tube that has a 0.6-mm focal spot and anode rotation of 10,000 rpm requires technique factors of 95 kVp, 150 mAs. What is the shortest possible exposure time for this examination?

Answer: Locate the proper radiographic rating chart (upper right in Figure 7-26) and the 95-kVp line (horizontal line near middle of chart). Beginning from the left (shorter exposure times), determine the mAs for the intersection of each mA curve with the 95 kVp level.
1. The first intersection is approximately 350 mA at 0.03 s = 10.5 mAs. Not enough.
2. The next intersection is approximately 300 mA at 0.2 s = 60 mAs. Not enough.
3. The next intersection is approximately 250 mA at 0.6 s = 150 mAs. This is sufficient.

Consequently, 0.6 s is the minimum possible exposure time.

Anode Cooling Chart

The anode has a limited capacity for storing heat. Although heat is dissipated to the oil bath and x-ray tube housing, it is possible through prolonged use or multiple exposures to exceed the heat storage capacity of the anode.

Thermal energy is conventionally measured in units of calories, British thermal units (BTUs), or joules. In x-ray applications, thermal energy is measured in **heat units (HUs).** The capacity of the anode and the housing to store heat is measured in heat units. One heat unit is equal to the product of 1 kVp, 1 mA, and 1 s.

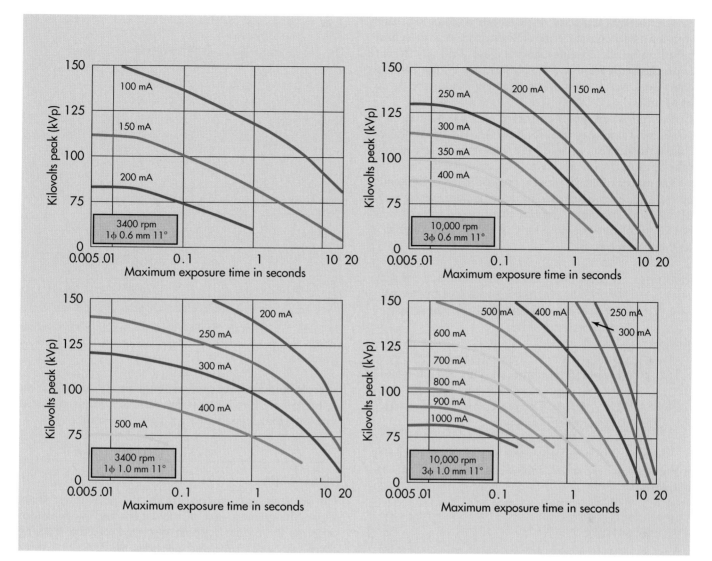

FIGURE 7-26 Representative radiographic rating charts for a given x-ray tube. Each chart specifies the conditions of operation under which it applies. (Courtesy General Electric Medical Systems.)

SINGLE-PHASE
$HU = kVp \times mA \times s$

Question: Radiographic examination of the lateral lumbar spine with a single-phase imaging system requires 98 kVp, 120 mAs. How many heat units are generated by this exposure?
Answer: Number of heat units = 98 kVp × 120 mAs
= 11,760 HU

Question: A fluoroscopic examination is performed with a single-phase imaging system at 76 kVp and 1.5 mA for 3.5 min. How many heat units are generated?
Answer: Number of heat units = 76 kVp × 1.5 mA
× 3.5 min × 60 s/min
= 23,940 HU

More heat is generated when three-phase equipment and high-frequency equipment are used than when single-phase equipment is used. A modification factor of 1.4 is necessary for calculating three-phase or high-frequency heat units.

THREE-PHASE/HIGH-FREQUENCY
$HU = 1.4 \times kVp \times mA \times s$

Question: Six sequential skull films are exposed with a three-phase generator operated at 82 kVp, 120 mAs. What is the total heat generated?
Answer:
Number of heat units/film = 1.4 × 82 kVp × 120 mAs
= 13,776 HU
Total HU = 6 × 13,776 HU
= 82,656 HU

The thermal capacity of an anode and its heat dissipation characteristics are contained in a rating chart called an **anode cooling chart** (Figure 7-27). Different from the radiographic rating chart, the anode cooling chart does not depend on the filament size or the speed of rotation.

The tube represented in Figure 7-27 has a maximum anode heat capacity of 350,000 HU. The chart shows that if the maximum heat load were attained, it would take 15 min for the anode to cool completely.

The rate of cooling is rapid at first and slows as the anode cools. In addition to determining the maximum heat capacity of the anode, the anode cooling chart is used to determine the length of time required for complete cooling after any level of heat input.

Question: A particular examination results in delivery of 50,000 HU to the anode in a matter of seconds. How long will it take the anode to cool completely?

Answer: The 50,000-HU level intersects the anode cooling curve at approximately 6 min. From that point on, the curve to complete cooling requires an additional 9 min (15 − 6 = 9). Therefore, 9 min is required for complete cooling.

Although the heat generated in producing x-rays is expressed in heat units, joules are the equivalent. By definition:

$$1 \text{ watt} = 1 \text{ volt} \times 1 \text{ amp}$$
$$= 1 \text{ J/C} \times 1 \text{ C/s}$$
$$= 1 \text{ J/s}$$
$$\text{Therefore: } 1 \text{ J/s} = 1 \text{ kV} \times 1 \text{ mA}$$
$$\text{and } 1 \text{ J} = 1 \text{ kV} \times 1 \text{ mA} \times 1 \text{ s}$$
$$\text{and since } 1 \text{ HU} = 1 \text{ kVp} \times 1 \text{ mA} \times 1 \text{ s}$$
$$1 \text{ HU} = 1.4 \text{ J (3Ø, HF)}$$
$$1 \text{ J} = 0.7 \text{ HU (3Ø, HF)}$$

Question: How much heat energy (in joules) is produced during a single high-frequency mammographic exposure of 25 kVp, 200 mAs?

Answer: 25 kVp × 200 mAs = 5000 HU
5000 HU × 1.4 J/HU = 7000 J
= 7 kJ

Housing Cooling Chart

The cooling chart for the housing of the x-ray tube has a shape similar to that of the anode cooling chart and is used in precisely the same way. Radiographic x-ray tube housings usually have maximum heat capacities in the range of several million heat units. Complete cooling

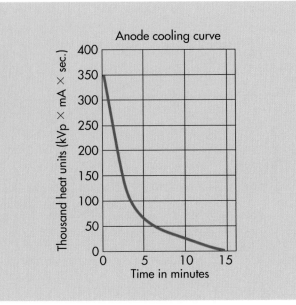

FIGURE 7-27 Anode cooling chart shows time required for heated anode to cool. (Courtesy General Electric Medical Systems.)

after maximum heat capacity requires from 1 to 2 hr. Approximately twice that amount of time is required without auxiliary fan–powered air circulation.

SUMMARY

The primary support structure for the x-ray tube, which allows the greatest ease of movement and range of position, is the ceiling support system. Protective housing covers the x-ray tube and provides the following three functions: (1) It reduces leakage radiation to less than 100 mR/hr at 1 m, (2) it provides mechanical support, thereby protecting the tube from damage, and (3) it serves as a way to conduct heat away from the x-ray tube target.

The glass or metal enclosure surrounds the cathode (−) and the anode (+), which are the electrodes of the vacuum tube. The cathode contains the tungsten filament, which is the source of electrons. The rotating anode is the tungsten-rhenium disc, which serves as a target for electrons accelerated from the cathode. The line-focus principle results from angled targets. The heel effect is the variation in x-ray intensity across the x-ray beam that results from absorption of x-rays in the heel of the target.

Safe operation of the x-ray tube is the responsibility of the radiographer. Tube failure can be prevented. The causes of tube failure are threefold:

- A single excessive exposure causes pitting or cracking of the anode.
- Long exposure time causes excessive heating of the anode, resulting in damage to the bearings in the rotor assembly. Bearing damage causes warping and rotational friction of the anode.

• Even with normal use, vaporization of the filament causes tungsten to coat the glass or metal enclosure; this eventually causes arcing.

Tube rating charts printed by manufacturers of x-ray tubes aid the radiographer in using acceptable exposure levels to maximize x-ray tube life.

CHALLENGE QUESTIONS

1. Define or otherwise identify the following:
   a. Housing cooling chart
   b. Leakage radiation
   c. Heat unit (HU)
   d. Focusing cup
   e. Anode rotation speed
   f. Thoriated tungsten
   g. X-ray tube current
   h. Grid-controlled x-ray tube
   i. Convection
   j. Space charge
2. List the three methods used to support the x-ray tube and briefly describe each.
3. Where in an x-ray imaging system is thoriated tungsten used?
4. What is saturation current?
5. Why are arcing and tube failure no longer a problem in modern x-ray tube design?
6. Explain the phenomenon of thermionic emission.
7. Describe the principal cause of x-ray tube failure. What addition to the filament material prolongs tube life?
8. What is the reason for the filament to be embedded in the focusing cup?
9. Why are x-ray tubes manufactured with two focal spots?
10. Is the anode or the cathode the negative side of the x-ray tube?
11. List and describe the two types of anodes.
12. What are the three functions the anode serves in an x-ray tube?
13. How do atomic number, thermal conductivity, and melting point affect the selection of anode target material?
14. Draw diagrams of a stationary and a rotating anode.
15. How does the anode rotate inside a glass enclosure with no mechanical connection to the outside?
16. Draw the difference between the actual focal spot and the effective focal spot.
17. Define the heel effect and describe how it can be used advantageously.
18. Explain the three causes of x-ray tube failure.
19. What happens when an x-ray tube is space charge limited?
20. What is a detent position?

The answers to the Challenge Questions can be found by logging on to our website at http://evolve.elsevier.com.

X-ray Production

OBJECTIVES

At the completion of this chapter, the student should be able
to do the following:

1. Discuss the interactions between projectile electrons and the x-ray
   tube target
2. Identify characteristic and bremsstrahlung x-rays
3. Describe the x-ray emission spectrum
4. Explain how mAs, kVp, added filtration, target material, and
   voltage ripple affect the x-ray emission spectrum

OUTLINE

Electron Target Interactions
   Anode Heat
   Characteristic Radiation
   Bremsstrahlung Radiation
X-ray Emission Spectrum
   Characteristic X-ray Spectrum
   Bremsstrahlung X-ray Spectrum
Factors Affecting the X-ray Emission Spectrum
   Effect of mA and mAs
   Effect of kVp
   Effect of Added Filtration
   Effect of Target Material
   Effect of Voltage Waveform

CHAPTER 7 discussed the internal components of the x-ray tube—the cathode and the anode—within the evacuated glass or metal enclosure. This chapter explains the interactions of the projectile electrons that are accelerated from the cathode to the x-ray tube target. Those interactions produce two types of x-rays—characteristic and bremsstrahlung; these are described by the x-ray emission spectrum. Various conditions that affect the x-ray emission spectrum are discussed.

ELECTRON TARGET INTERACTIONS

The x-ray imaging system description in Chapter 7 emphasized that its primary function is to accelerate electrons from the cathode to the anode in the x-ray tube. The three principal parts of an x-ray imaging system—the operating console, the high-voltage generator, and the x-ray tube—are designed to provide a large number of electrons with high kinetic energy focused toward a small spot on the anode.

 Kinetic energy is the energy of motion.

Stationary objects have no kinetic energy; objects in motion have kinetic energy proportional to their mass and to the square of their velocity. The kinetic energy equation follows.

KINETIC ENERGY

$$KE = \frac{1}{2}mv^2$$

where m is the mass in kilograms, v is velocity in meters per second, and KE is kinetic energy in joules.

For example, a 1000-kg automobile has four times the kinetic energy of a 250-kg motorcycle traveling at the same speed (Figure 8-1). If the motorcycle were to double its velocity, however, it would have the same kinetic energy as the automobile.

In determining the magnitude of the kinetic energy of a projectile, velocity is more important than mass. In an x-ray tube, the projectile is the electron. All electrons have the same mass; therefore, electron kinetic energy is increased by raising the kVp. As electron kinetic energy is increased, both the intensity (quantity) and the energy (quality) of the x-ray beam are increased.

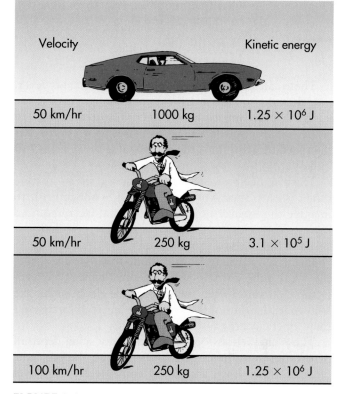

Velocity		Kinetic energy
50 km/hr	1000 kg	1.25×10^6 J
50 km/hr	250 kg	3.1×10^5 J
100 km/hr	250 kg	1.25×10^6 J

FIGURE 8-1 Kinetic energy is proportional to the product of mass and velocity squared.

The modern x-ray imaging system is remarkable. It conveys to the x-ray tube target an enormous number of electrons at a precisely controlled kinetic energy. At 100 mA, for example, 6×10^{17} electrons travel from the cathode to the anode of the x-ray tube every second.

In an x-ray imaging system operating at 70 kVp, each electron arrives at the target with a maximum kinetic energy of 70 keV. Because there are 1.6×10^{-16} J per keV, this energy is equivalent to the following:

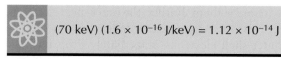

$$(70 \text{ keV}) (1.6 \times 10^{-16} \text{ J/keV}) = 1.12 \times 10^{-14} \text{ J}$$

When this energy is inserted into the expression for kinetic energy and calculations are performed to determine the velocity of the electrons, the result is as follows:

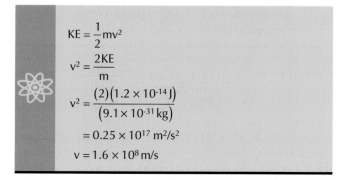

$$KE = \frac{1}{2}mv^2$$

$$v^2 = \frac{2KE}{m}$$

$$v^2 = \frac{(2)(1.2 \times 10^{-14} \text{ J})}{(9.1 \times 10^{-31} \text{ kg})}$$

$$= 0.25 \times 10^{17} \text{ m}^2/\text{s}^2$$

$$v = 1.6 \times 10^8 \text{ m/s}$$

Question: At what fraction of the velocity of light do 70-keV electrons travel?

Answer:
$$\frac{v}{c} = \frac{1.6 \times 10^8 \text{ m/s}}{3.0 \times 10^8 \text{ m/s}} = 0.53$$

These calculations are not precisely correct; however, they do serve to illustrate the point and demonstrate the use of the preceding equation. According to the theory of relativity, an electron's mass increases as it approaches the speed of light; thus, the actual value of v/c is 0.47 at 70 keV.

The distance between the filament and the x-ray tube target is only approximately 1 cm. It is not difficult to imagine the intensity of the accelerating force required to raise the velocity of electrons from zero to half the speed of light in so short a distance.

Electrons traveling from cathode to anode constitute the x-ray tube current and are sometimes called **projectile electrons.** When these projectile electrons hit the heavy metal atoms of the x-ray tube target, they transfer their kinetic energy to the target atoms.

These interactions occur within a very small depth of penetration into the target. As they occur, the projectile electrons slow down and finally come nearly to rest, at which time they are conducted through the x-ray anode assembly and out into the associated electronic circuitry.

The projectile electron interacts with the orbital electrons or the nuclear field of target atoms. These interactions result in the conversion of electron kinetic energy into thermal energy (heat) and electromagnetic energy in the form of infrared radiation (also heat) and x-rays.

Anode Heat

Most of the kinetic energy of projectile electrons is converted into heat (Figure 8-2). The projectile electrons interact with the outer-shell electrons of the target atoms but do not transfer sufficient energy to these outer-shell electrons to ionize them. Rather, the outer-shell electrons are simply raised to an excited, or higher, energy level.

The outer-shell electrons immediately drop back to their normal energy level with the emission of infrared radiation. The constant excitation and return of outer-shell electrons are responsible for most of the heat generated in the anodes of x-ray tubes.

 Approximately 99% of the kinetic energy of projectile electrons is converted to heat.

Only approximately 1% of projectile electron kinetic energy is used for the production of x-radiation. Therefore, sophisticated as it is, the x-ray imaging system is very inefficient.

The production of heat in the anode increases directly with increasing x-ray tube current. Doubling the x-ray tube current doubles the heat produced. Heat

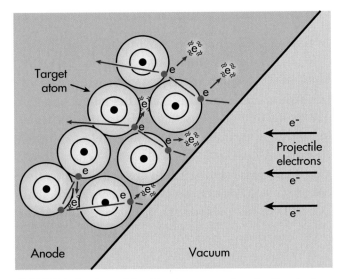

FIGURE 8-2 Most of the kinetic energy of projectile electrons is converted to heat by interactions with outer-shell electrons of target atoms. These interactions are primarily excitations rather than ionizations.

production also increases directly with increasing kVp, at least in the diagnostic range. Although the relationship between varying kVp and varying heat production is approximate, it is sufficiently exact to allow the computation of heat units for use with anode cooling charts.

The efficiency of x-ray production is independent of the tube current. Consequently, regardless of what mA is selected, the efficiency of x-ray production remains constant.

The efficiency of x-ray production increases with increasing kVp. At 60 kVp, only 0.5% of the electron kinetic energy is converted to x-rays. At 100 kVp, approximately 1% is converted to x-rays, and at 20 MV, 70% is converted.

Characteristic Radiation

If the projectile electron interacts with an inner-shell electron of the target atom rather than with an outer-shell electron, **characteristic x-rays** can be produced. Characteristic x-rays result when the interaction is sufficiently violent to ionize the target atom through total removal of an inner-shell electron.

 Characteristic x-rays are emitted when an outer-shell electron fills an inner-shell void.

Figure 8-3 illustrates how characteristic x-rays are produced. When the projectile electron ionizes a target atom by removing a K-shell electron, a temporary electron void is produced in the K shell. This is a highly unnatural state for the target atom, and it is corrected when an outer-shell electron falls into the void in the K shell.

The transition of an orbital electron from an outer shell to an inner shell is accompanied by the emission of

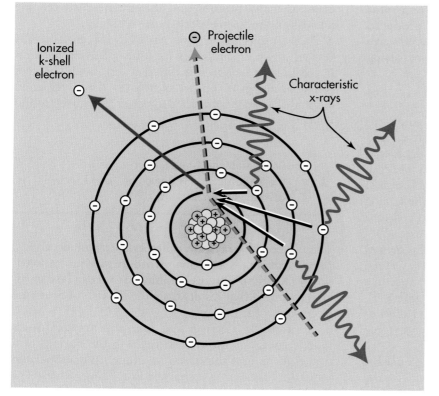

FIGURE 8-3 Characteristic x-rays are produced after ionization of a K-shell electron. When an outer-shell electron fills the vacancy in the K shell, an x-ray is emitted.

an x-ray. The x-ray has energy equal to the difference in the binding energies of the orbital electrons involved.

Question: A K-shell electron is removed from a tungsten atom and is replaced by an L-shell electron. What is the energy of the characteristic x-ray that is emitted?

Answer: Reference to Figure 8-4 shows that for tungsten, K-shell electrons have binding energies of 69 keV, and L-shell electrons are bound by 12 keV. Therefore, the characteristic x-ray emitted has energy of 69 − 12 = 57 keV.

By the same procedure, the energy of x-rays resulting from M-to-K, N-to-K, O-to-K, and P-to-K transitions can be calculated. Tungsten, for example, has electrons in shells out to the P shell, and when a K-shell electron is ionized, its position can be filled with electrons from any of the outer shells. All these x-rays are called *K x-rays* because they result from electron transitions into the K shell.

Similar characteristic x-rays are produced when the target atom is ionized by removal of electrons from shells other than the K shell. Note that Figure 8-3 does not show the production of x-rays resulting from ionization of an L-shell electron.

Such a diagram would show the removal of an L-shell electron by the projectile electron. The vacancy in the L shell would be filled by an electron from any of the outer shells. X-rays resulting from electron transitions to

the L shell are called *L x-rays* and have much less energy than K x-rays because the binding energy of an L-shell electron is much lower than that of a K-shell electron.

> Only the K-characteristic x-rays of tungsten are useful for imaging.

Similarly, M-characteristic x-rays, N-characteristic x-rays, and even O-characteristic x-rays can be produced in a tungsten target. Figure 8-4 illustrates the electron configuration and Table 8-1 summarizes the production of characteristic x-rays in tungsten.

Although many characteristic x-rays can be produced, these can be produced only at specific energies, equal to the differences in electron-binding energies for the various electron transitions.

Except for K x-rays, all the characteristic x-rays have very low energy. The L x-rays, with approximately 12 keV of energy, penetrate only a few centimeters into soft tissue. Consequently, they are useless as diagnostic x-rays, as are all the other low-energy characteristic x-rays. The last column in Table 8-1 shows the effective energy for each of the characteristic x-rays of tungsten.

> This type of x-radiation is called *characteristic* because it is characteristic of the target element.

Because the electron binding energy for every element is different, the energy of characteristic x-rays produced in the various elements is also different. The effective energy of characteristic x-rays increases with increasing atomic number of the target element.

Bremsstrahlung Radiation

The production of heat and characteristic x-rays involves interactions between the projectile electrons and the electrons of x-ray tube target atoms. A third type of interaction in which the projectile electron can lose its kinetic energy is an interaction with the nuclear field of a target atom. In this type of interaction, the kinetic energy of the projectile electron is also converted into electromagnetic energy.

A projectile electron that completely avoids the orbital electrons as it passes through a target atom may come sufficiently close to the nucleus of the atom to come under the influence of its electric field (see Figure 8-5). Because the electron is negatively charged and the nucleus is positively charged, there is an electrostatic force of attraction between them.

The closer the projectile electron gets to the nucleus, the more it is influenced by the electric field of the nucleus. This field is very strong because the nucleus

contains many protons and the distance between the nucleus and projectile electron is very small.

As the projectile electron passes by the nucleus, it is slowed down and changes its course, leaving with reduced kinetic energy in a different direction. This loss of kinetic energy reappears as an x-ray. This interaction is somewhat analogous to a comet in its course around the sun.

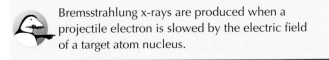

Bremsstrahlung x-rays are produced when a projectile electron is slowed by the electric field of a target atom nucleus.

These types of x-rays are called **bremsstrahlung x-rays.** *Bremsstrahlung* is a German word that means "sloweddown radiation." Bremsstrahlung x-rays can be considered radiation that results from the braking of projectile electrons by the nucleus.

A projectile electron can lose any amount of its kinetic energy in an interaction with the nucleus of a target atom, and the bremsstrahlung x-ray associated with the loss can take on corresponding values. For example, when an x-ray imaging system is operated at 70 kVp, projectile electrons have kinetic energies up to 70 keV.

An electron with kinetic energy of 70 keV can lose all, none, or any intermediate level of that kinetic energy in a bremsstrahlung interaction. Therefore, the bremsstrahlung x-ray produced can have any energy up to 70 keV.

This is different from the production of characteristic x-rays, which have very specific energies. Figure 8-5 illustrates how one can consider the production of such a wide range of energies through the bremsstrahlung interaction.

A low-energy bremsstrahlung x-ray results when the projectile electron is barely influenced by the nucleus. A maximum-energy x-ray occurs when the projectile electron loses all its kinetic energy and simply drifts away from the nucleus. Bremsstrahlung x-rays with energies between these two extremes occur more frequently.

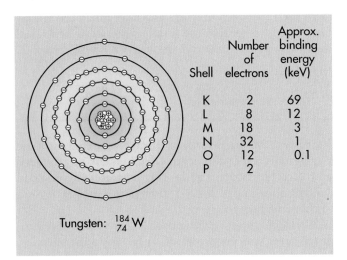

Shell	Number of electrons	Approx. binding energy (keV)
K	2	69
L	8	12
M	18	3
N	32	1
O	12	0.1
P	2	

Tungsten: $^{184}_{74}$W

FIGURE 8-4 Atomic configuration and electron binding energies for tungsten.

Table 8-1	**Characteristic X-rays of Tungsten and Their Effective Energies (keV)**					
	ELECTRON TRANSITION FROM SHELL					
Characteristic	**L-Shell**	**M-Shell**	**N-Shell**	**O-Shell**	**P-Shell**	**Effective Energy of X-ray**
K	57.4	66.7	68.9	69.4	69.5	69
L		9.3	11.5	12.0	12.1	12
M			2.2	2.7	2.8	3
N				0.52	0.6	0.6
O					0.08	0.1

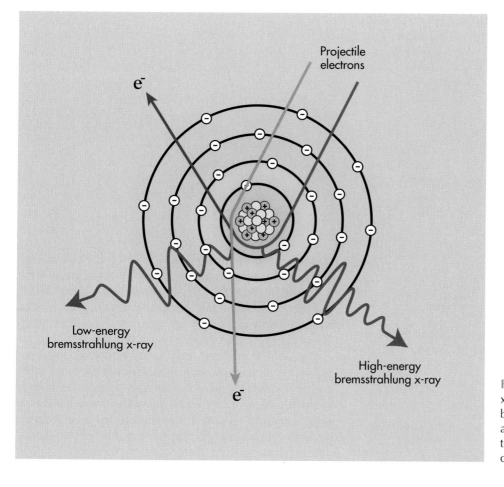

Projectile
electrons

e⁻

Low-energy
bremsstrahlung x-ray

High-energy
bremsstrahlung x-ray

e⁻

FIGURE 8-5 Bremsstrahlung x-rays result from the interaction between a projectile electron and a target nucleus. The electron is slowed and its direction is changed.

 In the diagnostic range, most x-rays are bremsstrahlung x-rays.

Bremsstrahlung x-rays can be produced at any projectile electron energy. K-characteristic x-rays require an x-ray tube potential of at least 69 kVp. At 65 kVp, for example, no useful characteristic x-rays are produced; therefore, the x-ray beam is all bremsstrahlung. At 100 kVp, approximately 15% of the x-ray beam is characteristic, and the remaining is bremsstrahlung.

X-RAY EMISSION SPECTRUM

Most people have seen or heard of pitching machines (the devices used by baseball teams for batting practice so that pitchers do not get worn out). Similar machines are used to automatically eject bowling balls, tennis balls, and even ping-pong balls.

Suppose there was a device that could eject all these types of balls at random. The most straightforward way to determine how often each type of ball was ejected on average would be to catch each ball as it was ejected and then identify it and drop it into a basket; at the end of the observation period, the total number of each type of ball could be counted.

Let us suppose that the results obtained for a given period are those shown in Figure 8-6. A total of 600 balls were ejected. Perhaps the easiest way to represent these results graphically would be to plot the total number of each type of ball emitted during the observation period and represent each total by a bar (Figure 8-7).

Such a bar graph can be described as a discrete ball ejection spectrum that is representative of the automatic pitching machine. It is a plot of the number of balls ejected as a function of the type of ball. It is called discrete because only five distinct types of balls are involved.

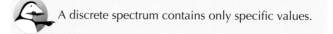 A discrete spectrum contains only specific values.

Connecting the bars with a dashed curve as shown would indicate a large number of different types of balls. Such a curve is called a **continuous** ejection spectrum. The word **spectrum** refers to the range of types of balls or values of any quantity such as x-rays. The total number of balls ejected is represented by the sum of the areas under the bars in the case of the discrete spectrum and the area under the curve in the case of the continuous spectrum.

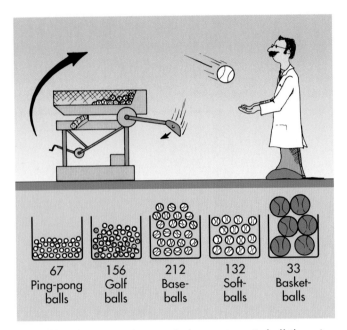

FIGURE 8-6 Over a given period, an automatic ball-throwing machine might eject 600 balls, distributed as shown.

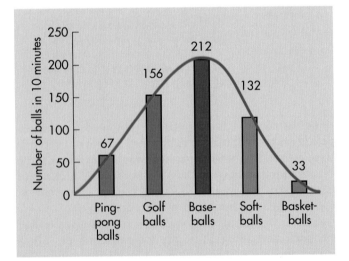

FIGURE 8-7 Bar graph representing the results of observation of balls ejected by the automatic pitching machine in Figure 8-6. When the height of each bar is joined, a smooth emission spectrum is created.

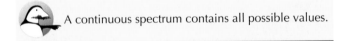

A continuous spectrum contains all possible values.

Without regard for the absolute number of balls emitted, Figure 8-7 also could be identified as a relative ball ejection spectrum because at a glance, one can tell the relative frequency with which each type of ball was ejected. Relatively speaking, baseballs are ejected most frequently and basketballs least frequently.

This type of relationship is fundamental to describing the output of an x-ray tube. If one could stand in the

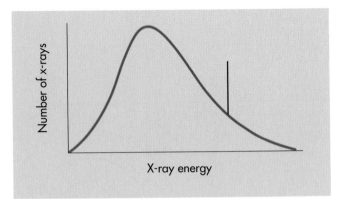

FIGURE 8-8 General form of an x-ray emission spectrum.

middle of the useful x-ray beam, catch each individual x-ray, and measure its energy, one could describe what is known as the **x-ray emission spectrum** (Figure 8-8).

Here, the relative number of x-rays emitted is plotted as a function of the energy of each individual x-ray. X-ray energy is the variable that is considered.

Although we cannot catch and identify each individual x-ray, instruments are available that allow us to do essentially that. X-ray emission spectra have been measured for all types of x-ray imaging systems. Data on x-ray emission spectra are needed if one is to gain an understanding of how changes in voltage, kVp, mA, and added filtration affect the quality of an image.

Characteristic X-ray Spectrum

The discrete energies of characteristic x-rays are characteristic of the differences between electron binding energies in a particular element. A characteristic x-ray from tungsten, for example, can have 1 of 15 different energies (see Table 8-1) and no others. A plot of the frequency with which characteristic x-rays are emitted as a function of their energy would look similar to that shown for tungsten in Figure 8-9.

Such a plot is called the *characteristic x-ray emission spectrum*. Five vertical lines representing K x-rays and four vertical lines representing L x-rays are included. The lower-energy lines represent characteristic emissions from the outer electron shells.

Characteristic x-rays have precisely fixed (discrete) energies and form a discrete emission spectrum.

The relative intensity of the K x-rays is greater than that of the lower-energy characteristic x-rays because of the nature of the interaction process. K x-rays are the only characteristic x-rays of tungsten with sufficient energy to be of value in diagnostic radiology. Although there are five K x-rays, it is customary to represent them as one, as has been done in this figure with a single vertical line, at 69 keV (Figure 8-10). Only this line will be shown in later graphs.

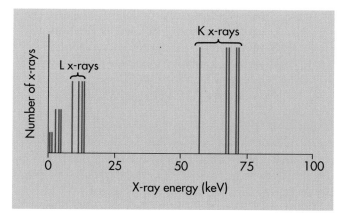

FIGURE 8-9 Characteristic x-ray emission spectrum for tungsten contains 15 different x-ray energies.

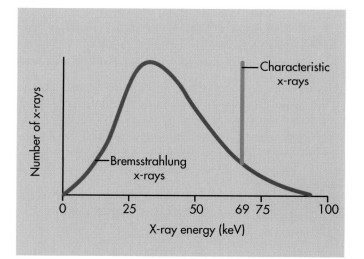

FIGURE 8-10 Bremsstrahlung x-ray emission spectrum extends from zero to maximum projectile electron energy, with the highest number of x-rays having approximately one-third the maximum energy. The characteristic x-ray emission spectrum is represented by a line at 69 keV.

Bremsstrahlung X-ray Spectrum

If it were possible to measure the energy contained in each bremsstrahlung x-ray emitted from an x-ray tube, one would find that these energies range from the peak electron energy all the way down to zero. In other words, when an x-ray tube is operated at 90 kVp, bremsstrahlung x-rays with energies up to 90 keV are emitted. A typical bremsstrahlung x-ray emission spectrum is shown in Figure 8-10.

 Bremsstrahlung x-rays have a range of energies and form a continuous emission spectrum.

Question: At what kVp was the x-ray imaging system presented in Figure 8-10 operated?

Answer: Because the bremsstrahlung spectrum intersects the energy axis at approximately 90 keV, the imaging system must have been operated at approximately 90 kVp.

The general shape of the bremsstrahlung x-ray spectrum is the same for all x-ray imaging systems. The maximum energy (in keV) of a bremsstrahlung x-ray is numerically equal to the kVp of operation.

The greatest number of x-rays is emitted with energy approximately one third of the maximum energy. The number of x-rays emitted decreases rapidly at very low energies.

Question: What would be the expected emission spectrum for an x-ray imaging system with a pure molybdenum target (effective energy of K x-ray = 19 keV) operated at 95 kVp?

Answer: The spectrum should look something like Figure 8-8. The curve intersects the energy axis at 0 and 95 keV and has the general shape shown in Figure 8-10. The bremsstrahlung spectrum is much lower because the atomic number of Mo is low, and x-ray production is much less efficient. A line extends above the curve at 19 keV to represent the K-characteristic x-rays of molybdenum.

As described in Chapter 5, the energy of an x-ray is equal to the product of its frequency *(f)* and Planck's constant *(h)*. X-ray energy is inversely proportional to its wavelength. As x-ray wavelength increases, x-ray energy decreases.

Maximum x-ray energy is associated with the minimum x-ray wavelength (λ_{min}).

The minimum wavelength of x-ray emission corresponds to the maximum x-ray energy, and the maximum x-ray energy is numerically equal to the kVp.

FACTORS AFFECTING THE X-RAY EMISSION SPECTRUM

The total number of x-rays emitted from an x-ray tube could be determined by adding together the number of x-rays emitted at each energy over the entire spectrum, a process called **integration**. Graphically, the total number of x-rays emitted is equivalent to the area under the curve of the x-ray emission spectrum.

The general shape of an emission spectrum is always the same, but its relative position along the energy axis can change. The farther to the right a spectrum is, the higher the effective energy or **quality** of the x-ray beam.

The larger the area under the curve, the higher is the x-ray intensity or **quantity**. A number of factors under the control of the radiologic technologist influence the size and shape of the x-ray emission spectrum, and therefore, the quality and quantity of the x-ray beam. These factors are summarized in Table 8-2.

Effect of mA and mAs

If one changes the current from 200 to 400 mA while all other conditions remain constant, twice as many electrons will flow from cathode to anode, and the mAs will be doubled. This operating change will produce twice as many x-rays at every energy. In other words, the x-ray emission spectrum will be changed in amplitude but not in shape (Figure 8-11).

Each point on the curve labeled 400 mA is precisely two times higher than the associated point on the 200-mA curve. This relationship also is true for changes in mAs. Thus, the area under the x-ray emission spectrum varies in proportion to changes in mA or mAs, as does the x-ray quantity.

 A change in mA or mAs results in a proportional change in the amplitude of the x-ray emission spectrum at all energies.

FOUR PRINCIPAL FACTORS INFLUENCING THE SHAPE OF AN X-RAY EMISSION SPECTRUM

1. The projectile electrons accelerated from cathode to anode do not all have peak kinetic energy. Depending on the types of rectification and high-voltage generation, many of these electrons may have very low energies when they strike the target. Such electrons can produce only heat and low-energy x-rays.
2. The target of a diagnostic x-ray tube is relatively thick. Consequently, many of the bremsstrahlung x-rays emitted result from multiple interactions of the projectile electrons, and for each successive interaction, a projectile electron has less energy.
3. Low-energy x-rays are more likely to be absorbed in the target.
4. External filtration is always added to the x-ray tube assembly. This added filtration serves selectively to remove low-energy x-rays from the beam.

Question: Suppose the area under the 200-mA curve in Figure 8-11 totals 4.2 cm^2 and the x-ray quantity is 325 mR (3.25 mGy$_a$). What would the area under the curve and the x-ray quantity be if the tube current were increased to 400 mA, while other operating factors remain constant?

Answer: In going from 200 to 400 mA, the tube current has been increased by a factor of two. The area under the curve and the x-ray quantity are increased proportionately:
Area = 4.2 cm^2 × 2 = 8.4 cm^2
Intensity = 325 mR × 2 = 650 mR

Effect of kVp

As the kVp is raised, the area under the curve increases to an area approximating the square of the factor by which kVp was increased. Accordingly, the x-ray quantity increases with the square of this factor.

When kVp is increased, the relative distribution of emitted x-ray energy shifts to the right, to a higher average x-ray energy. The maximum energy of x-ray emission always remains numerically equal to the kVp.

A change in kVp affects both the amplitude and the position of the x-ray emission spectrum.

Figure 8-12 demonstrates the effect of increasing the kVp while other factors remain constant. The lower spectrum represents x-ray operation at 72 kVp, and the upper spectrum represents operation at 82 kVp—a 10-kVp (or 15%) increase.

Table 8-2	Factors That Affect the Size and Relative Position of X-ray Emission Spectra	
Factor	**Effect**	
Tube current	Amplitude of spectrum	
Tube voltage	Amplitude and position	
Added filtration	Amplitude, most effective at low energy	
Target material	Amplitude of spectrum and position of line spectrum	
Voltage waveform	Amplitude, most effective at high energy	

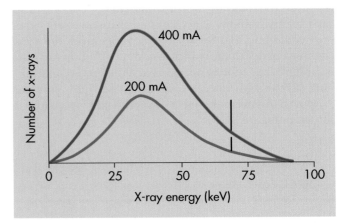

FIGURE 8-11 Change in mA results in a proportionate change in the amplitude of the x-ray emission spectrum at all energies.

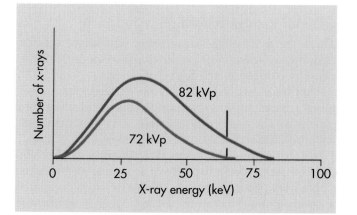

FIGURE 8-12 Change in kVp results in an increase in the amplitude of the emission spectrum at all energies, but a greater increase at high energies than at low energies. Therefore, the spectrum is shifted to the right, or high-energy side.

The area under the curve has approximately doubled, while the relative position of the curve has shifted to the right, the high-energy side. More x-rays are emitted at all energies during operation at 82 kVp than during operation at 72 kVp. The increase, however, is relatively greater for high-energy x-rays than for low-energy x-rays.

A change in kVp has no effect on the position of the discrete x-ray emission spectrum.

Question: Suppose the curve labeled 72 kVp in Figure 8-12 covers a total area of 3.6 cm² and represents an x-ray quantity of 125 mR (1.25 mGy_a). What area under the curve and x-ray quantity would be expected for operations at 82 kVp?

Answer: The area under the curve and the output intensity are proportional to the *square* of the ratio of the kVp change. A ratio can be established.

$$\left(\frac{82}{72}\right)^2 \left(3.6\ cm^2\right) = (1.3)\left(3.6\ cm^2\right) = 4.7\ cm^2$$

and

$$(1.3)(125\ mR) = 163\ mR$$

This example partially explains the rule of thumb used by radiologic technologists to relate the kVp and mAs changes necessary to produce a constant optical density (OD) on a radiograph. The rule states that a 15% increase in kVp is equivalent to doubling the mAs. At low kVp, such as 50 to 60 kVp, approximately a 7-kVp increase is equivalent to doubling the mAs. At tube potentials above about 100 kVp, a 15-kVp change may be necessary.

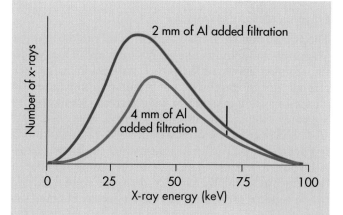

FIGURE 8-13 Adding filtration to an x-ray tube results in reduced x-ray intensity but increased effective energy. The emission spectra represented here resulted from operation at the same mA and kVp but with different filtration.

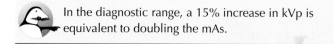

In the diagnostic range, a 15% increase in kVp is equivalent to doubling the mAs.

A 15% increase in kVp does not double the x-ray intensity but is equivalent to doubling the mAs to obtain a given OD on the radiograph. To double the output intensity by increasing kVp, one would have to raise the kVp by as much as 40%.

Radiographically, only a 15% increase in kVp is necessary, because with increased kVp, the penetrability of the x-ray beam is increased. Therefore, less radiation is absorbed by the patient, leaving a proportionately greater number of x-rays to expose the image receptor.

Effect of Added Filtration

Adding filtration to the useful x-ray beam reduces x-ray beam intensity while increasing average energy. This effect is shown in Figure 8-13, where an x-ray tube is operated at 95 kVp with 2-mm aluminum (Al) added filtration, compared with the same operation with 4-mm Al added filtration. Added filtration more effectively absorbs low-energy x-rays than high-energy x-rays; therefore, the bremsstrahlung x-ray emission spectrum is reduced further on the left than on the right.

The result of added filtration is an increase in the average energy of the x-ray beam with an accompanying reduction in x-ray quantity.

Adding filtration is sometimes called **hardening** the x-ray beam because of the relative increase in average energy. The characteristic spectrum is not affected, nor is the maximum energy of x-ray emission. There is no simple method for calculating the precise changes that occur in x-ray quality and quantity with a change in added filtration.

Effect of Target Material

The atomic number of the target affects both the number (quantity) and the effective energy (quality) of x-rays. As the atomic number of the target material increases, the efficiency of the production of bremsstrahlung radiation increases and high-energy x-rays increase in number to a greater extent than low-energy x-rays.

The change in the bremsstrahlung x-ray spectrum is not nearly as pronounced as the change in the characteristic spectrum. After an increase in the atomic number of the target material, the characteristic spectrum is shifted to the right, representing the higher-energy characteristic radiation. This phenomenon is a direct result of the higher electron binding energies associated with increasing atomic number.

 Increasing target atomic number enhances the efficiency of x-ray production and the energy of characteristic and bremsstrahlung x-rays.

These changes are shown schematically in Figure 8-14. Tungsten is the primary component of x-ray tube targets, but some specialty x-ray tubes use gold as target material. The atomic numbers for tungsten and gold are 74 and 79, respectively.

Molybdenum (Z = 42) and rhodium (Z = 45) are target elements used for mammography. In many dedicated mammography imaging systems, these elements are incorporated separately into the target.

The x-ray quantity from such targets is low owing to the inefficiency of x-ray production. This occurs because of the low atomic number of these target elements. Elements of low atomic number also produce low-energy characteristic x-rays.

Effect of Voltage Waveform

There are five voltage waveforms: half-wave rectification, full-wave rectification, three-phase/six-pulse, three-phase/twelve-pulse, and high-frequency.

Half-wave–rectified and full-wave–rectified voltage waveforms are the same except for the frequency of x-ray pulse repetition. There are twice as many x-ray pulses per cycle with full-wave rectification as with half-wave rectification.

The difference between three-phase/six-pulse and three-phase/twelve-pulse power is simply the reduced ripple obtained with twelve-pulse generation compared with six-pulse generation. High-frequency generators are based on fundamentally different electrical engineering principles. They produce the lowest voltage ripple of all high-voltage generators.

Figure 8-15 shows an exploded view of a full-wave–rectified voltage waveform for an x-ray imaging system operated at 100 kVp. Recall that the amplitude of the waveform corresponds to the applied voltage, and that the horizontal axis represents time.

At t = 0, the voltage across the x-ray tube is zero, indicating that at this instant, no electrons are flowing and no x-rays are being produced. At t = 1 ms, the voltage across the x-ray tube has increased from 0 to approximately 60,000 V. The x-rays produced at this instant are of relatively low intensity and energy; none exceeds 60 keV. At t = 2.1 ms, the tube voltage has increased to approximately 80,000 V and is rapidly approaching its peak value.

At t = 4.2 ms, the maximum tube voltage is obtained, and the maximum energy and intensity of x-ray emission are produced. For the following one-quarter cycle between 4.2 and 8.3 ms, the x-ray quantity and quality decrease again to zero.

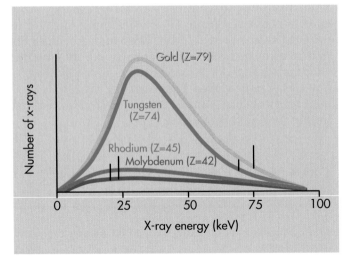

FIGURE 8-14 Discrete emission spectrum shifts to the right with an increase in the atomic number of the target material. The continuous spectrum increases slightly in amplitude, particularly to the high-energy side, with an increase in target atomic number.

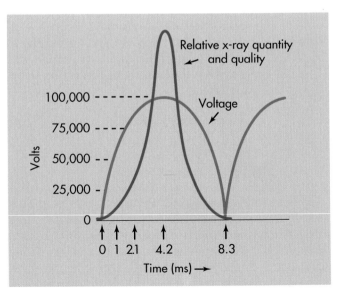

FIGURE 8-15 As the voltage across the x-ray tube increases from zero to its peak value, x-ray intensity and energy increase slowly at first and then rapidly as peak voltage is obtained.

The number of x-rays emitted at each instant through a cycle is not proportional to the voltage. The number is low at lower voltages and increases at higher voltages. The quantity of x-rays is much greater at peak voltages than at lower voltages. Consequently, voltage waveforms of three-phase or high-frequency operation result in considerably more intense x-ray emission than those of single-phase operation.

The relationship between x-ray quantity and type of high-voltage generator provides the basis for another rule of thumb used by radiologic technologists. If a radiographic technique calls for 72 kVp on single-phase equipment, then on three-phase equipment, approximately 64 kVp—a 12% reduction—will produce similar results. High-frequency generators produce approximately the equivalent of a 16% increase in kVp, or slightly more than a doubling of mAs over single-phase power.

> Because of reduced ripple, operation with three-phase power or high frequency is equivalent to an approximate 12% increase in kVp, or almost a doubling of mAs over single-phase power.

This discussion is summarized in Figure 8-16, where an x-ray emission spectrum from a full-wave–rectified unit is compared with that from a three-phase, twelve-pulse generator and a high-frequency generator, all operated at 92 kVp and at the same mAs. The x-ray emission spectrum that results from high-frequency operation is more efficient than that produced with a single-phase or a three-phase generator. The area under the curve is considerably greater, and the x-ray emission spectrum is shifted to the high-energy side.

The characteristic x-ray emission spectrum remains fixed in its position on the energy axis but increases slightly in magnitude as a result of the increased number of projectile electrons available for K-shell electron interactions.

Question: What would be the difference in the x-ray emission spectra between a full-wave–rectified operation and a half-wave–rectified operation if the kVp and the mAs are held constant?

Answer: Under constant conditions of kVp and mAs, there should be no difference in the x-ray emission spectra. The x-ray quantity and quality will remain the same for both modes of operation. Exposure time will double for the half-wave–rectified operation.

Table 8-3 presents a summary of the effect on x-ray quantity and quality produced by each of the factors that influence the x-ray emission spectrum. Although

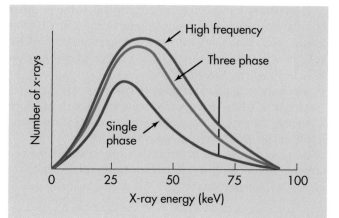

FIGURE 8-16 Three-phase and high-frequency operation are considerably more efficient than single-phase operation. Both the x-ray intensity (area under the curve) and the effective energy (relative shift to the right) are increased. Shown are representative spectra for 92-kVp operation at constant mAs.

Table 8-3	Changes in X-ray Beam Quality and Quantity Produced by Factors That Influence the Emission Spectrum
An Increase in	**Results in**
Current (mAs)	An increase in quantity. No change in quality.
Voltage (kVp)	An increase in quantity and quality.
Added filtration	A decrease in quantity. An increase in quality.
Target atomic number (Z)	An increase in quantity and quality.
Voltage ripple	A decrease in quantity and quality.

five factors are listed, only the first two, mAs and kVp, are routinely controlled by the radiologic technologist. Occasionally, the added filtration is changed if the imaging system design permits.

SUMMARY

When electrons are accelerated from the cathode to the target of the anode, three effects take place: the production of heat, the formation of characteristic x-rays, and the formation of bremsstrahlung x-rays.

Characteristic x-rays are produced when an electron ionizes an inner-shell electron of a target atom. As the inner-shell void is filled, a characteristic x-ray is emitted.

Bremsstrahlung x-rays are produced by the slowing down of an electron by the target atom's electrostatic nuclear field. Most x-rays in the diagnostic range (20 to 150 kVp) are bremsstrahlung x-rays.

X-ray emission spectra can be graphed as the number of x-rays for each increment of energy in keV. Characteristic x-rays of tungsten have a discrete energy of 69 keV. Bremsstrahlung x-rays have a range of energies up to X keV, where X is the kVp.

The following four factors influence the x-ray emission spectrum: (1) Low-energy electrons interact to produce low-energy x-rays, (2) successive interactions of electrons result in the production of x-rays with lower energy, (3) low-energy x-rays are most likely to be absorbed by the target material, and (4) added filtration preferentially removes low-energy x-rays from the useful beam.

CHALLENGE QUESTIONS

1. Define or otherwise identify the following:
   a. Projectile electron
   b. Binding energy
   c. Characteristic x-rays
   d. Bremsstrahlung x-rays
   e. X-ray quantity
   f. X-ray quality
   g. Effective energy
   h. Added filtration
   i. Emission spectrum
   j. Molybdenum
2. Calculate the energy and wavelength of the characteristic x-ray produced when a K-shell electron is replaced by an M-shell electron in tungsten.
3. At what fraction of the velocity of light do 90-keV electrons travel?
4. What does the discrete x-ray spectrum represent?
5. Draw the x-ray emission spectrum for an x-ray imaging system with a tungsten-targeted x-ray tube operated at 90 kVp.
6. When an x-ray imaging system is operated at 80 kVp, its emission spectrum represents an output intensity of 3.5 mR/mAs. What will be the output intensity if the voltage is increased to 90 kVp? How will the emission spectrum change?

7. Discuss the effect on the x-ray emission spectrum if a single-phase x-ray imaging system is changed to a three-phase system.
8. Explain the effect the addition of filtration to an x-ray tube has on the discrete and continuous x-ray emission spectra.
9. How is the kinetic energy of the projectile electrons streaming across the x-ray tube increased?
10. At 80 kVp, what is the energy in joules of electrons arriving at the x-ray tube target?
11. Why is the x-ray tube considered an inefficient device?
12. Draw the diagram and write a description of the formation of characteristic radiation.
13. What is the importance of K-characteristic x-rays in forming a diagnostic radiograph?
14. What is the range of energies of bremsstrahlung x-rays?
15. What is the minimum wavelength associated with x-rays emitted from an x-ray tube operated at 90 kVp?
16. List three factors that affect the shape of the x-ray emission spectrum and briefly describe each.
17. Define and explain the 15% kVp rule.
18. What is the diagnostic range of x-rays?
19. What type of radiation is useful for mammography and not useful for general diagnostic exposures?
20. In your clinical setting, observe or ask what filtration is used on the x-ray tubes. Why is filtration important?

The answers to the Challenge Questions can be found by logging on to our website at http://evolve.elsevier.com.

X-ray Emission

OBJECTIVES

**At the completion of this chapter, the student should be able
to do the following:**

1. Define radiation quantity and its relation to x-ray intensity
2. List and discuss the factors that affect the intensity of the x-ray beam
3. Explain x-ray quality and penetrability
4. List and discuss the factors that affect the quality of the x-ray beam

OUTLINE

X-ray Quantity
  X-ray Intensity
  Factors That Affect X-ray Quantity
X-ray Quality
  Penetrability
  Half-Value Layer
  Factors That Affect X-ray Quality
  Types of Filtration

X-RAYS ARE emitted through a window in the glass or metal enclosure to form a beam of varied energies. The x-ray beam is characterized by quantity (the number of x-rays in the beam) and quality (the penetrability of the beam). This chapter discusses the numerous factors that affect x-ray beam quantity and quality.

X-RAY QUANTITY

X-ray Intensity

The intensity of the x-ray beam of an x-ray imaging system is measured in roentgens (R) or milliroentgens (mR) (mGy$_a$) and is called the **x-ray quantity.** Another term, **radiation exposure,** is often used instead of x-ray intensity or x-ray quantity. All have the same meaning and all are measured in roentgens.

The roentgen (mGy$_a$) is a measure of the number of ion pairs produced in air by a quantity of x-rays. Ionization of air increases as the number of x-rays in the beam increases. The relationship between the x-ray quantity as measured in roentgens and the number of x-rays in the beam is not always one-to-one. Some small variations are related to the effective x-ray energy.

Exposure rate expressed as mR/s, mR/min, or mR/mAs can also be used to express x-ray intensity.

> X-ray quantity is the number of x-rays in the useful beam.

These variations are unimportant over the x-ray energy range used in radiology, and we can therefore assume that the number of x-rays in the useful beam is the radiation quantity. Most general purpose radiographic tubes, when operated at approximately 70 kVp, produce x-ray intensities of approximately 5 mR/mAs (50 µGy$_a$/mAs) at a 100-cm source-to-image receptor distance (SID).

Figure 9-1 is a nomogram for estimating x-ray intensity for a wide range of techniques. These curves apply only for single-phase, full-wave–rectified apparatus.

Factors That Affect X-ray Quantity

A number of factors affect x-ray quantity. Most were discussed briefly in Chapter 8; consequently, this section may serve primarily as a review. The factors that affect x-ray quantity affect exposure of the image receptor similarly and are nearly the same as those that control optical density on a radiograph. These relationships are summarized in Table 9-1.

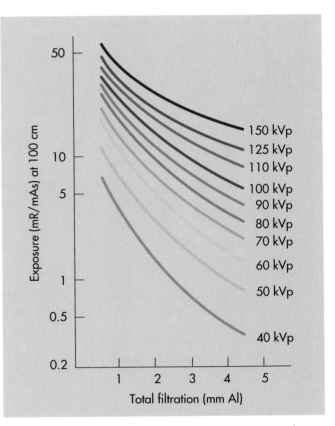

FIGURE 9-1 Nomogram for estimating the intensity of x-ray beams. From the position on the x-axis corresponding to the filtration of the imaging system, draw a vertical line until it intersects with the appropriate voltage (kVp). A horizontal line from that point will intersect the y-axis at the approximate x-ray intensity for the imaging system. (Courtesy Edward McCullough, University of Wisconsin.)

TABLE 9-1	Factors That Affect X-ray Quantity and Image Receptor Exposure	
The Effect of Increasing	**X-ray Quantity Is**	**Image Receptor Exposure Is**
mAs	Increased proportionately	Increased
kVp	Increased by $\left(\dfrac{kVp_2}{kVp_1}\right)^2$	Increased
Distance	Reduced by $\left(\dfrac{d_1}{d_2}\right)^2$	Reduced
Filtration	Reduced	Reduced

Milliampere-Seconds (mAs). X-ray quantity is directly proportional to the mAs. When mAs is doubled, the number of electrons striking the tube target is doubled, and therefore the number of x-rays emitted is doubled.

X-RAY QUANTITY AND mAs

$$\frac{I_1}{I_2} = \frac{mAs_1}{mAs_2}$$

where I_1 and I_2 are the x-ray intensities at mAs_1 and mAs_2, respectively.

Question: A lateral chest technique calls for 110 kVp, 10 mAs, which results in an x-ray intensity of 32 mR (0.32 mGy$_a$) at the position of the patient. If the mAs is increased to 20 mAs, what will the x-ray intensity be?

Answer:
$$\frac{x}{32\ mR} = \frac{20\ mAs}{10\ mAs}$$

$$x = \frac{(32\ mAs)(20\ mR)}{10\ mAs} = 64\ mR$$

 X-ray quantity is proportional to mAs.

Question: The radiographic technique for a KUB (kidneys, ureters, and bladder) examination uses 74 kVp/60 mAs. The result is a patient exposure of 250 mR (2.5 mGy$_a$). What will be the exposure if the mAs can be reduced to 45 mAs?

Answer:
$$\frac{x}{250\ mR} = \frac{45\ mAs}{60\ mAs}$$

$$x = \frac{(250\ mR)(45\ mAs)}{60\ mAs} = 187.5\ mR$$

Remember that mAs is just a measure of the total number of electrons that travel from cathode to anode to produce x-rays.

mAs = mA × s
= mC/s × s
= mC

where C (coulomb) is a measure of electrostatic charges and 1 C = 6.25 × 10^{18} electrons.

Question: A radiograph is made at 74 kVp/100 mAs. How many electrons interact with the target?

Answer: 100 mAs = 100 mC
= 6.25 × 10^{17} electrons

Question: If the radiographic output intensity is 6.2 mR/mAs (62 μGy$_a$/mAs), how many electrons are required to produce 1.0 mR?

Answer: 6.2 mR/mAs = 6.2 mR/6.25 × 10^{15} electrons
Stated inversely, 6.25 × 10^{15} electrons/6.2 mR = 1 × 10^{15} electrons/mR

Kilovolt Peak (kVp). X-ray quantity varies rapidly with changes in kVp. The change in x-ray quantity is proportional to the square of the ratio of the kVp; in other words, if kVp were doubled, the x-ray intensity would increase by a factor of four. Mathematically, this is expressed as follows:

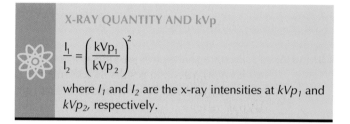

X-RAY QUANTITY AND kVp

$$\frac{I_1}{I_2} = \left(\frac{kVp_1}{kVp_2}\right)^2$$

where I_1 and I_2 are the x-ray intensities at kVp_1 and kVp_2, respectively.

Question: A lateral chest technique calls for 110 kVp, 10 mAs and results in an x-ray intensity of 32 mR (0.32 mGy$_a$). What will be the intensity if the kVp is increased to 125 kVp and the mAs remains fixed?

Answer:
$$\frac{32\ mR}{I_2} = \left(\frac{110\ kVp}{125\ kVp}\right)^2$$

$$I_2 = (32\ mR)\left(\frac{125\ kVp}{110\ kVp}\right)^2$$
$$= (32\ mR)(1.14)^2$$
$$= (32\ mR)(1.29) = 41.3\ mR$$

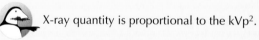 X-ray quantity is proportional to the kVp^2.

Question: An extremity is examined through a technique of 58 kVp/8 mAs, resulting in an entrance skin exposure (ESE) of 24 mR. If the technique is changed to 54 kVp/8 mAs to improve contrast, what will be the x-ray quantity?

Answer:
$$\frac{1}{24\ mR} = \left(\frac{54\ kVp}{58\ kVp}\right)^2$$

$$I = (24\ mR)\left(\frac{54\ kVp}{58\ kVp}\right)^2$$
$$= (24\ mR)(0.93)^2$$
$$= (24\ mR)(0.867) = 20.8\ mR$$

In practice, a slightly different situation prevails. Radiographic technique factors must be selected from a relatively narrow range of values, from approximately 40 to 150 kVp. Theoretically, doubling the x-ray intensity by kVp manipulation alone requires an increase of 40% in kVp.

This relationship is not adopted clinically because as kVp is increased, the penetrability of the x-ray beam is increased and relatively fewer x-rays are absorbed in the patient. More x-rays go through the patient and interact with the image receptor. Consequently, to maintain a constant exposure of the image receptor and constant radiographic optical density (OD) would require that an increase of 15% in kVp should be accompanied by a reduction of one half in mAs.

Question: A radiographic technique calls for 80 kVp/30 mAs and results in 135 mR (1.4 mGy$_a$). What is the expected ESE if the kVp is increased to 92 kVp (+15%) and the mAs reduced by one half to 15 mAs?

Answer:

$$\frac{1}{135 \text{ mR}} = \left(\frac{15 \text{ mAs}}{30 \text{ mAs}}\right)\left(\frac{92 \text{ kVp}}{80 \text{ kVp}}\right)^2$$

$$I = 135 \text{ mR}\left(\frac{15 \text{ mAs}}{30 \text{ mAs}}\right)\left(\frac{92 \text{ kVp}}{80 \text{ kVp}}\right)^2$$

$$= 135 \text{ mR}(0.5)(1.32) = 89 \text{ mR}$$

Note that by increasing kVp and reducing mAs so that optical density remains constant, patient dose is reduced significantly. The disadvantage of such a technique adjustment is reduced image contrast.

Distance. X-ray intensity varies inversely with the square of the distance from the x-ray tube target. This relationship is known as the **inverse square law** (see Chapter 4).

X-RAY QUANTITY AND DISTANCE

$$\frac{I_1}{I_2} = \left(\frac{d_2}{d_1}\right)^2$$

where I_1 and I_2 are the x-ray intensities at distances d_1 and d_2, respectively.

Question: Mobile radiography is conducted at 100 cm SID and results in an exposure of 12.5 mR (0.13 mGy$_a$) at the image receptor. If 91 cm is the maximum SID that can be obtained for a particular situation, what will be the image receptor exposure?

Answer:

$$\frac{1.25 \text{ mR}}{I_2} = \left(\frac{91 \text{ cm}}{100 \text{ cm}}\right)^2$$

$$I_2 = (1.25 \text{ mR})\left(\frac{100 \text{ cm}}{91 \text{ cm}}\right)^2$$

$$= (12.5 \text{ mR})(1.1)^2$$

$$= (12.5 \text{ mR})(1.1) = 13.8 \text{ mR}$$

X-ray quantity is inversely proportional to the square of the distance from the source.

Question: A posteroanterior (PA) chest examination (120 kVp/3 mAs) with a dedicated x-ray imaging system is taken at an SID of 300 cm. The exposure at the image receptor is 12 mR (0.12 mGy$_a$). If the same technique is used at a SID of 100 cm, what will be the x-ray exposure?

Answer:

$$\frac{1}{12 \text{ mR}} = \left(\frac{300 \text{ cm}}{100 \text{ cm}}\right)^2$$

$$I = 12 \text{ mR}\left(\frac{300 \text{ cm}}{100 \text{ cm}}\right)^2$$

$$= (12 \text{ mR})(3)^2$$

$$= (12 \text{ mR})(9) = 108 \text{ mR}$$

When SID is increased, mAs must be increased by SID^2 to maintain constant exposure to the image receptor.

Compensating for a change in SID by changing mAs by the factor SID^2 is known as the **square law**, a corollary to the **inverse square law.**

THE SQUARE LAW

$$\frac{\text{mAs}_1}{\text{mAs}_2} = \frac{\text{SID}_1^2}{\text{SID}_2^2}$$

where mAs_1 is the technique at SID_1, and mAs_2 is the technique at SID_2.

In practical terms, this can be rewritten as follows:

$$\frac{\text{Old mAs}}{\text{New mAs}} = \frac{\text{Old distance squared}}{\text{New distance squared}}$$

Question: What should be the new mAs in the previous question to reduce the x-ray quantity to 12 mR at 100 cm?

Answer:

$$\frac{\text{x mAs}}{3 \text{ mAs}} = \frac{12 \text{ mR}}{108 \text{ mR}}$$

$$\text{x mAs} = (3 \text{ mAs})\left(\frac{12 \text{ mR}}{108 \text{ mR}}\right) = (3 \text{ mAs})(0.111)$$

$$= 0.3 \text{ mAs}$$

Filtration. X-ray imaging systems have metal filters, usually of 1 to 5 mm of aluminum (Al), positioned in the useful beam. The purpose of these filters is to reduce the number of low-energy x-rays.

Low-energy x-rays contribute nothing useful to the image. They only increase patient dose unnecessarily because they are absorbed in superficial tissues and do not penetrate to reach the image receptor.

 Adding filtration to the useful x-ray beam reduces patient dose.

When filtration is added to the x-ray beam, patient dose is reduced because fewer low-energy x-rays are found in the useful beam. Calculation of the reduction in exposure requires knowledge of half-value layer (HVL), which is discussed in the following section.

An estimate of exposure reduction can be made from the nomogram in Figure 9-1, where it is shown that the reduction is not proportional to the thickness of the added filter but is related in a complex way. The disadvantage of x-ray beam filtration is reduced image contrast caused by beam hardening. Beam hardening increases the number of high energy x-rays in the beam by removing the lower-energy nonpenetrating x-rays.

X-RAY QUALITY
Penetrability

As the energy of an x-ray beam is increased, penetrability is also increased. **Penetrability** refers to the ability of x-rays to penetrate deeper in tissue. High-energy x-rays are able to penetrate tissue more deeply than low-energy x-rays.

The penetrability of an x-ray beam is called the **x-ray quality.** X-rays with high penetrability are termed *high-quality x-rays.* Those with low penetrability are *low-quality x-rays.*

 Penetrability is one description of the ability of an x-ray beam to pass through tissue.

Factors that affect x-ray beam quality also influence radiographic contrast. Distance and mAs do not affect radiation quality; they do affect radiation quantity.

Half-Value Layer

Although x-rays are attenuated exponentially, high-energy x-rays are more penetrating than low-energy x-rays. Whereas 100-keV x-rays are attenuated at the rate of approximately 3%/cm of soft tissue, 10-keV x-rays are attenuated at approximately 15%/cm of soft tissue. X-rays of any given energy are more penetrating in material of low atomic number than in material of high atomic number.

 Attenuation is the reduction in x-ray intensity that results from absorption and scattering.

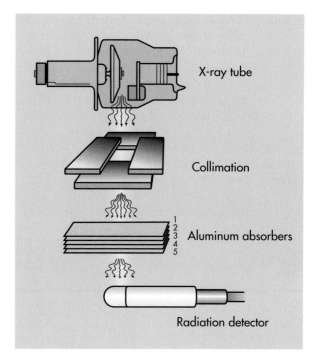

FIGURE 9-2 Typical experimental arrangement for determination of half-value layer.

In radiography, the quality of x-rays is measured by the HVL. Therefore, HVL is a characteristic of the useful x-ray beam. A diagnostic x-ray beam usually has an HVL in the range of 3 to 5 mm Al or 3 to 6 cm of soft tissue.

 The HVL of an x-ray beam is the thickness of absorbing material necessary to reduce the x-ray intensity to half of its original value.

The HVL is determined experimentally, with a setup similar to that shown in Figure 9-2. This setup consists of three principal parts: the x-ray tube, a radiation detector, and graded thicknesses of filters, usually aluminum.

First, a radiation measurement is made with no filter between the x-ray tube and the detector. Then, measurements of radiation intensity are made for successively thicker sections of filter. The thickness of filtration that reduces the x-ray intensity to half of its original value is the HVL.

Several methods can be used to determine the HVL of an x-ray beam. Perhaps the most straightforward way is to graph the results of x-ray intensity measurements made with an experimental setup, like that in Figure 9-2. The graph in Figure 9-3 and the boxed graph below it show how this can be done when the following steps are completed.

Question: The following data were obtained with the radiographic tube operated at 70 kVp, while the detector was positioned 100 cm from the target with 1.0-mm Al filters inserted between the target and the detector. Estimate the HVL from a simple observation of this data. Then, plot the data to see how close you were.

mm Al	0	1.0	2.0	3.0	4.0	5.0
mR	118	82	63	51	38	29

Answer: One half of 118 is 59; therefore, the HVL must be between 2 and 3 mm of Al. A plot of the data shows the HVL to be 2.4 mm Al.

HVL is the best method for specifying x-ray quality.

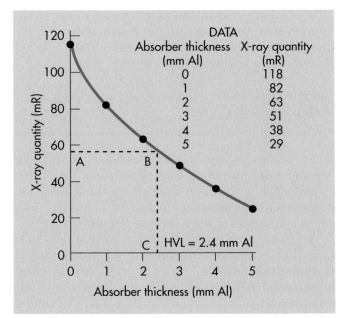

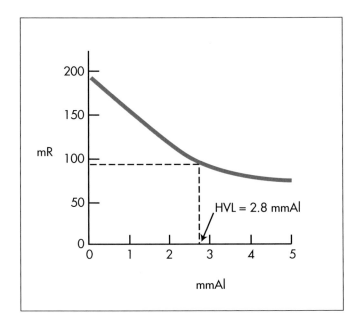

FIGURE 9-3 Data in the table are typical for half-value layer (HVL) determination. The plot of these data shows an HVL of 2.4 mm Al.

STEPS TO DETERMINE THE HVL

1. Determine the x-ray beam intensity with no absorbing material in the beam and then with different known thicknesses of an absorber.
2. Plot the ordered pairs of data (thickness of absorber, x-ray quantity).
3. Determine the x-ray quantity equal to half the original quantity, and locate this value on the y-or vertical axis of the graph in Figure 9-3.
4. Draw a horizontal line parallel to the x-axis from point A in step 3 until it intersects the curve (B).
5. From point B, drop a vertical line to the x-axis.
6. On the x-axis, read the thickness of the absorber required to reduce the x-ray intensity to half of its original value point (C). This is the HVL.

Question: The boxed graph at right was plotted from measurements designed to estimate HVL. What does this graph suggest the HVL to be?

Answer: At zero filtration, x-ray quantity appears to be approximately 190 mR. One half of 190 mR is 95 mR. At the level of 95 mR, a horizontal line is drawn from the y-axis until it intersects the plotted curve. From that intersection, a vertical line is dropped to the x-axis, where it intersects at 2.8 mm Al, the HVL.

X-ray beam penetrability changes in a complex way with variations in kVp and filtration. Different combinations of added filtration and kVp can result in the same x-ray beam HVL. For example, measurements may show that a single x-ray imaging system has the same HVL when operated at 90 kVp with 2-mm Al total filtration as when operated at 70 kVp with 4-mm Al total filtration. In this case, x-ray penetrability remains constant, as does the HVL.

X-ray beam quality can be identified by voltage or filtration, but HVL is most appropriate.

Factors That Affect X-ray Quality

Some of the factors that affect x-ray quantity have no effect on x-ray quality. Other factors affect both x-ray quantity and x-ray quality. These relationships are summarized in Table 9-2.

Kilovolt Peak (kVp). As the kVp is increased, so is x-ray beam quality and therefore the HVL. An increase in kVp results in a shift of the x-ray emission spectrum toward the high-energy side, indicating an increase in the effective energy of the beam. The result is a more penetrating x-ray beam.

> Increasing the kVp peak increases the quality of an x-ray beam.

Table 9-3 shows the measured change in HVL as kVp is increased from 50 to 150 kVp for a representative x-ray imaging system. The total filtration of the beam is 2.5 mm of Al.

Filtration. The primary purpose of adding filtration to an x-ray beam is to remove selectively low-energy x-rays that have little chance of getting to the image receptor. Figure 9-4 shows the emission spectrum of an unfiltered x-ray beam and an x-ray beam with normal filtration.

The ideally filtered x-ray beam would be monoenergetic because such a beam would further reduce patient dose. It is desirable to remove totally all x-rays below a certain energy determined by the type of x-ray examination. To improve image contrast, it is also desirable to remove x-rays with energies above a certain level. Unfortunately, such removal of regions of an x-ray beam is not normally possible.

> Increasing filtration increases the quality of an x-ray beam.

Almost any material could serve as an x-ray filter. Aluminum (Z = 13) is chosen because it is efficient in removing low-energy x-rays through the photoelectric effect, and because it is readily available, inexpensive, and easily shaped. Copper (Z = 29), tin (Z = 50), gadolinium (Z = 64), and holmium (Z = 67) have been used sparingly in special situations. As filtration is increased, so is beam quality, but quantity is decreased.

Types of Filtration

Filtration of diagnostic x-ray beams has two components: inherent filtration and added filtration.

Inherent Filtration. The glass or metal enclosure of an x-ray tube filters the emitted x-ray beam. This type of filtration is called **inherent filtration.** Inspection of an x-ray tube reveals that the part of the glass or metal enclosure

TABLE 9-2	Factors That Affect X-ray Quality and Quantity	
An Increase in	**EFFECT ON**	
	X-ray Quality	**X-ray Quantity**
mAs	None	Increased
kVp	Increased	Increased
Distance	None	Reduced
Filtration	Increased	Reduced

TABLE 9-3	Approximate Relationship Between kVp and HVL
kVp	**HVL (mm Al)**
50	1.9
75	2.8
100	3.7
125	4.6
150	5.4

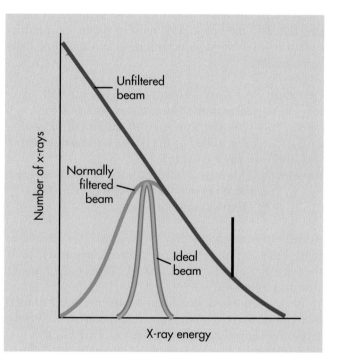

FIGURE 9-4 Filtration is used selectively to remove low-energy x-rays from the useful beam. Ideal filtration would remove all low-energy x-rays.

through which x-rays are emitted—**the window**—is very thin. This provides for low inherent filtration.

The inherent filtration of a general purpose x-ray tube is approximately 0.5 mm Al equivalent. With age, inherent filtration tends to increase because some of the tungsten metal of both target and filament is vaporized and is deposited on the inside of the window.

Special purpose tubes, such as those used in mammography, have very thin x-ray tube windows. They are sometimes made of beryllium (Z = 4) rather than glass and have an inherent filtration of approximately 0.1 mm Al.

Added Filtration. A thin sheet of aluminum positioned between the protective x-ray tube housing and the x-ray beam collimator is the usual form of added filtration.

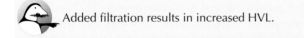

Added filtration results in increased HVL.

The addition of a filter to an x-ray beam attenuates x-rays of all energies emitted, but it attenuates a greater number of low-energy x-rays than high-energy x-rays. This shifts the x-ray emission spectrum to the high-energy side, resulting in an x-ray beam with higher energy, greater penetrability, and better quality. The HVL increases, but the extent of increase in the HVL cannot be predicted even when the thickness of added filtration is known.

Because added filtration attenuates the x-ray beam, it affects x-ray quantity. This value can be predicted if the HVL of the beam is known. The addition of filtration equal to the beam HVL reduces the beam quantity to half its prefiltered value and results in a **higher** x-ray beam quality.

Question: An x-ray imaging system has an HVL of 2.2 mm Al. The exposure is 2 mR/mAs (20 μGy$_a$/mAs) at 100 cm SID. If 2.2 mm Al is added to the beam, what will be the x-ray exposure?

Answer: This is an addition of one HVL; therefore, the x-ray exposure will be 1 mR/mAs (10 μGy$_a$/mAs).

Added filtration usually has two sources. First, 1-mm or more sheets of aluminum are permanently installed in the port of the x-ray tube housing, between the housing and the collimator.

With a conventional light-localizing variable-aperture collimator, the collimator contributes an additional 1 mm Al equivalent added filtration. This filtration results from the silver surface of the mirror in the collimator (Figure 9-5).

Compensating Filters One of the most difficult tasks that faces the radiologic technologist is producing an image with a uniform intensity when a body part is examined that varies greatly in thickness or tissue composition. When a filter is used in this fashion, it is called a **compensating filter** because it compensates for differences in subject radiopacity.

Compensating filters can be fabricated for many procedures; therefore, they come in various sizes and shapes. They are nearly always constructed of aluminum, but plastic materials also can be used. Figure 9-6 shows some common compensating filters.

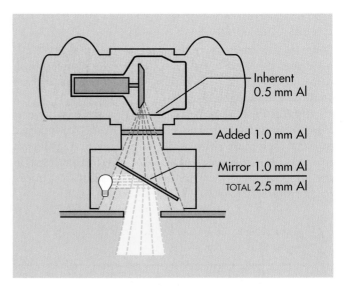

FIGURE 9-5 Total filtration consists of the inherent filtration of the x-ray tube, an added filter, and filtration achieved by the mirror of the light-localizing collimator.

During film-screen PA chest radiography, for instance, if the left chest is relatively radiopaque because of fluid, consolidation, or mass, the image would appear with very low OD (see Chapter 17) on the left side of the chest and very high OD on the right side of the chest. One could compensate for this OD variation by inserting a wedge filter so that the thin part of the wedge is positioned over the left side of the chest.

The wedge filter is principally used during radiography of a body part, such as the foot, that varies considerably in thickness (Figure 9-7). During an AP projection of the foot, the wedge would be positioned with its thick portion shadowing the toes and the thin portion toward the heel.

A bilateral wedge filter, or a trough filter, is sometimes used in chest radiography (Figure 9-8). The thin central region of the wedge is positioned over the mediastinum, while the lateral thick portions shadow the lung fields. The result is a radiograph with more uniform OD or signal intensity. Specialty compensating wedges of this type usually are used with dedicated apparatus, such as an x-ray imaging system used exclusively for chest radiography.

Special "bow-tie"–shaped filters are used with computed tomography (CT) imaging systems to compensate for the shape of the head or body. Conic filters, either concave or convex, find application in digital fluoroscopy, where the image receptor, the image intensifier tube, is round.

A step-wedge filter is an adaptation of the wedge filter (Figure 9-9). It is used in some special procedures, usually when long sections of the anatomy are imaged with the use of two or three separate image receptors.

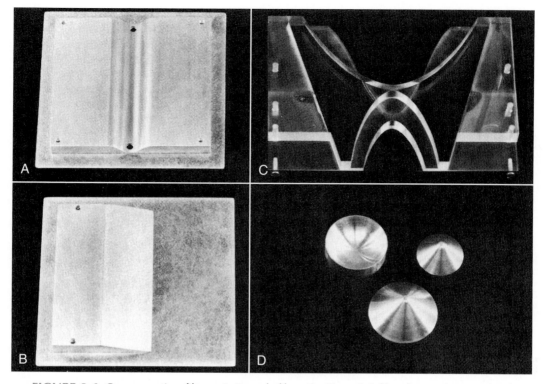

FIGURE 9-6 Compensating filters. **A,** Trough filter. **B,** "Bow-tie" filter for use in computed tomography. **C,** Wedge filter. **D,** Conic filters for use in digital fluoroscopy.

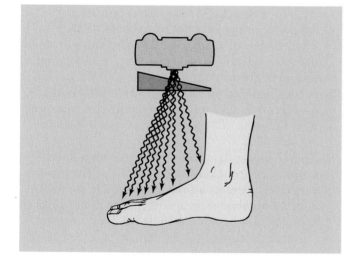

FIGURE 9-7 Use of a wedge filter for examination of the foot.

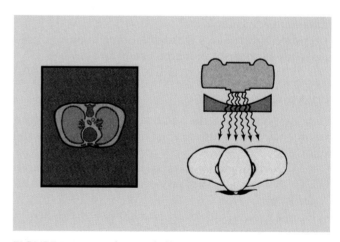

FIGURE 9-8 Use of a trough filter for examination of the chest.

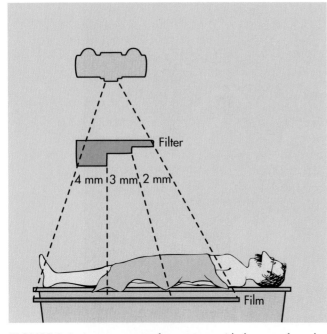

FIGURE 9-9 Arrangement of apparatus with the use of an aluminum step-wedge for serial radiography of the abdomen and lower extremities.

A common application of a step-wedge filter involves a three-step aluminum wedge and three 14 × 17-in (35 × 43-cm) films in a rapid changer for translumbar and femoral arteriography and venography. These procedures call for careful selection of screens, grids, and radiographic technique.

Compensating filters are useful for maintaining image quality. They are not radiation protection devices.

SUMMARY

Radiation quantity is the number of x-rays in the useful beam. Factors that affect radiation quantity include the following:

- mAs: X-ray quantity is directly proportional to mAs.
- kVp: X-ray quantity is proportional to the square of the kVp.
- Distance: X-ray quantity varies inversely with distance from the source.
- Filtration: X-ray quantity is reduced by filtration, which absorbs low-energy x-rays in the beam.

Radiation quality is the penetrating power of the x-ray beam. The penetrability is quantified by the HVL, which is the thickness of additional filtration that reduces x-ray intensity to half its original value. Factors that affect beam penetrability or radiation quality include the following:

- kVp: X-ray penetrability is increased as kVp is increased.
- Filtration: X-ray penetrability is increased when filtration is added to the beam.

Following are the three types of filtration: (1) inherent filtration of the glass or metal enclosure, (2) added filtration in the form of aluminum sheets, and (3) compensating filters, which provide variation in intensity across the x-ray beam.

CHALLENGE QUESTIONS

1. Define or otherwise identify the following:
   a. Inherent filtration
   b. The unit of x-ray quantity
   c. A filtered x-ray spectrum
   d. A kVp change equal to twice the mAs
   e. Three filter materials used with diagnostic x-ray beams
   f. Half-value layer
   g. Wedge filter
   h. The unit of x-ray quality
   i. The approximate HVL of your x-ray imaging system
   j. X-ray intensity
2. Graph the change in HVL with changing kVp (from 50 to 120 kVp) for an x-ray imaging system that has total filtration of 2.5 mm Al. Check your answer by plotting the data in Table 9-3.
3. An abdominal radiograph taken at 84 kVp, 150 mAs results in patient radiation exposure of 650 mR. The image is too light and is repeated at 84 kVp, 250 mAs. What is the exposure?
4. An image of the lateral skull taken at 68 kVp, 20 mAs has sufficient optical density but too much contrast. If the kVp is increased to 78 kVp, what should be the new mAs?
5. A chest radiograph taken at 180 cm SID results in an exposure of 12 mR. What would the exposure be if the same radiographic factors were used at 100 cm SID?
6. The following data were obtained with a fluoroscopic x-ray tube operated at 80 kVp. The exposure levels were measured 50 cm above the patient couch with aluminum absorbers positioned on the surface of the couch. Estimate the HVL through visual inspection of the data; then, plot the data and determine the precise value of the HVL.

Added mm Al	mR
None	65
1	48
3	30
5	21
7	16
9	13.0

7. When operated at 74 kVp, 100 mAs with 2.2 mm Al added filtration and 0.6 mm Al inherent filtration, the HVL of an x-ray imaging system is 3.2 mm Al and its output intensity at 100 cm SID is 350 mR. How much additional filtration is necessary to reduce the x-ray intensity to 175 mR?

8. The following technique factors have been shown to produce good-quality radiographs of the cervical spine with an x-ray imaging system that has 3 mm Al total filtration. Refer to Figure 9-1 and estimate the x-ray intensity at 100 cm SID for each.
   a. 62 kVp, 70 mAs
   b. 70 kVp, 40 mAs
   c. 78 kVp, 27 mAs
9. A radiographic exposure is 80 kVp at 50 mAs. How many electrons will interact with the target?
10. An extremity is radiographed at 60 kVp, 10 mAs, resulting in an x-ray intensity of 28 mR. If the technique is changed to 55 kVp, 10 mAs, what is the resultant x-ray intensity?
11. What is the square law, and how is it used?
12. What is the primary purpose of x-ray beam filtration?
13. The kVp is reduced from 78 to 68 kVp. What, if anything, should be done with mAs to maintain exposure of the image receptor constant?
14. What is the relationship between x-ray quantity and mAs?
15. Define half-value layer.
16. List the two ways an x-ray beam can be shifted to a higher average energy.
17. Why is aluminum used for x-ray beam filtration?
18. Describe the use of a wedge filter during radiography of a foot.
19. Does adding filtration to the x-ray beam affect the quantity of x-rays reaching the image receptor?
20. Fill in the following chart:

Increasing	Effect on X-ray Quality	Effect on X-ray Quantity
mAs	_____	_____
kVp	_____	_____
Distance	_____	_____
Filtration	_____	_____

The answers to the Challenge Questions can be found by logging on to our website at http://evolve.elsevier.com.

CHAPTER 100

X-ray Interaction With Matter

OBJECTIVES

At the completion of this chapter, the student should be able to do the following:

1. Describe each of the five x-ray interactions with matter
2. Define differential absorption and describe its effect on image contrast
3. Explain the effect of atomic number and mass density of tissue on differential absorption
4. Discuss why radiologic contrast agents are used to image some tissues and organs
5. Explain the difference between absorption and attenuation

OUTLINE

Five X-ray Interactions With Matter
    Coherent Scattering
    Compton Effect
    Photoelectric Effect
    Pair Production
    Photodisintegration
Differential Absorption
    Dependence on Atomic Number
    Dependence on Mass Density
Contrast Examination
Exponential Attenuation

X-RAYS INTERACT with matter in the following five ways: (1) by coherent scattering, (2) through the Compton effect, (3) through the photoelectric effect, (4) by pair production, and (5) by photodisintegration. Only the Compton effect and the photoelectric effect are important in making an x-ray image. The conditions that govern these two interactions control differential absorption, which determines the degree of contrast of an x-ray image.

FIVE X-RAY INTERACTIONS WITH MATTER

In Chapter 4, the interaction between electromagnetic radiation and matter was described briefly. This interaction was said to have wavelike and particle-like properties. Electromagnetic radiation interacts with structures that are similar in size to the wavelength of the radiation.

X-rays have very short wavelengths, no larger than approximately 10^{-8} to 10^{-9} m. The higher the energy of an x-ray, the shorter is its wavelength. Consequently, low-energy x-rays tend to interact with whole atoms, which have diameters of approximately 10^{-9} to 10^{-10} m;

moderate-energy x-rays generally interact with electrons, and high-energy x-rays generally interact with nuclei.

X-rays interact at these various structural levels through five mechanisms: coherent scattering, Compton effect, photoelectric effect, pair production, and photodisintegration. Two of these—Compton effect and photoelectric effect—are of particular importance to diagnostic radiology. They are discussed in some detail here.

Coherent Scattering

X-rays with energies below approximately 10 keV interact with matter by coherent scattering, sometimes called classical scattering or Thompson scattering (Figure 10-1). J. J. Thompson was the physicist to first describe coherent scattering.

In coherent scattering, the incident x-ray interacts with a target atom, causing it to become excited. The target atom immediately releases this excess energy as a scattered x-ray with wavelength equal to that of the incident x-ray ($\lambda = \lambda'$), and therefore of equal energy. However, the direction of the scattered x-ray is different from that of the incident x-ray.

The result of coherent scattering is a change in direction of the x-ray without a change in its energy. There is no energy transfer, and therefore no ionization. Most coherently scattered x-rays are scattered in the forward direction.

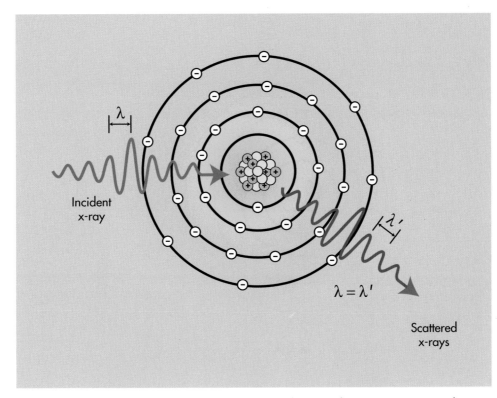

FIGURE 10-1 Classical scattering is an interaction between low-energy x-rays and atoms. The x-ray loses no energy but changes direction slightly. The wavelength of the incident x-ray is equal to the wavelength of the scattered x-ray.

Coherent scattering is of little importance to diagnostic radiology.

Coherent scattering primarily involves low-energy x-rays, which contribute little to the medical image. Some coherent scattering, however, occurs throughout the diagnostic range. At 70 kVp, a few percent of the x-rays undergo coherent scattering, which contributes slightly to **image noise,** the general graying of an image that reduces image contrast.

Compton Effect

X-rays throughout the diagnostic range can undergo an interaction with outer-shell electrons that not only scatters the x-ray but reduces its energy and ionizes the atom as well. This interaction is called the **Compton effect** or **Compton scattering** (Figure 10-2).

In the Compton effect, the incident x-ray interacts with an outer-shell electron and ejects it from the atom, thereby ionizing the atom. The ejected electron is called a Compton electron or a secondary electron. The x-ray continues in a different direction with less energy.

The energy of the Compton-scattered x-ray is equal to the difference between the energy of the incident x-ray and the energy of the ejected electron. The energy of the ejected electron is equal to its binding energy plus the kinetic energy with which it leaves the atom. Mathematically, this energy transfer is represented as follows:

> **COMPTON EFFECT**
>
> $E_i = E_s (E_b + E_{KE})$
>
> where E_i is energy of the incident x-ray, E_s is energy of the scattered x-ray, E_b is electron binding energy, and E_{KE} is kinetic energy of the electron.

Question: A 30-keV x-ray ionizes an atom of barium by ejecting an O-shell electron with 12 keV of kinetic energy. What is the energy of the scattered x-ray?

Answer: Figure 3-9 shows that the binding energy of an O-shell electron of barium is 0.04 keV; therefore,

$$30 \text{ keV} = E_s + (0.04 \text{ keV} + 12 \text{ keV})$$
$$E_s = 30 \text{ keV} - (0.04 \text{ keV} + 12 \text{ keV})$$
$$= 30 \text{ keV} - (12.04 \text{ keV})$$
$$= 17.96 \text{ keV}$$

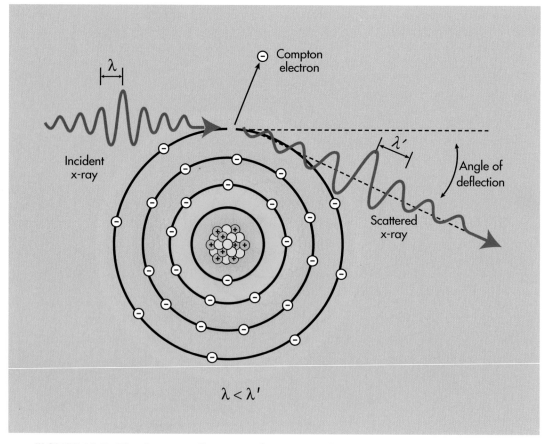

FIGURE 10-2 The Compton effect occurs between moderate-energy x-rays and outer-shell electrons. It results in ionization of the target atom, change in x-ray direction, and reduction in x-ray energy. The wavelength of the scattered x-ray is greater than that of the incident x-ray.

During a Compton interaction, most of the energy is divided between the scattered x-ray and the Compton electron. Usually, the scattered x-ray retains most of the energy. Both the scattered x-ray and the Compton electron may have sufficient energy to undergo additional ionizing interactions before they lose all their energy.

Ultimately, the scattered x-ray is absorbed photoelectrically. The Compton electron loses all of its kinetic energy through ionization and excitation and drops into a vacancy in an electron shell previously created by some other ionizing event.

Compton-scattered x-rays can be deflected in any direction, including 180 degrees from the incident x-ray. At a deflection of 0 degrees, no energy is transferred. As the angle of deflection increases to 180 degrees, more energy is transferred to the Compton electron, but even at 180 degrees of deflection, the scattered x-ray retains at least approximately two thirds of its original energy.

X-rays scattered back in the direction of the incident x-ray beam are called **backscatter radiation.** In diagnostic radiography, backscatter radiation is responsible for the cassette-hinge image sometimes seen on a radiograph even though the hinge was on the back side of the cassette. In such situations, the x-radiation has backscattered from the wall or the examination table, not from the patient.

The probability that a given x-ray will undergo the Compton effect is a complex function of the energy of the incident x-ray. In general, the probability of the Compton effect decreases as x-ray energy increases.

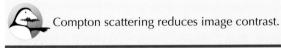

The probability of the Compton effect is inversely proportional to x-ray energy (1/E) and independent of atomic number.

The probability of the Compton effect does not depend on the atomic number of the atom involved. Any given x-ray is just as likely to undergo the Compton effect with an atom of soft tissue as with an atom of bone (Figure 10-3). Table 10-1 summarizes Compton scattering.

Compton scattering reduces image contrast.

Compton scattering in tissue can occur with all x-rays and therefore is of considerable importance in x-ray imaging. However, its importance involves a negative sense. Scattered x-rays provide no useful information on the radiograph. Rather, they produce a uniform optical density on the film radiograph and uniform intensity on the digital radiograph that results in

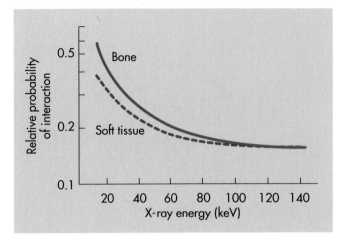

FIGURE 10-3 The probability that an x-ray will interact through the Compton effect is about the same for atoms of soft tissue and those of bone. This probability decreases with increasing x-ray energy.

Table 10-1	Features of Compton Scattering
Most likely to occur	With outer-shell electrons With loosely bound electrons
As x-ray energy increases	Increased penetration through tissue without interaction Increased Compton scattering relative to photoelectric effect Reduced Compton scattering ($\approx 1/E$)
As atomic number of absorber increases	No effect on Compton scattering
As mass density of absorber increases	Proportional increase in Compton scattering

reduced image contrast. Ways of reducing this scattered radiation are discussed later, but none is totally effective.

The scattered x-rays from Compton interactions can create a serious radiation exposure hazard in radiography and particularly in fluoroscopy. A large amount of radiation can be scattered from the patient during fluoroscopy. Such radiation is the source of most of the occupational radiation exposure that radiologic technologists receive.

During radiography, the hazard is less severe because no one but the patient is usually in the examining room. Nevertheless, scattered radiation levels are sufficient to necessitate protective shielding of the x-ray examining room.

Photoelectric Effect

X-rays in the diagnostic range also undergo ionizing interactions with inner-shell electrons. The x-ray is not scattered, but it is totally absorbed. This process is called the **photoelectric effect** (Figure 10-4).

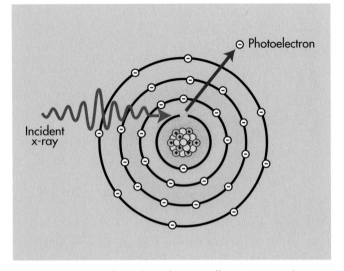

FIGURE 10-4 The photoelectric effect occurs when an incident x-ray is totally absorbed during the ionization of an inner-shell electron. The incident photon disappears, and the K-shell electron, now called a *photoelectron*, is ejected from the atom.

Table 10-2 | **Atomic Number and K-Shell Electron Binding Energy of Radiologically Important Elements**

Element	Atomic Number	K-Shell Electron Binding Energy (keV)
Hydrogen	1	0.02
Carbon	6	0.3
Nitrogen	7	0.4
Oxygen	8	0.5
Aluminum	13	1.6
Calcium	20	4.1
Molybdenum	42	19
Rhodium	45	23
Iodine	53	33
Barium	56	37
Tungsten	74	69
Rhenium	75	72
Lead	82	88

The electron removed from the atom, called a *photoelectron*, escapes with kinetic energy equal to the difference between the energy of the incident x-ray and the binding energy of the electron. Mathematically, this is shown as follows:

PHOTOELECTRIC EFFECT

$E_i = E_b + E_{KE}$

where E_i is the energy of the incident x-ray, E_b is the electron-binding energy, and E_{KE} is the kinetic energy of the electron.

The photoelectric effect is total x-ray absorption.

For low atomic number atoms, such as those found in soft tissue, the binding energy of even K-shell electrons is low (e.g., 0.3 keV for carbon). Therefore, the photoelectron is released with kinetic energy nearly equal to the energy of the incident x-ray.

For higher atomic number target atoms, electron binding energies are higher (37 keV for barium K-shell electrons). Therefore, the kinetic energy of the photoelectron from barium is proportionately lower. Table 10-2 shows the approximate K-shell binding energy for elements of radiologic importance.

Characteristic x-rays are produced after a photoelectric interaction in a manner similar to that described in Chapter 8. Ejection of a K-shell photoelectron by the incident x-ray results in a vacancy in the K shell. This unnatural state is immediately corrected when an outer-shell electron, usually from the L shell, drops into the vacancy.

This electron transition is accompanied by the emission of an x-ray whose energy is equal to the difference between binding energies of the shells involved. These characteristic x-rays consist of secondary radiation and behave in the same manner as scattered radiation. They contribute nothing of diagnostic value and fortunately have sufficiently low energy that they do not penetrate to the image receptor.

Question: A 50-keV x-ray interacts photoelectrically with (a) a carbon atom and (b) a barium atom. What is the kinetic energy of each photoelectron and the energy of each characteristic x-ray if an L-to-K transition occurs (see Figure 3-9)?

Answer:
a. $E_{KE} = K_i - K_b$
   $= 50 \text{ keV} - 0.3 \text{ keV}$
   $= 49.7 \text{ keV}$
   $E_x = 0.3 \text{ keV} - 0.006 \text{ keV}$
   $= 0.294 \text{ keV}$
b. $E_{KE} = E_i - E_b$
   $= 50 \text{ keV} - 37 \text{ keV}$
   $= 13 \text{ keV}$
   $E_x = 37 \text{ keV} - 5.989 \text{ keV}$
   $= 31.011 \text{ keV}$

The probability that a given x-ray will undergo a photoelectric interaction is a function of both the x-ray energy and the atomic number of the atom with which it interacts.

The probability of the photoelectric effect is inversely proportional to the third power of the x-ray energy $(1/E)^3$.

A photoelectric interaction cannot occur unless the incident x-ray has energy equal to or greater than the electron binding energy. A barium K-shell electron bound to the nucleus by 37 keV cannot be removed by a 36-keV x-ray.

If the incident x-ray has sufficient energy, the probability that it will undergo a photoelectric effect decreases with the third power of the photon energy ($1/E^3$). This relationship is shown graphically in Figure 10-5 for soft tissue and bone.

 The probability of photoelectric effect is directly proportional to the third power of the atomic number of the absorbing material (Z^3).

As the relative vertical displacement between the graphs of soft tissue and bone demonstrates, a photoelectric interaction is much more likely to occur with high-Z atoms than with low-Z atoms (see Figure 10-5). Table 10-3 presents the effective atomic numbers of materials of radiologic importance.

Question: If an 80-keV x-ray has a relative chance of one photoelectric effect with soft tissue, what is its relative probability of interacting with
   a. Fat? (Z = 6.3)
   b. Barium? (Z = 56)

Answer:

$$a. \left(\frac{6.3}{7.4}\right)^3 = 0.62$$

$$b. \left(\frac{56}{7.4}\right)^3 = 433$$

Semilogarithmic Graphs. Figure 10-5 is an example of a graph with a logarithmic (log, for short) scale along the vertical axis. A review of Table 2-1 shows that whole-log values represent orders of magnitude in power of 10 notation. Therefore, the difference between log 4 and log 2 is two orders of magnitude, or $10^4 - 10^2 = 10^2 = 100$.

A log scale is a power of 10 scale used to plot data that cover several orders of magnitude. In Figure 10-5, for example, the relative probability of photoelectric interaction with soft tissue varies from approximately 2 to less than 0.01 over the energy range from 10 to 60 keV.

A plot of these data in conventional arithmetic form appears in Figure 10-6. Clearly, this type of graph is unacceptable because all probability values above 30 keV are so close to zero.

On a linear scale, equal intervals have equal numeric value, but on a log scale, equal intervals represent equal ratios. This difference in scales is shown in Figure 10-7.

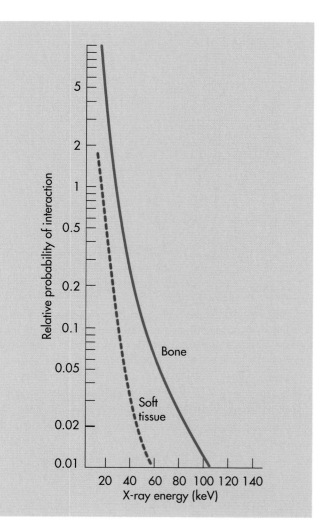

FIGURE 10-5   The relative probability that a given x-ray will undergo a photoelectric interaction is inversely proportional to the third power of the x-ray energy and directly proportional to the third power of the atomic number of the absorber.

Table 10-3	Effective Atomic Number of Materials Important to Radiologic Science
Type of Substance	**Effective Atomic Number**
HUMAN TISSUE	
Fat	6.3
Soft tissue	7.4
Lung	7.4
Bone	13.8
CONTRAST MATERIAL	
Air	7.6
Iodine	53
Barium	56
OTHER	
Concrete	17
Molybdenum	42
Tungsten	74
Lead	82

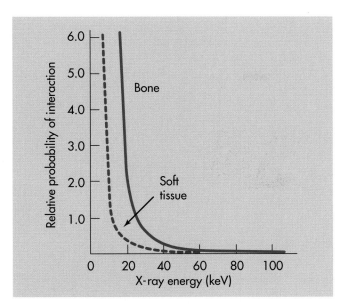

FIGURE 10-6 Relative probability for photoelectric interaction ranges over several orders of magnitude. If it is plotted in the conventional linear fashion, as here, one cannot estimate its value above an energy of approximately 30 keV.

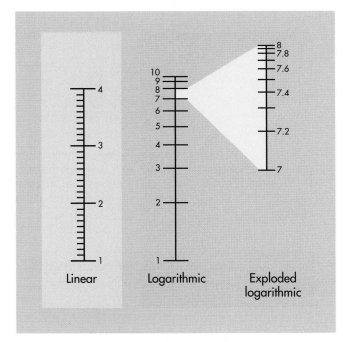

FIGURE 10-7 Graphic scales can be linear or logarithmic. The log scale is used to plot wide ranges of values.

All major intervals on the linear scale have a value of 1, and the subintervals a value of 0.1. On the other hand, the log scale contains major intervals that each equal one order of magnitude, with subintervals that are not equal in length. Figure 10-7 also shows an exploded view of one major log interval.

Cubic Relationships. The probability of interaction proportional to the third power changes rapidly. For the photoelectric effect, this means that a small variation in atomic number of the tissue atom or in x-ray energy results in a large change in the chance of photoelectric interaction. This is unlike the situation that exists for the Compton interaction.

Question: If the relative probability of photoelectric interaction with soft tissue for a 20-keV x-ray is 1, how much less likely will an interaction be for a 50-keV x-ray? How much more likely is interaction with iodine (Z = 53) than with soft tissue (Z = 7.4) for a 50-keV x-ray?

Answer:
$$\left(\frac{20 \text{ keV}}{50 \text{ keV}}\right)^3 = \left(\frac{2}{5}\right)^3 = 0.064$$

$$\left(\frac{53}{7.4}\right)^3 = 368$$

Table 10-4 summarizes the photoelectric effect.

Pair Production

If an incident x-ray has sufficient energy, it may escape interaction with electrons and come close enough to the nucleus of the atom to be influenced by the strong nuclear force field. The interaction between the x-ray and the nuclear field causes the x-ray to disappear, and in its place, two electrons appear, one positively charged (**positron**) and one negatively charged. This process is called **pair production** (Figure 10-8).

> Pair production does not occur during x-ray imaging.

Table 10-4	Features of Photoelectric Effect
Most likely to occur	With inner-shell electrons
	With tightly bound electrons
	When x-ray energy is just higher than electron binding energy
As x-ray energy increases	Increased penetration through tissue without interaction
	Less photoelectric effect relative to Compton effect
	Reduced absolute photoelectric effect (~ $1/E^3$)
As atomic number of absorber increases	Increases proportionately with the cube of the atomic number (Z^3)
As mass density of absorber increases	Proportional increase in photoelectric absorption

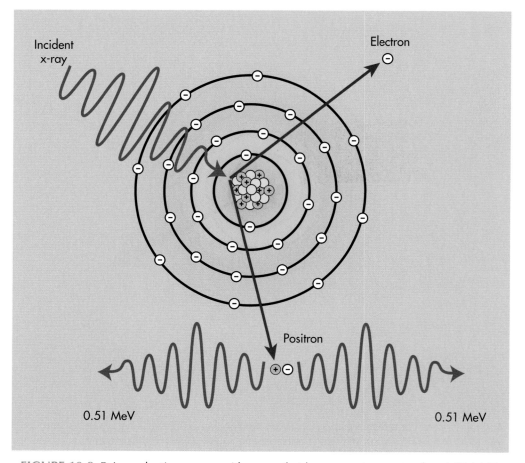

Incident x-ray

Electron

Positron

0.51 MeV

0.51 MeV

FIGURE 10-8 Pair production occurs with x-rays that have energies greater than 1.02 MeV. The x-ray interacts with the nuclear force field, and two electrons that have opposite electrostatic charges are created.

In Chapter 4, we calculated the energy equivalence of the mass of an electron to be 0.51 MeV. Because two electrons are formed in a pair production interaction, the incident photon must have at least 1.02 MeV of energy.

An x-ray with less than 1.02 MeV cannot undergo pair production. Any of the x-ray's energy in excess of 1.02 MeV is distributed equally between the two electrons as kinetic energy.

The electron that results from pair production loses energy through excitation and ionization and eventually fills a vacancy in an atomic orbital shell. The positron unites with a free electron, and the mass of both particles is converted to energy in a process called **annihilation radiation.**

Because pair production involves only x-rays with energies greater than 1.02 MeV, it is unimportant in x-ray imaging, but it is very important for positron emission tomography (PET) imaging in nuclear medicine.

Photodisintegration

X-rays with energy above approximately 10 MeV can escape interaction with electrons and the nuclear force field and be absorbed directly by the nucleus. When this happens, the nucleus is raised to an excited state and

instantly emits a nucleon or other nuclear fragment. This process is called **photodisintegration** (Figure 10-9).

 Photodisintegration does not occur in diagnostic radiology.

DIFFERENTIAL ABSORPTION

Of the five ways an x-ray can interact with tissue, only two are important to radiology: the Compton effect and the photoelectric effect. Similarly, only two methods of x-ray production (see Chapter 8)—bremsstrahlung x-rays and characteristic x-rays—are important.

More important than interaction of the x-ray by Compton or photoelectric effect, however, is the x-ray transmitted through the body without interacting. Figure 10-10 shows schematically how each of these types of x-ray contributes to an image.

Differential absorption occurs because of Compton scattering, photoelectric effect, and x-rays transmitted through the patient.

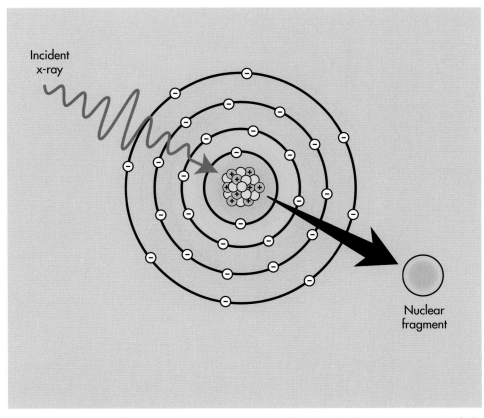

FIGURE 10-9 Photodisintegration is an interaction between high-energy x-rays and the nucleus. The x-ray is absorbed by the nucleus, and a nuclear fragment is emitted.

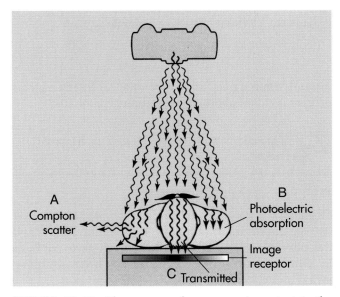

FIGURE 10-10 Three types of x-rays are important to the making of a radiograph: those scattered by Compton interaction (**A**); those absorbed photoelectrically (**B**); and those transmitted through the patient without interaction (**C**).

The **Compton-scattered x-ray contributes no useful information** to the image. When a Compton-scattered x-ray interacts with the image receptor, the image receptor assumes that the x-ray came straight from the x-ray tube target (Figure 10-11). The image receptor does not

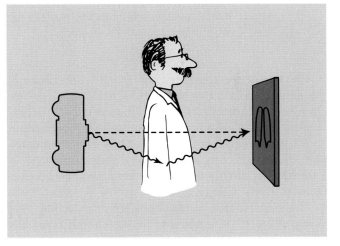

FIGURE 10-11 When an x-ray is Compton scattered, the image receptor thinks it came straight from the source.

recognize the scattered x-ray as representing an interaction off the straight line from the target.

These scattered x-rays result in image noise, a generalized dulling of the image by x-rays not representing diagnostic information. To reduce this type of noise, we use techniques and apparatus to reduce the number of scattered x-rays that reach the image receptor.

X-rays that undergo photoelectric interaction provide diagnostic information to the image receptor. Because they do not reach the image receptor, these x-rays are representative of anatomical structures with high x-ray absorption characteristics; such structures are radiopaque. The photoelectric absorption of x-rays produces the light areas in a radiograph, such as those corresponding to bone.

Other x-rays penetrate the body and are transmitted to the image receptor with no interaction whatsoever. They produce the dark areas of a radiograph. The anatomical structures through which these x-rays pass are radiolucent.

Basically, an x-ray image results from the difference between those x-rays absorbed photoelectrically in the patient and those transmitted to the image receptor. This difference in x-ray interaction is called *differential absorption*.

Approximately 1% of the x-rays incident on a patient reach the image receptor. Less than half of those that reach the image receptor interact to form an image. Thus, the radiographic image results from approximately 0.5% of the x-rays emitted by the x-ray tube. Consequently, careful control and selection of the x-ray beam are necessary to produce high-quality radiographs.

> Differential absorption increases as the kVp is reduced.

Producing a high-quality radiograph requires the proper selection of kVp, so that the effective x-ray energy results in maximum differential absorption. Unfortunately, reducing the kVp to increase differential absorption and therefore image contrast results in increased patient dose. A compromise is necessary for each examination.

Dependence on Atomic Number

Consider the image of an extremity (Figure 10-12). An image of the bone is produced because many more x-rays are absorbed photoelectrically in bone than in soft tissue. Recall that the probability of an x-ray undergoing photoelectric effect is proportional to the third power of the atomic number of the tissue.

Bone has an atomic number of 13.8, and soft tissue has an atomic number of 7.4 (see Table 10-3). Consequently, the probability that an x-ray will undergo a photoelectric interaction is approximately seven times greater in bone than in soft tissue.

Question: How much more likely is an x-ray to interact with bone than with muscle?

Answer: $\left(\dfrac{13.8}{7.4}\right)^3 = \dfrac{2628}{405} = 6.5$

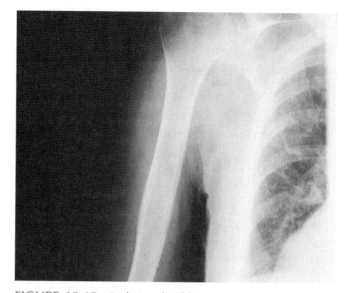

FIGURE 10-12 Radiograph of bony structures results from differential absorption between bone and soft tissue.

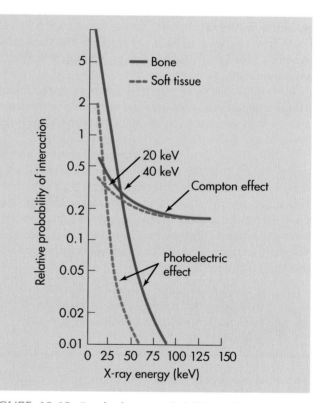

FIGURE 10-13 Graph shows probabilities of photoelectric and Compton interactions with soft tissue and bone. The interactions of these curves indicate those x-ray energies at which the chance of photoelectric absorption equals the chance of Compton scattering.

These relative values of interaction are apparent in Figure 10-13, when one pays particular attention to the logarithmic scale of the vertical axis. Note that the relative probability of interaction between bone and soft tissue (differential absorption) remains constant, whereas the

absolute probability of each decreases with increasing energy. With higher x-ray energy, fewer interactions occur, so more x-rays are transmitted without interaction.

Question: What is the relative probability that a 20-keV x-ray will undergo photoelectric interaction in bone compared with fat?

Answer: $Z_{bone} = 13.8$, $Z_{fat} = 6.8$

$$\left(\frac{13.8}{6.8}\right)^3 = 8.36$$

The Compton effect is independent of the atomic number of tissue. The probability of Compton scattering for bone atoms and for soft tissue atoms is approximately equal and decreases with increasing x-ray energy.

This decrease in scattering, however, is not as rapid as the decrease in photoelectric effect with increasing x-ray energy. The probability of the Compton effect is inversely proportional to x-ray energy ($1/E$). The probability of the photoelectric effect is inversely proportional to the third power of the x-ray energy ($1/E^3$).

At low energies, most x-ray interactions with tissue are photoelectric. At high energies, Compton scattering predominates.

Of course, as x-ray energy is increased, the chance of any interaction at all decreases. As kVp is increased, more x-rays penetrate to the image receptor; therefore, a lower x-ray quantity (lower mAs) is required.

Factor 10-13 combines all these factors into a single graph. At 20 keV, the probability of photoelectric effect equals the probability of Compton effect in soft tissue. Below this energy, most x-rays interact with soft tissue photoelectrically. Above this energy, the predominant interaction with soft tissue is Compton effect. Low kVp resulting in increased differential absorption provides the basis for mammography.

> To image small differences in soft tissue, one must use low kVp to get maximum differential absorption.

The relative frequency of Compton interaction compared with photoelectric interaction increases with increasing x-ray energy. The crossover point between photoelectric effect and Compton effect for bone is approximately 40 keV. Nevertheless, low-kVp technique is usually appropriate for bone radiography to maintain image contrast.

High-kVp technique is usually used for examination of barium studies and chest radiography, in which intrinsic contrast is high, resulting in much lower patient dose.

When high-kVp technique is used in this manner, the amount of scattered radiation from surrounding soft tissue contributes little to the image. When the amount

of scattered radiation becomes too great, grids are used (see Chapter 14). Grids do not affect the magnitude of the differential absorption.

Differential absorption in bone and soft tissue results from photoelectric interactions, which greatly depend on the atomic number of tissue. The loss of contrast is due to noise caused by Compton scattering. Two other factors are important in making an x-ray image: x-ray emission spectrum and mass density of patient tissue.

The crossover energies of 20 keV and 40 keV refer to a **monoenergetic** x-ray beam, that is, a beam containing x-rays that all have the same energy. In fact, as we saw in Chapter 8, clinical x-rays are **polyenergetic.** They are emitted over an entire spectrum of energies.

The correct selection of voltage for optimum differential absorption depends on the other factors discussed in Chapter 9 that affect the x-ray emission spectrum. For instance, in AP radiography of the lumbar spine at 110 kVp, a greater number of x-rays are emitted with energy above the 40-keV crossover for bone than below it. Less filtration or a grid may then be necessary.

Dependence on Mass Density

Intuitively, we know that we could image bone even if differential absorption were not Z-related because bone has a higher mass density than soft tissue. **Mass density** is not to be confused with optical density. Mass density is the quantity of matter per unit volume, specified in units of kilograms per cubic meter (kg/m^3). Sometimes, mass density is reported in grams per cubic centimeter (g/cm^3).

Question: How many g/cm^3 are there in $1 \ kg/m^3$?

Answer: $1 \ kg/m^3 = \dfrac{1000 \ g}{(100 \ cm)^3} = \dfrac{10^3 \ g}{10^6 \ cm^3} = 10^{-3} \ g/cm^3$

Table 10-5 gives the mass densities of several radiologically important materials. Mass density is related to the mass of each atom and basically tells how tightly the atoms of a substance are packed.

Water and ice are composed of precisely the same atoms, but ice occupies greater volume. The mass density of ice is $917 \ kg/m^3$ compared with $1000 \ kg/m^3$ for water. Ice floats in water because of this difference in mass density. Ice is lighter than water.

> The interaction of x-rays with tissue is proportional to the mass density of the tissue regardless of the type of interaction.

When mass density is doubled, the chance for x-ray interaction is doubled because twice as many electrons are available for interaction. Therefore, even without the Z-related photoelectric effect, nearly twice as many

Table 10-5	Mass Density of Materials Important to Radiologic Science
Substance	**Mass Density (kg/m³)**
HUMAN TISSUE	
Lung	320
Fat	910
Soft tissue, muscle	1000
Bone	1850
CONTRAST MATERIAL	
Air	1.3
Barium	3500
Iodine	4930
OTHER	
Calcium	1550
Concrete	2350
Molybdenum	10,200
Lead	11,350
Rhenium	12,500
Tungstate	19,300

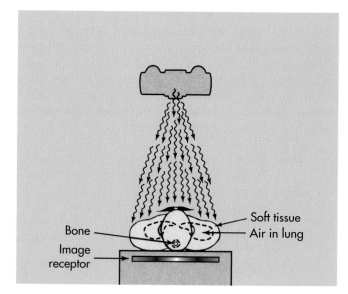

FIGURE 10-14 Even if x-ray interaction were not related to atomic number (Z), differential absorption would occur because of differences in mass density.

x-rays would be absorbed and scattered in bone as in soft tissue. The bone would be imaged.

Question: What is the relative probability that 60-keV x-rays will undergo Compton scattering in bone compared with soft tissue?

Answer: Mass density of bone = 1850 kg/m³
Mass density of soft tissue = 1000 kg/m³

$$\frac{1850}{1000} = 1.85$$

Lungs are imaged in chest radiography primarily because of differences in mass density. According to Table 10-5, the mass density of soft tissue is 770 times that of air (1000/1.3) and three times that of lung (1000/320). Therefore, for the same thickness, we can expect almost three times as many x-rays to interact with the soft tissue as with lung tissue.

The Z values of air and soft tissue are about the same: 7.4 for soft tissue and 7.6 for air; thus, differential absorption in air-filled soft tissue cavities is due primarily to differences in mass density. Figure 10-14 demonstrates differential absorption in air, soft tissue, and bone caused by mass density differences. Table 10-6 summarizes the various relationships of differential absorption.

Question: Assume that all x-ray interactions during mammography are photoelectric. What is the differential absorption of x-rays in microcalcifications (Z=20, ϱ=1550 kg/m³) relative to fatty tissue (Z=6.3, ϱ=910 kg/m³)?

Table 10-6	Characteristics of Differential Absorption
As x-ray energy increases	Fewer Compton interactions
	Many fewer photoelectric interactions
	More transmission through tissue
As tissue atomic number increases	No change in Compton interactions
	Many more photoelectric interactions
	Less x-ray transmission
As tissue mass density increases	Proportional increase in Compton interactions
	Proportional increase in photoelectric interactions
	Proportional reduction in x-ray transmission

Answer: Differential absorption due to atomic number:

$$\left(\frac{20}{6.3}\right)^3 = \frac{8000}{250} = 32:1$$

Differential absorption due to mass density

$$= \frac{1550}{910} = 1.7:1$$

Total differential absorbtion

$$= 32 \times 1.7 = 54.4:1$$

CONTRAST EXAMINATION

Barium and iodine compounds are used as an aid for imaging internal organs with x-rays. The atomic number of barium is 56; that of iodine is 53. Each has a much higher atomic number and greater mass density than soft tissue. When used in this fashion, they are called **contrast agents,** and because of their high atomic numbers, they are positive contrast agents.

Question: What is the probability that an x-ray will interact with iodine rather than soft tissue?

Answer: Differential absorption as a result of atomic number:

$$\left(\frac{53}{7.4}\right)^3 = 367:1$$

Differential absorbtion due to mass density

$$= \frac{4.93}{1.0} = 4.93:1$$

Total differential absorbtion

$$= 367 \times 4.93 = 1809:1$$

When an iodinated compound fills the internal carotid artery, or when barium fills the colon, these internal organs are readily visualized on a radiograph. Low-kVp technique (e.g., below 80 kVp) produces excellent, high-contrast radiographs of the organs of the gastrointestinal tract. Higher-kVp operation (e.g., above 90 kVp) often can be used in these examinations not only to outline the organ under investigation but to penetrate the contrast medium so the lumen of the organ can be visualized more clearly.

Air was used at one time as a contrast medium in procedures such as pneumoencephalography and ventriculography. Air is still used for contrast in some examinations of the colon along with barium; this is called a **double-contrast examination.** When used in this fashion, air is a negative contrast agent.

EXPONENTIAL ATTENUATION

When x-rays are incident on any type of tissue, they can interact with the atoms of that tissue through any of these five mechanisms: coherent scattering, Compton effect,

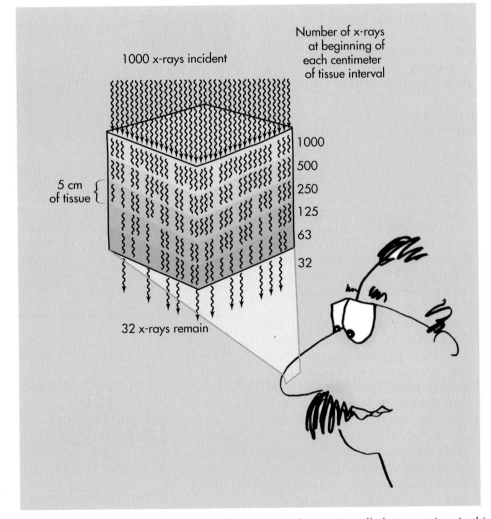

FIGURE 10-15 Interaction of x-rays by absorption and scatter is called *attenuation*. In this example, the x-ray beam has been attenuated 97%; 3% of the x-rays have been transmitted.

photoelectric effect, pair production, and photodisintegration. The relative frequency of interaction through each mechanism depends on the atomic number of the tissue atoms, the mass density, and the x-ray energy.

An interaction such as the photoelectric effect is called an *absorption process* because the x-ray disappears. **Absorption** is an all-or-none condition for x-ray interaction.

Interactions in which the x-ray is only partially absorbed, such as the Compton effect, are scattering processes. Coherent scattering is also a scattering event because the x-ray that emerges from the interaction travels in a direction that is different from that of the incident x-ray. Pair production and photodisintegration are absorption processes.

The total reduction in the number of x-rays remaining in an x-ray beam after penetration through a given thickness of tissue is called **attenuation.** When a broad beam of x-rays is incident on any tissue, some of the x-rays are absorbed and some are scattered. The result is a reduced number of x-rays, a condition referred to as *x-ray attenuation.*

> Attenuation is the product of absorption and scattering.

X-rays are attenuated exponentially, which means that they do not have a fixed range in tissue. They are reduced in number by a given percentage for each incremental thickness of tissue they go through.

Consider the situation diagrammed in Figure 10-15. One thousand x-rays are incident on a 25-cm-thick abdomen. The x-ray energy and the atomic number of the tissue are such that 50% of the x-rays are removed by the first 5 cm. Therefore, in the first 5 cm, 500 x-rays are removed, leaving 500 available to continue penetration.

By the end of the second 5 cm, 50% of the 500 or 250 additional x-rays have been removed, leaving 250 x-rays to continue. Similarly, entering the fourth 5-cm thickness are 125 x-rays, and entering the fifth and last 5 cm thickness are 63. Half of the 63 x-rays will be attenuated in the last 5 cm of tissue; therefore, only 32 will be transmitted to interact with the image receptor. The total effect of these interactions is 97% attenuation and 3% transmission of the x-ray beam.

A plot of this hypothetical x-ray beam attenuation, which closely resembles the actual situation, appears in Figure 10-16. Is it obvious that the assumed HVL in soft tissue was 5 cm? It should be clear that, theoretically at least, the number of x-rays emerging from any thickness of absorber will never reach zero. Each succeeding thickness can attenuate the x-ray beam only by a fractional amount, and a fraction of any positive number is always greater than zero.

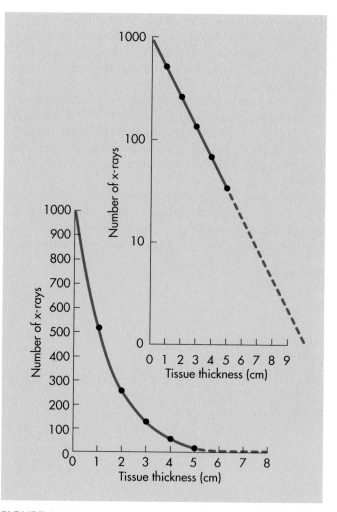

FIGURE 10-16 Linear and semilog plots of exponential x-ray attenuation data in Figure 10-15.

This is not the way that alpha particles and beta particles interact with matter. Regardless of the energy of the particle and the type of tissue, these particulate radiations can penetrate only so far before they are totally absorbed. For example, beta particles with 2 MeV of energy have a range of approximately 1 cm in soft tissue.

SUMMARY

Following are five fundamental interactions between x-rays and matter:
1. Coherent scattering is a change in the direction of an incident x-ray without a loss of energy.
2. The Compton effect occurs when incident x-rays ionize atoms and the x-ray then changes direction with a loss of energy.
3. The photoelectric effect occurs when the incident x-ray is absorbed into one of the inner electron shells and emits a photoelectron.

4. Pair production occurs when the incident x-ray interacts with the electric field of the nucleus. The x-ray disappears and two electrons appear—one positively charged (positron) and one negatively charged (electron).

5. Photodisintegration occurs when the incident x-ray is directly absorbed by the nucleus. The x-ray disappears and nuclear fragments are released.

The interactions that are important to diagnostic x-ray imaging are the Compton effect and the photoelectric effect.

Differential absorption controls the contrast of an x-ray image. The x-ray image results from the difference between those x-rays absorbed by photoelectric interaction and those x-rays that pass through the body as image-forming x-rays. Attenuation is the reduction in x-ray beam intensity as it penetrates through tissue. Differential absorption and attenuation of the x-ray beam depend on the following factors:

- The atomic number (Z) of the atoms in tissue
- The mass density of the atoms in tissue
- The x-ray energy

Radiologic contrast agents, such as iodine and barium, use the principles of differential absorption to image soft tissue organs. Iodine is used in vascular, renal, and biliary imaging. Barium is used for gastrointestinal imaging. Both elements have high atomic numbers (iodine is 53, barium is 56) and mass density much greater than that of soft tissue.

CHALLENGE QUESTIONS

1. Define or otherwise identify the following:
   a. Differential absorption
   b. Classical scattering
   c. Mass density
   d. 1.02 MeV
   e. Contrast agent
   f. Compton effect
   g. Attenuation
   h. Monoenergetic
   i. Secondary electron
   j. Photoelectric effect
2. What are the two factors of importance to differential absorption?
3. A 28-keV x-ray interacts photoelectrically with a K-shell electron of a calcium atom. What is the kinetic energy of the secondary electron (see Table 3-3)?
4. 1000 x-rays with energy of 140 keV are incident on bone and soft tissue of equal thickness. If 87 are scattered in soft tissue, approximately how many are scattered in bone?
5. Why are iodinated compounds such excellent agents for vascular contrast examinations?
6. Diagram the Compton interaction; identify the incident x-ray, positive ion, negative ion, secondary x-ray, and scattered x-ray.
7. Describe backscatter radiation. Can you think of examples in diagnostic radiology?
8. Tungsten is sometimes alloyed into the beam-defining collimators of an x-ray imaging system. If a 63-keV x-ray undergoes a Compton interaction with an L-shell electron and ejects that electron with 12 keV of energy, what is the energy of the scattered x-ray (see Figure 3-9)?
9. Of the five basic mechanisms of x-ray interaction with matter, three are not important to diagnostic radiology. Which are they, and why are they not important?
10. On average, 33.7 eV is required for each ionization in air. How many ion pairs would a 22-keV x-ray probably produce in air, and approximately how many of these would be produced photoelectrically?
11. How is the energy of the Compton-scattered x-ray computed?
12. Does the probability of the Compton effect depend on the atomic number of the target atom?
13. When the kVp is increased, is Compton scattering increased or reduced?
14. Describe the photoelectric effect.
15. When the kVp is increased, what happens to the absolute probability of the photoelectric effect versus the Compton effect?
16. How much more likely is it that an x-ray will interact with bone than with muscle?
17. What is the relationship between atomic number (Z) and differential absorption?
18. What is the relationship between mass density and differential absorption?
19. In a contrast radiographic examination with iodine, what is the relative probability that x-rays will interact with iodine rather than with soft tissue?
20. What kVp is used to penetrate barium in a contrast examination?

The answers to the Challenge Questions can be found by logging on to our website at http://evolve.elsevier.com.

PART III

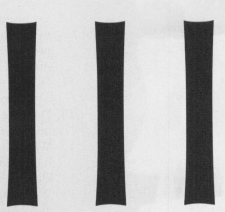

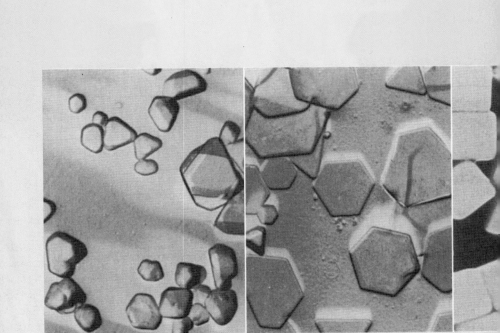

THE
RADIOGRAPH

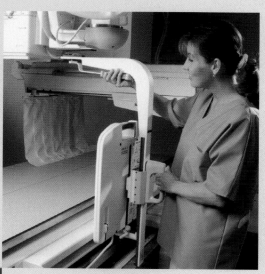

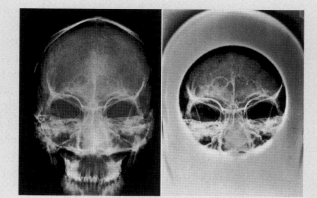

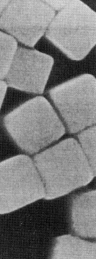

Radiographic Film

OBJECTIVES

At the completion of this chapter, the student should be able to do the following:

1. Discuss the construction of radiographic film
2. Describe the formation of the latent image
3. List and define the characteristics of x-ray film
4. Identify the types of film used in medical imaging
5. Explain proper film handling and storage

OUTLINE

Film Construction
    Base
    Emulsion
Formation of the Latent Image
    Silver Halide Crystal
    Photon Interaction With Silver Halide Crystal
    Latent Image
Types of Film
    Screen-Film
    Direct-Exposure Film
    Mammography Film
    Laser Film
    Specialty Film
Handling and Storage of Film
    Heat and Humidity
    Light
    Radiation
    Shelf Life

MAGE-FORMING x-rays exit the patient and expose the radiographic intensifying screen placed in the protective radiographic cassette. The radiographic intensifying screen emits light, which exposes the radiographic film placed between the two screens.

This chapter discusses the construction and various types of radiographic film, the use of x-rays to form a latent image, and tips for handling and storing film.

The primary purpose of diagnostic radiologic apparatus and techniques is to transfer information from an x-ray beam to the eye-brain complex of the radiologist. The x-ray beam that emerges from the x-ray tube is nearly uniformly distributed in space. After interaction with the patient, the beam of **image-forming x-rays** (see Chapter 10) is not uniformly distributed in space but varies in intensity according to the characteristics of the tissue through which it has passed.

> Image-forming x-rays are those that exit the patient and interact with the image receptor.

The **exit beam** refers to the x-rays that remain as the useful beam exits the patient. It consists of x-rays scattered away from the image receptor and image-forming x-rays.

The diagnostically useful information in this exit beam must be transferred to a form that is intelligible to the radiologist. X-ray film is one such medium. Other media include the fluoroscopic image intensifier, the television monitor, the laser imaging system, and solid-state detectors, all of which are discussed later. The medium that converts the x-ray beam into a visible image is called the **image receptor (IR)**. The most common IR is still photographic film, although solid-state digital IRs are finding increased application.

Photography has its origins in the early 19th century. By the time of the American Civil War (1860 to 1865), photography was professionally used. Amateur photography surfaced early in the 20th century.

The construction and characteristics of radiographic film are similar to those of regular photographic film. Radiographic film is manufactured with rigorous quality control and has a spectral response different from that of photographic film; however, its mechanism of operation is much the same. The following discussion concerns radiographic film, but with very few modifications, it could be applied to photographic film.

FILM CONSTRUCTION

The manufacture of radiographic film is a precise procedure that requires tight quality control. Manufacturing facilities are extremely clean because the slightest bit of dirt or other contaminant in the film limits the film's ability to reproduce information from the x-ray beam.

During the early 1960s, at the height of nuclear weapons testing, x-ray film manufacturers took extraordinary precautions to ensure that contamination from radioactive fallout did not invade their manufacturing environment. Such contamination could seriously **fog** the film.

Radiographic film basically has two parts: the **base** and the **emulsion** (Figure 11-1). In most x-ray film, the emulsion is coated on both sides; therefore, it is called **double-emulsion film.** Between the emulsion and the base is a thin coating of material called the **adhesive layer,** which ensures uniform adhesion of the emulsion to the base. This adhesive layer allows the emulsion and the base to maintain proper contact and integrity during use and processing.

The emulsion is enclosed by a protective covering of gelatin called the *overcoat*. This overcoat protects the emulsion from scratches, pressure, and contamination during handling, processing, and storage and allows for relatively rough manipulation of x-ray film before exposure. Processed film may be handled with even less regard for damage. The thickness of radiographic film is approximately 150 to 300 μm.

Base

The base is the foundation of radiographic film. Its primary purpose is to provide a rigid structure onto which the emulsion can be coated. The base is flexible and fracture resistant to allow easy handling but is rigid enough to be snapped into a viewbox.

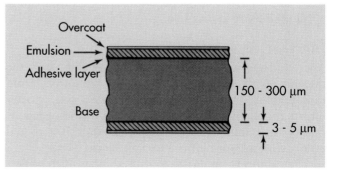

FIGURE 11-1 Cross section of radiographic film. The bulk of the film is the base. The emulsion contains the medical image.

Conventional photographic film has a much thinner base than radiographic film and therefore is not as rigid. Can you imagine attempting to snap a 14 × 17-inch photographic negative into a viewbox?

The base of radiographic film is 150 to 300 μm thick, semirigid, lucent, and made of polyester.

The base of radiographic film maintains its size and shape during use and processing so that it does not contribute to image distortion. This property of the base is known as **dimensional stability.** The base is of uniform **lucency** and is nearly transparent to light, so no unwanted pattern or shading is found on the image.

During manufacturing, however, dye is added to the base of most radiographic film to slightly tint the film blue. Compared with untinted film, this coloring reduces eyestrain and fatigue, enhancing the radiologist's diagnostic efficiency and accuracy.

The original radiographic film base was a glass plate. Radiologists used to refer to radiographs as x-ray plates. During World War I, high-quality glass became largely unavailable while medical applications of x-rays, particularly by the military, were increasing rapidly.

A substitute material, **cellulose nitrate,** soon became the standard base. Cellulose nitrate, however, had one serious deficiency. It was flammable. Improper storage and handling of some x-ray film files resulted in severe hospital fires during the 1920s and early 1930s.

By the mid-1920s, film with a "safety base," **cellulose triacetate,** was introduced. Cellulose triacetate has properties similar to those of cellulose nitrate but is not as flammable.

In the early 1960s, a **polyester** base was introduced. Polyester has taken the place of cellulose triacetate as the film base of choice. Polyester is more resistant to warping from age and is stronger than cellulose triacetate, permitting easier transport through automatic processors. Its dimensional stability is superior. Polyester bases are thinner than triacetate bases (approximately 175 μm) but are just as strong.

Emulsion

The emulsion is the heart of the x-ray film. It is the material with which x-rays or light photons from radiographic intensifying screens interact and transfer information. The emulsion consists of a homogeneous mixture of **gelatin** and **silver halide crystals.** It is coated evenly with a layer that is 3 to 5 μm thick.

The gelatin is similar to that used in salads and desserts but is of much higher quality. It is clear, so it transmits light, and it is sufficiently porous for processing chemicals to penetrate to the crystals of silver halide.

Its principal function is to provide mechanical support for silver halide crystals by holding them uniformly dispersed in place.

The silver halide crystal is the active ingredient of the radiographic emulsion. In the typical emulsion, 98% of the silver halide is **silver bromide;** the remainder is usually **silver iodide.** These atoms have relatively high atomic numbers ($Z_{Br} = 35$, $Z_{Ag} = 47$, $Z_I = 53$) compared with the gelatin and the base (for both, $Z \approx 7$). The interaction of x-ray and light photons with these high-Z atoms ultimately results in the formation of a latent image on the radiograph.

Depending on the intended imaging application, silver halide crystals may have tabular, cubic, octahedral, polyhedral, or irregular shapes. Tabular grains are used in most radiographic films.

Tabular silver halide crystals are flat and typically 0.1 μm thick, with a triangular, hexagonal, or higher-order polygonal cross section. The crystals are approximately 1 μm in diameter. The arrangement of atoms in a crystal is cubic, as shown in Figure 11-2.

The crystals are made by dissolving metallic silver (Ag) in nitric acid (HNO_3) to form silver nitrate ($AgNO_3$). Light-sensitive silver bromide (AgBr) crystals are formed by mixing silver nitrate with potassium bromide (KBr) in the following reaction:

> **SILVER HALIDE CRYSTAL FORMATION**
> $AgNO_3 + KBr \rightarrow AgBr \downarrow + KNO_3$
> The arrow ↓ indicates that the silver bromide is precipitated while the potassium nitrate, which is soluble, is washed away.

The entire process takes place in the presence of gelatin and with precise control of temperature, pressure, and the rate at which ingredients are mixed.

The shape and lattice structure of silver halide crystals are not perfect, and some of the imperfections result in the imaging property of the crystals. The type of imperfection thought to be responsible is a chemical contaminant, usually silver sulfide, which is introduced by chemical sensitization into the crystal lattice, usually at or near the surface.

This contaminant has been given the name **sensitivity center.** During exposure, photoelectrons and silver ions are attracted to these sensitivity centers, where they combine to form a **latent image center** of metallic silver.

Differences in speed, contrast, and resolution among various radiographic films are determined by the process by which silver halide crystals are manufactured and by the mixture of these crystals into the gelatin. The number of sensitivity centers per crystal, the concentration of crystals in the emulsion, and the size and distribution

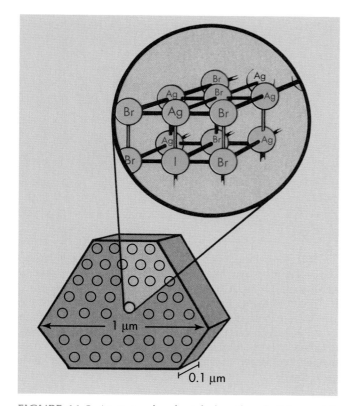

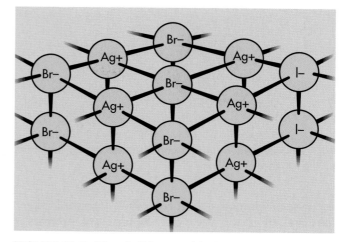

FIGURE 11-3 Silver halide crystal lattice contains ions. Electrons from Ag atoms have been loaned to Br and I atoms.

FIGURE 11-2 An example of a tabular silver halide crystal. The arrangement of atoms in the crystal is cubic.

of the crystals affect the performance characteristics of radiographic film.

Direct-exposure film contains a thicker emulsion with more silver halide crystals than screen-film. The size and concentration of silver halide crystals primarily affect film speed. The composition of the radiographic emulsion is a proprietary secret that is closely guarded by each manufacturer.

Radiographic film is manufactured in total darkness. From the moment the emulsion ingredients are brought together until final packaging, no light is present.

FORMATION OF THE LATENT IMAGE

The image-forming x-rays exiting the patient and incident on the radiographic intensifying screen-film deposit visible light energy in the emulsion primarily through photoelectric interaction with atoms of the silver halide crystal. This energy is deposited in a pattern that is representative of the object or anatomical part that is being radiographed.

Immediately after exposure, no image can be observed on the film. An invisible image is present, however, and is called a **latent image**. With proper chemical processing, the latent image becomes a **visible image**.

 The latent image is the invisible change that is induced in the silver halide crystal.

The interaction between photons and silver halide crystals is fairly well understood, as is the processing of the latent image into the visible image. However, the formation of the latent image, sometimes called the **photographic effect**, is not well understood and continues to be the subject of considerable research. The following discussion is an extraction of the Gurney-Mott theory, the accepted, although incomplete, explanation of latent image formation.

Silver Halide Crystal

The silver, bromine, and iodine atoms are fixed in the **crystal lattice** in ion form (Figure 11-3). Silver is a positive ion, and bromide and iodide are negative ions. When a silver halide crystal is formed, each silver atom releases an outer-shell electron, which becomes attached to a halide atom (either bromine or iodine).

The silver atom is missing an electron and therefore is a positively charged ion, identified as Ag^+. The bromine and iodine atoms each have one extra electron and therefore are negatively charged ions, identified as bromide and iodide (Br^- and I^-), respectively.

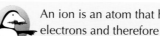 An ion is an atom that has too many or too few electrons and therefore has electric charge.

The silver halide crystal is not as rigid as some crystals such as diamonds. Under certain conditions, atoms and electrons are free to migrate within the silver halide crystal.

The halide ions, bromide and iodide, are generally found in greatest concentration along the surface of the crystal. Therefore, the crystal takes on a negative surface charge, which is matched by the positive charge of the **interstitial** silver ions, the silver ions inside the crystal. An inherent defect in the structure of silver halide

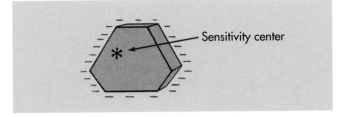

FIGURE 11-4 Model of a silver halide crystal emphasizing the sensitivity center and the concentration of negative ions on the surface.

crystals, the **Frankel defect,** consists of interstitial silver ions and silver ion vacancies. Figure 11-4 presents a model of the silver halide crystal.

Photon Interaction With Silver Halide Crystal

When radiation interacts with film, it is the interaction with the silver and halide atoms (Ag, Br, I) that forms the latent image. If the x-ray is totally absorbed, its interaction is photoelectric (Figure 11-5, *A*). If it is partially absorbed, its interaction is Compton.

In both cases, a secondary electron—either a photoelectron or a Compton electron—is released with sufficient energy to travel a large distance within the crystal (Figure 11-5, *B*). While crossing the crystal, the secondary electron may have sufficient energy to dislodge additional electrons from the crystal lattice.

Consequently, as a result of one x-ray interaction, a number of electrons are released and travel through the crystal lattice. The release of these secondary electrons is represented as follows:

SECONDARY ELECTRON FORMATION
$Br^- + photon \rightarrow Br + e^-$

Because light photons have lower energy, more of them are needed to produce a number of migrating secondary electrons equal to the number produced by a single x-ray.

 The result is the same whether the interaction involves visible light from an intensifying screen or direct exposure by x-rays.

Secondary electrons liberated by the absorption event migrate to the sensitivity center and are trapped. Once a sensitivity center captures a photoelectron and becomes more negatively charged, the center is attractive to mobile interstitial silver ions (Figure 11-5, *C*). The interstitial silver ion combines with the electron trapped at the sensitivity center to form metallic silver atoms.

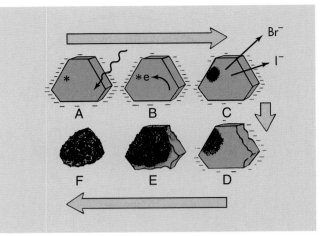

FIGURE 11-5 Production of the latent image and conversion of the latent image into a manifest image require several simultaneous steps. **A,** Radiation interaction releases electrons. **B,** These electrons migrate to the sensitivity center. **C,** At the sensitivity center, atomic silver is formed by attraction of an interstitial silver ion. **D,** This process is repeated many times, resulting in the buildup of silver atoms. **E,** The remaining silver halide is converted to silver during processing. **F,** The silver grain results.

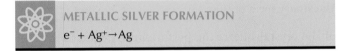

METALLIC SILVER FORMATION
$e^- + Ag^+ \rightarrow Ag$

Most of these electrons come from the bromide and iodide ions because these negative ions have one extra electron. These negative ions therefore are converted to neutral atoms, and the loss of ionic charge results in disruption of the crystal lattice.

The bromine and iodine atoms are now free to migrate because they no longer are bound by ionic forces. They migrate out of the crystal into the gelatin portion of the emulsion. The deterioration of crystalline structure also makes it easier for remaining silver ions to migrate.

Latent Image

The concentration of electrons at the sensitivity center produces a region of negative electrification. As halide atoms are removed from the crystal, the positive silver ions are electrostatically attracted to the sensitivity center. After migrating to the sensitivity center, the silver ions are neutralized by electrons and are converted to metallic silver.

In an optimally exposed film, most developable silver halide crystals have collected 4 to 10 silver atoms at a sensitivity center (Figure 11-5, *D*). Consequently, this silver deposition is not observable, even microscopically.

This group of silver atoms is called a **latent image center.** It is here that visible quantities of silver form during processing to create the radiographic image (Figure 11-5, *E*).

Crystals with silver deposited at the sensitivity center are developed into black grains (Figure 11-5, *F*). Crystals that have not been irradiated remain crystalline and inactive. The unobservable information contained in radiation-activated and -inactivated silver halide crystals constitutes the latent image.

Processing is the term applied to the chemical reactions that transform the latent image into a visible image. Because of its importance, processing is dealt with separately in the next chapter.

TYPES OF FILM

Medical imaging is becoming extremely technical and sophisticated, and this is reflected in the number and variety of films that are now available. Each major film manufacturer produces many different films for medical imaging. When combined with the various film formats offered, more than 500 selections are possible (Table 11-1).

In addition to screen-film, direct-exposure film, sometimes called nonscreen film and special application film (such as that used in mammography, video recording, duplication, subtraction, cineradiography, and dental radiology), is available. Each has particular characteristics that become more familiar to the radiologic technologist with use.

Table 11-2 shows standard film sizes in English and SI (Le Système International d'Unités) units. In most cases, the sizes are not exactly equivalent, but they are usually interchangeable. By far, the most commonly used film is that customarily called **screen-film**. Screen-film is the type of film that is used with radiographic intensifying screens.

Screen-Film

As was previously stated, screen-film is the most widely used IR in radiology. Several characteristics must be considered when one is selecting screen-film: contrast, speed, spectral matching, anticrossover/antihalation dyes, and requirement for a safelight.

Contrast. Most manufacturers offer screen-film with multiple contrast levels. High-contrast film produces a very black-and-white image, whereas a low-contrast image is more gray. Contrast is discussed in greater detail in Chapter 16.

The contrast of an IR is inversely proportional to its exposure **latitude,** that is, the range of exposure techniques that produce an acceptable image. Consequently, screen-film is available in multiple latitudes. Usually, the manufacturer identifies the contrast of these films as medium, high, or higher.

The difference depends on the **size and distribution of the silver halide crystals.** A high-contrast emulsion contains smaller silver halide grains with a relatively uniform grain size. Low-contrast films, on the other hand, contain larger grains that have a wider range of sizes.

Speed. Screen-film IRs are available with different speeds. Speed is the sensitivity of the screen-film combination to x-rays and light. Usually, a manufacturer offers several different IRs of different speeds that result from different film emulsions and different intensifying screen phosphors.

For direct-exposure film, speed is principally a function of the concentration and the total number of silver halide crystals. For screen-film, silver halide grain size and shape are the principal determinants of film speed.

Large-grain emulsions are more sensitive than small-grain emulsions.

To optimize speed, screen-films are almost always **double emulsion,** that is, an emulsion is layered on either side of the base. This double-layering is due primarily to the efficiency conferred by the use of two screens to expose the film from both sides. This produces twice the speed that could be attained with a single-emulsion film, even if the single emulsion were made twice as thick.

Table 11-1	Types of Film Used in Medical Imaging		
Type	**Emulsions**	**Characteristics**	**Applications**
Intensifying screen	Two	Blue or green sensitive	General radiography
Laser printing	Single with antihalation backing	Matches laser used (about 630 nm)	Laser printers attached to CT, MRI, ultrasound, etc.
Copy or duplicating	Single with antihalation backing	Pre-exposed to Dmax	Duplicating radiographs
Dental	Two packed in sealed envelope	Has lead foil to reduce back scatter	Dentistry
Radiation monitoring	Two packed in sealed envelope	One emulsion can be sloughed off to increase OD scale	Radiation monitoring
Dry transfer	One	Thermally sensitive	"Dry" printers

Film speed is limited, however, because the light from the radiographic intensifying screen is absorbed very rapidly in the superficial layers of the emulsion. If the emulsion is too thick, that portion next to the film base remains largely unexposed.

Compared with earlier technology, current emulsions contain less silver yet produce the same optical density per unit exposure. This more efficient use of silver in the emulsion is called the **covering power** of the emulsion.

The reported speed of a film is nearly always that for the IR: the film and two radiographic screens. When radiographic intensifying screens and film are properly matched, the reported speed is accurate. Mismatch can cause significant exposure error.

Crossover. Until recently, silver halide crystals were usually fat and three-dimensional (Figure 11-6, *A*). Most emulsions now (Figure 11-6, *B*) contain tabular grains, which are flat silver halide crystals, and provide a large surface area/volume ratio. The result is improved covering power and significantly lower crossover.

When light is emitted by a radiographic intensifying screen, it not only exposes the adjacent emulsion, it can also expose the emulsion on the other side of the base.

Table 11-2	Standard Film Sizes	
English Units	**SI Units**
7 × 7 in	18 × 18 cm
8 × 10 in	20 × 25 cm
10 × 12 in	24 × 30 cm
14 × 14 in	35 × 35 cm
14 × 17 in	35 × 43 cm

When light crosses over the base, it causes increased blurring of the image (Figure 11-7).

> Crossover is the exposure of an emulsion caused by light from the opposite radiographic intensifying screen.

Tabular grain emulsions reduce crossover because the covering power is increased, which relates not only to light absorption from the screen (which is increased) but also to light transmitted through the emulsion to cause crossover (which is reduced).

The addition of a light-absorbing dye in a **crossover control layer** reduces crossover to near zero (Figure 11-8). The crossover control layer has three critical characteristics: (1) It absorbs most of the crossover light, (2) it does not diffuse into the emulsion but remains as a separate layer, and (3) it is completely removed during processing.

Crossover can be reduced or eliminated by the use of radiographic intensifying screens that emit short-wavelength light (blue or ultraviolet). Such light is more strongly absorbed by silver halide crystals. Also, the polyester base is not transparent to ultraviolet light, so no crossover with ultraviolet-emitting screens occurs.

Spectral Matching. Perhaps the most important consideration in the selection of modern screen-film is its spectral absorption characteristics. Since the introduction of **rare Earth screens** in the early 1970s, radiologic technologists must be particularly careful to use a film whose sensitivity to various colors of light—its **spectral response**—is properly matched to the spectrum of light emitted by the screen.

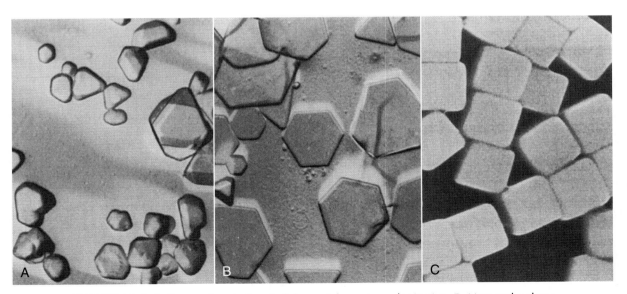

FIGURE 11-6 **A,** Conventional silver halide crystals are irregular in size. **B,** New technology produces flat, tablet-like grains. **C,** Cubic grains (Courtesy Eastman Kodak.)

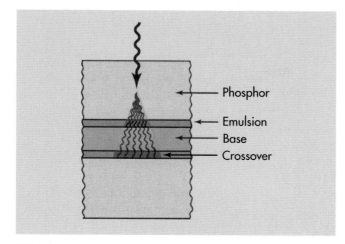

FIGURE 11-7 Crossover occurs when screen light crosses the base to expose the opposite emulsion.

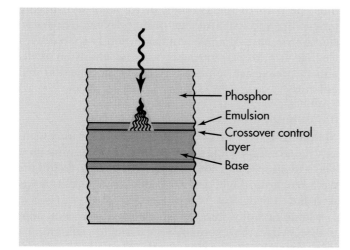

FIGURE 11-8 Crossover is reduced by adding a dye to the base; this is called a *crossover control layer.*

 Rare Earth screens are made with rare Earth elements—those with atomic numbers of 57 to 71.

Calcium tungstate screens, which emit blue and blue-violet light, have been largely replaced with rare Earth screens, which are faster. Now, many rare Earth phosphors emit ultraviolet, blue, green, and red. All silver halide films respond to violet and blue light but not to green, yellow, or red unless they are spectrally sensitized with dyes.

If green-emitting screens are used, they should be matched with a film that is sensitive not only to blue light but also to green light. Such film is **orthochromatic** and is called green-sensitive film. This is distinct from **panchromatic film,** which is used in photography and is sensitive to the entire visible light spectrum.

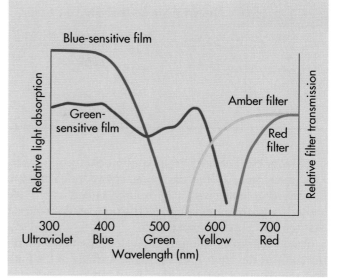

FIGURE 11-9 Radiographic films are blue-sensitive or green-sensitive, and they require amber- and red-filtered safelights, respectively.

Figure 11-9 shows the spectral response of blue-sensitive and green-sensitive films. Blue-sensitive film should be used only with blue- or ultraviolet-emitting screens. Green-sensitive film usually is exposed with green-emitting screens.

If films with sensitivity only in the ultraviolet and blue regions of the spectrum are used with green-emitting screens, then the IR speed is greatly reduced and patient dose increases. Proper spectral matching results in selection of the correct screen-film combination.

Reciprocity Law. One would expect that the total exposure of a film would not depend on the time taken to expose it. That is the definition of the **reciprocity law,** which also can be stated as follows:

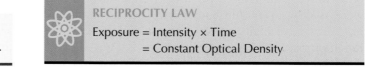

RECIPROCITY LAW

Exposure = Intensity × Time
= Constant Optical Density

The reciprocity law is true for film exposed directly to x-rays. Industrial radiographers do not have to compensate for this effect. The reciprocity law fails when film is exposed to light from radiographic intensifying screens.

Very long or very short exposure times produce a lower optical density than that predicted by the reciprocity law. Radiographers must be aware of this.

Reciprocity law failure is important when exposure times are long (as in mammography) or short (as in angiography). The result of long or short exposures is reduced speed. An increase in radiographic technique may be required. Table 11-3 shows approximate speed loss as a function of exposure time.

Table 11-3	Approximate Reciprocity Law Failure
Exposure Time	**Relative Speed (%)**
1 ms	95
10 ms	100
100 ms	100
1 s	90
10 s	60

Safelights. The use of radiographic film requires certain precautions in the darkroom. Most **safelights** are incandescent lamps with a color filter; safelights provide enough light to illuminate the darkroom while ensuring that the film remains unexposed.

Proper darkroom illumination depends not only on the color of the filter but also on the wattage of the bulb and the distance between the lamp and the work surface. A 15 W bulb should be no closer than 5 ft (1.5 m) from the work surface.

With blue-sensitive film, an **amber filter** is used. The amber filter transmits light that has wavelengths longer than approximately 550 nm, which is above the spectral response of blue-sensitive film.

The use of an amber filter would fog green-sensitive film; therefore, a **red filter,** which transmits only light above approximately 600 nm, must be used in this case. A red filter is suitable for both green- and blue-sensitive film. Figure 11-9 shows the approximate transmission characteristics for amber and red safelight filters.

Direct-Exposure Film

The use of radiographic intensifying screens with film allows reduced technique and therefore reduced patient dose. However, the image is more blurred than it would be after exposure without screens. In the past, certain films were manufactured for use without screens; they were used to image thin body parts, such as hands and feet, that have high subject contrast and present low radiation risk.

Most extremity examinations now use fine-grain, high-detail screens and double-emulsion film as the IR. Until the early 1970s, such film was also used for mammography, but patient dose was much too high. This film typically requires 10 to 100 times more radiation than screen-film and is rarely used today.

This type of film is identified as **direct-exposure film.** The emulsion of a direct-exposure film is thicker than that of screen-film, and it contains higher concentrations of silver halide crystals to improve direct x-ray interaction.

After processing, double-emulsion film is flat because the expansion and contraction characteristics of the two emulsion layers compensate for one another. With single-emulsion film, however, special attention

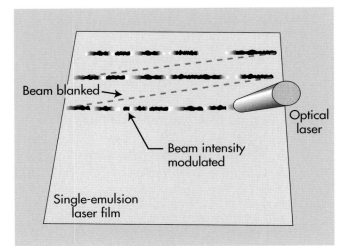

FIGURE 11-10 The laser beam writes in raster fashion.

must be paid to the swelling of the emulsion during processing and its shrinkage during drying. The backside of the base of single-emulsion film is coated with clear gelatin, so that during processing, emulsion swells and shrinkage are balanced, ensuring that the film will not curl.

Mammography Film

Mammography was originally performed with an industrial-grade, double-emulsion, direct-exposure film. The radiation doses associated with such a technique were much too high, and consequently, specialty films were developed.

Mammography film is single-emulsion film that is designed to be exposed with a single radiographic intensifying screen. All currently available mammography screen-film systems use green-emitting terbium-doped gadolinium oxysulfide screens with green-sensitive film.

The surface of the base opposite the screen is coated with a special light-absorbing dye to reduce reflection of screen light, which is transmitted through the emulsion and base. This effect is called **halation,** and the absorbing dye is an **antihalation coating.** Such an antihalation coating is used on all single-emulsion screen-film, not just mammography film. The coating is removed during processing for better viewing.

Laser Film

A laser printer uses the digital electronic signal from an imaging device. The intensity of the laser beam is varied in direct proportion to the strength of the image signal. This process is called laser beam **modulation.** While being modulated, the laser beam writes in raster fashion over the entire film (Figure 11-10).

Laser printers provide exceptionally consistent image quality for multiple film sizes and multiple image formats per film. These printers can be electronically

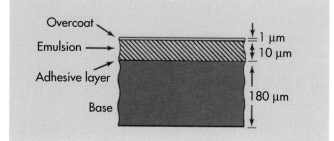

FIGURE 11-11 Cross section of single-emulsion mammography and laser film.

interfaced with multiple digital imaging modalities such as computed tomography (CT), magnetic resonance imaging (MRI), and computed radiology. For even greater productivity, laser printers can be docked to an automatic film processor.

Laser film is silver halide film that has been sensitized to the red light emitted by the laser in much the same way that blue- and green-sensitive screen-film is sensitized. Different types of lasers are used in laser printers and laser film is light-sensitive; therefore, laser film must be handled in total darkness.

Figure 11-11 presents a cross section of single-emulsion film, such as that used for mammography and laser imaging.

Specialty Film

Cinefluorography is a special examination that is reserved almost exclusively for the cardiac catheterization laboratory. The radiologic technologist who becomes involved in such procedures uses **cine film.**

Cine film is 35 mm and is supplied in rolls of 100 and 500 ft. Because of acceleration to all digital imaging, the use of cine film is declining rapidly.

Spot films from 70 to 105 mm in width are used in a number of different types of spot film cameras. These films are similar in composition to cine film but are larger than cine film; therefore, spot film can be viewed directly on a conventional viewbox without resorting to a projector. Figure 11-12 shows the format of the more popular sizes of cine and roll-type spot films.

Processing of cine film and spot film is critical for providing a quality image. Roll-type spot film usually can be adequately processed in the automatic processor used for conventional radiographs. Cine film, on the other hand, should be processed with specially designed movie film processing equipment because artifacts are magnified along with the image during projection.

When a radiograph is copied with the use of conventional film, a film with a positive image is produced first. This "positive" film is overlaid on top of another sheet of film to produce a negative image similar to the original radiograph. This double process results in loss of image quality.

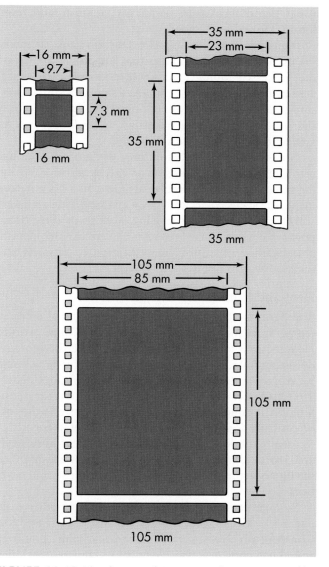

FIGURE 11-12 The format of 16-mm and 35-mm cine film and of 105-mm spot film.

Duplicating or **copy film** has already been exposed to maximum optical density by the manufacturer, so further exposure occurs in the region of solarization of the characteristic curve, and the film behaves opposite to normal.

Note that the orientation of single-sided emulsions is important. Manufacturers place a small notch in one corner of the film. In the darkroom, feel for the notch with the forefinger.

HANDLING AND STORAGE OF FILM

Radiographic film is a sensitive radiation detector and must be handled accordingly. Improper handling and storage result in poor radiographs with artifacts that interfere with diagnosis. For this reason, it is essential that anyone who handles radiographic film should be careful not to bend, crease, or otherwise subject it to rough handling. Clean hands are a must, and hand lotions should be avoided.

Improper handling or processing can cause **artifacts,** the marks or spurious images that sometimes appear on the processed radiograph. Artifacts also can be generated by the useful x-ray beam. Radiographic film is pressure sensitive, so rough handling or the imprint of any sharp object, such as a fingernail, is reproduced as an artifact on the processed radiograph.

Creasing of the film before processing produces a line artifact. Dirt on the hands or on radiographic intensifying screens produces specular artifacts. In a dry environment, static electricity can cause characteristic artifacts.

During automatic processing, a worn or dirty transport system can cause artifacts that are usually identifiable by their repetition. Identification of artifacts and their causes are discussed in Chapter 17.

Heat and Humidity

Radiographic film is sensitive to the effects of elevated temperature and humidity, especially for long periods. Heat increases the fog of a radiograph and therefore reduces contrast. Consequently, radiographic film should be stored at temperatures lower than approximately 20 °C (68 °F). With higher storage temperatures, the longer the time of storage, the more severe is the loss of contrast that results from the increase in fog.

Ideally, radiographic films should be kept in refrigerated storage. Storage for a year or longer is acceptable if the film is maintained at 10 °C (50 °F). Film should never be stored near steam pipes or other sources of heat.

Storage under conditions of elevated humidity (e.g., over 60%) also reduces contrast because of increased fog. Consequently, before use, radiographic film should be stored in a cool, dry place, ideally in a climate-controlled environment. Storage in an area that is too dry can be equally objectionable. Static artifacts are possible when the relative humidity dips to below about 40%.

Light

Radiographic film must be stored and handled in the dark. Any light at all can expose the emulsion before processing. If low-level, diffuse light exposes the film, fog is increased. If bright light exposes or partially exposes the film, a gross, obvious artifact is produced.

Control of light is ensured by a well-sealed darkroom and a light-proof storage bin for film that has been opened but not clinically exposed. The storage bin should have an electrical interlock that prevents it from being opened while the door to the darkroom is ajar or open.

Radiation

Ionizing radiation, other than the useful beam, creates an image artifact by increasing fog and reducing contrast. Film fog is the dull, uniform optical density that appears if the film has been inadvertently exposed to light, x-rays, heat, or humidity.

Darkrooms usually are located next to x-ray rooms and are lined with lead. However, this is not always necessary. It is usually acceptable to lead-line only the storage shelf and the film bin.

> The fog level for unprocessed film is approximately 0.2 mR (2 μ Gy$_a$).

Radiographic film is more sensitive after an exposure than before. This is so because some of the original exposure is used to raise the optical density to above the toe of the characteristic curve. A subsequent exposure on the same film does not have to do this and has an immediate effect on optical density.

Radiographic film is far more sensitive to x-ray exposure than are people; therefore, more lead is required to protect film than people. The thickness of the lead barrier is designed to keep the total exposure of unprocessed film below 0.2 mR. This, of course, requires some assumptions about the storage time of the film. Monthly turnover of film requires four times the lead shielding than is required for weekly turnover.

Care should be taken to ensure that the receiving area for radiographic film is not the same as that for the radioactive material used in nuclear medicine. Even though the packaging of radioactive material ensures the safety of those who handle it, the low-level radiation emitted can fog radiographic film if the radioactive material and film are stored together for even a short time.

Shelf Life

Most radiographic film is supplied in boxes of 100 sheets. Some film is packaged in an interleaved fashion, with chemically treated protective paper between sheets of film. Each box contains an expiration date, which indicates the maximum shelf life of the film.

Under no circumstances should film be stored for periods longer than the stated shelf life. Film must be used before its expiration date, which is usually a year or so after purchase. Aging results in loss of speed and contrast and an increase in fog.

It is always wise to store boxes of film on edge rather than laying them flat. When stored on edge, they are less likely to warp and, in the case of noninterleaved packaging, are less likely to stick to one another, or to suffer from pressure artifacts caused by the weight of boxes on top.

The storage of film should be sequenced so that the oldest film is used first. Rotation of the film, much like the rotation of perishables in a supermarket, is appropriate.

Many imaging facilities now use a method of stock control that requires films to be stored on specific shelves adjacent to a bar code on the edge of the shelf. Using a device the size of a large calculator, the stock controller swipes the bar code for each size/type of film and enters the number of boxes on the shelf. This exercise tells the supply staff how many new boxes to issue and places an order with the film supplier to replenish stocks.

 It is bad practice to store film and boxes of chemistry in the same cupboard.

Most hospitals receive film each month and purchase enough film for 5 weeks of use. The extra few days beyond monthly use are necessary to cover civil emergencies that require an unexpectedly large number of x-ray examinations. Given a 5-week supply schedule and the first-in, first-out rule, **30 days is a reasonable maximum storage time for radiographic film.**

SUMMARY

Image-forming x-radiation is that part of the x-ray beam that exits a patient and exposes the IR. The conventional image radiographic IR is a cassette that contains radiographic film sandwiched between two radiographic intensifying screens. Radiographic film is made up of a polyester base that is covered on both sides with a film emulsion.

The film emulsion contains light-sensitive silver bromide crystals that are made from the mixture of silver nitrate and potassium bromide. During manufacture, the emulsion is spread onto the base in darkness or under red lights because the AgBr molecule is sensitive to light.

The invisible latent image is formed in the film emulsion when light photons interact with the silver halide crystals. Processing of radiographic film converts the latent image to a visible image.

Following are some important characteristics of radiographic film:

- **Contrast.** High-contrast film produces black-and-white images. Low-contrast film produces images with shades of gray.
- **Latitude.** Latitude is the range of exposure techniques (kVp and mAs) that produce an acceptable image.
- **Speed.** Speed is the sensitivity of the screen-film combination to x-rays and light. Fast screen-film combinations need fewer x-rays to produce a diagnostic image.
- **Crossover.** When light is emitted from a radiographic intensifying screen, it exposes not only the adjacent film emulsion but also the emulsion on the other side of the base. The light crosses over the base and blurs the radiographic image.
- **Spectral Matching.** The x-ray beam does not directly expose the x-ray film. Radiographic intensifying screens emit light when exposed to x-rays and the emitted light then exposes the radiographic film. The color of light emitted must match the response of the film.
- **Reciprocity Law.** When exposed to the light of radiographic intensifying screens, radiographic film speed is less if the exposure time is very short or very long.

Film should be handled carefully and stored at specific temperatures and humidities to reduce artifacts. Artifacts on radiographic film can also be caused by rough handling.

CHALLENGE QUESTIONS

1. Define or otherwise identify the following:
   a. Polyester
   b. Sensitivity center
   c. Latent image
   d. Emulsion covering power
   e. Orthochromatic film
   f. Silver halide
   g. Spectral matching
   h. Artifact
   i. Radiation fog
   j. Shelf life
2. Diagram the cross-sectional view of a radiographic film designed for use with a pair of radiographic intensifying screens.
3. What does the term **dimensional stability** mean when applied to radiographic film? Which part of the film is responsible for this characteristic?
4. List the principal ingredients in the radiographic emulsion with their respective atomic numbers (Z).
5. Silver bromide crystals are made from silver nitrate and potassium bromide. After exposure, some of the silver bromide is reduced to metallic silver. What chemical equations represent these interactions?
6. Describe the process whereby a latent image is created in one crystal of the film emulsion.
7. What is the difference between panchromatic film and orthochromatic film?
8. What determines proper darkroom safelight selection?
9. What precautions are necessary when films are used that are designed specifically for screen-film mammography?
10. What precautions are necessary when radiographic film is used and stored?
11. Briefly discuss the historical development of x-ray film.

12. Write the silver halide crystal reaction. What does the arrow pointing down represent?
13. What determines the speed of radiographic film?
14. What is the term for closely guarded information held by film manufacturers?
15. Explain the Gurney-Mott theory of latent image formation.
16. What is the importance of spectral matching in selection of screen-film combinations?
17. Why do radiographers need to be aware of reciprocity law failure?
18. An amber filter on a safelight is used under what conditions? A red filter on a safelight is used under what conditions?
19. Discuss the difference between regular screen-film and mammography screen-film.
20. List the proper film storage conditions in terms of (a) temperature, (b) humidity, and (c) shelf life.

The answers to the Challenge Questions can be found by logging on to our website at http://evolve.elsevier.com.

CHAPTER 12

Processing the Latent Image

OBJECTIVES

At the completion of this chapter, the student should be able to do the following:

1. Discuss historical development from hand processing to automatic processing
2. List the chemicals used in each processing step
3. Discuss the use of each chemical
4. Explain the systems of the automatic processor
5. Describe alternative processing methods

OUTLINE

Film Processing
   Automatic Processing
   Processing Sequence
Processing Chemistry
   Wetting
   Developing
   Fixing
   Washing
   Drying
Automatic Processing
   Transport System
   Temperature Control System
   Circulation System
   Replenishment System
   Dryer System
Alternative Processing Methods
   Rapid Processing
   Extended Processing
   Daylight Processing
   Dry Processing

PROCESSING THE invisible latent image creates the visible image. Processing causes the silver ions in the silver halide crystal that have been exposed to light to be converted into microscopic black grains of silver. The processing sequence comprises the following steps: (1) wetting, (2) developing, (3) rinsing in stop bath, (4) fixing, (5) washing, and (6) drying.

These processing steps are completed in an automatic processor. This chapter discusses automatic processor design and use, as well as alternative processing methods.

FILM PROCESSING

The latent image is invisible because only a few silver ions have been changed to metallic silver and deposited at the sensitivity center. Processing the film magnifies this action many times until all the silver ions in an exposed crystal are converted to atomic silver, thus converting the latent image into a visible radiographic image.

The exposed crystal becomes a black grain that is visible microscopically. The silver contained in fine jewelry and tableware would also appear black except that it has been highly polished, which smoothes the surface and makes it reflective.

Processing is as important as technique and positioning in preparing a quality radiograph. A change in recommended processing conditions should never be a substitute for a poor radiographic exposure because the result is always a higher patient dose.

Before the introduction of automatic film processing, x-ray films were processed manually. It took approximately 1 hour to prepare a completely dry and ready-to-read radiograph.

Automatic Processing

The first automatic x-ray film processor was introduced by Pako in 1942 (Figure 12-1). The first commercially available model could process 120 films/hr with the use of special film hangers. These film hangers were dunked from one tank to another. The total cycle time for processing one film was approximately 40 minutes.

Automatic x-ray film processing advanced significantly in 1956, when the Eastman Kodak Company introduced the first roller transport system for processing medical radiographs. The roller transport automatic processor shown in Figure 12-2 was about 10 feet long, weighed nearly three quarters of a ton, and sold for approximately $350,000 in today's dollars.

Automatic processing revolutionized busy departments. Finished radiographs became available in 6 minutes, and the variability in results caused by the human element was eliminated. Departmental efficiency, work flow, and radiographic quality all improved.

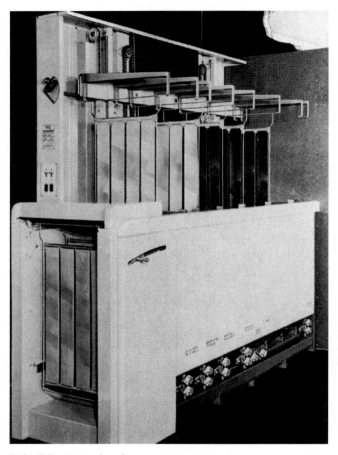

FIGURE 12-1 The first automatic processor, circa 1942. (Courtesy Art Haus, Columbus, Ohio.)

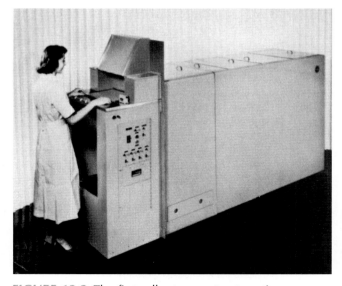

FIGURE 12-2 The first roller transport automatic processor, circa 1956. (Courtesy Eastman Kodak Company.)

Another significant breakthrough was Eastman Kodak's introduction of 90-second rapid processing in 1965. Rapid processing was possible because of the development of new chemistry and emulsions, as well as the faster drying permitted by a polyester film base. With this processor, the dry-to-drop time is 90 seconds. This type of automatic film processing system remains the standard.

In 1987, Konica introduced an automatic film processor with a processing cycle of approximately 45 seconds. This processor requires special films and chemicals, however.

Processing Sequence

Radiographic film processing involves several steps; these are summarized in Table 12-1.

All radiographic processing is automatic today; therefore, the following discussion does not cover manual processing. The chemicals involved in both are basically the same. In automatic processing, the time for each step is shorter, and the chemical concentration and temperature is higher.

The first step in the processing sequence involves **wetting** the film to swell the emulsion, so that subsequent chemical baths can reach all parts of the emulsion uniformly. In automatic processing, this step is omitted and the wetting agent is incorporated into the second step, **developing.**

 Developing is the stage of processing during which the latent image is converted to a visible image.

The developing stage is very short and highly critical. After developing, the film is rinsed in an acid solution designed to stop the developing process and remove excess developer chemicals from the emulsion. Photographers call this step the **stop bath.** In radiographic processing, the stop bath is included in the next step, **fixing.**

 Fixing the silver halide that was not exposed to radiation is the process of clearing it from the emulsion and hardening the emulsion to preserve the image.

The gelatin portion of the emulsion is **hardened** at the same time to increase its structural soundness. Fixing is followed by vigorous **washing** of the film to remove any remaining chemicals from the previous processing steps.

Finally, the film is **dried** to remove the water used to wash it and to make the film acceptable for handling and viewing.

Developing, fixing, and washing are important steps in the processing of radiographic film. The precise chemical reactions involved in these steps are not completely understood. However, a review of the general action is in order because of the importance of **processing** in a high-quality radiograph.

PROCESSING CHEMISTRY

The chemicals used to process films are designed to penetrate an emulsion and cause an effect. Those used in automatic processors do this very efficiently in the very short time the film is immersed.

Thus, when one is mixing solutions, cleaning a processor, or participating in any activity with or near processing solutions, these steps should be followed:

- Wear a proper mask that reduces inhalation of fumes—not the standard surgical mask that only guards against particles and bugs.
- Wear nitrile gloves. Do not use surgical gloves; they only protect against biologic matter. Remember that photographic chemicals are designed to penetrate, and thin rubber gloves provide no guarantee of safety.
- Wear protective glasses. Chemical splashes in the eyes are painful.

TABLE 12-1	**Sequence of Events in Processing a Radiograph**			
			APPROXIMATE TIME	
Event	Purpose		Manual	Automatic
Wetting	Swells the emulsion to permit subsequent chemical penetration		15 s	—
Developing	Produces a visible image from the latent image		5 min	22 s
Rinsing in stop bath	Terminates development and removes excess chemical from the emulsion		30 s	—
Fixing	Removes remaining silver halide from emulsion and hardens gelatin		15 min	22 s
Washing	Removes excess chemicals		20 min	20 s
Drying	Removes water and prepares radiograph for viewing		30 min	26 s

Wetting

A **solvent** is a liquid into which various solids and powders can be dissolved. The **universal solvent** is water, which is the solvent for all the chemicals used in processing a radiograph.

For these chemicals to penetrate the emulsion, the radiograph must first be treated by a **wetting agent.** The wetting agent is water, and it penetrates the gelatin of the emulsion, causing it to swell. In automatic processing, the wetting agent is in the developer.

Developing

The principal action of developing is to change the silver ions of exposed crystals into metallic silver. The **developer** is the chemical that performs this task. The developer provides electrons to the sensitivity center of the crystal to change the silver ions to silver.

In addition to the solvent, the developer contains a number of other ingredients. The composition of the developer and the function of each ingredient are outlined in Table 12-2.

For the ionic silver to be changed to metallic silver, an electron must be supplied to the silver ion. Chemically, the reaction is described as follows:

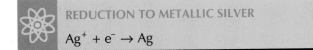

REDUCTION TO METALLIC SILVER

$$Ag^+ + e^- \rightarrow Ag$$

When an electron is given up by a chemical, in this case the **developing agent,** to neutralize a positive ion, the process is called **reduction.** The silver ion is said to be **reduced** to metallic silver, and the chemical responsible for this is called a **reducing agent.**

The opposite of reduction is **oxidation,** a reaction that produces an electron. Oxidation and reduction occur simultaneously and are called **redox** reactions. To help recall the proper association, think of **EUR/OPE:** electrons are **used** in reduction/oxidation **produces** electrons.

The principal component of the developing agent is **hydroquinone.** Secondary constituents of the developing agent are **Phenidone** and **Metol.**

Usually, hydroquinone and Phenidone are combined for rapid processing. As reducing agents, each of these molecules has an abundance of electrons that can be easily released to reduce silver ions. Chapter 16 discusses various aspects of film sensitometry.

The optical density of a processed radiograph results from the development of crystals that contain a latent image (Figure 12-3).

 Synergism occurs when the action of two agents working together is greater than the sum of the action of each agent working independently.

The characteristic curve of a radiograph is shaped by the synergistic action of developing agents. Hydroquinone acts rather slowly but is responsible for the very

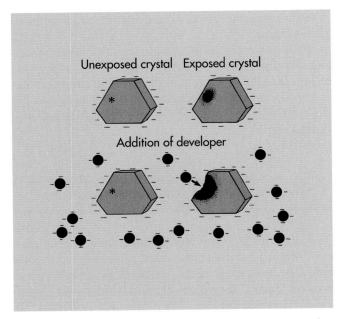

FIGURE 12-3 Development is the chemical process that amplifies the latent image. Only crystals that contain a latent image are reduced to metallic silver by the addition of developing agents.

TABLE 12-2	Components of the Developer and Their Functions	
Component	**Chemical**	**Function**
Developing agent	Phenidone	Reducing agent; produces shades of gray rapidly
	Hydroquinone	Reducing agent; produces black tones slowly
Activator	Sodium carbonate	Helps swell gelatin; produces alkalinity; controls pH
Restrainer	Potassium bromide	Antifog agent; protects unexposed crystals from chemical "attack"
Preservative	Sodium sulfite	Controls oxidation; maintains balance among developer components
Hardener	Glutaraldehyde	Controls emulsion swelling and enhances archival quality
Sequestering agent	Chelates	Removes metallic impurities; stabilizes developing agent
Solvent	Water	Dissolves chemicals for use

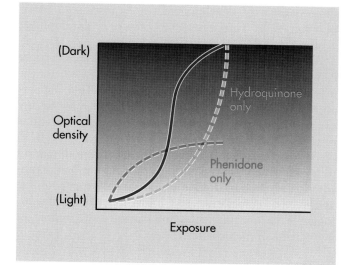

FIGURE 12-4 The shape of the characteristic curve is controlled by the developing agents. Phenidone controls the toe, and hydroquinone controls the shoulder.

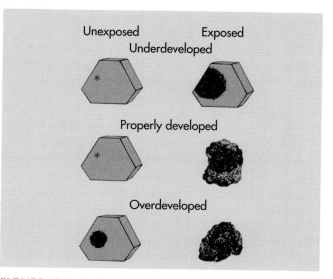

FIGURE 12-5 Underdevelopment results in a dull radiograph because the crystals that contain a latent image have not been completely reduced. Overdevelopment produces a similar radiograph because of the partial reduction of unexposed crystals. Proper development results in maximum contrast.

blackest shades. Phenidone acts rapidly and influences the lighter shades of gray. Phenidone controls the toe of the characteristic curve, and hydroquinone controls the shoulder (Figure 12-4).

An unexposed silver halide crystal has a negative electrostatic charge distributed over its entire surface. An exposed silver halide crystal, on the other hand, has a negative electrostatic charge distributed over its surface, except at the sensitivity center. The similar electrostatic charges on the developing agent and the silver halide crystal make it difficult for the developing agent to penetrate the crystal surface, except in the region of the sensitivity center in an exposed crystal.

In such an exposed crystal, the developing agent penetrates the crystal through the sensitivity center and reduces the remaining silver ions to atomic silver. The sensitivity center can be considered a metallic conducting electrode through which electrons are transferred from the developing agent into the crystal. Development of exposed and unexposed crystals results in the types of differences illustrated in Figure 12-5.

Development occurs over time and depends on factors such as crystal size, developer concentration, and temperature. Initially, metallic silver slowly builds up at the site of the sensitivity center. After complete development has occurred, exposed crystals are destroyed and a grain of black metallic silver is all that remains. Unexposed crystals remain unaffected.

The reduction of a silver ion is accompanied by the liberation of a bromide ion. The bromide ion migrates through the remnant of the crystal into the gelatin portion of the emulsion. From there, the ion is dissolved into the developer and is removed from the film.

The developer contains alkali compounds, such as **sodium carbonate** and **sodium hydroxide**. These **buffering agents** enhance the action of the developing agent by controlling the concentration of hydrogen ions: **the pH.**

These alkali compounds are caustic, that is, they are very corrosive and can cause a skin burn. Sodium hydroxide, the strongest alkali, is commonly called **lye.** Be very cautious if you mix a developer solution that contains sodium hydroxide. You should wear rubber gloves and, of course, never let it get near your mouth or eyes.

Potassium bromide and **potassium iodide** are added to the developer as **restrainers.** Restrainers restrict the action of the developing agent to only those silver halide crystals that have been irradiated. Without the restrainer, even those crystals that have not been exposed are reduced to metallic silver. This results in an increased fog that is called **development fog.**

A **preservative** is also included in the developer to control the oxidation of the developing agent by air. Air is introduced into the chemistry when it is mixed, handled, and stored; such oxidation is called **aerial oxidation.** By controlling aerial oxidation, the preservative helps maintain the proper development rate.

Mixed chemicals last only a couple of weeks; thus, replenishment tanks require close-fitting floating lids for the control of aerial oxidation. Hydroquinone is particularly sensitive to aerial oxidation. It is easy to tell when the developing agent has been oxidized because it turns brownish. The addition of a preservative causes the developer to remain clear. **Sodium sulfite** is the usual preservative.

Developers used in automatic processors contain a **hardener,** usually glutaraldehyde. If the emulsion swells too much or becomes too soft, the film will not be transported properly through the system because of the very close tolerances of the transport system.

The hardener controls swelling and softening of the emulsion. When films that drop from the processor are damp, the usual cause is depletion of the hardener.

 Lack of sufficient glutaraldehyde may be the biggest cause of problems with automatic processing.

The developer may contain metal impurities and soluble salts. Such impurities can accelerate the oxidation of hydroquinone, rendering the developer unstable. **Chelates** are introduced as **sequestering agents** that form stable complexes with these metallic ions and salts.

With proper development, all exposed crystals that contain a latent image are reduced to metallic silver, and unexposed crystals are unaffected. The development process, however, is not perfect: Some crystals that contain a latent image remain undeveloped (unreduced), but other crystals that are unexposed may be developed. Both of these actions reduce the quality of the radiograph.

Film development is basically a chemical reaction. Similar to all chemical reactions, it is governed by three physical characteristics: time, temperature, and concentration (of the developer). Long development time increases reduction of the silver in each grain and promotes the development of the total number of grains. High developer temperature has the same effect.

Similarly, silver reduction is controlled by the concentrations of developing chemicals. With increased developer concentrations, the reducing agent becomes more powerful and can more readily penetrate both exposed and unexposed silver halide crystals.

Manufacturers of x-ray film and of developing chemicals have very carefully determined the optimal conditions of time, temperature, and concentration for proper development. Optimal conditions of contrast, speed, and fog can be expected if the manufacturer's recommendations for development are followed.

Deviation from the manufacturer's recommendations can result in loss of image quality. Figure 12-5 illustrates three degrees of development for exposed and unexposed crystals. The importance of proper development is obvious.

The image on a fogged film is gray and lacks proper contrast. The causes of fog are many, but perhaps the most important are those just mentioned—time, temperature, and developer concentration. An increase in any of these factors beyond manufacturer recommendations results in increased development fog.

Fog also can be produced by chemical contamination of the developer (**chemical fog**), by unintentional exposure to radiation (**radiation fog**), or by improper storage at elevated temperature and humidity. Chemical antifoggants, such as indozoles and triazoles, are important ingredients in the developer.

Fixing

Once development is complete, the film must be treated so that the image will not fade but will remain permanently. This stage of processing is **fixing**. The image is said to be fixed on the film, and this produces film of **archival quality**.

Archival quality refers to the permanence of the radiograph: The image does not deteriorate with age but remains in its original state.

When the film is removed from the developer, some developer is trapped in the emulsion and continues its reducing action. If developing is not stopped, development fog results. As was discussed earlier, the step in manual processing that follows development is called **stop bath**, and its function is just that—to neutralize the residual developer in the emulsion and stop its action. The chemical used in the stop bath is **acetic acid.**

In automatic processing, a stop bath is not used because the rollers of the transport system squeeze the film clean. Furthermore, the fixer contains acetic acid that behaves as a stop bath. This acetic acid, however, is called an **activator**. An activator neutralizes the pH of the emulsion and stops developer action. Table 12-3 lists the chemical components of the fixer.

TABLE 12-3	Components of the Fixer and Their Functions	
Component	**Chemical**	**Function**
Activator	Acetic acid	Neutralizes the developer and stops its action
Fixing agent	Ammonium thiosulfate	Removes undeveloped silver bromine from emulsion
Hardener	Potassium alum	Stiffens and shrinks emulsion
Preservative	Sodium sulfite	Maintains chemical balance
Buffer	Acetate	Maintains proper pH
Sequestering agent	Boric acids/salts	Removes aluminum ions
Solvent	Water	Dissolves other components

The terms **clearing agent, hypo,** and **thiosulfate** often are used interchangeably in reference to the fixing agent. Fixing agents remove unexposed and undeveloped silver halide crystals from the emulsion. Sodium thiosulfate is the agent classically known as hypo, but ammonium thiosulfate is the fixing agent that is used in most fixer chemistries.

Areas in the image-forming x-ray beam where x-rays have been removed by photoelectric absorption result in unexposed silver halide crystals. These unexposed crystals will be removed by the fixer.

Hypo retention is the term used to describe the undesirable retention of the fixer in the emulsion. Excess hypo slowly oxidizes and causes the image to discolor to brown over a long time. Fixing agents retained in the emulsion combine with silver to form silver sulfide, which appears yellow-brown.

 Silver sulfide stain is the most common cause of poor archival quality.

The fixer also contains a chemical called a **hardener.** As the developed and unreduced silver bromide is removed from the emulsion during fixation, the emulsion shrinks. The hardener accelerates this shrinking process and causes the emulsion to become more rigid or hardened.

The purpose of hardeners is to ensure that the film is transported properly through the wash-and-dry section and that rapid and complete drying occurs. The chemicals commonly used as hardeners are **potassium alum, aluminum chloride,** and **chromium alum.** Normally, only one is used in a given formulation.

The fixer also contains a **preservative** that is of the same composition and that serves the same purpose as the preservative in the developer. The preservative is **sodium sulfite,** and it is needed to maintain the chemical balance, because of the carryover of developer and fixer from one tank to another.

The alkalinity/acidity—the pH—of the fixer must remain constant. This is helped by adding a **buffer,** usually acetate, to the fixer.

In the same way that metallic ions are sequestered in the developer, so must they be sequestered in the fixer. Aluminum ions represent the principal impurity at this stage. Boric acids and boric salts are used for sequestering.

Finally, the fixer contains water as the solvent. Other chemicals might be applicable as a solvent, but they are thicker and are more likely to gum up the transport mechanism of the automatic processor.

Washing

The next stage in processing is to wash away any residual chemicals remaining in the emulsion, particularly hypo that clings to the surface of the film. Water is used as the

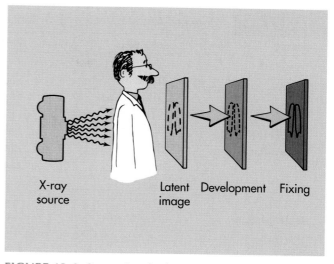

FIGURE 12-6 Converting the latent image to a visible image requires a three-step process.

wash agent. In automatic processing, **the temperature of the wash water should be maintained at approximately 3° C (5° F) below the developer temperature.**

In this way, the wash bath also serves to stabilize developer temperature. Inadequate washing leads to excessive hypo retention and the production of an image that will fade, turn brown with time, and be of generally poor archival quality.

Drying

For the final step in processing, drying the radiograph, warm dry air is blown over both surfaces of the film as it is transported through the drying chamber.

The total sequence of events involved in manual processing takes longer than 1 hour to be completed. Most automatic processors are 90-second processors and require a total time from start to finish—the **dry-to-drop time**—of just that, 90 seconds.

The process of converting the latent image to a visible image can be summarized as a three-step process within the emulsion (Figure 12-6). First, the latent image is formed by exposure of silver halide grains. Next, the exposed grains and only the exposed grains are made visible by development. Finally, fixing removes the unexposed grains from the emulsion and makes the image permanent.

AUTOMATIC PROCESSING

With the introduction of roller transport automatic processing in 1956, the efficiency of radiologic services was increased considerably. Additionally, automatic processing has resulted in better image quality because each radiograph is processed in exactly the same way. The opportunity for human variation and error is nearly absent.

The principal components of an automatic processor are the transport system, the temperature control

TABLE 12-4		Principal Components of an Automatic Processor
System	**Subsystem**	**Purpose**
Transport		Transports film through various stages at precise intervals
	Roller	Supports film movement
	Transport rack	Moves and changes direction of film via rollers and guide shoes
	Drive	Provides power to turn rollers at a precise rate
Temperature		Monitors and adjusts temperature at each stage
Circulation		Agitates fluids
	Developer	Continuously mixes, filters
	Fixer	Continuously mixes
	Wash	Single-pass water flows at constant rate
Replenishment	Developer	Meters and replaces
	Fixer	Meters and replaces
Dryer		Removes moisture, vents exhaust

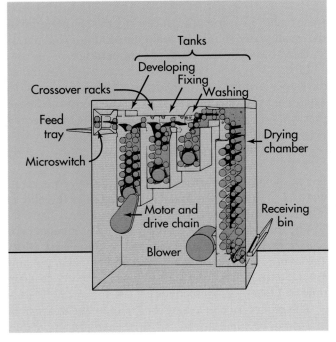

FIGURE 12-7 A cutaway view of an automatic processor. Major components are identified.

system, the circulation system, the replenishment system, and the dryer system (Table 12-4). Figure 12-7 is a cutaway view of an automatic processor.

Transport System

The transport system begins at the **feed tray,** where the film to be processed is inserted into the automatic processor in the darkroom. There, **entrance rollers** grip the film to begin its trip through the processor. A **microswitch** is engaged to control the replenishment rate of the processing chemicals.

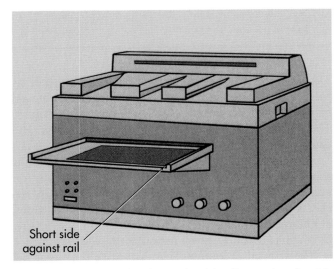

FIGURE 12-8 Place the short side of the film against the side rail of the feed tray.

Always feed the film evenly, using the side rails of the feed tray, and **alternate sides from film to film** (Figure 12-8). This ensures even wear of the transport system components. From the entrance rollers, the film is transported by rollers and racks through the wet chemistry tanks and the drying chamber, and is finally deposited in the receiving bin.

> The shorter dimension of the film should always be against the side rail, so the proper replenishment rate is maintained.

The transport system not only transports the film, it also controls processing by controlling the time the film is immersed in each wet chemical. Timing for each step

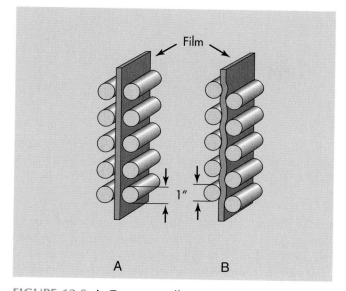

FIGURE 12-9 A, Transport rollers positioned opposite each other. **B,** Transport rollers positioned offset from one another.

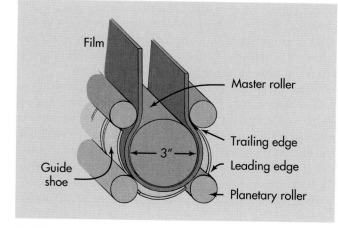

FIGURE 12-10 A master roller with planetary rollers and guide shoes is used to reverse the direction of film in a processor.

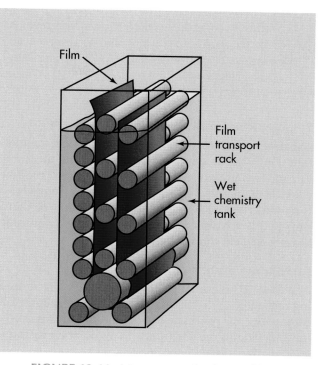

FIGURE 12-11 A transport rack subassembly.

in processing is governed by careful control of the rate of film movement through each stage. The transport system consists of the following three principal subsystems: **rollers, transport racks,** and **drive motor.**

Roller Subassembly. Three types of rollers are used in the transport system. **Transport rollers,** with a diameter of 1 inch, convey the film along its path. They are positioned opposite one another in pairs or are offset from one another (Figure 12-9).

A **master roller** (or solar roller), with a diameter of 3 inches, is used when the film makes a turn in the processor (Figure 12-10). A number of **planetary rollers** and metal or plastic guide shoes are usually positioned around the master roller.

Transport Rack Subassembly. Except for the entering rollers at the feed tray, most of the rollers in the transport system are positioned on a rack assembly (Figure 12-11).

These racks are easily removable and provide for convenient maintenance and efficient cleaning of the processor.

When the film is transported in one direction along the rack assembly, only 1-inch (25-mm) rollers are required to guide and propel it. At each bend, however, a curved metal lip with smooth grooves guides the film around the bend. These are called **guide shoes.** For a 180-degree bend, the film is positioned for the turn by the leading guide shoe, is propelled around the curve by the master roller and its planetary rollers, and leaves the curve by entering the next straight run of rollers through the trailing guide shoe.

Such a system consisting of a master roller, planetary rollers, and guide shoes is called a **turnaround assembly.** The turnaround assembly is located at the bottom of the transport rack assembly. For each chemistry cycle, a transport rack assembly is positioned in the tank.

When the film exits the top of the rack assembly, it is guided to the adjacent rack assembly through a **crossover rack.** The crossover rack is a smaller rack assembly that is composed of rollers and guide shoes.

Drive Subsystem. Power for the transport system is provided by a fractional horsepower drive motor. The shaft of the drive motor is usually reduced to 10 to 20 rpm through a gear reduction assembly. A chain, pulley, or gear assembly transfers power to the transport rack and drives the rollers. Figure 12-12 illustrates the three principal mechanical devices: a belt and pulley, a chain and sprocket, and gears. These devices connect the mechanical energy of the drive motor to the drive motor mechanism of the rack assembly.

The speed of the transport system is controlled by the speed of the motor and the gear reduction system used. The tolerance on this mechanical assembly is rigid.

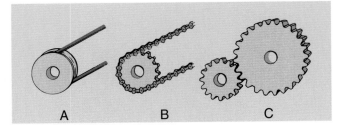

FIGURE 12-12 The three means of transferring power to the transport rack. **A,** Belt and pulley. **B,** Chain and sprocket. **C,** Gears.

Temperature Control System

The developer, fixer, and wash require precise temperature control. The developer temperature is most critical, and it is usually maintained at 35° C (95° F). Wash water is maintained at 3° C (5° F) lower. Temperature is monitored at each stage by a thermocouple or thermistor and is controlled thermostatically by a controlled heating element in each tank.

Circulation System

Agitation is necessary to continually mix the processing chemicals, to maintain a constant temperature throughout the processing tank, and to aid exposure of the emulsion to the chemicals. In automatic processing, a circulation system continuously pumps the developer and the fixer, thus maintaining constant agitation within each tank.

The developer circulation system requires a filter that traps particles as small as approximately 100 μm to trap flecks of gelatin that are dislodged from the emulsion. The particles thus have less chance of becoming attached to the rollers, where they can produce artifacts. These filters are not 100% efficient; therefore, sludge can build up on the rollers.

 Cleaning the tanks and the transport system should be a part of the routine maintenance of any processor.

Filtration in the fixer circulation system is normally unnecessary because the fixer hardens and shrinks the gelatin so that the rollers are not coated. Furthermore, the fixer neutralizes the developer; therefore, the products of this reaction do not affect the final radiograph.

Water must be circulated through the wash tank to remove all of the processing chemicals from the surface of the film before drying; this ensures archival quality. An open system, rather than a closed circulation system, usually is used. Fresh tap water is piped into the tank at the bottom and overflows out the top, where it is collected and discharged directly to the sewer system. The minimum flow rate for the wash tank in most processors is 12 L/min (3 gal/min).

Replenishment System

Each time a film makes its way through the processor, it uses some of the processing chemicals. Some developer is absorbed into the emulsion and then is neutralized during fixing. The fixer, likewise, is absorbed during that stage of processing, and some is carried over into the wash tank.

If neither the developer nor the fixer is replenished, each quickly loses chemical balance and the level of solution in each tank drops, resulting in short contact times of the film with the chemicals.

The replenishment system meters the proper quantities of chemicals into each tank to maintain volume and chemical activity. Although replenishment of the developer is more important, the fixer also has to be replenished. Wash water is not recirculated and therefore is continuously and completely replenished.

When a film is inserted onto the feed tray with its widest dimension gripped by the leading rollers and its narrow side against the side rail, a microswitch is activated and turns on the replenishment for as long as film travels through the microswitch. Replenishment rates are approximately 60 to 70 ml of developer and 100 to 110 ml of fixer for every 14 inches (35 cm) of film.

Exact film response to overreplenishment or underreplenishment depends on many emulsion variables, making it difficult to make accurate statements. Usually, if the replenishment rate is increased, radiographic contrast is slightly increased. If the rate is too low, contrast decreases significantly.

Dryer System

A wet or damp finished radiograph easily picks up dust particles that can result in artifacts. Furthermore, a wet or damp film is difficult to handle in a viewbox. When stored, it can become sticky and may be destroyed.

The dryer system consists of a blower, ventilation ducts, drying tubes, and an exhaust system. The dryer system extracts all residual moisture from the processed radiograph, so it drops into the receiving bin dry.

A processor should be run at a negative internal air pressure so that air is continually being sucked in and the fume-laden moist air vented externally. Ideally, the receiving bin, which obviously faces the adjacent work area, should have a lid on it to prevent escape of fumes.

The blower is a fan that sucks in room air and blows it across heating coils through ductwork to the drying tubes. Therefore, room air should be low in humidity and free of dust. Sometimes, as many as three heating coils of approximately 2500 W capacity are used. The temperature of the air entering the drying chamber is thermostatically regulated.

 Most processing faults leading to damp film are due to depletion of glutaraldehyde, the hardener in the developer.

The drying tubes are long, hollow cylinders with slitlike openings that extend the length of the cylinder and face the film. They are positioned on both sides of the film as it is transported through the drying chamber.

The hot, moist air is vented from the drying chamber to the outside, in much the same way as the air in a clothes dryer is vented. Some fraction of the exhaust air may be recirculated within the dryer system.

A finished radiograph that is damp easily picks up dust particles that could result in artifacts.

When damp films drop into the receiving bin, the radiologic technologist should immediately suspect a malfunction of the dryer system, although developer and fixer replenishment also should be checked. Underreplenishment reduces the concentration of hardener and is a common cause of damp films.

ALTERNATIVE PROCESSING METHODS

We tend to think that most of the recent advances in medical x-ray imaging are associated with the imaging devices. This is certainly true. We forget, however, the excellent progress made by radiographic film manufacturers in improving image quality and enhancing the efficiency of radiology departments.

Rapid processing and extended processing are attractive alternatives in many imaging facilities. Daylight processing is fast becoming standard in medical imaging.

Rapid Processing

No matter what the task, today we want to do it faster. Medical imaging is no exception. The manufacturers of radiographic film have developed microprocessor-controlled equipment and specially formulated processing chemicals for this task. Processing can now be as rapid as 30 seconds.

These rapid processors are useful in angiography, special procedures, surgery, and emergency rooms, where time is most critical. Here, it is important to make radiographic images available for physicians as soon as possible. When used with proper chemistry, rapid processing produces images with sensitometric properties similar to those of 90-second processing.

For rapid processing, the chemicals are more concentrated and the developer and fixer temperatures are higher. Consequently, it is not possible to switch from standard to rapid processing between films.

Extended Processing

Extended processing is particularly useful in mammography. Whereas the standard processing time is 90 seconds, extended processing may take as long as 3 minutes. Developer immersion time is nearly doubled, but it is not necessary to alter developer temperature. Furthermore, standard chemicals may be used. The only significant disadvantage is the longer dry-to-drop time.

Two principal advantages are associated with extended processing: greater image contrast and lower patient dose. Contrast is increased by approximately 15%. Image receptor sensitivity is increased by at least 30%. Thus, patient radiation dose is reduced by at least 30%.

Improvements in extended processing in terms of contrast and patient dose occur only with single-emulsion film. Extended processing is not recommended for double-emulsion films because improvement in contrast or dose is insignificant with such films.

Daylight Processing

Aside from the speed with which images are developed, another change is quietly taking place in radiology department darkrooms. They are disappearing! Consequently, the position of the darkroom technologist also is disappearing.

Daylight systems are being adopted. When a daylight system is used (Figure 12-13), the radiologic technologist needs only position a cassette with an exposed film into the appropriate slot of this system. The film is automatically extracted from the cassette and is sent to the processor.

The processor may be an integral part of the daylight system, or it may be a separate unit docked to the daylight system. The cassette is reloaded with unexposed film of proper size before it is released by the system for the next exposure.

Speed is the quality that makes the daylight system attractive. It takes only about 15 seconds for the radiologic technologist to insert the exposed cassette into the daylight loader and retrieve a fresh cassette. Total load, unload, and processing time is approximately 2 minutes. Multiple film sizes are automatically accommodated.

Microprocessor technology makes daylight systems possible. The microprocessor automatically monitors and controls unloading and reloading of the cassette by sensing the cassette size and the film consumption rate.

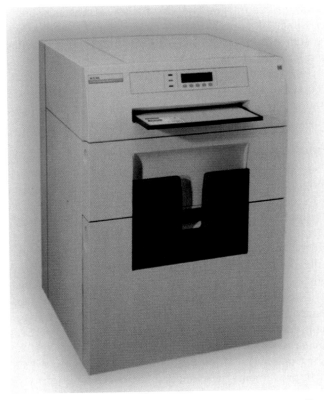

FIGURE 12-13 A daylight processing system. (Courtesy Eastman Kodak.)

Most daylight systems can accommodate up to 1000 sheets of radiographic film of various sizes. Some units also can annotate the radiograph with data such as the date, time, and other examination characteristics. System status is continuously indicated with light-emitting diodes (LEDs) or liquid crystal displays (LCDs). Some models are on rollers for even greater flexibility.

Dry Processing

Dry processing refers to the development of images without the use of wet chemistry. Many advantages are associated with dry processing, and these are driving its use in replacing wet chemistry processing:

- Elimination of handling, maintenance, and disposal of chemicals
- No darkroom required (space saved)
- No plumbing required
- Less environmental impact
- Reduced capital cost
- Reduced operating cost
- Higher throughput

Although dry processing can be performed through several approaches, two technologies prevail at this time: photothermography (PTG) and thermography (TG).

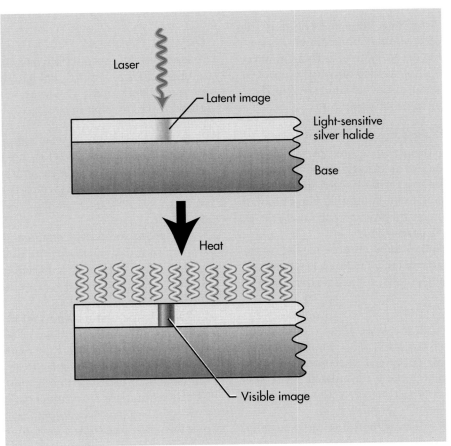

FIGURE 12-14 This photothermograph method of dry processing uses a laser to form a latent image and heat to process the image.

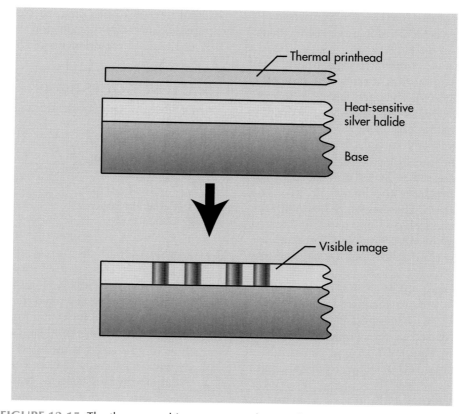

FIGURE 12-15 The thermographic process uses heat to directly produce a visible image.

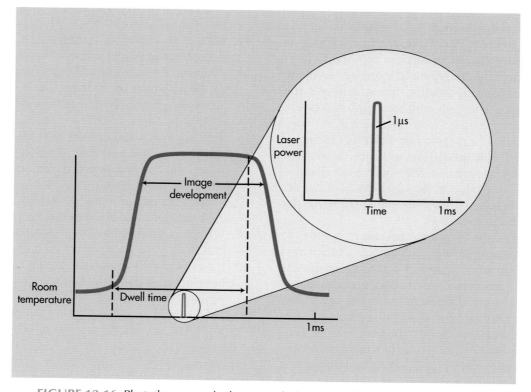

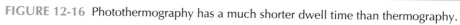

FIGURE 12-16 Photothermography has a much shorter dwell time than thermography.

The basic difference between the two is in the manner in which the latent image is recorded and the visible image processed onto the film media.

PTG uses a low-power modulated laser beam to record the image signal on the film, thereby generating the latent image (Figure 12-14). The latent image so formed on the sensitized silver halide emulsion is subsequently developed by a thermal process at 125°C that takes approximately 15 seconds—the so-called **dwell time.**

TG technology, on the other hand, uses a modulated heat source, referred to as a "print head," that heats the film and produces the image directly. The print head converts electrical energy into heat with the use of resistive elements. No latent image is created in the TG technology because organic silver salts are directly developed by the application of localized heat (Figure 12-15).

One of the advantages of PTG is that the laser beam can be modulated in a more accurate fashion over a very short interval (1 μs) compared with heat in the print head of a TG-based system (1 ms). This characteristic is shown in Figure 12-16 and can result in increased image blur in TG systems compared with PTG systems.

Because of the discrete size of the print head and its physical contact with the film media, the TG technique may result in a pixilated image. Furthermore, dust accumulated between the print head and the film media can cause loss of image.

SUMMARY

Converting the latent image to a visible image requires a three-step process. First, the latent image is formed when silver halide grains are exposed to light or x-rays. Next, only the grains so exposed are made visible by development. Finally, fixing removes the unexposed grains from the emulsion and makes the image permanent.

The 90-second radiographic film processor is the industry standard. The processing sequence consists of (1) wetting, (2) developing, (3) stop bath, (4) fixing, (5) washing, and (6) drying. Tables 12-2 and 12-3 list the chemicals and their functions as they are used in the developing and fixing processes.

Components of the automatic processor include (1) the transport system, (2) the temperature control system, (3) the circulation system, (4) the replenishment system, and (5) the dryer system. Diagnostic imaging departments may have alternative processing systems as well. Extended processing is used to develop specialty films such as single-emulsion mammography screen-film. Daylight processing allows radiographers to provide uninterrupted patient care. The daylight system commonly is used in critical care areas such as the emergency department.

Photothermography and thermography are image processing methods that do not require chemistry and all the attendant requirements of chemistry.

CHALLENGE QUESTIONS

1. Define or otherwise identify the following:
   a. Solvent
   b. Glutaraldehyde
   c. Reducing agent
   d. Synergism
   e. Archival quality
   f. Planetary roller
   g. Guide shoe
   h. Extended processing
   i. LED
   j. Dry-to-drop
2. Identify the steps involved in the automatic processing of a radiograph and the time required for each step when a 90-second processor is used.
3. Describe the actions of Phenidone and hydroquinone in producing optical density on a radiograph.
4. By what other name is fixer known?
5. What are the characteristic features of daylight processing?
6. During the wash cycle, what restrictions are placed on temperature and flow rate?
7. What is a redox reaction?
8. When did automatic processing begin?
9. Which company invented the first roller transport processing system?
10. What types of processors are used at the clinical sites you visit?
11. What is the universal wetting agent?
12. What is the principal action of development?
13. What is the process of making a latent image visible with laser light? How does it work?
14. Name the principal component of developer solutions.
15. Why are gloves and goggles recommended for persons who mix or handle developer solutions?
16. What happens over time if the preservative is not added to the developer?
17. If a film is damp or wet when it drops into the receiving bin, what is the problem and the probable cause?
18. Why does the film have to go through the fixer tank?
19. If a radiographic film turns brown once it has been stored in the file room, what may be the problem?
20. How should each x-ray film be fed onto the feed tray of the automatic processor? Why is this important?

The answers to the Challenge Questions can be found by logging on to our website at http://evolve.elsevier.com.

CHAPTER 13

Radiographic Intensifying Screens

OBJECTIVES

At the completion of this chapter, the student should be able
to do the following:

1. Describe the component layers of a radiographic intensifying screen
2. Discuss luminescence and its relationship to phosphorescence and fluorescence
3. Define and use the term *intensification factor*
4. Identify how detective quantum efficiency (DQE) and conversion efficiency (CE) affect radiographic intensifying screen speed
5. Describe image noise and image blur
6. Discuss the various screen-film combinations
7. Describe the handling and cleaning of radiographic intensifying screens

OUTLINE

Screen Construction
  Protective Coating
  Phosphor
  Reflective Layer
  Base
Luminescence
Screen Characteristics
  Screen Speed
  Image Noise
  Spatial Resolution
Screen-Film Combinations
  Cassette
  Carbon Fiber Material
  Direct Film Exposure versus Screen-Film Exposure
  Rare Earth Screens
Care of Screens

RADIOGRAPHIC INTENSIFYING screens are part of the conventional image receptor. The image receptor (IR) includes the cassette (which is the protective holder), the radiographic intensifying screens, and the radiographic film.

Although some x-rays reach the film emulsion, it is actually visible light from the radiographic intensifying screens that exposes the radiographic film. Visible light is emitted from the phosphor of the radiographic intensifying screens, which is activated by the image-forming x-rays exiting the patient.

This chapter discusses the components of a radiographic intensifying screen, how these components contribute to a screen's performance characteristics, the properties of rare Earth screens, and the importance of spectral matching.

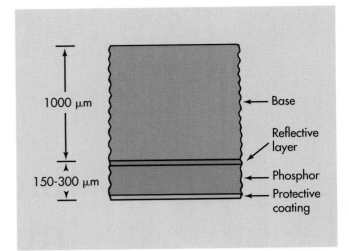

FIGURE 13-1 Cross-sectional view of an intensifying screen, showing its four principal layers.

SCREEN CONSTRUCTION

Use of film to detect x-rays and to image anatomical structures is inefficient. In fact, less than 1% of the x-rays incident on radiographic film interact with the film and contribute to the latent image.

Most radiographs are made with the film in contact with a radiographic intensifying screen because the use of film alone requires a high patient dose. A radiographic intensifying screen is a device that converts the energy of the x-ray beam into visible light. This visible light then interacts with the radiographic film, forming the latent image.

Approximately 30% of the x-rays that strike a radiographic intensifying screen interact with the screen. For each such interaction, a large number of visible light photons are emitted.

 The radiographic intensifying screen amplifies the effect of image-forming x-rays that reach the screen-film cassette.

On the one hand, use of a radiographic intensifying screen lowers patient dose considerably; on the other hand, the image is slightly blurred. With modern screens, however, such image blur is not serious.

Radiographic intensifying screens resemble flexible sheets of plastic or cardboard. They come in sizes that correspond to film sizes.

Usually, the radiographic film is sandwiched between two screens. The film used is called **double-emulsion film** because it has an emulsion coating on both sides of the base. Most screens have four distinct layers; these are shown in cross section in Figure 13-1.

Protective Coating

The layer of the radiographic intensifying screen closest to the radiographic film is the **protective coating**. It is 10 to 20 µm thick and is applied to the face of the screen to make the screen resistant to the abrasion and damage caused by handling. This layer also helps to eliminate the buildup of static electricity and provides a surface for routine cleaning without disturbing the active phosphor. The protective layer is transparent to light.

Phosphor

The active layer of the radiographic intensifying screen is the **phosphor.** The phosphor emits light during stimulation by x-rays. Phosphor layers vary in thickness from 50 to 300 µm, depending on the type of screen. The active substance of most phosphors before about 1980 was crystalline **calcium tungstate** embedded in a polymer matrix. The **rare Earth** elements gadolinium, lanthanum, and yttrium are the phosphor material in newer, faster screens.

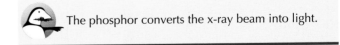 The phosphor converts the x-ray beam into light.

The action of the phosphor can be seen by viewing an opened cassette in a darkened room through the protective window of the control booth. The radiographic intensifying screen glows brightly when exposed to x-rays.

Many materials react in this way, but radiography requires that materials possess the characteristics given in Box 13-1. Through the years, several materials have been used as phosphors because they exhibit these characteristics. These materials include **calcium tungstate, zinc sulfide, barium lead sulfate,** and oxysulfides of the rare Earths **gadolinium, lanthanum,** and **yttrium.**

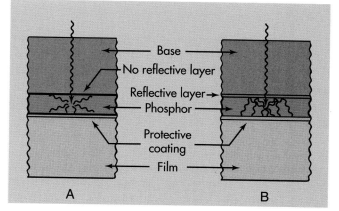

FIGURE 13-2 **A,** Screen without reflective layer. **B,** Screen with reflective layer. Screens without reflective layers are not as efficient as those with reflective layers because fewer light photons reach the film.

Roentgen discovered x-rays quite by accident. He observed the luminescence of **barium platinocyanide,** a phosphor that was never successfully applied to diagnostic radiology. Within a year of Roentgen's discovery of x-rays, the American inventor Thomas A. Edison developed calcium tungstate. Although Edison demonstrated the use of radiographic intensifying screens before the beginning of the 20th century, screen-film combinations did not come into general use until about the time of World War I. With improved manufacturing techniques and quality control procedures, calcium tungstate proved superior for nearly all radiographic techniques and, until the 1970s, was used almost exclusively as the phosphor.

Since then, rare Earth screens have been used in diagnostic radiology. These screens are faster than those made of calcium tungstate, rendering them more useful for most types of radiographic imaging. Use of rare Earth screens results in lower patient dose, less thermal stress on the x-ray tube, and reduced shielding for x-ray rooms.

Differences in screen imaging characteristics are primarily due to differences in phosphor composition. The thickness of the phosphor layer and the concentration and size of the phosphor crystals also influence the action of intensifying screens. The thickness of the phosphor layer is approximately 50 to 300 μm; individual phosphor crystals are 5 to 15 μm thick.

Reflective Layer

Between the phosphor and the base is a reflective layer, approximately 25 μm thick, that is made of a shiny substance such as magnesium oxide or titanium dioxide (Figure 13-2). When x-rays interact with the phosphor, light is emitted isotropically.

Less than half of this light is emitted in the direction of the film. The reflective layer intercepts light headed in other directions and redirects it to the film. The reflective layer enhances the efficiency of the radiographic

intensifying screen, nearly doubling the number of light photons that reach the film.

Isotropic emission refers to radiation emitted with equal intensity in all directions.

Some radiographic intensifying screens incorporate special dyes in the phosphor layer to selectively absorb those light photons emitted at a large angle to the film. These light photons increase image blur. Because they must travel a longer distance in the phosphor than those emitted perpendicular to the film, these photons are more easily absorbed by the dye. Unfortunately, this addition reduces screen speed somewhat.

Base

The layer farthest from the film is the **base.** The base is approximately 1 mm thick and serves principally as a mechanical support for the active phosphor layer. Polyester is the popular base material in radiographic intensifying screens, just as it is for radiographic film. Box 13-2 presents the requirements for a base material of high quality.

LUMINESCENCE

Any material that emits light in response to some outside stimulation is called a **luminescent material,** or a **phosphor,** and the emitted visible light is called **luminescence.** A number of stimuli, including electric current (the fluorescent light), biochemical reactions (the lightning bug), visible light (a watch dial), and x-rays (a radiographic intensifying screen), cause luminescence in materials.

Luminescence is similar to characteristic x-ray emission. However, luminescence involves **outer-shell electrons** (Figure 13-3). In a radiographic intensifying screen, absorption of a single x-ray causes emission of thousands of light photons.

When a luminescent material is stimulated, the outer-shell electrons are raised to excited energy levels. This effectively creates a hole in the outer-shell electron, which is an unstable condition for the atom. The hole is filled when the excited electron returns to its normal state. This transition is accompanied by the emission of a visible light photon.

The range of excited energy states for an outer-shell electron is narrow, and these states depend on the structure of the luminescent material. The wavelength of emitted light is determined by the level of excitation to which the electron was raised and is characteristic of a given luminescent material. In other words, luminescent materials emit light of a characteristic color.

Two types of luminescence have been identified. If visible light is emitted only while the phosphor is stimulated, the process is called **fluorescence.** If, on the other hand, the phosphor continues to emit light after stimulation, the process is called **phosphorescence.**

Some materials can phosphoresce for long periods after stimulation. For example, a light-stimulated watch dial will fade slowly in a dark closet. Radiographic intensifying screens fluoresce. Phosphorescence in an intensifying screen is called **screen lag** or **afterglow** and is undesirable.

SCREEN CHARACTERISTICS

The radiologic technologist is concerned with three primary characteristics of radiographic intensifying screens: screen speed, image noise, and spatial resolution.

Because screens are used to reduce patient dose, one characteristic is the magnitude of dose reduction. This property is called the **intensification factor** and is a measure of the **speed** of the screen.

With some exceptions, an increase in screen speed can result in increased **image noise.** Image noise, the speckled appearance on some images, has several sources (see Chapter 16).

Unfortunately, when image-forming x-rays are converted to visible light and the visible light in turn produces the latent image, the image is blurred somewhat. The **spatial resolution** of the screen is its ability to produce an accurate and clear image. Resolution usually is measured by the minimum line spacing that can be detected and imaged. See Chapter 25 for a discussion of spatial resolution measured in terms of line pairs per millimeter (lp/mm).

Screen Speed

Many types of radiographic intensifying screens are available, and each manufacturer uses different names to identify them. Collectively, however, screens usually are identified by their relative speed expressed numerically. Screen speeds range from 100 (slow, detail) to 1200 (very fast).

Screen speed is a relative number that describes how efficiently x-rays are converted into light. Par-speed calcium tungstate screens are assigned a value of 100 and serve as the basis for comparison of all other screens. Calcium tungstate screens seldom are used anymore. High-speed rare Earth screens have speeds up to 1200; detail screens have speeds of approximately 50 to 80. These and other characteristics are summarized in Table 13-1.

The speed of a radiographic intensifying screen conveys no information regarding patient dose. This information is related by the intensification factor (IF). The IF is defined as the ratio of the exposure required to produce the same optical density with a screen to the exposure required to produce an optical density without a screen.

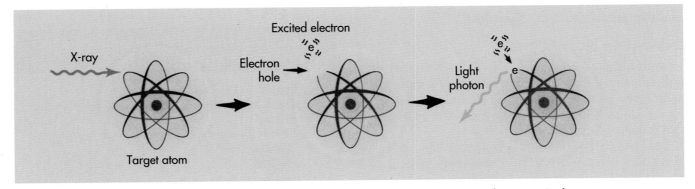

FIGURE 13-3 Luminescence occurs when an outer-shell electron is raised to an excited state and returns to its normal state with the emission of a light photon.

Table 13-1	Characteristics of Typical Radiographic Intensifying Screens	
	TYPE OF SCREEN	
Characteristic Type of Phosphor	**Calcium Tungstate**	**Oxysulfides and Oxybromides of Y, La, Gd**
Color of emission	Blue	Green or blue
Approximate speed	50-200	80-1200
Intensification factor	20-100	40-400
Resolution (lp/mm)	8-15	8-15

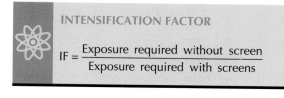

INTENSIFICATION FACTOR

$$IF = \frac{\text{Exposure required without screen}}{\text{Exposure required with screens}}$$

The optical density chosen for comparison of one radiographic intensifying screen versus another is usually 1.0. The value of the IF can be used to determine the dose reduction accompanying the use of a screen.

Question: A pelvic examination performed with a 100 speed radiographic intensifying screen is taken at 75 kVp, 50 mAs and results in an entrance skin exposure (ESE) of 200 mR (2 mGy$_a$). A similar examination taken without screens would result in an ESE of 6400 mR (64 mGy$_a$). What is the approximate IF of the screen-film combination?

Answer: $IF = \dfrac{6400}{200} = 32$

Several factors influence radiographic intensifying screen speed; some of these are controlled by the radiologic technologist. Ultimately, the screen speed is determined by the relative number of x-rays that interact with the phosphor, and how efficiently x-ray energy is converted into the visible light that interacts with the film.

Box 13-3 gives the properties of radiographic intensifying screens that affect screen speed and **cannot be controlled by the radiologic technologist.** They are listed in their relative order of importance.

Several conditions that affect radiographic intensifying screen speed **are controlled by the radiologic technologist.** These include radiation quality, image processing, and temperature.

Radiation Quality. As x-ray tube potential is increased, the IF also increases (Figure 13-4). Although this

BOX 13-3   Properties of Radiographic Intensifying Screens That Are Not Controlled by the Radiologic Technologist

- **Phosphor composition.** Rare earth phosphors efficiently convert x-rays into usable light.
- **Phosphor thickness.** The thicker the phosphor layer, the higher is the DQE. High-speed screens have thick phosphor layers; fine-detailed screens have thin phosphor layers.
- **Reflective layer.** The presence of a reflective layer increases screen speed but also increases image blur.
- **Dye.** Light-absorbing dyes are added to some phosphors to control the spread of light. These dyes improve spatial resolution but reduce speed.
- **Crystal size.** Larger individual phosphor crystals produce more light per x-ray interaction. The crystals of detail screens are approximately half the size of the crystals of high-speed screens.
- **Concentration of phosphor crystals.** Higher crystal concentration results in higher screen speed.

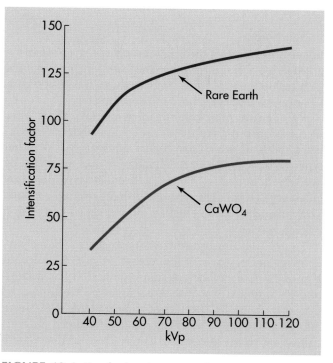

FIGURE 13-4 Graph showing approximate variation of the intensification factor (IF) with kVp.

may seem contrary to the discussion of x-ray absorption in Chapter 10, it is not.

In Chapter 10, x-ray absorption was shown to decrease with increasing kVp. Remember, however, that the IF is the ratio of x-ray absorption in a radiographic intensifying screen to that in radiographic film alone.

Screens have higher effective atomic numbers than films; therefore, although true absorption in the screen decreases with increasing kVp, relative absorption compared with that in film increases. At 70 kVp, the IF for a typical par-speed screen is 60, whereas that for a rare Earth screen is 150.

Image Processing. Only the superficial layers of the emulsion are affected when radiographic film is exposed to light. However, the emulsion is affected uniformly throughout when the film is exposed to x-rays.

Therefore, excessive developing time for screen-film results in lowering of the IF because the emulsion nearest the base contains no latent image, yet it can be reduced to silver if the developer is allowed sufficient time to penetrate the emulsion to the depth. This too is relatively unimportant because films manufactured for use with screens have thinner emulsion layers than those produced for direct exposure.

Temperature. Radiographic intensifying screens emit more light per x-ray interaction at low temperatures than at high temperatures. Consequently, the IF is lower at higher temperatures. This characteristic, although it is relatively unimportant in a clinic with a controlled environment, can be significant in field work in hot or cold climates.

Image Noise

Image noise appears on a radiograph as a speckled background. It occurs most often when fast screens and high-kVp techniques are used. Noise reduces image contrast. Chapter 16 discusses noise more completely.

Rare Earth radiographic intensifying screens have increased speed because of two important characteristics, both of which are higher compared with other types of screens. The percentage of x-rays absorbed by the screen is higher. This is called **detective quantum efficiency (DQE).** The amount of light emitted for each x-ray absorbed also is higher. This is called **conversion efficiency (CE).**

Figure 13-5 illustrates why an increase in CE increases image noise, whereas an increase in DQE does not. In Figure 13-5, *A,* a calcium tungstate screen has a DQE of 20% and a CE of 5%. A radiographic technique of 10 mAs results in 1000 x-rays incident on the screen, 200 of which are absorbed, resulting in light photons equivalent to 10 x-rays. We could say that this system has a speed of 100.

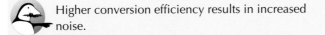

Higher conversion efficiency results in increased noise.

If phosphor thickness is doubled as in Figure 13-5, *B,* the DQE increases to 40%, so the mAs can be reduced to 5 mAs. The speed is now 200, but there is no increase in noise because the same number of x-rays is absorbed.

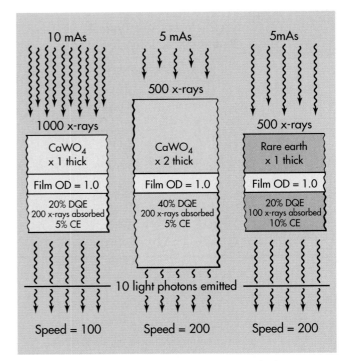

FIGURE 13-5 Image noise increases with higher conversion efficiency (CE) but not with higher detective quantum efficiency (DQE).

However, if the phosphor is changed to one with a CE of 10%, the speed is doubled at the expense of increased noise (Figure 13-5, *C,*). A 200-speed screen is attained because twice as much light is emitted per x-ray absorption. Only half as many x-rays are required, and this results in increased **quantum mottle,** a principal component of image noise.

$$DQE = \frac{\#x\text{-rays absorbed}}{\#\text{incident x-rays}} \times 100$$

$$CE = \frac{\text{emitted light}}{\text{x-rays absorbed}} \times 100$$

Quantum mottle often is a direct result of use of very fast speed screen-film systems that require very small amounts of exposure and result in a grainy, mottled, or splotchy image.

In practice, rare Earth screens of the same spatial resolution are at least twice as fast as calcium tungstate, with no significant increase in noise. Rare Earth screens have higher DQE and CE, but the gain in speed is principally due to DQE.

Spatial Resolution

Radiographers often use the term **image detail** or **visibility of detail** when describing image quality. These qualitative terms combine the quantitative measures of spatial resolution and contrast resolution. *Spatial resolution* refers to how small an object can be imaged. *Contrast resolution* refers to the ability to image similar tissues, such as liver and pancreas or gray matter and white matter.

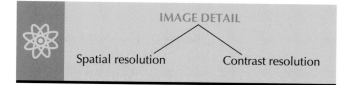

The use of radiographic intensifying screens adds one more step to the process of imaging with x-rays. Radiographic intensifying screens have the disadvantage of lower spatial resolution compared with direct-exposure radiographs.

Spatial resolution is measured in a number of ways and can be assigned a numeric value. Spatial resolution is limited principally by effective focal spot size. For our purposes, a general description should be sufficient.

A photograph in focus shows good spatial resolution; one out of focus shows poor spatial resolution and therefore much image blur. Figure 13-6 shows the differences in spatial resolution between a direct-exposure film and a par-speed screen-film combination obtained when an x-ray test pattern is imaged.

Such a test pattern is called a line-pair test pattern. It consists of lead lines separated by interspaces of equal size. As is discussed more completely in Chapter 25, spatial resolution may be expressed by the number of line pairs per millimeter (lp/mm) that are

imaged. The higher this number, the smaller is the object that can be imaged and the better is the spatial resolution.

Very fast screens can resolve 7 lp/mm, and fine-detail screens can resolve 15 lp/mm (see Table 13-1). Direct-exposure film can resolve 50 lp/mm. The unaided eye can resolve about 10 lp/mm.

When x-rays interact with the screen's phosphor, the area of the film emulsion that is activated by the emitted light is larger than it would be with direct x-ray exposure. This situation results in reduced spatial resolution or increased image blur.

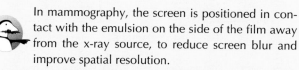

Generally, those conditions that increase the IF reduce spatial resolution.

High-speed screens have low spatial resolution, and fine-detail screens have high spatial resolution. Spatial resolution improves with smaller phosphor crystals and thinner phosphor layers. Figure 13-7 shows how these factors affect image resolution. Unfortunately, these factors are not controlled by the radiologic technologist.

In mammography, the screen is positioned in contact with the emulsion on the side of the film away from the x-ray source, to reduce screen blur and improve spatial resolution.

In both parts of Figure 13-7, the x-ray is shown to interact with the phosphor soon after entry; this results in screen blur. Screen blur is reduced in thinner screens.

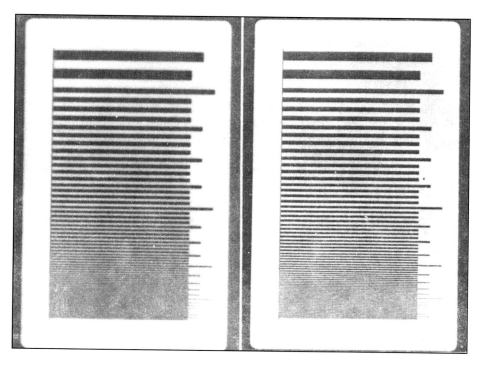

FIGURE 13-6 Radiographs of an x-ray test pattern made with direct-exposure film *(right)* and a par-speed screen-film combination *(left)*. The difference in image blur is obvious.

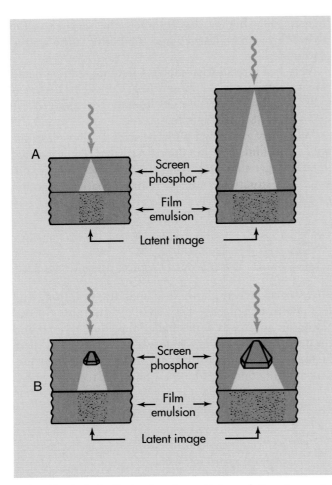

FIGURE 13-7 **A,** Reduction in spatial resolution is greater when phosphor layers are thick. **B,** Reduction also is greater when crystal size is large. These same conditions increase screen speed and reduce patient dose by producing a greater number of light photons per incident x-ray.

Figure 13-8 illustrates how spatial resolution is improved in mammography by placing the single-emulsion film on the tube side of the cassette (see Chapter 22 for a more complete discussion).

SCREEN-FILM COMBINATIONS

Screens and films are manufactured for compatibility; this helps to ensure good results.

Radiographic intensifying screens are nearly always used in pairs. Figure 13-9 is a cross section of a properly loaded cassette that contains front and back screens with a double-emulsion film. Production of the latent image is nearly evenly divided between front and back screens, with less than 1% being contributed directly by x-ray interaction. Each screen exposes the emulsion it contacts.

 Screen-film compatibility is essential; use only those films for which the screens are designed.

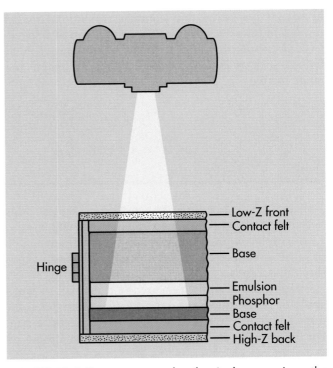

FIGURE 13-8 For mammography, the single screen is on the far side of the emulsion to reduce screen blur.

In addition to reduced patient dose, use of radiographic intensifying screens in an image receptor offer several advantages (Box 13-4). Attaining these advantages requires proper selection, handling, and use of a screen-film combination.

Cassette

The **cassette** is the rigid holder that contains the film and radiographic intensifying screens. The front cover, the side facing the x-ray source, is made of material with a low atomic number such as plastic. It is thin, yet sturdy. The front cover of the cassette is designed for minimum attenuation of the x-ray beam.

Attached to the inside of the front cover is the front screen, and attached to the back cover is the back screen. The radiographic film is sandwiched between the two screens.

Between each screen and the cassette cover is some sort of **compression device,** such as radiolucent plastic foam, which maintains close screen-film contact when the cassette is closed and latched.

The back cover is usually made of heavy metal to minimize backscatter. The x-rays transmitted through the screen-film combination to the back cover more readily undergo photoelectric effect in a high-Z material than in a low-Z material.

X-rays can be transmitted through the entire cassette, and some might be scattered back to the film by the cassette-holding device or a nearby wall. This is called **backscatter** radiation and results in image fog.

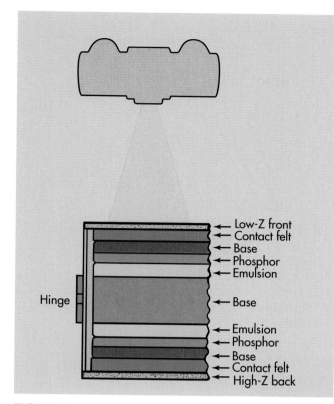

FIGURE 13-9 Cross-sectional view of cassette containing front and back screens and loaded with double-emulsion film.

BOX 13-4 Advantages of Proper Screen-Film Use

INCREASED
- Flexibility of kVp selection
- Adjustment of radiographic contrast
- Spatial resolution when smaller focal spots are used
- Capacity for magnification radiography

DECREASED
- Patient dose
- Occupational exposure
- X-ray tube heat production
- X-ray exposure time
- X-ray tube mA
- Focal spot size

Sometimes, the cassette hinges or hold-down clamps on the back cover are imaged. This occurs because of backscatter radiation, normally only during high-kVp radiography when the x-ray beam is sufficiently penetrating.

Carbon Fiber Material

One of the materials developed early in the space exploration program was **carbon fiber.** This material was developed for nose cone applications because of its superior strength and heat resistance. It consists principally of graphite fibers ($Z_C = 6$) in a plastic matrix that can be formed to any shape or thickness.

In radiology, this material now is used widely in devices designed to reduce patient exposure. A cassette with a front that consists of carbon fiber material absorbs only approximately half the number of x-rays that an aluminum or plastic cassette does.

Carbon fiber also is used as pallet material for fluoroscopic examination tables and computed tomography beds.

Carbon fiber not only reduces patient exposure, it also may produce longer x-ray tube life because of the lower-demand radiographic techniques required.

Direct Film Exposure versus Screen-Film Exposure

The principal advantage associated with the use of radiographic intensifying screens is that fewer x-rays are needed than in direct-exposure techniques. Indeed, there is no reason to avoid using radiographic intensifying screens, except in dental radiography.

Table 13-2 shows the relative number of x-rays and light photons at various stages for radiographs taken directly and with a par-speed screen-film combination. This table assumes an IF of 50.

The major differences are due to the interaction of x-rays with the screen phosphor and to the large number of visible-light photons produced by each of these interactions. Unfortunately, the number of latent image centers formed is less than 1% of the number of light photons produced.

From its introduction in 1896 by Thomas Edison until the 1970s, calcium tungstate ($CaWO_4$) was used almost exclusively as the phosphor for radiographic intensifying screens. Such screens, however, exhibit only 5% CE.

One reason why calcium tungstate is a useful screen phosphor is that it emits light in the violet-to-blue region. The sensitivity of conventional radiographic

TABLE 13-2	Comparison of Relative Numbers of X-rays and Light Photons at Various Stages for Direct and Screen-Film Exposure*	
	TYPE OF EXPOSURE	
Stage	**Direct**	**Screen-Film**
Incident x-rays	1000	20
X-rays absorbed by film	10	1
X-rays absorbed by screens	—	5
Light photons produced	—	5000
Light photons incident on film	—	3000
Light photons absorbed by film	—	1000
Latent images formed	10	10

*Intensification factor = 1000/20 = 50.

film is highest in the violet-blue region of the spectrum. Consequently, the light emitted by calcium tungstate screens is readily absorbed in radiographic film (Figure 13-10).

If the screen phosphor emitted green or red light, its IF would be greatly reduced because it would require a greater number of light photons to produce a latent image. The light of the screen emission would be mismatched to the light sensitivity of the film.

Rare Earth Screens

Newer phosphor materials have become the material of choice for most radiographic applications. Table 13-3 lists these phosphors and the general identification of screens into which they have been incorporated. Except for barium- and zinc-based phosphors, the other new phosphors are identified as rare Earth; therefore, all these screens have come to be known as **rare Earth screens.**

The term *rare Earth* describes those elements of group IIIa in the periodic table (see Figure 3-4) that have atomic numbers of 57 to 71. These elements are transitional metals that are scarce in nature. Those used in rare Earth screens are principally **gadolinium, lanthanum, and yttrium.** The compositions of the four principal rare Earth phosphors are terbium-activated gadolinium oxysulfide (Gd_2O_2S: Tb), terbium-activated lanthanum oxysulfide (La_2O_2S: Tb), terbium-activated yttrium oxysulfide (Y_2O_2S: Tb), and lanthanum oxybromide (LaOBr).

> Rare Earth radiographic intensifying screens have the principal advantage of speed.

Rare Earth radiographic intensifying screens are manufactured to perform at several speed levels, up to 1200. This increase in speed is attained without loss of spatial or contrast resolution; however, with the fastest rare Earth screens, the effects of **quantum mottle** (image noise) are noticeable and can become bothersome (see Chapter 16).

Because rare Earth radiographic intensifying screens are faster, lower radiographic techniques can be used, and this results in lower patient dose. Rare Earth screens provide a general reduction in the radiation environment and, when used exclusively, can influence the design of radiographic facilities and reduce the need for protective lead shielding. The lower radiographic technique also results in increased x-ray tube life.

Rare Earth radiographic intensifying screens obtain their increased sensitivity through higher x-ray absorption (DQE) and more efficient conversion of x-ray energy into light (CE). The light emitted by these screens, however, differs from that emitted by other screens; therefore, rare Earth screens require specially matched film.

Higher X-ray Absorption. When diagnostic x-rays interact with a calcium tungstate screen, approximately

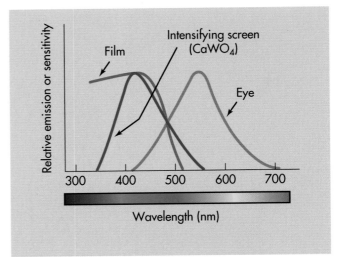

FIGURE 13-10 Importance of spectral matching is demonstrated by showing the relative emission spectrum for a radiographic intensifying screen and the relative sensitivity of radiograph film to light from that screen.

TABLE 13-3	Composition and Emulsion of Radiographic Intensifying Screens	
Phosphor	**Activator**	**Emission**
Barium fluorochloride	Europium	Ultraviolet
Barium strontium sulfate	Europium	Ultraviolet
Barium sulfate	Lead	Ultraviolet
Zinc sulfide	Silver	Blue-ultraviolet
Calcium tungstate	Lead	Blue
Lanthanum oxybromide	Thulium	Blue
Yttrium oxysulfide	Terbium	Blue
Gadolinium oxysulfide	Terbium	Green
Lanthanum oxysulfide	Terbium	Green
Zinc cadmium sulfide	Silver	Yellow-green

30% of the x-rays are absorbed. The mechanism of absorption is almost entirely the photoelectric effect. Recall that photoelectric absorption occurs readily with the inner electrons of atoms of high atomic number.

The tungsten atom determines the absorption properties of a calcium tungstate screen. Tungsten has an atomic number of 74 and a K-shell electron binding energy of 69 keV. In the diagnostic range, x-ray absorption in tungsten follows the relationship shown in Figure 13-11.

At very low energies, photoelectric absorption is very high, but as the x-ray energy increases, the probability of absorption decreases rapidly until the x-ray energy is equal to the binding energy of the K-shell electrons. At x-ray energies below the K-shell electron binding energy, the incident x-ray has too little energy to ionize K-shell electrons.

When the x-ray energy equals the K-shell electron binding energy, the two K-shell electrons become available for photoelectric interaction. Consequently, at this energy, the probability of photoelectric absorption increases abruptly.

This abrupt increase in absorption at this energy level is called the K-shell absorption edge, and it is followed by another rapid reduction in photoelectric absorption with increasing x-ray energy.

The rare Earth materials used for radiographic intensifying screens all have atomic numbers less than that for tungsten. Consequently, each has lower K-shell electron binding energy. Table 13-4 lists the important physical characteristics of the elements included in radiographic intensifying screens.

Figure 13-12 shows that the probability of x-ray absorption in rare Earth screens is lower than that in calcium tungstate screens at all x-ray energies except those between respective K-shell electron binding energies.

Below the K-shell absorption edge for the rare Earth elements, x-ray absorption is higher in tungsten. At an x-ray energy equal to the K-shell electron binding energy of the rare Earth elements, however, the probability of photoelectric absorption is considerably higher than that for tungsten.

As with tungsten, the absorption probability of the rare Earth elements decreases with increasing x-ray energy. At x-ray energies above the K-shell absorption edge for tungsten, the rare Earth elements again exhibit lower absorption than that for tungsten.

Each of the rare Earth radiographic intensifying screens has an absorption curve characteristic of the phosphor that determines the speed of the screen and how it changes with kVp. Figure 13-13 shows the x-ray absorption in two phosphors relative to calcium tungstate. For instance, barium strontium sulfate has a higher DQE at a lower kVp than is the case with gadolinium oxysulfide.

The result of this complex interaction process is that in the x-ray energy range between the K-shell absorption edge for the rare Earth elements and that for tungsten, a rare Earth screen absorbs approximately five times more x-rays than a calcium tungstate screen. Furthermore, for each x-ray absorbed, more light is emitted by the rare Earth screens.

Rare Earth radiographic intensifying screens exhibit better absorption properties than calcium tungstate screens only in the energy range between the respective K-shell absorption edges. This energy range extends from approximately 35 to 70 keV and corresponds to

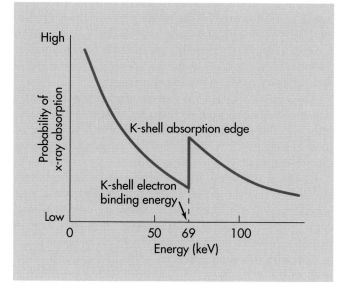

FIGURE 13-11 Probability of x-ray absorption in a calcium tungstate screen as a function of the incident x-ray energy.

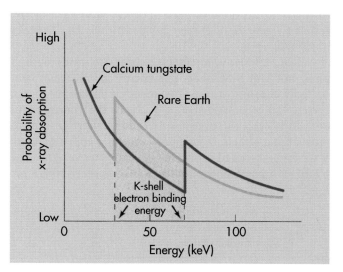

FIGURE 13-12 X-ray absorption probability in a rare Earth screen compared with that in a calcium tungstate screen. In the energy interval between respective K-shell electron binding energies, absorption in a rare Earth screen is greater.

TABLE 13-4	Atomic Number and K-Shell Electron Binding Energy of High-Z Elements in Radiographic Intensifying Screen Phosphors		
Element	Chemical Symbol	Atomic Number (Z)	K-Shell Electron Binding Energy (keV)
Yttrium	Y	39	17
Barium	Ba	56	37
Lanthanum	La	57	39
Gadolinium	Gd	64	50
Tungsten	W	74	69

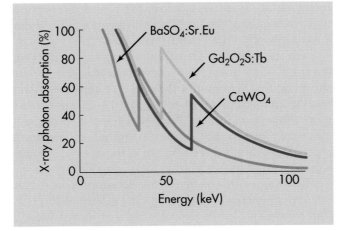

FIGURE 13-13 X-ray absorption for three intensifying screen phosphors.

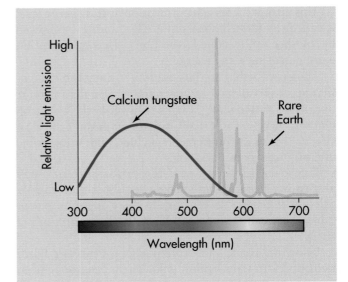

FIGURE 13-14 Calcium tungstate emits a broad spectrum of light centered in the blue region. With rare Earth screens, discrete emissions are centered near the green-yellow region.

most of the useful x-rays emitted during routine x-ray examinations. Outside this energy range, calcium tungstate radiographic intensifying screens absorb more x-rays than rare Earth screens.

Higher Conversion Efficiency. An additional property of the rare Earth phosphors, the CE, contributes to their extraordinary speed. The CE is defined as the ratio of visible light energy emitted to the x-ray energy absorbed.

When an x-ray interacts photoelectrically with a phosphor and is absorbed, its energy reappears as heat or light through a rearrangement of electrons in the crystal lattice of the phosphor. If all the energy reappeared as heat, the phosphor would be worthless as an intensifying screen. In calcium tungstate, approximately 5% of the absorbed x-ray energy reappears as light. **The CE of rare Earth phosphors is approximately 20%.**

> The combination of improved CE and higher DQE results in the increased speed of rare Earth radiographic intensifying screens.

Faster Speed. Rare Earth radiographic intensifying screens are available in many combinations with different films, resulting in varying relative speeds. Rare Earth screen-film combinations have relative speeds from 200 to 1200.

When rare Earth screen-film systems with relative speeds as high as 1200 are used, image quality may be degraded somewhat by increased quantum mottle, but this may be acceptable for some types of examinations in view of the significantly reduced patient dose.

Spectrum Matching. To be fully effective, rare Earth radiographic intensifying screens must be used only in conjunction with film emulsions whose light absorption characteristics are matched to the light emission of the screen. This is called spectrum matching. Calcium tungstate screens emit light in a rather broad continuous spectrum centered

in the violet-to-blue region, with a maximum intensity at approximately 430 nm (Figure 13-14).

The spectral emission of rare Earth phosphors is more discrete, as indicated by the many peaks in the spectrum (see Figure 13-14). The spectral emission is centered in the green region of the visible spectrum at approximately 540 mm. Terbium activation is responsible for the shape and intensity of this emission spectrum.

The emission spectrum can be altered somewhat by various concentrations of terbium atoms in the phosphor, by the addition of activators, and by the use of light-absorbing dyes. Phosphors are available that emit ultraviolet, blue, green, and red light.

Conventional x-ray film is sensitive to blue and blue-violet light and is rather insensitive to light of longer wavelengths. Such blue-sensitive films are used with calcium tungstate screens because their absorption spectrum matches the emission spectrum of calcium tungstate.

Specially designed green-sensitive film must be used with rare Earth screens (Figure 13-15). If a green-emitting screen were used with blue-sensitive film, the strong emission in the green region would go undetected, and system speed would be sharply reduced. To obtain maximum advantage and speed from rare Earth screens, the film must be sensitized for emission of the screen.

Safelights. Green-sensitive film creates problems in the darkroom. Safelight filters that are satisfactory for regular x-ray film fog film manufactured for use with rare Earth screens. Rare Earth screen-film requires the use of safelights that are colored even more toward the red portion of the spectrum.

Asymmetric Screen-Film. Consider the double-emulsion screen-film combination depicted in Figure 13-16. If each screen has a DQE of 50%, only 50% of

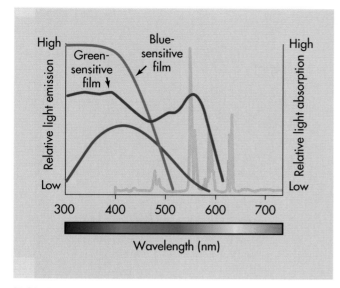

FIGURE 13-15 Blue-sensitive film must be used with blue-emitting screens and green-sensitive film with green-emitting screens.

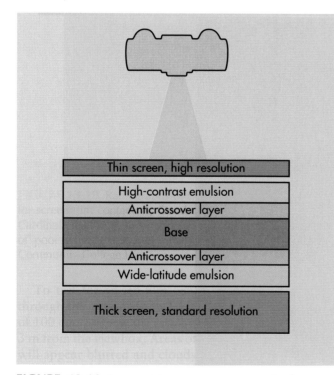

FIGURE 13-16 Asymmetric screens compensate for x-ray absorption in the front screen.

the x-rays are transmitted to the back screen. Therefore, the back screen absorbs only 25% of the x-rays incident on the cassette, resulting in only one half of the exposure of the back emulsion as the front emulsion.

This difference in exposure can be remedied by thickening the back radiographic intensifying screen. Another remedy is to use a different screen, thereby exposing a different emulsion. Such screens and/or emulsions are

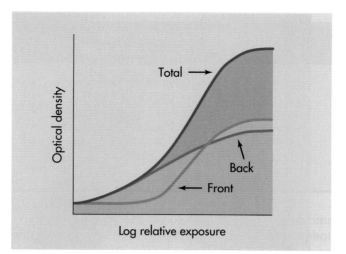

FIGURE 13-17 Characteristic curves from an asymmetric screen emulsion image receptor.

called **asymmetric** and are used to great advantage in some applications, such as chest, pediatric, and mobile radiography.

In chest radiography, for example, the front screen/emulsion is slower and higher in contrast, and the back screen/emulsion is faster and lower in contrast (Figure 13-17). The result is a more balanced image of wide latitude and high contrast over the lung fields and the mediastinum (Figure 13-18).

CARE OF SCREENS

High-quality radiographs require that radiographic intensifying screens receive proper care. Screen handling requires the utmost care because even a small fingernail scratch can produce artifacts and degrade the radiographic image. Screens should be handled only when they are new and are being installed in cassettes, and when they are being cleaned. When screens are mounted in a cassette, the manufacturer's instructions must be followed carefully.

When loading cassettes, do not slide the film in. A sharp corner or the edge can scratch the screen. Place the film inside the cassette. Remove the film by rocking the cassette on the hinged edge and letting it fall to your fingers. Do not dig the film out of the cassette with your fingernails. Do not leave cassettes open because the screens can be damaged by whatever might fall on them, be it dust or darkroom chemicals.

Radiographic intensifying screens must be cleaned periodically. The frequency of cleaning is determined primarily by two factors: the amount of use and the level of dust in the work environment. In a busy radiology department, it may be necessary to clean screens once each month or even more often. Under other circumstances, the cleaning frequency may be extended safely to 2 to 3 months.

Special screen cleaning materials are used, and the manufacturer's instructions should be followed carefully. One advantage of the use of these commercial

CONTRAST AND contrast resolution are important characteristics of image quality. Contrast arises from the areas of light, dark, and shades of gray on the x-ray image. These variations make up the radiographic image. Contrast resolution is the ability to image adjacent similar tissues. Scatter radiation produced by the Compton effect produces noise, reducing image contrast and contrast resolution. It makes the image less visible.

Three factors contribute to increased scatter radiation: increased kVp, increased x-ray field size, and increased patient thickness. Beam-restricting devices are designed to control and minimize scatter radiation by limiting the x-ray field size to only the anatomy of interest. The three principal types of beam-restricting devices are aperture diaphragm, cones or cylinders, and collimators. By removing scattered x-rays from the remnant beam, the grid removes a major source of noise, thus improving image contrast.

The two principal characteristics of any image are *spatial resolution* and *contrast resolution*. Some refer to these together as *image detail* or *visibility of detail*. In fact, these qualities are quite distinct and are influenced by different links of the imaging chain.

Spatial resolution is determined by focal-spot size and other factors that contribute to blur. Contrast resolution is determined by scatter radiation and other sources of image noise. Two principal tools are used to control scatter radiation: beam-restricting devices and grids.

PRODUCTION OF SCATTER RADIATION

Two types of x-rays are responsible for the optical density and contrast on a radiograph: those that pass through the patient without interacting, and those that are scattered within the patient through Compton interaction. X-rays that exit from the patient are remnant x-rays and those that exit and interact with the image receptor are called **image-forming x-rays** (Figure 14-1).

Proper collimation of the x-ray beam has the primary effect of reducing patient dose by restricting the volume of irradiated tissue. Proper collimation also improves image contrast. Ideally, only those x-rays that do not interact with the patient should reach the image receptor.

 Collimation reduces patient dose and improves contrast resolution.

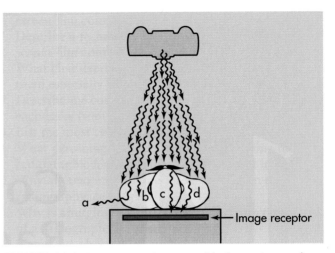

FIGURE 14-1 Some x-rays interact with the patient and are scattered away from the image receptor *(a)*. Others interact with the patient and are absorbed *(b)*. X-rays that arrive at the image receptor are those transmitted through the patient without interacting *(c)* and those scattered in the patient *(d)*. X-rays of types *c* and *d* are called *image-forming x-rays.*

As scatter radiation increases, the radiograph loses contrast and appears gray and dull. Three primary factors influence the relative intensity of scatter radiation that reaches the image receptor: kVp, field size, and patient thickness.

kVp

As x-ray energy is increased, the absolute number of Compton interactions decreases, but the number of photoelectric interactions decreases much more rapidly. Therefore, the relative number of x-rays that undergo Compton interaction increases.

Table 14-1 shows the percentage of x-rays incident on a 10-cm thickness of soft tissue that will undergo photoelectric interaction and Compton interaction at selected kVp levels. Kilovoltage, which is one of the factors that affect the level of scatter radiation, can be controlled by the radiologic technologist.

It would be easy enough to say that all radiographs should be taken at the lowest reasonable kVp because this technique would result in minimum scatter and thus higher image contrast. Unfortunately, it is not that simple.

Figure 14-2 shows the relative contributions of photoelectric effect and Compton effect to the radiographic image. The increase in photoelectric absorption results in a considerable increase in patient dose.

Also, fewer x-rays reach the image receptor at low kVp—a phenomenon that is usually compensated for by increasing the mAs. The result is still higher patient dose.

Approximately 1% of x-rays incident on the patient reach the image receptor.

Table 14-1	Percent Interaction of X-rays by Photoelectric and Compton Processes and Percent Transmission Through 10 cm of Soft Tissue			
	PERCENT INTERACTION			
kVp	Photoelectric	Compton	Total	Percent Transmission
50	79	21	>99	<1
60	70	30	>99	<1
70	60	40	>99	<1
80	46	52	98	2
90	38	59	97	3
100	31	63	94	6
110	23	70	93	7
120	18	83	91	9

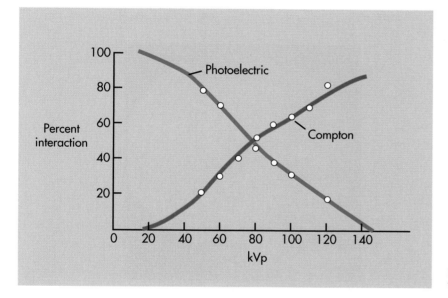

FIGURE 14-2 The relative contributions of photoelectric effect and Compton scattering to the radiographic image.

With large patients, kVp must be high to ensure adequate penetration of the portion of the body that is being radiographed. If, for example, the normal technique factors for an AP examination of the abdomen are inadequate, the technologist has the choice of increasing mAs or kVp.

Increasing the mAs usually generates enough x-rays to provide a satisfactory image but may result in an unacceptably high patient dose. On the other hand, a much smaller increase in kVp is usually sufficient to provide enough x-rays, and this can be done at a much lower patient dose. Unfortunately, when kVp is increased, the level of scatter radiation also increases, leading to decreased image contrast.

Collimators and grids are used to reduce the level of scatter radiation. Figure 14-3 shows a series of radiographs of a skull phantom taken at 70, 80, and 90 kVp with the use of appropriate collimation and grids, with the mAs adjusted to produce radiographs of equal optical density (OD).

Most radiologists would accept any of these radiographs. Notice that the patient dose at 90 kVp is approximately one third that at 70 kVp. In general, because of this reduction in patient dose, a high-kVp technique is preferred to a low-kVp technique.

Field Size

Another factor that affects the level of scatter radiation and is controlled by the radiologic technologist is x-ray beam field size. As field size is increased, scatter radiation also increases (Figure 14-4).

Scatter radiation increases as the field size of the x-ray beam increases.

Figure 14-5 shows two AP views of the lumbar spine. Figure 14-5, *A*, was taken on a full-frame, 35 × 43-cm film; in Figure 14-5, *B*, field size is restricted to the spinal

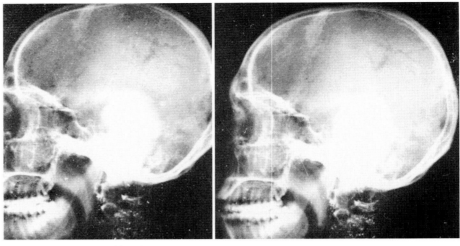

70 kVp / 120 mAs
665 mR

80 kVp / 60 mAs
545 mR

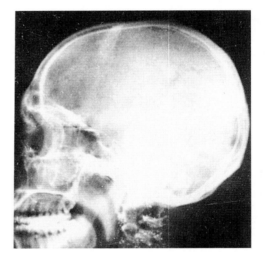

90 kVp / 30 mAs
230 mR

FIGURE 14-3 Each of these skull radiographs is of acceptable quality. The technique factors for each are shown, along with the resultant patient exposure. (Courtesy Donald Sommers, Lincoln Land Community College.)

FIGURE 14-4 Collimation of the x-ray beam results in less scatter radiation, reduced dose, and improved contrast resolution.

column. Contrast is noticeably lower in the full-frame radiograph because of the increased scatter radiation that accompanies larger field size.

Compared with a large field size, radiographic exposure factors may have to be increased for the purpose of maintaining the same OD when the exposure is made with a smaller field size. Reduced scatter radiation results in lower radiographic OD, which must be raised by increasing technique.

Patient Thickness

Imaging thick parts of the body results in more scatter radiation than imaging thin parts does. Compare a radiograph of the bony structures in an extremity with a radiograph of the bony structures of the chest or pelvis. Even when the two are taken with the same screen-film combination, the extremity radiograph will be much

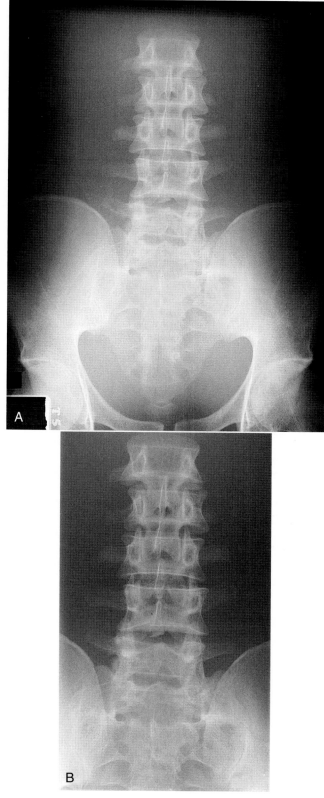

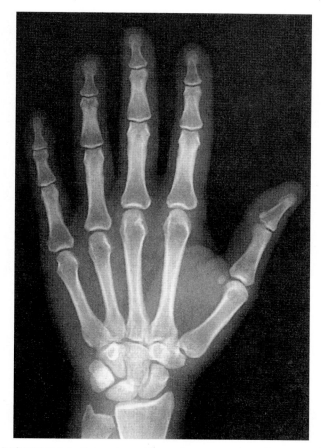

FIGURE 14-6 Extremity radiographs appear sharp because of less tissue and, hence, less scatter radiation. Posterior-anterior view of the hand. (Courtesy Rees Stuteville, Oregon Institute of Technology.)

sharper because of the reduced amount of scatter radiation (Figure 14-6).

The types of tissue (muscle, fat, bone) and pathology, such as a fluid-filled lung, also play a part in the production of scatter radiation.

Figure 14-7 shows the relative intensity of scattered x-rays as a function of the thickness of soft tissue for a 20 × 25-cm field. Exposure of a 3-cm-thick extremity at 70 kVp produces about 45% scatter radiation. Exposure of a 30-cm-thick abdomen causes nearly 100% of the x-rays to exit the patient as scattered x-rays. With increasing patient thickness, more x-rays undergo multiple scattering, so that the average angle of scatter in the remnant beam is greater.

Normally, patient thickness is not controlled by the radiologic technologist. If you recognize that more x-rays are scattered with increasing patient thickness, you can produce a high-quality radiograph by choosing the proper technique factors, and by using devices that reduce scatter radiation to the image receptor, such as a compression paddle (Figure 14-8).

FIGURE 14-5 The recommended technique for lumbar spine radiography calls for collimation of the beam to the vertebral column. The full-field technique results in reduced image contrast. **A,** Full-field technique. **B,** Preferred collimated technique. (Courtesy Mike Enriquez, Merced Community College.)

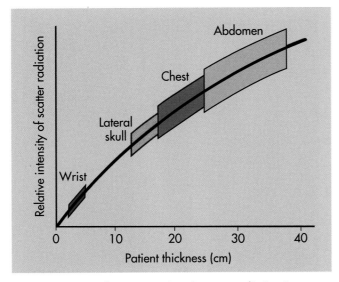

FIGURE 14-7 Relative intensity of scatter radiation increases with increasing thickness of anatomy.

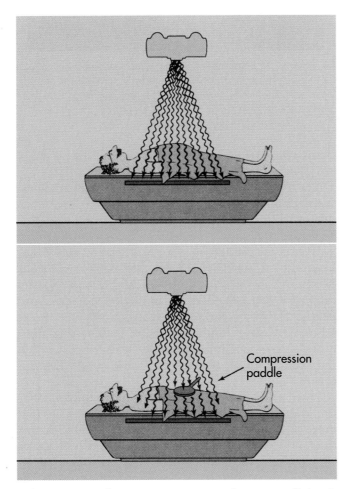

FIGURE 14-8 When tissue is compressed, scatter radiation is reduced, resulting in lower dose and improved contrast resolution.

Compression of anatomy improves spatial resolution and contrast resolution and lowers patient dose.

Compression devices improve spatial resolution by reducing patient thickness and bringing the object closer to the image receptor. Compression also reduces patient dose and improves contrast resolution. Compression is particularly important during mammography.

CONTROL OF SCATTER RADIATION
Effect of Scatter Radiation on Image Contrast

One of the most important characteristics of image quality is **contrast,** the visible difference between the light and dark areas of an image. Contrast is the degree of difference in OD between areas of a radiographic image. Contrast resolution is the ability to image and distinguish soft tissues.

Even under the most favorable conditions, most **remnant x-rays** are scattered. Figure 14-9 illustrates that scattered x-rays are emitted in all directions from the patient.

If you could image a long bone in cross section using only transmitted, unscattered x-rays, the image would be very sharp (Figure 14-10, *A*). The change in OD from dark to light, corresponding to the bone–soft tissue interface, would be very abrupt; therefore, image contrast would be high.

Reduced image contrast results from scattered x-rays.

On the other hand, if the radiograph were taken with only scatter radiation and no transmitted x-rays reached the image receptor, the image would be dull gray (Figure 14-10, *B*). The radiographic contrast would be very low.

In the normal situation, however, x-rays arriving at the image receptor consist of both transmitted and scattered

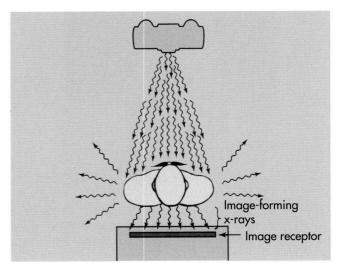

FIGURE 14-9 When primary x-rays interact with the patient, x-rays are scattered from the patient in all directions.

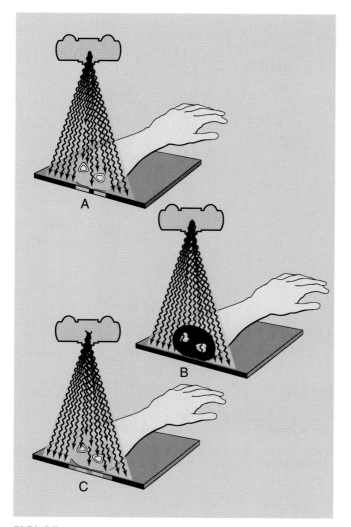

FIGURE 14-10 Radiographs of a cross section of long bone. **A,** High contrast would result from the use of only transmitted, unattenuated x-rays. **B,** No contrast would result from the use of only scattered x-rays. **C,** Moderate contrast results from the use of both transmitted and scattered x-rays.

x-rays. If the radiograph were properly exposed, the image in cross-sectional view would appear as in Figure 14-10, *C.* This image would have moderate contrast. The loss of contrast results from the presence of scattered x-rays.

Two types of devices reduce the amount of scatter radiation that reaches the image receptor: **beam restrictors** and **grids.**

Beam Restrictors

Basically, three types of beam-restricting devices are used: the aperture diaphragm, cones or cylinders, and the variable-aperture collimator (Figure 14-11).

Aperture Diaphragm. An aperture is the simplest of all beam-restricting devices. It is basically a lead or lead-lined metal diaphragm that is attached to the x-ray tube head. The opening in the diaphragm usually is designed to cover just less than the size of the image receptor used. Figure 14-12 shows how the x-ray tube, the aperture diaphragm, and the image receptor are related.

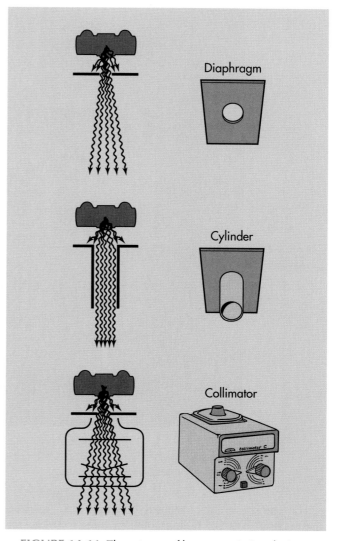

FIGURE 14-11 Three types of beam-restricting devices.

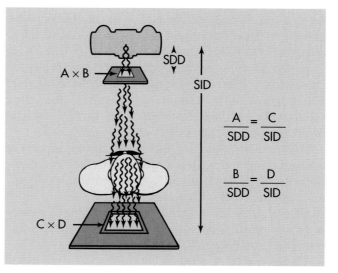

FIGURE 14-12 Aperture diaphragm is a fixed lead opening designed for a fixed image receptor size and constant source-to-image receptor distance (SID). *SDD,* Source-to-diaphragm distance.

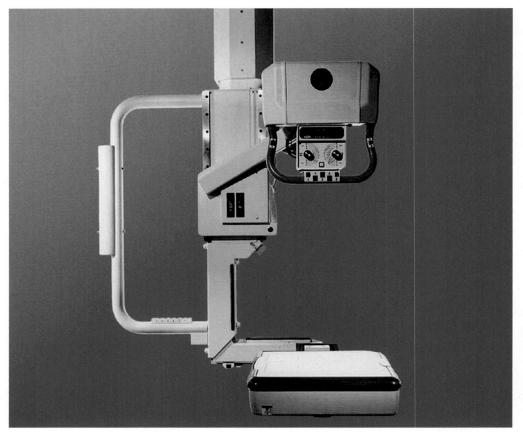

FIGURE 14-13 Typical trauma radiographic imaging system used for imaging the skull, spine, and extremities. Such units are flexible and adaptable for examination of many body parts. (Courtesy Fischer Imaging.)

The most familiar clinical example of aperture diaphragms may be radiographic imaging systems for trauma. The typical trauma system has a fixed source-to-image receptor distance (SID) and is equipped with diaphragms designed to accommodate film sizes of 13 × 18 cm, 20 × 25 cm, and 25 × 30 cm. Radiographic imaging systems for trauma can be positioned to image all parts of the body (Figure 14-13).

X-ray imaging systems dedicated specifically to chest radiography can be supplied with fixed-aperture diaphragms. Such aperture diaphragms for chest radiography are designed to expose all of a 35 × 43-cm image receptor, except for a 1-cm border.

Dental radiography represents another application of aperture diaphragms. Dental radiographs are customarily obtained at 20 or 40 cm SID. Most dental imaging systems are supplied with rectangular collimation, which requires that the dental radiologic technologist precisely align and position the x-ray tube head, the patient, and the image receptor.

Cones and Cylinders. Radiographic extension cones and cylinders are considered modifications of the aperture diaphragm. Figure 14-14 presents a diagram of a typical extension cone and cylinder. In both, an extended metal structure restricts the useful beam to the

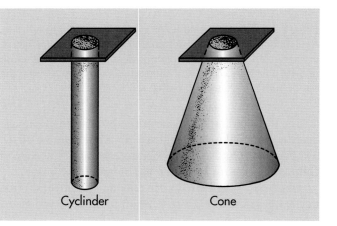

FIGURE 14-14 Radiographic cones and cylinders produce restricted useful x-ray beams of circular shape.

required size. The position and size of the distal end act as an aperture and determine field size.

In contrast to the beam produced by an aperture diaphragm, the useful beam produced by an extension cone or cylinder is usually circular. Both of these beam restrictors are routinely called *cones*, even though the most commonly used type is actually a cylinder.

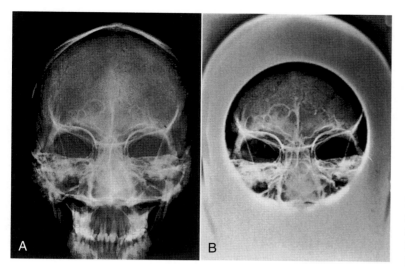

FIGURE 14-15 Radiographs of the frontal and maxillary sinuses without a cone (**A**) and with a cone (**B**). Cones reduce scatter radiation and improve contrast resolution. (Courtesy Lynne Davis, Houston Community College.)

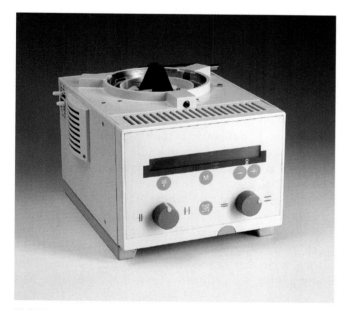

FIGURE 14-16 Automatic variable-aperture collimator. (Courtesy Huestis Medical.)

One difficulty with using cones is alignment. If the x-ray source, cone, and image receptor are not aligned on the same axis, one side of the radiograph may not be exposed because the edge of the cone may interfere with the x-ray beam. Such interference is called *cone cutting*.

At one time, cones were used extensively in diagnostic radiology. Today, they are reserved primarily for examinations of selected areas. Figure 14-15 shows how a cone improves image contrast when used in examination of the frontal sinuses.

Variable Aperture Collimator. The light-localizing variable-aperture collimator is the most commonly used beam-restricting device in radiography. The photograph in Figure 14-16 shows an example of a modern automatic variable-aperture collimator. Figure 14-17 identifies the principal parts of such a collimator.

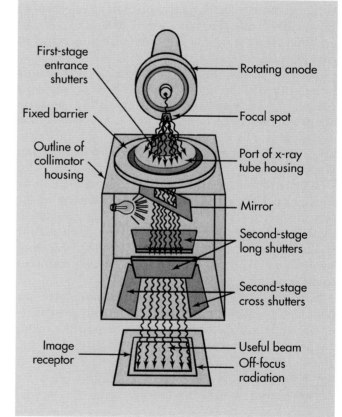

FIGURE 14-17 Simplified schematic of a variable-aperture light-localizing collimator.

Collimation reduces patient dose and improves contrast resolution.

Not all x-rays are emitted precisely from the focal spot of the x-ray tube. Some x-rays are produced when projectile electrons stray and interact at positions on the anode other than the focal spot. Such radiation, which is called **off-focus radiation**, increases image blur.

To control off-focus radiation, a first-stage entrance-shuttering device that has multiple collimator blades protrudes from the top of the collimator into the x-ray tube housing.

The leaves of the second-stage collimator shutter are usually made of lead that is at least 3 mm thick. They work in pairs and are independently controlled, thereby allowing for both rectangular and square fields.

Light localization in a typical variable-aperture collimator is accomplished with a small lamp and mirror. The mirror must be far enough on the x-ray tube side of the collimator leaves to project a sufficiently sharp light pattern through the collimator leaves when the lamp is on.

The collimator lamp and the mirror must be adjusted so that the projected light field coincides with the x-ray beam. If the light field and the x-ray beam do not coincide, the lamp or the mirror must be adjusted. Such coincidence checking is a necessary evaluation of any quality control program. Misalignment of the light field and x-ray beam can result in collimator cutoff of anatomical structures.

Today, nearly all light-localizing collimators manufactured in the United States for fixed radiographic equipment are automatic. They are called **positive-beam–limiting (PBL)** devices. Positive beam limitation was mandated by the U. S. Food and Drug Administration in 1974. That regulation was removed in 1994, but PBL prevails.

When a film-loaded cassette is inserted into the Bucky tray and is clamped into place, sensing devices in the tray identify the size and alignment of the cassette. A signal transmitted to the collimator housing actuates the synchronous motors that drive the collimator leaves to a precalibrated position, so the x-ray beam is restricted to the image receptor size in use.

Even with PBL devices, when appropriate, the radiologic technologist should manually collimate more tightly to reduce patient dose and improve image quality.

 Under no circumstances should the x-ray beam exceed the size of the image receptor.

Depending on the tube potential, additional **collimator filtration** may be necessary to produce high-quality radiographs with minimum patient exposure. Some collimator housings are designed to allow easy changing of the added filtration. Filtration stations of 0, 1, 2, and 3 mm Al are the most common.

 TOTAL FILTRATION

Total Filtration = Inherent Filtration + Added Filtration

Even in the zero position, however, the added filtration to the x-ray tube is not zero because collimator structures intercept the beam. In addition to the inherent filtration of the tube, the exit port, usually plastic, and the reflecting mirror provide filtration. The added filtration of the collimator assembly is usually equivalent to approximately 1 mm Al.

Grids

Scattered x-rays that reach the image receptor are part of the image-forming process; indeed, the x-rays that are scattered forward do contribute to the image. An extremely effective device for reducing the level of scatter radiation that reaches the image receptor is the **grid,** a carefully fabricated series of sections of radiopaque material (**grid strips**) alternating with sections of radiolucent material (**interspace material**). The grid is positioned between the patient and the image receptor.

This technique for reducing the amount of scatter radiation that reaches the image receptor was first demonstrated in 1913 by Gustave Bucky. Over the years, Bucky's grid has been improved by more precise manufacturing, but the basic principle has not changed.

The grid is designed to transmit only those x-rays whose direction is on a straight line from the source to the image receptor. Scatter radiation is absorbed in the grid material. Figure 14-18 is a schematic representation of how a grid "cleans up" scatter radiation.

X-rays that exit the patient and strike the radiopaque grid strips are absorbed and do not reach the image receptor. For instance, a typical grid may have grid strips 50 μm wide that are separated by interspace material 350 μm wide. Consequently, up to 12.5% of all x-rays

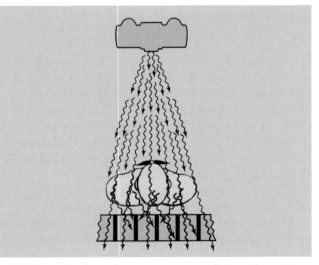

FIGURE 14-18 The only x-rays transmitted through a grid are those that travel in the direction of the interspace. X-rays scattered obliquely through the interspace are absorbed.

that strike the grid interact with the radiopaque grid strips and are absorbed.

GRID SURFACE X-RAY ABSORPTION

% x-ray absorption

$$= \frac{width\ of\ grid\ strip}{width\ of\ grid\ strip + width\ of\ interspace} \times 100$$

Question: A grid is constructed with 50-μm strips and a 350-μm interspace. What percentage of x-rays incident on the grid will be absorbed by its entrance surface?

Answer: $\dfrac{50\,\mu m}{350\,\mu m + 50\,\mu m} = 0.125 = 12.5\%$

Primary beam x-rays incident on the interspace material are transmitted to the image receptor. Scattered x-rays incident on the interspace material may or may not be absorbed, depending on their angle of incidence and the physical characteristics of the grid.

If the angle of a scattered x-ray is great enough to cause it to intersect a lead grid strip, it will be absorbed. If the angle is slight, the scattered x-ray will be transmitted similarly to a primary x-ray. Laboratory measurements show that high-quality grids can attenuate 80% to 90% of the scatter radiation. Such a grid is said to exhibit good "cleanup."

Question: When viewed from the top, a particular grid shows a series of lead strips 40 μm wide separated by interspaces 300 μm wide. How much of the radiation incident on this grid should be absorbed?

Answer: If 300 + 40 represents the total surface area, and 40 the surface area of absorbing material, then the percentage absorption is as follows:
$\dfrac{40\,\mu m}{340\,\mu m} = 0.118 = 11.8\%$

Grid Ratio. A grid consists of three important dimensions: the thickness of the grid strip (T), the width of the interspace material (D), and the height of the grid (h). The **grid ratio** is the height of the grid divided by the interspace width (Figure 14-19).

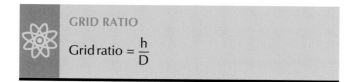

GRID RATIO

$Grid\ ratio = \dfrac{h}{D}$

High-ratio grids are more effective in cleaning up scatter radiation than are low-ratio grids. This is because the angle of scatter allowed by high-ratio grids is less than that permitted by low-ratio grids (Figure 14-20).

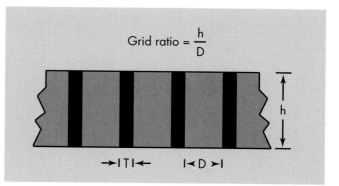

FIGURE 14-19 Grid ratio is defined as the height of the grid strip *(h)* divided by the thickness of the interspace material *(D)*. *T,* Width of grid strip.

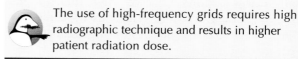

High-ratio grids increase patient radiation dose.

In general, grid ratios range from 5:1 to 16:1; higher-ratio grids are used most often in high-kVp radiography. An 8:1 to 10:1 grid is frequently used with general-purpose x-ray imaging systems. A 5:1 grid cleans up approximately 85% of the scatter radiation, whereas a 16:1 grid may clean up as much as 97%.

Question: A grid is fabricated of 30-μm lead grid strips sandwiched between interspace material that is 300 μm thick. The height of the grid is 2.4 mm. What is the grid ratio?

Answer:

$$Grid\ ratio = \frac{h}{D} = \frac{2400\,\mu m}{300\,\mu m} = 8:1$$

Grid Frequency. The number of grid strips per centimeter is called the *grid frequency*. Grids with high frequency show less distinct grid lines on a radiograph compared with grids with low frequency.

If grid strip width is held constant, the higher the frequency of a grid, the thinner its interspace must be and the higher the grid ratio.

The use of high-frequency grids requires high radiographic technique and results in higher patient radiation dose.

As grid frequency increases, relatively more grid strip is available to absorb x-rays; therefore, the patient dose is high because a higher radiographic technique is required. The disadvantage of the increased patient dose associated with high-frequency grids can be overcome by reducing the width of the grid strips, but this effectively reduces the grid ratio and therefore the cleanup.

Most grids have frequencies in the range of 25 to 45 lines per centimeter. Grid frequency can be calculated

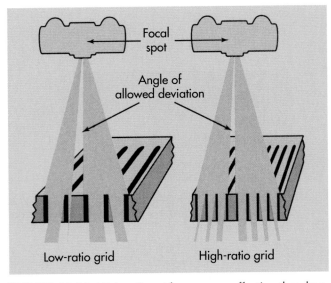

FIGURE 14-20 High-ratio grids are more effective than low-ratio grids because the angle of deviation is smaller.

if the widths of the grid strip and of the interspace are known. Grid frequency is computed by dividing the thickness of one line pair (T + D), expressed in μm, into 1 cm:

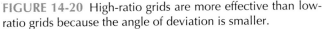

GRID FREQUENCY

$$Grid\ frequency = \frac{10,000\ \mu m/cm}{(T+D)\ \mu m/line\ pair}$$

Question: What is the grid frequency of a grid that has a grid strip width of 30 μm and an interspace width of 300 μm?

Answer: If one line pair = 300 μm + 30 μm = 330 μm, how many line pairs are in 10,000 μm (10,000 μm = 1 cm)?

$$\frac{10,000\ \mu m/cm}{330\ \mu m/line\ pair} = 30.3\ lines/cm$$

Specially designed grids are used for mammography. Usually, a 4:1 or a 5:1 ratio grid is used. These low-ratio grids have grid frequencies of approximately 80 lines/cm.

Interspace Material. The purpose of the interspace material is to maintain a precise separation between the delicate lead strips of the grid. The interspace material of most grids consists of **aluminum** or **plastic fiber;** reports are conflicting as to which is better.

Aluminum has a higher atomic number than plastic and therefore may provide some selective filtration of scattered x-rays not absorbed in the grid strip. Aluminum also has the advantage of producing less visible grid lines on the radiograph.

On the other hand, use of aluminum as interspace material increases the absorption of primary x-rays in the interspace, especially at low kVp. The result is higher mAs and higher patient dose. Above 100 kVp, this property is unimportant, but at low kVp, the patient dose may be increased by approximately 20%. For this reason, fiber interspace grids usually are preferred to aluminum interspace grids.

Still, aluminum has two additional advantages over fiber. It is **nonhygroscopic,** that is, it does not absorb moisture as plastic fiber does. Fiber interspace grids can become warped if they absorb moisture. Also, aluminum interspace grids of high quality are easier to manufacture because aluminum is easier to form and roll into sheets of precise thickness.

Grid Strip. Theoretically, the grid strip should be infinitely thin and should have high absorption properties. These strips may be formed from several possible materials. Lead is most widely used because it is easy to shape and is relatively inexpensive. Its high atomic number and high mass density make lead the material of choice in the manufacture of grids. Tungsten, platinum, gold, and uranium all have been tried, but none has the overall desirable characteristics of lead.

GRID PERFORMANCE

Perhaps the largest single factor responsible for poor radiographic quality is scatter radiation. By removing scattered x-rays from the remnant beam, the radiographic grid removes the source of reduced contrast.

 The principal function of a grid is to improve image contrast.

Contrast Improvement Factor

The characteristics of grid construction previously described, especially the grid ratio, usually are specified when a grid is identified. Grid ratio, however, does not reveal the ability of the grid to improve image contrast. This property of the grid is specified by the **contrast improvement factor** *(k)*. A contrast improvement factor of 1 indicates no improvement.

Most grids have contrast improvement factors of between 1.5 and 2.5. In other words, the image contrast is approximately doubled when grids are used. Mathematically, the contrast improvement factor, *k*, is expressed as follows:

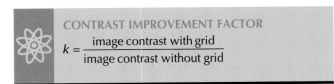

CONTRAST IMPROVEMENT FACTOR

$$k = \frac{image\ contrast\ with\ grid}{image\ contrast\ without\ grid}$$

Question: An aluminum step wedge is placed on a tissue phantom that is 20 cm thick and a radiograph is made. Without a grid, analysis of the radiograph shows an average gradient (a measure of contrast) of 1.1. With a 12:1 grid, radiographic contrast is 2.8. What is the contrast improvement factor of this grid?

Answer: $k = \dfrac{2.8}{1.1} = 2.55$

The contrast improvement factor usually is measured at 100 kVp, but it should be realized that k is a complex function of the x-ray emission spectrum, patient thickness, and the tissue irradiated.

> The contrast improvement factor is higher for high-ratio grids.

Bucky Factor

Although the use of a grid improves contrast, a penalty is paid in the form of patient dose. The quantity of image-forming x-rays transmitted through a grid is much less than that of image-forming x-rays incident on the grid. Therefore, when a grid is used, the radiographic technique must be increased to produce the same OD. The amount of this increase is given by the **Bucky factor (B)**, often called the **grid factor.**

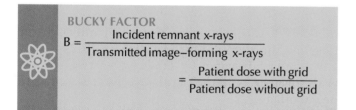

BUCKY FACTOR

$$B = \frac{\text{Incident remnant x-rays}}{\text{Transmitted image–forming x-rays}}$$

$$= \frac{\text{Patient dose with grid}}{\text{Patient dose without grid}}$$

The Bucky factor is named for Gustave Bucky, the inventor of the grid. It is an attempt to measure the penetration of primary and scatter radiation through the grid. Table 14-2 gives representative values of the Bucky factor for several popular grids.

Two generalizations can be made from the data presented in Table 14-2:

1. **The higher the grid ratio, the higher is the Bucky factor.** The penetration of primary radiation through a grid is fairly independent of grid ratio. Penetration of scatter radiation through a grid becomes less likely with increasing grid ratio; therefore, the Bucky factor increases.

2. **The Bucky factor increases with increasing kVp.** At high voltage, more scatter radiation is produced. This scatter radiation has a more difficult time penetrating the grid; thus, the Bucky factor increases.

> As the Bucky factor increases, radiographic technique and patient dose increase proportionately.

Whereas the contrast improvement factor measures improvement in image quality when grids are used, the Bucky factor measures how much of an increase in technique will be required compared with nongrid exposure. The Bucky factor also indicates how large an increase in patient dose will accompany the use of a particular grid.

GRID TYPES
Parallel Grid

The simplest type of grid is the parallel grid, which is diagrammed in cross section in Figure 14-21. In the parallel grid, all lead grid strips are parallel. This type of grid is the easiest to manufacture, but it has some properties that are clinically undesirable, namely **grid cutoff**, the undesirable absorption of primary x-rays by the grid.

The attenuation of primary x-rays becomes greater as the x-rays approach the edge of the image receptor. The lead strips in a 35 × 43-cm grid are 43 cm long. Across the 35-cm dimension, the OD reaches a maximum along the center line of the image receptor and decreases toward the sides.

Grid cutoff can be partial or complete. The term is derived from the fact that the primary x-rays are "cut off" from reaching the image receptor. Grid cutoff can occur with any type of grid if the grid is improperly positioned, but it is most common with parallel grids.

	BUCKY FACTOR AT			
Grid Ratio	**70 kVp**	**90 kVp**	**120 kVp**	**Average**
No grid	1	1	1	1
5:1	2	2.5	3	2
8:1	3	3.5	4	4
12:1	3.5	4	5	5
16:1	4	5	6	6

Table 14-2   Approximate Bucky Factor Values for Popular Grids

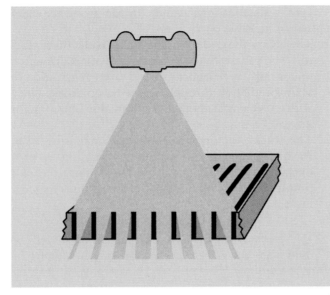

FIGURE 14-21 A parallel grid is constructed with parallel grid strips. At a short source-to-image receptor distance (SID), some grid cutoff may occur.

This characteristic of parallel grids is most pronounced when the grid is used at a short SID or with a large-area image receptor. Figure 14-22 shows the geometric relationship for attenuation of primary x-rays by a parallel grid. The distance from the central ray at which complete cutoff will occur is determined by the following:

> **GRID CUTOFF**
>
> $$\text{Distance to cutoff} = \frac{SID}{Grid\ ratio}$$

For instance, in theory, a 10:1 grid when used at 100 cm SID should absorb all primary x-rays farther than 10 cm from the central ray. When this grid is used with a 35 × 43-cm image receptor, OD should be apparent only over a 20 × 43-cm area of the image receptor.

The radiographs in Figure 14-23 were taken with a 6:1 parallel grid at 76 and 61 cm SID (**A** and **B**, respectively). They show increasing degrees of grid cutoff with decreasing SID.

Question: A 16:1 parallel grid is positioned for chest radiography at 180 cm SID. What is the distance from the central axis to complete grid cutoff? Will the image satisfactorily cover a 35 × 43-cm image receptor?

Answer:

$$\text{Distance to cutoff} = \frac{180}{16} = 11.3\ \text{cm}$$

$$\text{Distance to edge of image receptor}$$
$$= 35 \div 2 = 17.5\ \text{cm}$$

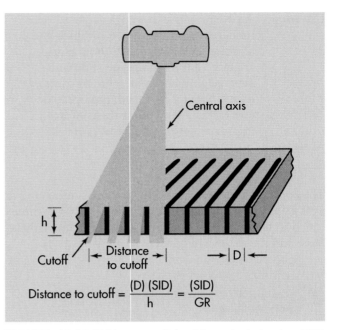

FIGURE 14-22 With a parallel grid, optical density (OD) decreases toward the edge of the image receptor. The distance to grid cutoff is the source-to-image receptor distance (SID) divided by the grid ratio.

No! Grid cutoff will occur on the lateral 6.2 cm (17.5 − 11.3) of the image receptor.

Crossed Grid

Parallel grids clean up scatter radiation in only one direction, along the axis of the grid. Crossed grids are designed to overcome this deficiency. Crossed grids have lead grid strips that run parallel to the long and short axes of the grid (Figure 14-24). They are usually fabricated by sandwiching two parallel grids together, with their grid strips perpendicular to one another.

They are not too difficult to manufacture and therefore are not excessively expensive. However, they have found restricted application in clinical radiology. (It is interesting to note that Bucky's original grid was crossed.)

Crossed grids are much more efficient than parallel grids in cleaning up scatter radiation. In fact, a crossed grid has a higher contrast improvement factor than a parallel grid of twice the grid ratio. A 6:1 crossed grid will clean up more scatter radiation than a 12:1 parallel grid.

This advantage of the crossed grid increases as the operating kVp is increased. A crossed grid identified as having a grid ratio of 6:1 is constructed with two 6:1 parallel grids.

 The main disadvantage of parallel and crossed grids is grid cutoff.

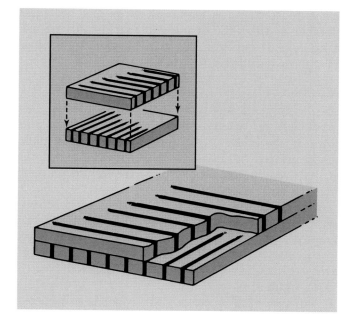

FIGURE 14-24 Crossed grids are fabricated by sandwiching two parallel grids together, so their grid strips are perpendicular.

FIGURE 14-23 **A,** Radiograph taken with a 6:1 parallel grid at a source-to-image receptor distance (SID) of 76 cm. **B,** Radiograph taken with 6:1 parallel grid at an SID of 61 cm. Optical density decreases from the center to the edge of the image and to complete cutoff. (Courtesy Dawn Stark, Mississippi State University.)

Three serious disadvantages are associated with the use of crossed grids. First, positioning the grid is critical; the central ray of the x-ray beam must coincide with the center of the grid. Second, tilt-table techniques are possible only if the x-ray tube and the table are properly aligned. Finally, the exposure technique required is substantial and results in higher patient dose.

Focused Grid

The focused grid is designed to minimize grid cutoff. The lead grid strips of a focused grid lie on the imaginary radial lines of a circle centered at the focal spot, so they coincide with the divergence of the x-ray beam. The x-ray tube target should be placed at the center of this imaginary circle when a focused grid is used (Figure 14-25).

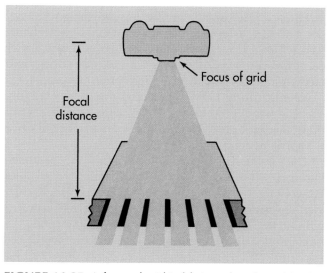

FIGURE 14-25 A focused grid is fabricated so that grid strips are parallel to the primary x-ray path across the entire image receptor.

Focused grids are more difficult to manufacture than parallel grids. They are characterized by all the properties of parallel grids, except that when properly positioned, they exhibit no grid cutoff. The radiologic technologist must take care when positioning focused grids because of their geometric limitations.

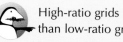 High-ratio grids have less positioning latitude than low-ratio grids.

Every focused grid is marked with its intended focal distance and the side of the grid that should face the x-ray tube. If radiographs are taken at distances other than those intended, grid cutoff occurs.

Moving Grid

An obvious and annoying shortcoming of the grids previously discussed is that they can produce **grid lines** on the image. Grid lines are the images made when primary x-rays are absorbed within the grid strips. Even though the grid strips are very small, their image is still observable.

The presence of grid lines can be demonstrated simply by radiographing a grid. Usually, high-frequency grids present less obvious grid lines compared with low-frequency grids. This is not always the case, however, because the visibility of grid lines is directly related to the width of the grid strips.

A major improvement in grid development occurred in 1920. Hollis E. Potter hit on a very simple idea: Move the grid while the x-ray exposure is being made. The grid lines disappear at little cost of increased radiographic technique. A device that does this is called a **moving grid** or a Potter-Bucky diaphragm ("Bucky" for short).

Focused grids usually are used as moving grids. They are placed in a holding mechanism that begins moving just before x-ray exposure and continues moving after the exposure ends. Two basic types of moving grid mechanisms are in use today: reciprocating and oscillating.

Reciprocating Grid. A reciprocating grid is a moving grid that is motor-driven back and forth several times during x-ray exposure. The total distance of drive is approximately 2 cm.

Oscillating Grid. An oscillating grid is positioned within a frame with a 2- to 3-cm tolerance on all sides between the frame and the grid. Delicate, springlike devices located in the four corners hold the grid centered within the frame. A powerful electromagnet pulls the grid to one side and releases it at the beginning of the exposure. Thereafter, the grid oscillates in a circular fashion around the grid frame, coming to rest after 20 to 30 seconds.

Disadvantages of Moving Grids. Moving grids require a bulky mechanism that is subject to failure. The distance between the patient and the image receptor is increased with moving grids because of this mechanism; this extra distance may create an unwanted increase in magnification and image blur. Moving grids can introduce motion into the cassette-holding device, which can result in additional image blur.

Fortunately, the advantages of moving grids far outweigh the disadvantages. The types of motion blur discussed are for descriptive purposes only. The motion blur generated by moving grids that are functioning properly is undetectable. Moving grids are usually the technique of choice and therefore are used widely.

GRID PROBLEMS

Most grids in diagnostic imaging are of the moving type. They are permanently mounted in the moving mechanism just below the tabletop or just behind the vertical chest board.

To be effective, of course, the grid must move from side to side. If the grid is installed incorrectly and moves in the same direction as the grid strips, grid lines will appear on the radiograph (Figure 14-26).

The most frequent error in the use of grids is improper positioning. For the grid to function correctly, it must be precisely positioned relative to the x-ray tube target and to the central ray of the x-ray beam. Four situations characteristic of focused grids must be avoided (Table 14-3). Only an off-level grid is a problem with parallel and crossed grids.

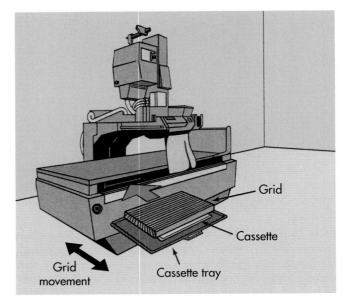

FIGURE 14-26 Proper installation of moving grid.

Table 14-3	Focused-Grid Misalignment
Type of Grid Misalignment	**Result**
Off-level	Grid cutoff across image; underexposed, light image
Off-center	Grid cutoff across image; underexposed, light image
Off-focus	Grid cutoff toward edge of image
Upside-down	Severe grid cutoff toward edge of image
Off-center, off-focus	Grid cutoff on one side of image

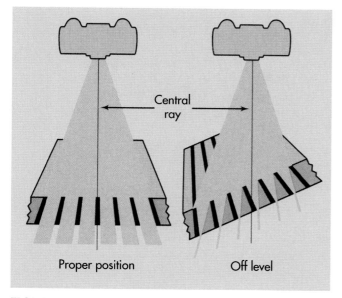

FIGURE 14-27 If a grid is off-level so that the central axis is not perpendicular to the grid, partial cutoff occurs over the entire image receptor.

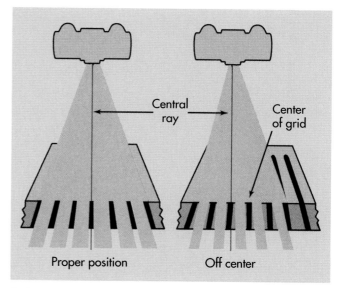

FIGURE 14-28 When a focused grid is positioned off-center, partial grid cutoff occurs over the entire image receptor.

Off-Level Grid

A properly functioning grid must lie in a plane perpendicular to the central ray of the x-ray beam (Figure 14-27). The **central ray** x-ray beam is the x-ray that travels along the center of the useful x-ray beam.

Despite its name, an **off-level grid** in fact is usually produced with an improperly positioned x-ray tube and not an improperly positioned grid. However, this can occur when the grid tilts during horizontal beam radiography or during mobile radiography when the image receptor sinks into the patient's bed.

If the central ray is incident on the grid at an angle, then all incident x-rays will be angled and grid cutoff will occur across the entire radiograph, resulting in lower OD.

Off-Center Grid

A grid can be perpendicular to the central ray of the x-ray beam and still produce grid cutoff if it is shifted laterally. This is a problem with focused grids, as shown in Figure 14-28, where an off-center grid is shown with a properly positioned grid.

The center of a focused grid must be positioned directly under the x-ray tube target, so the central ray of the x-ray beam passes through the centermost interspace of the grid. Any lateral shift results in grid cutoff across the entire radiograph, producing lower OD. This error in positioning is called **lateral decentering.**

As with an off-level grid, an off-center grid is more a result of positioning the x-ray tube than the grid. In practice, it means that the radiologic technologist must carefully line up the center of the light-localized field with the center of the cassette.

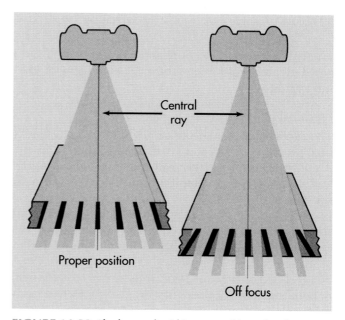

FIGURE 14-29 If a focused grid is not positioned at the specified focal distance, grid cutoff occurs and the optical density (OD) decreases with distance from the central ray.

Off-Focus Grid

A major problem with using a focused grid arises when radiographs are taken at SIDs unspecified for that grid. Figure 14-29 illustrates what happens when a focused grid is not used at the proper focal distance. The farther the grid is from the specified focal distance, the more severe will be the grid cutoff. Grid cutoff is not uniform across the image receptor but instead is more severe at the edges.

This condition is not usually a problem if all chest radiographs are taken at 180 cm SID and all table radiographs at 100 cm SID. Positioning the grid at the

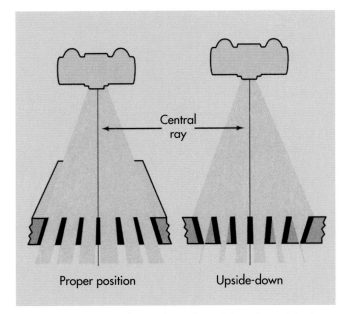

FIGURE 14-30 A focused grid positioned upside-down should be detected on the first radiograph. Complete grid cutoff occurs, except in the region of the central ray.

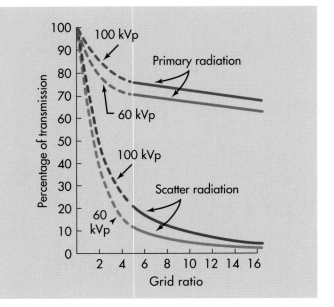

FIGURE 14-31 As grid ratio increases, transmission of scatter radiation decreases faster than transmission of primary radiation. Therefore, cleanup of scatter radiation increases.

proper focal distance is more important with high-ratio grids; greater positioning latitude is possible with low-ratio grids.

Upside-Down Grid

The explanation for an upside-down grid is obvious. It need occur only once, and it will be noticed immediately. A radiographic image taken with an upside-down focused grid shows severe grid cutoff on either side of the central ray (Figure 14-30).

Every focused grid has a clear label on one side and sometimes on both. It also has a line running down the center of the grid on the tube side in the same direction as the grid strips.

Labels indicate the tube side or the image receptor side, or both, and the prescribed focal distance. With even moderate attention, upside-down grids will not occur.

Combined Off-Center, Off-Focus Grid. Perhaps the most common improper grid position occurs if the grid is both off center and off focus. Without proper attention, this can occur easily during mobile radiography. It is an easily recognized grid-positioning artifact because the result is uneven exposure. The resultant radiograph appears dark on one side and light on the other.

GRID SELECTION

Modern grids are sufficiently well manufactured that many radiologists do not find the grid lines of stationary grids objectionable, especially for mobile radiography and horizontal views of an upright patient.

Moving grid mechanisms, however, rarely fail, and image degradation rarely occurs. Therefore, in most situations, it is appropriate to design radiographic procedures around moving grids. When moving grids are used, parallel grids can be used, but focused grids are more common.

Focused grids are in general far superior to parallel grids, but their use requires care and attention. When focused grids are used, the indicators on the x-ray apparatus must be in good adjustment and properly calibrated. The SID indicator, the source-to-tabletop distance (STD) indicator, and the light-localizing collimator all must be properly adjusted.

Selection of a grid with the proper ratio depends on an understanding of three interrelated factors: kVp, degree of cleanup, and patient dose. When a high kVp is used, high-ratio grids should be used as well. Of course, the choice of grid is also influenced by the size and shape of the anatomy that is being radiographed.

As grid ratio increases, the amount of cleanup also increases. Figure 14-31 shows the approximate percentage of scatter radiation and primary radiation transmitted as a function of grid ratio. Note that the difference between grid ratios of 12:1 and 16:1 is small.

The difference in patient dose is large, however; therefore, 16:1 grids are not often used. Many general-purpose x-ray examination facilities find that an 8:1 grid represents a good compromise between the desired levels of scatter radiation cleanup and patient dose.

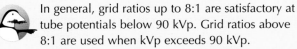

In general, grid ratios up to 8:1 are satisfactory at tube potentials below 90 kVp. Grid ratios above 8:1 are used when kVp exceeds 90 kVp.

Table 14-4	Approximate Entrance Skin Dose for Examination of the Adult Pelvis With a 400-Speed Image Receptor		
	ENTRANCE DOSE (mrad)		
Type of Grid	70 kVp	90 kVp	110 kVp
No grid	40	35	25
5:1	135	110	75
8:1	160	140	100
12:1	210	200	145
16:1	260	240	185
5:1 crossed	270	200	145
8:1 crossed	290	265	200

Table 14-5	Approximate Change in Radiographic Technique for Standard Grids	
Grid Ratio	Milliampere-Second (mAs) Increase	Voltage (kVp) Increase
No grid	1 ×	0
5:1	2 ×	+ 8 to 10
8:1	4 ×	+ 13 to 15
12:1	5 ×	+ 20 to 25
16:1	6 ×	+ 30 to 40

The use of one grid also reduces the likelihood of grid cutoff because improper grid positioning can easily accompany frequent changes of grids. In those facilities where high-kVp technique for dedicated chest radiography is used, 16:1 grids can be installed.

Patient Dose

One major disadvantage that accompanies the use of x-ray grids is increased patient dose. For any examination, use of a grid may result in several times more radiation to the patient than is provided when a grid is not used. The use of a moving grid instead of a stationary grid with similar physical characteristics requires approximately 15% more radiation to the patient. Table 14-4 is a summary of approximate patient doses for various grid techniques with a 400-speed image receptor.

Low-ratio grids are used during mammography. All dedicated mammographic imaging systems are equipped with a 4:1 or a 5:1 ratio moving grid. Even at the low kVp used for mammography, considerable scatter radiation occurs.

The use of such grids greatly improves image contrast, with no loss of spatial resolution. The only disadvantage is the increase in patient dose, which can be as much as twice that without a grid. However, with dedicated equipment and grid, patient dose still is very low.

Grid Selection Factors
1. Patient dose increases with increasing grid ratio.
2. High-ratio grids are used for high-kVp examinations.
3. Patient dose at high kVp is less than that at low kVp.

In general, compared with the use of low-kVp and low-ratio grids, the use of high-kVp and high-ratio grids results in lower patient doses and equal image quality.

One additional disadvantage of the use of grids is the increased radiographic technique required. When a grid is used, technique factors must be increased over what they were for nongrid examinations: The mAs or the kVp must be increased. Table 14-5 presents approximate changes in technique factors required by standards grids. Usually, the mAs rather than the kVp is increased. One exception to this is chest radiography, wherein increased exposure time can result in motion blur.

Table 14-6 summarizes the clinical factors that should be considered in the selection of various types of grids.

Air-Gap Technique

A clever technique that may be used as an alternative to the use of radiographic grids is the **air-gap technique**. The air-gap technique is another method of reducing scatter radiation, thereby enhancing image contrast.

When the air-gap technique is used, the image receptor is moved 10 to 15 cm from the patient (Figure 14-32). A portion of the scattered x-rays generated in the patient would be scattered away from the image receptor and not be detected. Because fewer scattered x-rays interact with the image receptor, the contrast is enhanced.

Usually, when an air-gap technique is used, the mAs is increased approximately 10% for every centimeter of air gap. The technique factors usually are about the same as those for an 8:1 grid. Therefore, the patient dose is higher than that associated with the nongrid technique and is approximately equivalent to that of an intermediate grid technique.

One disadvantage of the air-gap technique is image magnification with associated focal-spot blur.

The air-gap technique has found application particularly in the areas of chest radiography and cerebral angiography. The magnification that accompanies these techniques is usually acceptable.

Table 14-6	Clinical Considerations in Grid Selection

		POSITIONING LATITUDE			
Type of Grid	Degree of Scatter Removal	Off Center	Off Focus	Recommended Technique	Remarks
5:1, linear	+	Very wide	Very wide	Up to 80 kVp	It is the least expensive. It is the easiest to use.
6:1, linear	+	Very wide	Very wide	Up to 80 kVp	It is the least expensive. It is ideally suited for bedside radiography.
8:1, linear	+	Wide	Wide	Up to 100 kVp	It is used for general stationary grids.
10:1, linear	+++	Wide	Wide	Up to 100 kVp	Reasonable care is required for proper alignment.
5:1, crisscross	+++	Narrow	Very wide	Up to 100 kVp	Tube tilt is limited to 5 degrees.
12:1, linear	++++	Narrow	Narrow	Over 110 kVp	Extra care is required for proper alignment. It usually is used in fixed mount.
6:1, crisscross	++++	Narrow	Very wide	Up to 110 kVp	It is not suited for tilted-tube techniques.
16:1, linear	+++++	Narrow	Narrow	Over 100 kVp	Extra care is required for proper alignment. It usually is used in fixed mount.
8:1, crisscross	+++++	Narrow	Wide	Up to 120 kVp	It is not suited for tilted-tube techniques.

Adapted from *Characteristics and applications of x-ray grids*, Cincinnati, c. 1980, Liebel-Florsheim.

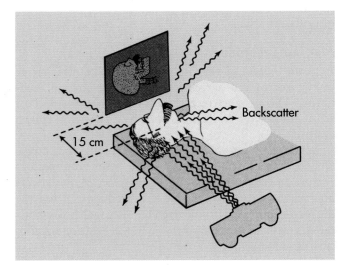

FIGURE 14-32 When the air-gap technique is used, the image receptor is positioned 10 to 15 cm from the patient. A large fraction of scattered x-rays do not interact with the image receptor.

In chest radiography, however, some radiologic technologists increase the SID from 180 to 300 cm. This results in very little magnification and a sharper image. Of course, the technique factors must be increased, but the patient dose is not increased (Figure 14-33).

The air-gap technique is not normally as effective with high-kVp radiography, in which the direction of the scattered x-rays is more forward. At tube potentials below approximately 90 kVp, the scattered

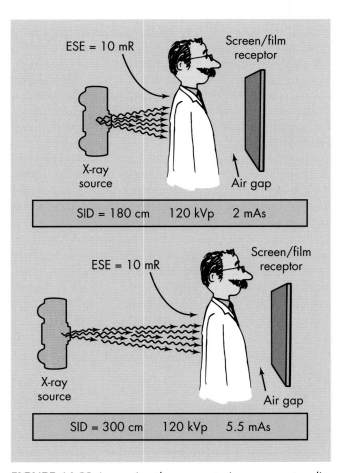

FIGURE 14-33 Increasing the source-to-image receptor distance (SID) to 300 cm from 180 cm improves spatial resolution with no increase in patient dose.

x-rays are directed more to the side; therefore, they have a higher probability of being scattered away from the image receptor. Nevertheless, at some centers, 120 to 140 kVp air-gap chest radiography is used with good results.

SUMMARY

Two types of image-forming x-rays exit the patient: (1) x-rays that pass through tissue without interacting, and (2) x-rays that are scattered in tissue by the Compton interaction and therefore contribute only noise to the image. The three factors that contribute to increased scatter radiation and ultimately to image noise are increasing kVp, increasing x-ray field size, and increasing anatomical thickness.

Although increased kVp increases scatter radiation, the trade-off is reduced patient exposure. Beam-restricting devices can be used to control and minimize the increase in scatter. Such devices include the aperture diaphragm, cones or cylinders, and the variable-aperture collimator. The variable-aperture collimator is the most commonly used beam-restricting device in diagnostic imaging.

Contrast is one of the most important characteristics of the radiographic image. Scatter radiation, the result of Compton interaction, is the primary factor that reduces image contrast. Grids reduce the amount of scatter that reaches the image receptor.

The two main components of grid construction are the interspace material (aluminum or plastic fiber) and the grid material (lead strips). The principal characteristic of a grid is grid ratio, that is, the height of the grid strip divided by the interspace width. Different grids are selected for use in particular situations. At less than 90 kVp, grid ratios of 8:1 and lower are used. At 90 kVp and above, grid ratios greater than 8:1 are used.

In all cases, the use of a grid increases patient dose. Table 14-5 summarizes the changes in grid ratio and changes in mAs or kVp that are required. Problems can arise with the use of grids, including off-level, off-center, and upside-down grid errors.

An alternative to use of a grid is the air-gap technique, in which the image receptor is moved 10 to 15 cm from the patient. Scatter is reduced with this technique because scatter that exits the patient escapes in the air space between the patient and the film.

CHALLENGE QUESTIONS

1. Define or otherwise identify the following:
   a. Three factors that affect scatter radiation
   b. Collimator filtration
   c. Image contrast
   d. Grid cutoff
   e. Collimation
   f. Off-focus radiation
   g. PBL device
   h. Air-gap technique
   i. Image-forming x-rays
   j. Contrast improvement factor
2. Why should a radiograph of the lumbar vertebrae be well collimated?
3. With particular references to materials used and dimensions, discuss the construction of a grid.
4. An acceptable IVP can be obtained with technique factors of (1) 74 kVp, 120 mAs, or (2) 82 kVp, 80 mAs. Discuss possible reasons for selecting one technique over the other.
5. Does the radiograph of a long bone in a wet cast result in more or less scatter than that of a long bone in a dry cast?
6. A focused grid has the following characteristics: 100 cm focal distance, 40 μm grid strips, 350 μm interspace, and 2.8 mm height. What is the grid ratio?
7. What happens to image contrast and patient dose as more filtration is added to the x-ray beam?
8. Why does tissue compression improve image contrast?
9. At the 80-kVp level, what percentage of the x-ray beam is scattered through Compton interaction?
10. Name the devices used to reduce the production of scatter radiation.
11. Compression of tissue is particularly important during what examination?
12. List two reasons for restricting the x-ray beam.
13. Compared with contact radiography, why does air-gap technique increase patient dose?
14. What is the reason why an unexposed border is shown on the edge of the radiograph?
15. Why does lowering kVp increase patient dose?
16. What is viewed in the light field of a variable-aperture light-localizing collimator?
17. Explain how grid cutoff can occur.
18. Does a light-localizing collimator add filtration to the x-ray beam?
19. If the light field and the radiation field do not coincide, what needs to be adjusted?
20. When should the x-ray field exceed the size of the image receptor?

The answers to the Challenge Questions can be found by logging on to our website at http://evolve.elsevier.com.

CHAPTER 15

Radiographic Technique

OBJECTIVES

At the completion of this chapter, the student should be able to do the following:

1. List the four prime exposure factors
2. Discuss mAs and kVp in relation to x-ray beam quantity and quality
3. Describe characteristics of the imaging system that affect x-ray beam quantity and quality
4. List the four patient factors and explain their effects on radiographic technique
5. Identify four image-quality factors and explain how they influence the characteristics of a radiograph
6. Discuss the three types of technique charts
7. Explain the three types of automatic exposure controls
8. Discuss the relationship between tomographic angle and section thickness
9. Describe magnification radiography and its uses

OUTLINE

Exposure Factors
  kVp
  mA
  Exposure Time
  Distance
Imaging System Characteristics
  Focal-Spot Size
  Filtration
  High-Voltage Generation
Patient Factors
  Thickness
  Composition
  Pathology

Image-Quality Factors
  Optical Density
  Contrast
  Detail
  Distortion
Exposure Technique Charts
Automatic Exposure Techniques
Tomography
Magnification Radiography

EXPOSURE FACTORS are a few of the tools that radiographers use to create high-quality radiographs. The prime exposure factors are kVp, mA, exposure time, and source-to-image receptor distance (SID).

Properties of the x-ray imaging system that influence the selection of exposure factors are reviewed, including focal-spot size, total x-ray beam filtration, and the source of high-voltage generation.

Radiographic technique usually is described as the combination of settings selected on the control panel of the x-ray imaging system to produce a high-quality image. The geometry and position of the x-ray tube, the patient, and the image receptor are included in this description.

Many areas of x-ray diagnosis require special equipment and specialized techniques to obtain the required information. Such procedures are designed to visualize more clearly a given anatomical structure, usually at the expense of nonvisualization of other structures.

The equipment and procedures discussed in this chapter include conventional tomography and magnification radiography. These x-ray examinations are not routine; therefore, the radiologic technologist must be specially trained to perform them.

TABLE 15-1	Factors That May Influence X-ray Quantity and Quality	
	WILL RESULT IN	
An Increase in	X-ray Quantity	X-ray Quality
Kilovolt peak	Increase	Increase
Milliampere	Increase	No change
Exposure time	Increase	No change
Milliampere-seconds	Increase	No change
Distance	Decrease	No change
Voltage ripple	Decrease	Decrease
Filtration	Decrease	Increase

EXPOSURE FACTORS

Proper exposure of a patient to x-radiation is necessary to produce a diagnostic radiograph. The factors that influence and determine the quantity and quality of x-radiation to which the patient is exposed are called **exposure factors** (Table 15-1). Recall from Chapter 9 that radiation quantity refers to radiation intensity measured in mR or mR/mAs, and radiation quality refers to x-ray beam penetrability, best measured by the half-value layer (HVL).

All of these factors, except those fixed by the design of the x-ray imaging system, are under the control of the radiologic technologist. For example, focal-spot size is limited to two selections. Sometimes, the added x-ray beam filtration is fixed. The high-voltage generator provides characteristic voltage ripple that cannot be changed.

The four prime exposure factors are kilovolt peak (kVp), current (given in milliampere [mA]), exposure time(s), and source-to-image receptor distance (SID). Of these, the most important are kVp and mAs, the factors principally

responsible for x-ray quality and quantity. Focal-spot size, distance, and filtration are secondary factors that may require manipulation for particular examinations.

kVp

To understand kVp as an exposure technique factor, assume that kVp is the primary control of x-ray beam quality, and therefore **beam penetrability.** A higher-quality x-ray beam is one with higher energy that is thus more likely to penetrate the anatomy of interest.

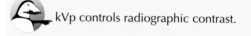 kVp controls radiographic contrast.

The kVp has more effect than any other factor on image receptor exposure because it affects beam quality and, to a lesser degree, influences beam quantity. With increasing kVp, more x-rays are emitted, and they have higher energy and greater penetrability. Unfortunately, because they have higher energy, they also interact more by Compton effect and produce more scatter radiation, which results in reduced image contrast.

The kVp selected greatly determines the number of x-rays in the image-forming beam, and hence the resulting average optical density (OD). Finally, and perhaps most important, the kVp controls the scale of contrast on the finished radiograph because as kVp increases, less differential absorption occurs. Therefore, high kVp results in reduced image contrast.

mA

The mA station selected determines the number of x-rays produced, and therefore the **radiation quantity.** Recall that the unit of electric current is the ampere (A). One ampere is equal to 1 coulomb (C) of electrostatic charge flowing each second in a conductor, as follows:

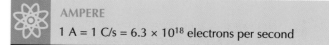
AMPERE
$1 \text{ A} = 1 \text{ C/s} = 6.3 \times 10^{18}$ electrons per second

Therefore, when the 100-mA station on the operating console is selected, 6.3×10^{18} electrons flow through the x-ray tube each second.

Question: What is the electron flow from cathode to anode when the 500-mA station is selected?

Answer: 500 mA = 0.5 A
= (0.5 A) (6.3 × 10^{18} electrons/s/A)
= 3.15 × 10^{18} electrons/second

As more electrons flow through the x-ray tube, more x-rays are produced. Assuming a constant exposure time, this relationship is directly proportional. A change from 200 mA to 400 mA would be a 100% increase or a doubling of the x-ray tube current, a doubling of the x-rays produced, and a doubling of patient dose.

 With a constant exposure time, mA controls x-ray quantity and therefore patient dose.

Question: At 200 mA, the entrance skin exposure (ESE) is 752 mR (7.5 mGy$_a$). What will be the ESE at 500 mA?

Answer:
$$ESE = 752\,mR \left(\frac{500\,mA}{200\,mA} \right) = 1880\,mR$$

A change in mA does not change the kinetic energy of electrons flowing from cathode to anode. It simply changes the number of electrons. Consequently, the energy of the x-rays produced is not changed, only the number is changed.

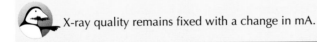 X-ray quality remains fixed with a change in mA.

Often, x-ray imaging systems are identified by the maximum x-ray tube current possible. Inexpensive radiographic imaging systems designed for private physicians' offices normally have a maximum capacity of 600 mA. Interventional radiology imaging systems may have a capacity of 1200 mA.

Exposure Time

Radiographic exposure times usually are kept as short as possible. The purpose is not to minimize patient radiation dose, but rather to minimize motion blur that can occur because of patient motion.

 Short exposure time reduces motion blur.

TABLE 15-2	Relationships Among Different Units of Exposure Time	
Fractional (s)	**Seconds (s)**	**Milliseconds (ms)**
1.0	1.0	1000
4/5	0.8	800
3/4	0.75	750
2/3	0.67	667
3/5	0.6	600
1/2	0.5	500
2/5	0.4	400
1/3	0.33	333
1/4	0.25	250
1/5	0.2	200
1/10	0.1	100
1/20	0.05	50
1/60	0.017	17
1/120	0.008	8

Producing a diagnostic image requires a certain radiation exposure of the image receptor. Therefore, when exposure time is reduced, the mA must be increased proportionately to provide the required x-ray intensity.

On older x-ray imaging systems, exposure time is expressed in fractional seconds, whereas current x-ray imaging systems identify exposure time in milliseconds (ms). Table 15-2 shows how the different units of time are related.

An easy way to identify an x-ray imaging system as single phase, three phase, or high frequency is to note the shortest exposure time possible. Single-phase imaging systems cannot produce an exposure time less than ½ cycle or its equivalent ¹/₁₂₀ second or 8 ms (10 ms on 50-Hz generators). Three-phase and high-frequency generators normally can provide an exposure as short as 1 ms.

mA and exposure time (in seconds) are usually combined and used as mAs. Indeed, many x-ray consoles do not allow the separate selection of mA and exposure time, and permit only mAs selection.

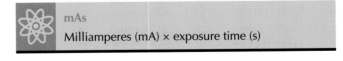 mAs
Milliamperes (mA) × exposure time (s)

Although the radiologic technologist may be required to select an exposure time, it is always selected with consideration of the mA station. The important parameter is the product of the exposure time and tube current.

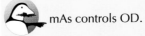 mAs controls OD.

The mAs value determines the number of x-rays in the primary beam; therefore, it principally controls radiation **quantity** in the same way that mA and exposure time, taken separately, do; it does not influence radiation quality. The mAs setting is the key factor in the control of OD on the radiograph.

EQUIVALENT EXPOSURES OF EQUAL mAs

$$mAs = mA \times Time$$

$$mA \text{ (first exposure)} \times time \text{ (first exposure)}$$
$$= mA \text{ (second exposure)} \times time \text{ (second exposure)}$$

$$\frac{mA \text{ (first exposure)}}{mA \text{ (second exposure)}} = \frac{Time \text{ (second exposure)}}{Time \text{ (first exposure)}}$$

Question: A radiographic technique calls for 600 mA at 200 ms. What is the mAs value?

Answer: 600 mA × 200 ms = 600 mA × 0.2 s
= 120 mAs

Time and mA can be used to compensate for each other in an indirect fashion. This is described by the following:

Question: A radiograph of the abdomen requires 300 mA and 500 ms. The patient is unable to breath-hold, which results in motion blur. A second exposure is made with an exposure time of 200 ms. Calculate the new mA that is required.

Answer:
$$\frac{x}{300\,mA} = \frac{500\,ms}{200\,ms}$$
$$(200\,ms)x = (500\,ms)(300\,mA)$$
$$(0.2\,s)x = (0.5\,s)(300\,ms)$$
$$(0.2\,s)x = 150\,mAs$$
$$x = \frac{150\,mAs}{0.2\,s} = 750\,mA$$

or

$$New\,mA = \frac{Original\,mAs}{New\,time}$$

$$New\,mA = \frac{0.5\,s \times 300\,mA}{0.2\,s} = 750\,mA$$

If the high-voltage generator is properly calibrated, the same mAs value and therefore the same OD can be produced with various combinations of mA and exposure time (Table 15-3). Because x-ray tube current is electron flow per unit time, the mAs value is therefore simply a measure of the total number of electrons conducted through the x-ray tube for a particular exposure.

TABLE 15-3		Products of Milliampere (mA) and Time (ms) for 10 mAs		
mA		ms		mAs
100	×	100	=	10
200	×	50	=	10
300	×	33	=	10
400	×	25	=	10
600	×	17	=	10
800	×	12	=	10
1000	×	10	=	10

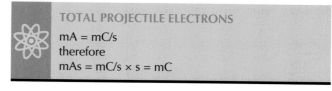

TOTAL PROJECTILE ELECTRONS

$$mA = mC/s$$
therefore
$$mAs = mC/s \times s = mC$$

Question: How many electrons are involved in x-ray production at 100 mAs?

Answer: 100 mAs = 0.1 As = 0.1 C/s × s = 0.1 C
1 C = 6.3×10^{18} electrons
Therefore, 0.1 C = 6.3×10^{17}
electrons = 100 mAs

mAs is one measure of electrostatic charge.

On an x-ray imaging system in which only mAs can be selected, exposure factors are adjusted automatically to the highest mA at the shortest exposure time allowed by the high-voltage generator. Such a design is called a **falling-load generator.**

Question: A radiologic technologist selects a technique of 200 mAs. The operating console is adjusted automatically to the maximum mA station, 1000 mA. What will be the exposure time?

Answer: $\dfrac{200\,mAs}{1000\,mA} = 0.2\,s = 200\,ms$

(The actual exposure time will be somewhat longer than 200 ms because the tube current falls as the anode heats up.)

Varying the mAs setting changes only the number of electrons conducted during an exposure—not the energy of those electrons. The relationship is directly proportional: Doubling of the mAs doubles the x-ray quantity.

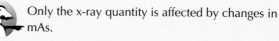

Only the x-ray quantity is affected by changes in mAs.

Question: A cervical spine examination calls for 68 kVp/30 mAs and results in an ESE of 114 mR (1.14 mGy$_a$). The next patient is examined at 68 kVp/25 mAs. What will be the ESE?

Answer: $\text{ESE} = 114\,\text{mR} \left(\dfrac{25\,\text{mAs}}{30\,\text{mAs}} \right) = 95\,\text{mR}$

Distance

Distance affects exposure of the image receptor according to the inverse square law, which was discussed in Chapter 4. The SID largely determines the intensity of the x-ray beam at the image receptor.

 Distance has no effect on radiation quality.

The following relationship, called the *direct square law,* is derived from the inverse square law. It allows a radiologic technologist to calculate the required change in mAs after a change in SID to maintain constant OD.

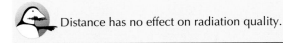

THE DIRECT SQUARE LAW

mAs versus SID

$$\frac{\text{mAs (second exposure)}}{\text{mAs (first exposure)}} =$$

$$\frac{(\text{SID})^2 \text{ (second exposure)}}{(\text{SID})^2 \text{ (first exposure)}}$$

$$\frac{\text{New mAs}}{\text{Old mAs}} = \frac{\text{New distance squared}}{\text{Old distance squared}}$$

Note that both the original mAs value and the original SID are in the denominator rather than reversed, as in the inverse square law.

Question: An examination requires 100 mAs at 180 cm SID. If the distance is changed to 90 cm SID, what should be the new mAs setting?

Answer: $\dfrac{x}{100} = \dfrac{90^2}{180^2}$

$$x = 100 \left(\frac{90}{180} \right)^2 = 100 \left(\frac{1}{2} \right)^2$$

$$= 100 \left(\frac{1}{4} \right) = 25\,\text{mAs}$$

 Distance (SID) affects OD.

When preparing to make a radiographic exposure, the radiologic technologist selects specific settings for each of the factors described: kVp, mAs, and SID. The control panel selections are based on an evaluation of the patient, the thickness of the anatomical part, and the type of accessories used.

Standard SIDs have been in use for many years. For tabletop radiography, 100 cm is common, whereas dedicated chest examination usually is conducted at 180 cm. With advances in generator design and image receptors, even larger SIDs are anticipated. Tabletop radiography at 120 cm and chest radiography at 300 cm are now in use.

The use of a longer SID results in less magnification, less focal spot blur, and improved spatial resolution. However, more mAs must be used because of the effects of the direct square law.

IMAGING SYSTEM CHARACTERISTICS
Focal-Spot Size

Most x-ray tubes are equipped with two focal-spot sizes. On the operating console, these usually are identified as small and large. Conventional tubes have two focal spots of normal size, that is, 0.5 mm/1.0 mm, 0.6 mm/1.2 mm, or 1.0 mm/2.0 mm. X-ray tubes used in angiointerventional procedures or magnification radiography may consist of 0.3 mm/1.0 mm focal spots.

Most mammography tubes have 0.1 mm/0.3 mm focal spots. These are called **microfocus tubes** and are designed specifically for imaging very small microcalcifications at relatively short SIDs.

For normal imaging, the large focal spot is used. This ensures that sufficient mAs can be used to image thick or dense body parts. The large focal spot also provides for a shorter exposure time, which minimizes motion blur.

One difference between large and small focal spots is the capacity to produce x-rays. Many more x-rays can be produced with the large focal spot because anode heat capacity is higher. With the small focal spot, electron interaction occurs over a much smaller area of the anode, and the resulting heat limits the capacity of x-ray production.

Changing the focal spot for a given kVp/mAs setting does not change x-ray quantity or quality.

A small focal spot is reserved for fine-detail radiography, in which the quantity of x-rays is relatively low. Small focal spots are always used for magnification radiography. These are normally used during extremity radiography and in examination of other thin body parts in which higher x-ray quantity is not necessary.

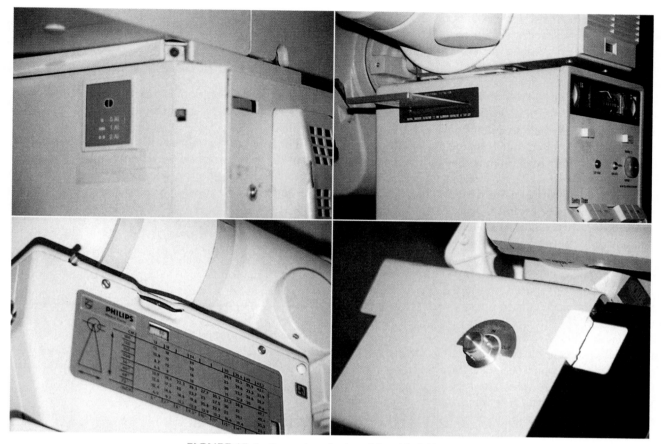

FIGURE 15-1   Examples of selectable added filtration.

Filtration

Three types of filtration are used: inherent, added, and compensating. All x-ray beams are affected by the **inherent filtration** properties of the glass or metal envelope of the x-ray tube. For general purpose tubes, the value of inherent filtration is approximately 0.5 mm Al equivalent.

The variable-aperture light-localizing collimator usually provides an additional 1.0 mm Al equivalent. Most of this is due to the reflective surface of the mirror of the collimator. To meet the required total filtration of 2.5 mm Al, an additional 1-mm Al filter is inserted between the x-ray tube housing and the collimator. The radiologic technologist has no control over these sources of filtration but may control stages of added filtration.

Some x-ray imaging systems have selectable **added filtration**, as shown in Figure 15-1. Usually, the imaging system is placed into service with the lowest allowable added filtration. Radiographic technique charts usually are formulated at the lowest filtration position. If a higher filter position is used, a radiographic technique chart must be developed at that position.

Figure 15-2 shows multiple layers of different filtration materials designed for specialty examinations and patient dose reduction. The two sets of collimator blades are open, showing the filters and the light field mirror.

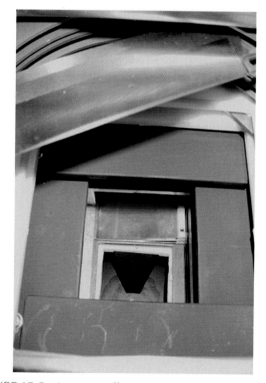

FIGURE 15-2   An open collimator showing the light field mirror and multiple layers of filtration. (Courtesy General Electric Medical Systems.)

Under normal conditions, it is unnecessary to change the filtration. Some facilities may be set for higher filtration during examinations of tissue with high subject contrast, such as extremities, joints, and chest. When properly used, higher filtration for these examinations results in lower patient dose. When added filtration is changed, **be sure to return it to its normal position before beginning the next examination.**

Compensating filters are shapes of aluminum mounted onto a transparent panel that slides in grooves beneath the collimator. These filters balance the intensity of the x-ray beam so as to deliver a more uniform exposure to the image receptor. For example, they may be shaped like a wedge for examination of the spine, or like a trough for chest examination.

As added filtration is increased, the result is increased x-ray beam quality and penetrability. The result on the image is the same as that for increased kVp, that is, more scatter radiation and reduced image contrast.

High-Voltage Generation

The radiologic technologist **cannot** select the type of high-voltage generator to be used for a given examination. That choice is fixed by the type of x-ray imaging system that is used. Still, it is important to understand how the various high-voltage generators affect radiographic technique and patient dose.

Three basic types of high-voltage generators are available: single phase, three phase, and high frequency. The radiation quantity and quality produced in the x-ray tube are influenced by the type of high-voltage generator that is used.

Review Figure 6-27 for the shape of the voltage waveform associated with each type of high-voltage generator. Table 15-4 lists the percentage ripple of various types of high-voltage generators, the variation in their output, and the change in radiographic technique used for two common examinations associated with each generator.

A **half-wave–rectified** generator has 100% voltage ripple. During exposure with a half-wave–rectified generator, x-rays are produced and emitted only half the time. During each negative half-cycle, no x-rays are emitted.

 Half-wave rectification results in the same radiation quality as is produced by full-wave rectification, but the radiation quantity is halved.

Half-wave rectification is used rarely today. Some mobile and dental x-ray imaging systems are half-wave rectified.

The voltage waveform for **full-wave rectification** is identical to that for half-wave rectification, except there is no dead time. During exposure, x-rays are emitted continually as pulses. Consequently, the required exposure time for full-wave rectification is only half that for half-wave rectification.

Radiation quality does not change when going from half-wave to full-wave rectification; however, radiation quantity doubles.

Three-phase power comes in two principal forms: 6 pulse or 12 pulse. The difference is determined by the manner in which the high-voltage step-up transformer is engineered.

Three-phase power results in higher x-ray quantity and quality.

The difference between the two forms is minor but does cause a detectable change in x-ray quantity and quality. Three-phase power is more efficient than single-phase power. More x-rays are produced for a given mAs setting, and the average energy of those x-rays is higher. The x-radiation emitted is nearly constant rather than pulsed.

High-frequency generators were developed in the early 1980s and are increasingly used. The voltage waveform is nearly constant, with less than 1% ripple.

High-frequency generation results in even greater x-ray quantity and quality.

TABLE 15-4	Characteristics of the Various Types of High-Voltage Generators				
				EQUIVALENT TECHNIQUE (kVp/mAs)	
Generator Type	**Percentage Ripple**	**Relative Quantity**		**Chest**	**Abdomen**
Half-wave	100	100		120/20*	74/40*
Full-wave	100	200		120/20	74/40
3-Phase, 6-pulse	14	260		115/6	72/34
3-Phase, 12-pulse	4	280		115/4	72/30
High-frequency	<1	300		112/3	70/24

*The milliampere-second value equals that for a full-wave generator; exposure time is doubled.

At present, high-frequency generators are used increasingly with dedicated mammography systems, computed tomography systems, and mobile x-ray imaging systems. It is likely that most high-voltage generators of the future will be of the high-frequency type, regardless of the required power levels.

PATIENT FACTORS

Radiographic techniques may be described by identifying three groups of factors. The first group includes **patient factors,** such as anatomical thickness and body composition. The second group consists of **image-quality factors,** such as optical density (OD), contrast, detail, and distortion. Also of importance is how these image-quality factors are influenced by the patient.

The final group includes the **exposure technique factors,** such as kilovolt peak, milliamperage, exposure time, and source-to-image receptor distance (SID), as well as grids, screens, focal-spot size, and filtration. These factors determine the basic characteristics of radiation exposure of the image receptor and patient dose, and they provide the radiologic technologist with a specific and orderly means of producing, evaluating, and comparing radiographs.

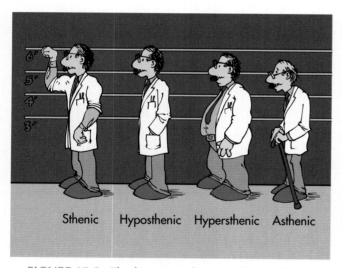

FIGURE 15-3 The four general states of body habitus.

An understanding of each of these factors is essential for the production of high-quality images.

Perhaps the most difficult task for the radiologic technologist involves evaluation of the patient. The patient's size, shape, and physical condition greatly influence the required radiographic technique.

The general size and shape of a patient is called **body habitus;** four such states have been described (Figure 15-3). The **sthenic**—meaning "strong, active"—patient is the average patient. The **hyposthenic** patient is thin but healthy appearing. Such a patient requires less radiographic technique. The **hypersthenic** patient is big in frame and usually overweight. The **asthenic** patient is small, frail, sometimes emaciated, and often elderly.

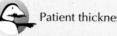 Radiographic technique charts are based on the sthenic patient.

Recognition of body habitus is essential to radiographic technique selection. Once this has been established, the thickness and composition of the anatomy being examined must be determined.

Thickness

The thicker the patient, the more x-radiation is required to penetrate the patient to expose the image receptor. For this reason, the radiologic technologist must use **calipers** to measure the thickness of the anatomy that is being irradiated.

Patient thickness should not be guessed.

Depending on the type of radiographic technique practiced, the mAs setting or the kVp will be altered as a function of the thickness of the part. Table 15-5 shows an example of how the mAs setting changes when the abdomen is imaged if a fixed-kVp technique is used. Table 15-6 reports the change in radiographic technique

TABLE 15-5	Fixed-kVp Technique for an Anterior-Posterior Abdominal Examination							
kVp	80	80	80	80	80	80	80	80
Patient thickness (cm)	16	18	20	22	24	26	28	30
mAs	12	15	22	30	45	60	90	120

TABLE 15-6	Variable-kVp Technique for an Anterior-Posterior Pelvis Examination							
mAs	100	100	100	100	100	100	100	100
Patient thickness (cm)	15	16	17	18	19	20	21	22
kVp	56	58	60	62	64	66	68	70

factors that occurs as a function of thickness of part when a variable-kVp technique is used.

Composition

Measurement of the thickness of the anatomical part does not release the radiologic technologist from exercising some additional judgment when selecting a proper radiographic technique. The thorax and the abdomen may have the same thickness, but the radiographic technique used for each will be considerably different. The radiologic technologist must estimate the mass density of the anatomical part and the range of mass densities involved.

In general, when only soft tissue is being imaged, low kVp and high mAs are used. With an extremity, however, which consists of soft tissue and bone, low kVp is used because the body part is thin.

When imaging the chest, the radiologic technologist takes advantage of the high subject contrast. Lung tissue has very low mass density, the bony structures have high mass density, and the mediastinal structures have intermediate mass density. Consequently, high kVp and low mAs can be used to good advantage. This results in an image with satisfactory contrast and low patient radiation dose.

> The chest has high subject contrast; the abdomen has low subject contrast.

These various tissues often are described by their degree of **radiolucency** or **radiopacity** (Figure 15-4). Radiolucent tissue attenuates few x-rays and appears black on the radiograph. Radiopaque tissue absorbs x-rays and appears white on the radiograph. Table 15-7 shows the relative degree of radiolucency for various types of body habitus and tissue.

Pathology

The type of pathology, its size, and its composition influence radiographic technique. In this case, the patient examination request form and previous images may be of some help. The radiologic technologist should not hesitate to seek more information from the referring physician, the radiologist, or the patient regarding the suspected pathology.

> Pathology can appear with increased radiolucency or radiopacity.

Some pathology is **destructive,** causing the tissue to be more radiolucent. Other pathology can **constructively** increase mass density or composition, causing the tissue to be more radiopaque. Practice and experience will

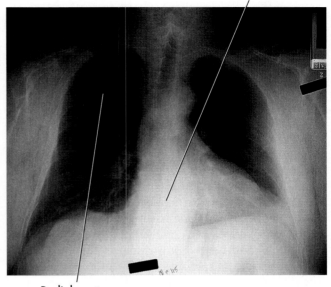

FIGURE 15-4 Relative radiolucency and optical density (OD) are shown on this radiograph. (Courtesy Bette Shans, Mesa State University.)

TABLE 15-7	Relative Degrees of Radiolucency		
	Radiographic Appearance	Body Habitus	Tissue Type
Radiolucent	Black	Asthenic	Lung
↓	↓	Hyposthenic	Fat
		Sthenic	Muscle
Radiopaque	White	Hypersthenic	Bone

guide the radiologic technologist's clinical judgment, but Box 15-1 presents a beginning classification scheme.

IMAGE-QUALITY FACTORS

The phrase *image-quality factors* refers to characteristics of the radiographic image; these include OD, contrast, image detail, and distortion. These factors provide a means for the radiologic technologist to produce, review, and evaluate radiographs. Image-quality factors are considered the "language" of radiography; often, it is difficult to separate one factor from another.

Optical Density

Optical density (OD) is the degree of blackening of the finished radiograph. OD has a numeric value (see Chapter 16) and can be present in varying degrees, from completely black, where no light is transmitted through the radiograph, to almost clear. Black is numerically

equivalent to an OD of 3 or greater, whereas clear is less than 0.2 (Figure 15-5). At an OD of 2, only 1% of viewbox light passes through the film.

In medical imaging, many problems involve an image being "too dark" or "too light." A radiograph that is too dark has a high OD caused by **overexposure.** This situation results when too much x-radiation reaches the image receptor. A radiograph that is too light has been exposed to too little x-radiation, resulting in **underexposure** and a low OD.

Overexposure and underexposure can result in unacceptable image quality, which may require that the examination be repeated. Figure 15-6 shows clinical examples of these two extremes of exposure.

OD can be controlled in radiography by two major factors: **mAs** and **SID.** A significant number of problems would arise if the SID were continually changed. Therefore, SID usually is fixed at 90 cm for mobile examinations, 100 cm for table studies, and 180 cm for upright chest examinations. Figure 15-7 illustrates the change in OD that occurs at these SIDs when other exposure technique factors remain constant.

When distance is fixed, however, as is usually the case, the mAs value becomes the primary variable technique factor used to control OD. OD increases directly with mAs, which means that if the OD is to be increased on a radiograph, the mAs setting must be increased accordingly.

> When the OD of the radiograph is the only characteristic that is to be changed, the appropriate factor to adjust would be the mAs.

OD can be affected by other factors, but the mAs value becomes the factor of choice for its control (Figure 15-8). A change in mAs of approximately 30% is required to produce a visible change in OD. As a general rule, when only the mAs setting is changed, it should be halved or doubled (Figure 15-9). If a significant change is not required, the repeat examination probably is not required.

BOX 15-1 Classifying Pathology

Radiolucent (destructive)	Radiopaque (constructive)
Active tuberculosis	Aortic aneurysm
Atrophy	Ascites
Bowel obstruction	Atelectasis
Cancer	Cirrhosis
Degenerative arthritis	Hypertrophy
Emphysema	Metastases
Osteoporosis	Pleural effusion
Pneumothorax	Pneumonia
	Sclerosis

Optical Density	Step Number
0.20	
0.22	
0.28	9
0.35	
0.50	6
0.73	
1.10	4
1.55	
2.05	2
2.57	

FIGURE 15-5 The amount of light transmitted through a radiograph is determined by the optical density (OD) of a film. The step-wedge radiograph shows a representative range of OD.

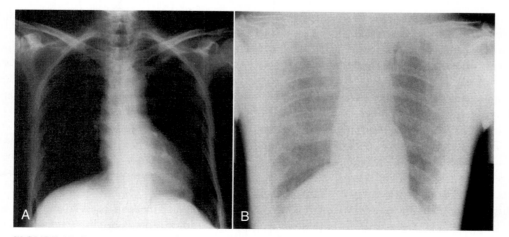

FIGURE 15-6 **A,** Overexposed radiograph of the chest is too black to be diagnostic. **B,** Likewise, an underexposed chest radiograph is unacceptable because no detail to the lung fields is apparent. (Courtesy Richard Bayless, University of Montana.)

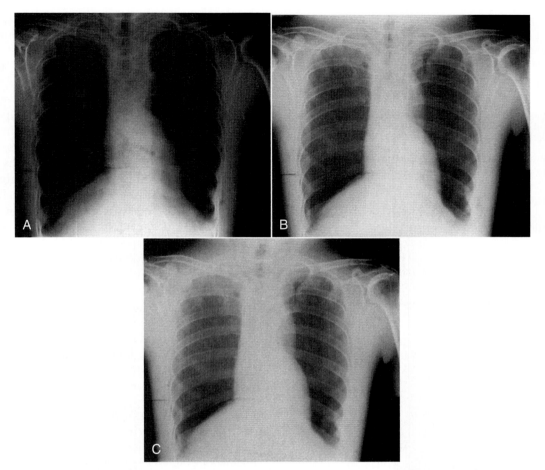

FIGURE 15-7   Normal chest radiograph taken at 100 cm source-to-image receptor distance (SID). **B,** If the exposure technique factors are not changed, a similar radiograph at 90 cm SID (**A**) will be overexposed, and at 180 cm SID (**C**) underexposed. (Courtesy Kurt Loveland, Southern Illinois University.)

> The mAs value must be changed by approximately 30% to produce a perceptible change in OD. The kVp setting must be changed by approximately 4% to produce a perceptible change in OD.

Because an increase in OD on the finished radiograph is accomplished with a proportionate increase in mAs, is the same true with kilovoltage? Yes, but the increase is not proportionate.

As kVp is increased, the quality of the beam is increased and more x-rays penetrate the anatomical part. This results in a greater number of image-forming x-rays. As discussed in Chapter 9, x-ray intensity at the patient is proportional to kVp^2 and at the image receptor to kVp^5.

Image contrast is affected when kVp is changed to adjust OD. This makes it much more difficult to optimize OD with kVp. It takes the eye of an experienced radiologic technologist to determine whether OD is the only factor to be changed, or if contrast also should be changed to optimize the radiographic image.

Technique changes involving kVp become complicated. A change in kVp affects penetration, scatter radiation, patient dose, and especially contrast. It is generally accepted that if the OD on the radiograph is to be increased with the use of kVp, an increase in kVp of 15% is equivalent to doubling the mAs. This is known as the **fifteen percent rule.**

Figure 15-10 illustrates the OD change when the fifteen percent rule is applied. If only OD is to be changed, the fifteen percent rule should not be used because such a large change in kVp would change image contrast.

> A 15% increase in kVp accompanied by a half reduction in mAs results in the same OD.

The simplest method used to increase or decrease OD on a radiograph is to increase or decrease the mAs. This reduces other possible factors that could affect the finished image. The various factors that affect OD are listed in Table 15-8.

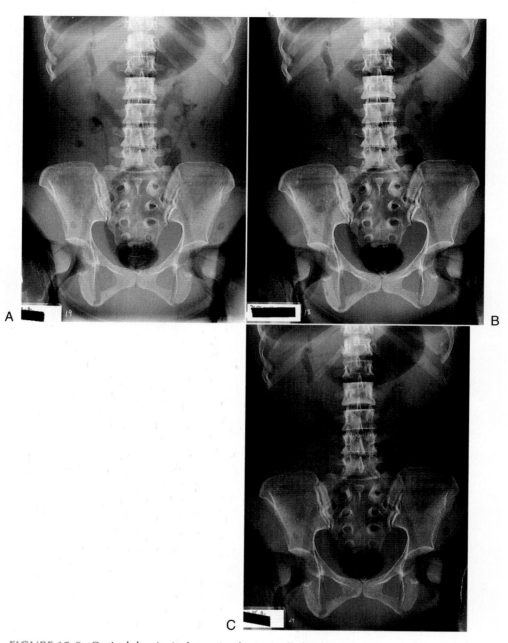

FIGURE 15-8 Optical density is determined principally by the mAs value, as shown by these phantom radiographs of the abdomen taken at 70 kVp. **A,** 10 mAs. **B,** Plus 25%, 12.5 mAs. **C,** Plus 50%, 15 mAs. (Courtesy Nancy Adams, Louisiana State University.)

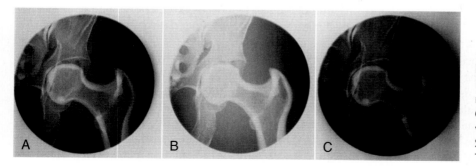

FIGURE 15-9 Changes in mAs value have a direct effect on OD. **A,** Original image. **B,** Decrease in OD when the mAs value is decreased by half. **C,** Increase in OD when the mAs value is doubled. (Courtesy Euclid Seeram, British Columbia Institute of Technology.)

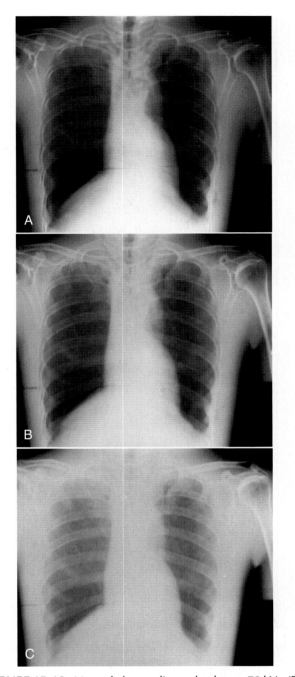

FIGURE 15-10 Normal chest radiograph taken at 70 kVp **(B)**. If the kilovoltage is increased by 15% to 80 kVp **(A)**, overexposure occurs. Similarly, at 15% less, 60 kVp **(C)**, the radiograph is underexposed. (Courtesy Euclid Seeram, British Columbia Institute of Technology.)

Contrast

The function of contrast in the image is to make anatomy more visible. Contrast is the difference in OD between adjacent anatomical structures, or the variation in OD on a radiograph. Contrast, therefore, is one of the most important factors in radiographic quality.

Contrast on a radiograph is necessary for the outline or border of a structure to be visible. Contrast is the result of differences in attenuation of the

TABLE 15-8	Technique Factors That May Affect Optical Density
Factor Increased	**Effect on Optical Density**
Milliampere-seconds (mAs)	Increase
Kilovoltage (kVp)	Increase
Source-to-image receptor distance (SID)	Decrease
Thickness of part	Decrease
Mass density	Decrease
Development time	Increase
Image receptor speed	Increase
Collimation	Decrease
Grid ratio	Decrease

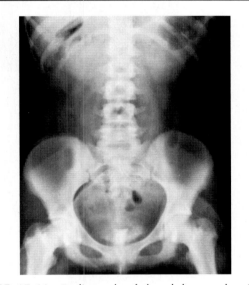

FIGURE 15-11 Radiograph of the abdomen showing the vertebral column with its inherent high contrast. The kidneys, liver, and psoas muscle are low-contrast tissues that are visualized better with low kVp. (Courtesy Euclid Seeram, British Columbia Institute of Technology.)

x-ray beam as it passes through various tissues of the body.

Figure 15-11 shows an image of the abdomen that illustrates the difference in OD between adjacent structures. High contrast is visible at the bone–soft tissue interface along the spinal column. The soft tissues of the psoas muscle and kidneys exhibit much less contrast, although details of these structures are readily visible. The contrast resolution of the soft tissues can be enhanced with reduced kVp, but at the expense of higher patient dose.

> kVp is the major factor used in controlling radiographic contrast.

The penetrability of the x-ray beam is controlled by kVp. Obtaining adequate contrast requires that the anatomical part be adequately penetrated; therefore,

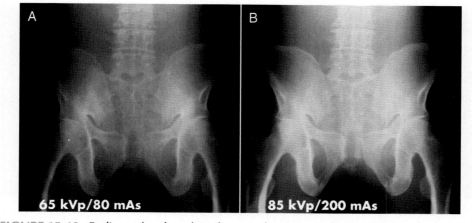

FIGURE 15-12 Radiographs of a pelvis phantom demonstrate short scale of contrast (**A**) and long scale of contrast (**B**). (Courtesy Kyle Thornton, City College of San Francisco.)

penetration becomes the key to understanding image contrast. Compare the radiographs shown in Figure 15-12: Figure 15-12, *A*, shows high contrast or "short gray scale," whereas Figure 15-12, *B*, shows low contrast or "long gray scale."

Gray scale of contrast refers to the range of ODs from the whitest to the blackest part of the radiograph. For example, think of using scissors to cut a small patch that represents each OD on the radiograph, then arranging the patches in order from lightest to darkest. The resulting OD range would be the gray scale of contrast.

High-contrast radiographs produce short gray scale. They exhibit black to white in just a few apparent steps. Low-contrast radiographs produce long gray scale and have the appearance of many shades of gray.

Figure 15-13 presents two radiographs of an aluminum step wedge—a penetrometer—that demonstrate scales of contrast. The one taken at 50 kVp shows that only five steps are visible. At 90 kVp, all 13 steps are visible because of the long scale of contrast.

To reduce contrast, the radiographer must produce a radiograph with longer gray scale contrast, and therefore with more grays. This is done by increasing the kVp. Normally, a change of approximately 4% in kVp is required visually to affect the scale of contrast in the 50- to 90-kVp range. At lower kVp, a 2-kVp change may be sufficient, whereas at higher kVp, a 10-kVp change may be required (Figure 15-14).

High contrast, "a lot of contrast," or a "short scale of contrast" is obtained by using low-kVp exposure techniques. **Low contrast** is the same as "long scale of contrast" and results from high-kVp exposure techniques. These relationships in radiographic contrast are summarized in Table 15-9.

In addition to kilovoltage, many other factors influence radiographic contrast. Although the mAs setting affects only x-ray quantity, not quality, it still influences contrast. If the mAs value is too high or too low, the

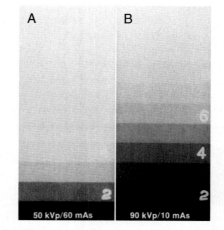

FIGURE 15-13 Images of a step wedge exposed at low kVp (**A**) and at high kVp (**B**) illustrate the meaning of short scale and long scale of contrast, respectively. (Courtesy Kyle Thornton, City College of San Francisco.)

predominant OD will fall on the shoulder or toe of the characteristic curve, respectively (see Chapter 16).

Radiographic contrast is low on the shoulder and toe regions because the gradient of the characteristic curve is low in these regions. The images of different structures will have similar ODs despite differences in subject contrast.

The use of radiographic intensifying screens results in shorter contrast scale compared with nonscreen exposures. Collimation removes some scatter radiation, producing a radiograph of shorter contrast scale. Grids also reduce the amount of scatter that reaches the film, thus also producing radiographs of shorter contrast scale. Grids with a high ratio increase the contrast. The exposure technique factors that affect contrast are summarized in Table 15-10.

A typical clinical problem faced by the radiologic technologist involves adjustment of radiographic contrast. An image is made, but the contrast scale may be too long (too many grays) or too short (too much black

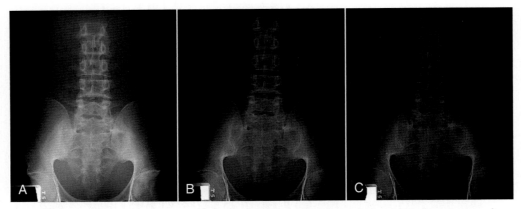

FIGURE 15-14 Radiographs of the pelvis and abdomen show that a 4-kVp increase results in a perceptible change in contrast. **A,** 75 kVp and 28 mAs. **B,** 79 kVp and 28 mAs. **C,** 81 kVp and 28 mAs. (Courtesy Mike Enriquez, Merced Community College.)

TABLE 15-9	Relationship Between kVp and Scale of Contrast
High kVp Produces	**Low kVp Produces**
Long scale	Short scale
Low contrast	High contrast
Less contrast	More contrast

TABLE 15-10	Exposure Technique Factors That May Affect Radiographic Contrast (in approximate order)
An Increase in This Factor	**Results in the Following Change in Contrast**
Kilovoltage	Decrease
Grid ratio	Increase
Beam restriction	Increase
Image receptor used	Variable
Development time	Decrease
Milliampere-seconds	Decrease (toe, shoulder)

and white). To solve such a problem, apply the fifteen percent rule. Change the kVp by 15%, while changing the mAs by one half or double.

Question: A patient's knee measures 14 cm and an exposure is made at 62 kVp/12 mAs. The resulting contrast scale is too short. What should the repeat technique be?

Answer: Increase kVp by 15%.
62 kVp × 0.15 = 9.3 kVp
Therefore, new kVp = 62 + 9 = 71 kVp
Reduce mAs to ½.
12 mAs × 0.5 = 6 mAs
Repeat technique = 71 kVp/6 mAs

A smaller technique compensation for a change in contrast scale may be required. An increase of 5% in kVp may be accompanied by a 30% reduction in mAs to produce the same OD at a slightly reduced contrast scale. This is known as the **five percent rule.**

Proper technique compensation by the radiologic technologist is a judgment call. The anatomical part, body habitus, suspected pathology, and x-ray image receptor characteristics all must be considered by the skillful radiologic technologist. With practice and experience, this will become routine.

Question: A modest reduction in image contrast is required for a knee exposed at 62 kVp/12 mAs. What technique should be tried?

Answer: Apply the five percent rule:
62 kVp × 0.05 = 3.1 kVp
62 + 3 = 65 kVp
12 mAs × 0.30 = 3.6 mAs
12 − 4 = 8 mAs
Repeat technique = 65 kVp/8 mAs

Detail

Detail describes the sharpness of appearance of small structures on the radiograph. With adequate detail, even the smallest parts of the anatomy are visible, and the radiologist can more readily detect tissue abnormalities. Image detail must be evaluated by two means—**recorded detail** and **visibility of image detail.**

Sharpness of image detail refers to the structural lines or borders of tissues in the image and the amount of blur of the image. Factors that generally control the sharpness of image detail are the geometric factors discussed in Chapter 16—focal spot size, SID, and object-to-image receptor distance (OID). Sharpness of image detail also is influenced by the type of intensifying screen used and the presence of motion.

Sharpness of image detail is best measured by spatial resolution.

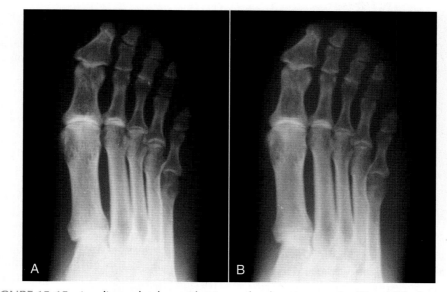

FIGURE 15-15   A radiograph taken with a 1-mm focal-spot x-ray tube **(A)** exhibits far greater detail than one taken with a 2-mm focal-spot x-ray tube **(B).** (Courtesy Mike Enriquez, Merced Community College.)

To produce the sharpest image detail, one should use the smallest appropriate focal spot and the longest SID and place the anatomical part as close to the image receptor as possible (i.e., minimize OID). Figure 15-15 shows two radiographs of a foot phantom. One was taken under optimum conditions and the other with poor technique. The difference in sharpness of image detail is obvious.

Visibility of image detail describes the ability to see the detail on the radiograph and is best measured by contrast resolution. Loss of visibility refers to any factor that causes deterioration or obscuring of image detail. For example, fog reduces the ability to see structural lines on the image.

An attempt to produce the best-defined image can be made by using all the correct factors, but if the film is fogged by light or radiation, the detail present will not be fully visible (Figure 15-16). You might conclude that good detail is still present but that its visibility is poor. Because kVp and the mAs value influence image contrast, these factors must be chosen with care for each examination.

> The visibility of image detail is best measured by contrast resolution.

The assumption is that any factor that affects OD and contrast affects the visibility of image detail. Key factors that provide the best visibility of image detail are collimation, use of grids, and other methods that prevent scatter radiation from reaching the image receptor.

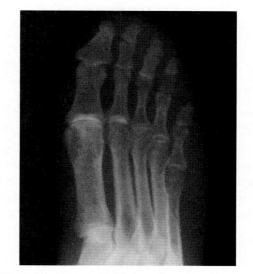

FIGURE 15-16   Same radiograph as shown in 15-15, *A*, except that visibility of image detail is reduced because of safelight fog. (Courtesy Mike Enriquez, Merced Community College.)

Distortion

The fourth image-quality factor is distortion, the misrepresentation of object size and shape on the radiograph. Because of the position of the x-ray tube, the anatomical part, and the image receptor, the final image may misrepresent the object.

Poor alignment of the image receptor or the x-ray tube can result in **elongation** of the image. *Elongation* means that the anatomical part of interest appears bigger than normal.

Poor alignment of the anatomical part may result in **foreshortening** of the image. *Foreshortening* means that the anatomical part appears smaller than

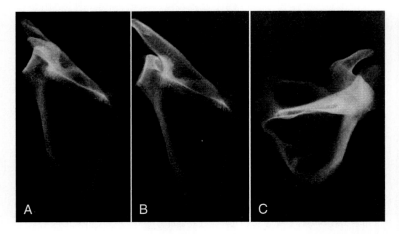

FIGURE 15-17 **A,** Normal projection of the scapula. **B,** Elongation of the scapula. **C,** Foreshortening of the scapula. (Courtesy Lynne Davis, Houston Community College.)

normal. Figure 15-17 provides examples of elongation and foreshortening. Many body parts are naturally foreshortened as a result of shape (e.g., ribs, facial bones).

Distortion can be minimized through proper alignment of the tube, the anatomical part, and the image receptor. This alignment is fundamentally important for **patient positioning.**

> Distortion is reduced by positioning the anatomical part of interest in a plane parallel to that of the image receptor.

Table 15-11 summarizes the principal radiographic image-quality factors. The primary controlling technique factor for each image-quality factor is given, as are secondary technique factors that influence each image-quality factor.

EXPOSURE TECHNIQUE CHARTS

kVp, mA, exposure time, and SID are the principal exposure technique factors. It is important for the radiologic technologist to know how to manipulate these exposure technique factors to produce the desired OD, radiographic contrast, image detail, and distortion on the finished radiograph.

It is not necessary, however, to become creative with each new patient. For each radiographic imaging system, a chart should be available that describes standard methods for consistently producing high-quality images. Such an aid is called a **radiographic technique chart.** Radiographic technique charts are tables that provide a means for determining the specific technical factors to be used in a given radiographic examination.

For a radiographic technique chart to meet with success, the radiologic technologist must understand its purpose, how it was constructed, and how it is to be used. Most important, the technologist must know how

TABLE 15-11	Principal Radiographic Image-Quality Factors	
Factor	**Controlled by**	**Influenced by**
Optical density	mAs	KVp
		Distance
		Thickness of part
		Mass density
		Development time/ temperature
		Image receptor speed
		Collimation
		Grid ratio
Contrast	kVp	mAs (toe, shoulder)
		Development time/ temperature
		Image receptor used
		Collimation
		Grid ratio
Detail	Focal-spot size	SID
		OID
		Motion
		All factors related to density and contrast
Distortion	Patient positioning	Alignment of tube, anatomical part, and image receptor

to make adjustments for body habitus and pathologic processes.

When used properly, the radiographic technique chart allows for consistently good diagnostic images. The scale of contrast and the OD are more predictable than if no chart is used.

Radiographic technique charts can be prepared to accommodate all types of facilities. The four principal types of charts are based on **variable kilovoltage, fixed kilovoltage, high kilovoltage,** and **automatic exposure.** Each chart provides the radiologic technologist with a guide to the selection of exposure factors for all patients and all examinations.

Most facilities select a particular type of chart for use and then prepare similar charts for each radiographic examination room. The type of chart selected usually depends on the technical director of radiology in place, the type of imaging systems available, the screen-film combination used, and the accessories available.

Radiographic technique charts and their use become an important issue in patient protection. Radiologic technologists are required to use their skills to produce the best possible image with a single exposure. Repeat examinations serve only to increase patient radiation dose.

A principal advantage of using technique charts is the consistency in exposure that occurs from one technologist to another and in comparison of examinations on the same patient on different dates and with different technologists.

Preparation of a technique chart does not require that it be created completely from scratch. Many authors have guides that can be used in preparation of specific charts. Each radiographic imaging system is unique in terms of its radiation characteristics. Therefore, a specific chart should be prepared and tested for each examination room.

Radiographic technique charts from books, pamphlets, and manufacturers should not be used as printed.

Before preparation of the radiographic technique chart begins, the x-ray equipment must be calibrated by a medical physicist and the processing system must be thoroughly evaluated. The total filtration should also be determined. Although 2.5 mm Al is the prescribed standard, 3 mm Al total filtration or more may be available on the collimator housing. This significantly alters contrast and makes a considerable difference in any technique chart.

The type of grid to be used should be known and the collimator or beam restrictor checked for accurate light field and x-ray beam coincidence. This is most important so that all variables are reduced to a minimum. When a radiographic technique chart is found to be inadequate, these factors should be checked first.

The **variable-kVp radiographic technique chart** uses a fixed mAs value and a kVp that varies according to the thickness of the anatomical part. The basic characteristic of the variable-kVp chart is an inherently short scale of contrast. In general, exposures made with this method provide radiographs of shorter contrast scale because of the use of lower kVp.

Exposure directed by the variable-kVp chart usually results in higher patient dose and less exposure latitude. For success, the radiologic technologist must be accurate in measuring the anatomical part before selecting exposure factors from the chart. Without such care and attention, the anatomical part may not be fully penetrated because of the lower kVp.

kVp varies with the thickness of the anatomical part by 2 kVp/cm.

A kVp can be established by approximate procedures, so a variable-kVp technique chart can be formulated. The beginning kVp depends on the voltage ripple as follows:

VARIABLE kVp
Beginning kVp (high frequency) =
2 × thickness of anatomy (cm) + 23

To begin preparation of a variable-kVp radiographic technique chart, select the body part for examination. For example, if the knee is chosen, use a knee phantom for test exposures.

First, measure the thickness of the knee phantom, using a caliper designed for that purpose. Multiply that thickness by 2, and add 23; this indicates a kVp with which to begin if the high-voltage generator is of high frequency. If the high-voltage generator is single phase or three phase, 30 or 25, respectively, is the additive factor.

Question: A phantom knee measures 14 cm thick. What single-phase kVp should be used to begin construction of a variable-kVp technique chart?

Answer: 14 cm × 2 = 28 + 30 = 58 kVp

The kilovoltage setting for examination of the knee is 58 kVp. The next task is to select the optimal mAs setting at this kVp. This depends on the image receptor characteristics and the effectiveness of scatter radiation control. For example, when using a 400-speed image receptor with an 8:1 grid, make test exposures at 58 kVp with 9 mAs, 12 mAs, and 20 mAs (Figure 15-18). Select the radiograph that produces the best OD, or make additional exposures at other mAs setting values if necessary.

The result of this exercise is the first line of the variable-kVp technique chart. The kVp and mAs settings to be used when a knee measuring 14 cm is radiographed

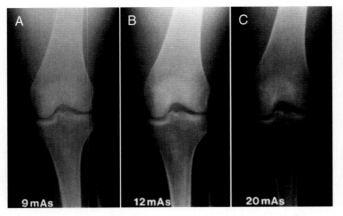

FIGURE 15-18 Radiographs of a knee phantom taken at 58 kVp. That obtained at 12 mAs **(B)** was selected to begin the variable-kilovoltage chart. (Courtesy Lynne Davis, Houston Community College.)

TABLE 15-12	Variable-kVp Chart for Examination of the Knee	
Knee—AP/Lat	**Part Thickness (cm)**	**kVp**
mAs: 12	8	50
SID: 100 cm	9	52
Grid: 12:1	10	54
Collimation: to part	11	56
Image receptor	**12**	**58**
Speed: 200	13	60
	14	62
	15	64
	16	66

AP, Anterior-posterior; *Lat,* lateral; *SID,* source-to-image receptor distance.

have been established at 58 kVp and 12 mAs, as shown in Table 15-12.

To prepare a variable-kVp radiographic technique chart for other anatomical parts, the same procedure is used. Because radiologists prefer similar contrast scales for examination of the same anatomy, the variable-kVp technique chart has been replaced largely by the fixed-kVp technique chart.

The **fixed-kVp radiographic technique chart** is the one used most often. Developed by Arthur Fuchs, it is a method of selecting exposures that produce radiographs with a longer scale of contrast. The kVp is selected as the optimum required for penetration of the anatomical part. This usually results in somewhat higher kVp values for most examinations than are produced by the variable-kVp technique.

 For each anatomical part, there is an optimum kVp.

TABLE 15-13	Fixed-kVp Chart for Examination of the Abdomen	
Abdomen—AP	**Part Thickness (cm)**	**Required mAs**
kVp: 80	Small: 14-20	56
SID: 100 cm	Medium: 21-25	80
Grid: 12:1	Large: 26-31	104
Collimation: to part		
Image receptor speed: 200		

AP, Anterior-posterior; *SID,* source-to-image receptor distance.

Once selected, the kVp is fixed at that level for each type of examination and does not vary according to different thicknesses of the anatomical part. The mAs value, however, is changed according to the thickness of the anatomical part, to provide the proper OD. For example, all examinations of the knee might require 60 kVp with mAs adjusted to accommodate for differences in thickness.

Because the fixed-kVp technique usually requires higher kVp, one benefit is lower patient dose. There is greater latitude and more consistency with exposures of the same anatomical part.

Measurement of the part is not critical because part size is grouped as small, medium, or large. For most x-ray examinations of the spine and trunk of the body, the optimal kVp is approximately 80 kVp. Approximately 70 kVp is appropriate for the soft tissue of the abdomen. For most extremities, the optimum would be approximately 60 kVp.

To prepare a fixed-kVp radiographic technique chart, the first step is to separate the anatomical part thickness into three groups—small, medium, and large—by identifying the range of thickness that is to be included in each group. With use of the abdomen as an example, small might be 14 to 20 cm; medium, 21 to 25 cm; and large, 26 to 32 cm.

For test exposures, use a medium-sized phantom and begin with 80 kVp. Produce radiographs at mAs increments of 40, 60, 80, and so forth, until the proper OD is attained (Figure 15-19). Again, the OD selected depends on the type of image receptor used and the scatter radiation control devices available.

Once the proper OD has been established, the chart then can be expanded to include small and large anatomical parts. For small anatomical parts, reduce the mAs by 30%. For large anatomical parts, increase the mAs by 30%. For a part that is swollen as a result of trauma, a 50% increase may be required. Table 15-13 presents the results of a representative procedure.

Fixed-kVp charts also can be calculated with specific mAs values for every 2-cm thickness. This approach is more accurate than is use of subjective small, medium, and large labels.

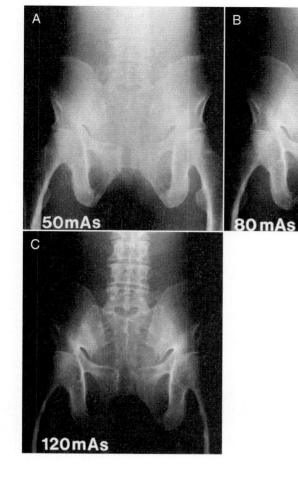

FIGURE 15-19 Radiographs of an abdomen phantom used to construct a fixed-kVp chart. All exposures were taken at 80 kVp. From this series, 80 mAs **(B)** was selected to begin the chart. (Courtesy Tammy Bauman, Banner Thunderbird Medical Center.)

The kVp selected for **high-kVp technique charts** is usually greater than 100. For example, overhead radiographs for procedures in which barium contrast medium is used would use 120 kVp for each exposure. High-kVp exposure techniques are ideal for barium work to ensure adequate penetration of the barium.

This type of exposure technique also could be used for routine chest radiography to attain improved visualization of the various tissue mass densities present in the lung fields and the mediastinum. Lower or more conventional kVp settings provide increased subject contrast between bone and soft tissue. When 120 kVp is selected for chest radiography, however, all skeletal tissue is penetrated, and visualization of the different soft tissue mass densities present is enhanced.

To prepare a high-kVp technique chart, the procedure is basically the same as for preparing the fixed-kVp technique chart. All exposures for a particular anatomical part would use the same kVp. Obviously, the mAs value would be much less.

Test exposures are made with the use of a phantom to determine the appropriate mAs setting for adequate OD. Figure 15-20 shows a chest radiograph made at 120 kVp. Note the improved visualization of the tissue markings of the bronchial tree and the mediastinal structures, compared with that of the low-kVp radiographs. An additional advantage of the high-kVp exposure technique is reduced patient dose.

AUTOMATIC EXPOSURE TECHNIQUES

The appearance of the operating console of x-ray imaging systems is changing in response to the ability to incorporate computer-assisted technology. Several automated exposure techniques are now available, but none relieves the radiologic technologist of the responsibility of identifying particular characteristics of the patient and the anatomical part to be imaged.

Computer-assisted automatic exposure systems use an electronic exposure timer, such as those described in Chapter 6. Radiation intensity is measured with a photocell or an ionization chamber, and exposure is terminated when the proper radiation exposure to the image receptor has been reached. The principles associated with automatic exposure systems have already been described, but the importance of using radiographic exposure charts with these systems has not.

Automatic control x-ray systems are not completely automatic. It is incorrect to assume that because the

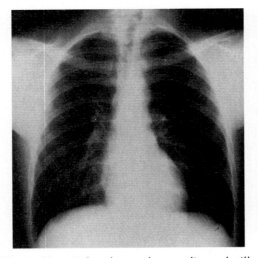

FIGURE 15-20 High-voltage chest radiograph illustrates improved visualization of mediastinal structures. (Courtesy Andrew Woodward, Wor-Wic Community College.)

TABLE 15-14	Factors to Consider When Constructing an Exposure Chart for Automatic Systems
Factor for Selection	**Rationale for Selection**
Kilovolt peak	To select for each anatomical part
Optical density control	To fine-tune for differences in field size or anatomical part
Collimation	To reduce patient dose and ensure proper response of automatic exposure control
Accessory selection	To optimize the radiation dose–image quality ratio

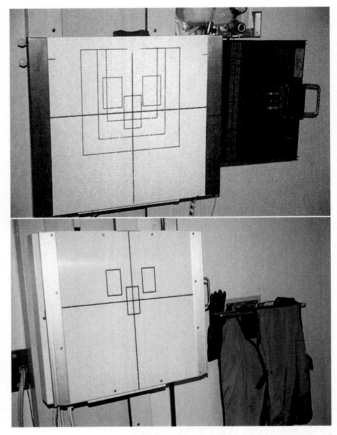

FIGURE 15-21 Vertical chest Bucky shows the position of automatic exposure control (AEC) sensors represented as three rectangles.

radiologic technologist does not have to select kVp and mAs settings and time for each examination, a less qualified or less skilled operator can use the system.

Usually, the radiologic technologist must use a guide for the selection of kVp that is similar to that used in the fixed-kVp method. OD selections are scaled numerically to allow for "tweaking" the calibration of the sensors for changes in field size or anatomy that require OD adjustment.

Patient positioning *must be absolutely accurate* because the specific body part must be placed over the phototiming device to ensure proper exposure.

The factors shown in Table 15-14 must be considered when one is preparing the radiographic exposure chart for an automatic x-ray system. The kVp is selected according to the specific anatomical part that is being examined.

Radiation exposure in most x-ray imaging systems is determined by an automatic exposure control (AEC) system. AEC incorporates a device that senses the amount of radiation incident on the image receptor. Through an electronic feedback circuit, radiation exposure is terminated when a sufficient number of x-rays has reached the image receptor to produce an acceptable OD.

To image with the use of an AEC, the radiologic technologist selects the appropriate kVp, mA, and backup time, as well as the proper sensors and OD. Exposure is terminated when the image receptor has received the appropriate radiation exposure to correspond with the acceptable OD.

With AEC devices, usually two or more exposure sensors are available for control (Figure 15-21). For instance, three radiation-sensing cells may be available, and the technologist is responsible for selecting which of the sensors should be used for the examination. During a chest examination, if the mediastinum is the region of interest, only the central sensing cell is used. If the lung fields are of principal importance, the two lateral cells are activated.

Regulations require that AECs have a 600-mAs safety override. If the AEC fails to terminate the exposure, the secondary safety circuit terminates it at 600 mAs, which is equivalent to a few seconds, depending on the mA.

In addition to selecting exposure cells, the radiologic technologist usually has a three- to seven-position dial labeled "OD" with numeric steps. Each step on the dial is calibrated to increase or decrease the preset average

OD of the image receptor by 0.1. This control can be used to accommodate any unusual patient characteristics or to overcome the slowly changing calibration or sensitivity of the AEC.

A technique chart for AEC may be helpful. Such a chart would include mA, kVp, backup time, sensor selection, and OD setting.

Microprocessors are being incorporated ever more frequently into operating consoles. A microprocessor allows the operator to select digitally any kVp or mAs setting; the microprocessor automatically activates the appropriate mA station and exposure time. With falling-load generators, the microprocessor begins the exposure at a maximum mA setting and then causes the tube current to be reduced during exposure. The overall objective is to minimize exposure time to reduce motion blur.

A widely used electronic technique for patient exposure control is referred to as **anatomically programmed radiography (APR)**. APR also uses microprocessor technology. Rather than have the radiologic technologist select a desired kVp and mAs, graphics on the console or on a video touch screen guide the technologist (Figure 15-22).

To produce an image, the radiologic technologist simply touches an icon or a written description of the anatomical part to be imaged and the body habitus. The microprocessor selects the appropriate kVp and mAs settings automatically. The whole process uses AEC, resulting in near-flawless radiographs and fewer repeats. However, precise patient positioning relative to the phototiming sensor is still critical for producing high-quality radiographs.

The principle of APR is similar to that of AEC, with the radiographic technique chart stored in the microprocessor of the control unit. The service engineer loads the controlling programs during installation and calibrates the exposure control circuit for the general conditions of the facility.

The radiologic technologist needs only to select the part and its relative size before each exposure. The programmed instructions, however, must be continuously adjusted by the radiologic technologist until the entire panel of examinations is optimized for best image quality.

Common to all AEC systems is the need for the radiographer to be very conscious of the possibility that scatter radiation may reach the sensing cells. These cells cannot tell the difference between primary beam and scatter radiation, so if a high proportion of scatter radiation reaches the cells, the exposure is terminated prematurely.

A classic example of a situation in which this can occur is the lateral lumbar spine examination. A piece of lead rubber on the tabletop behind the patient on the edge of the illuminated field absorbs scatter radiation, thereby correcting this problem.

TOMOGRAPHY

A conventional radiograph of the chest or abdomen images all structures contained in these parts of the body with approximately equal fidelity. Structures, however, are superimposed on one another, and often this superimposition results in masking of the structure of interest. When this occurs, a procedure called conventional **tomography** may be necessary.

The tomographic examination is designed to image only that anatomy that lies in a plane of interest, while blurring structures on either side of that plane. The radiographic contrast of the tissue of interest is enhanced by blurring of the anatomical structures above and below that tissue.

Most features of a tomographic x-ray imaging system appear similar to those of a conventional radiographic imaging system (Figure 15-23). Note the vertical rod that connects the x-ray tube above the table with the

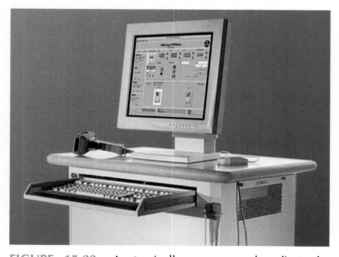

FIGURE 15-22 Anatomically programmed radiography (APR) operating console with lower ribs and automatic exposure control selected.

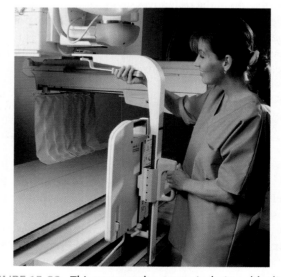

FIGURE 15-23 This tomography system is designed for linear movement with a general purpose imaging system. (Courtesy General Electric Medical Systems.)

TABLE 15-15	Representative Linear Tomography Techniques			
Examination	Projection	kVp	mAs*	Section Thickness
Cervical spine	Anterior-posterior	75	60	3-5 mm
	Lateral	77	60	2 mm
Thoracic spine	Anterior-posterior	77	80	5 mm
Lumbar spine	Anterior-posterior	77	140	5 mm
Chest	Anterior-posterior	96	80	2-5 cm
Intravenous pyelogram	Anterior-posterior	70	140	1 cm
Wrist	Anterior-posterior	48	20	2 mm

*Usually automatic exposure control.

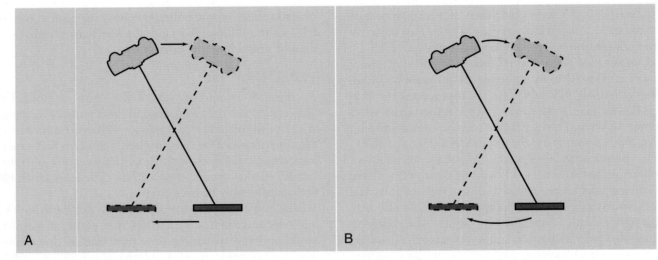

FIGURE 15-24   A, Image receptor and tube head of a general purpose x-ray imaging system designed to move tomographically within a plane. **B,** An imaging system designed for tomography to move within an arc.

image receptor below the patient to enable both to move in reciprocal fashion about the fulcrum. This feature is unique to tomography.

As the top of the rod moves in one direction, the bottom of the rod moves in the opposite direction. At one point, no movement is occurring in either direction. This is the fulcrum; all images at the level of the fulcrum are stationary, thus appearing with less blur and higher contrast.

 The principal advantage of tomography is improved contrast resolution.

Since the introduction of computed tomography (CT) and magnetic resonance imaging (MRI) with their excellent contrast resolution, conventional tomography is used less frequently. Conventional tomography is now applied principally to high-contrast procedures, such as imaging of calcified kidney stones. Table 15-15 lists the more common tomographic examinations and their representative techniques.

The simplest tomographic examination is linear tomography. During linear tomography (Figure 15-24),

the x-ray tube is attached mechanically to the image receptor and moves in one direction, while the image receptor moves in the opposite direction.

Other aspects of the linear tomographic examination are shown in Figure 15-25. The fulcrum is the imaginary pivot point about which the x-ray tube and the image receptor move. The position of the fulcrum determines the object plane, and only those anatomical structures lying within this plane are imaged clearly.

Figure 15-26 illustrates how anatomical structures in the object plane are imaged while structures above and below this plane are not. The examination begins with the x-ray tube and the image receptor positioned on opposite sides of the fulcrum. Exposure begins as the x-ray tube and the image receptor move simultaneously in opposite directions. The image of an anatomical structure lying in the object plane, such as the arrow, will have a fixed position on the image receptor throughout tube travel.

On the other hand, images of structures lying above or below the object plane, such as the ball and the box, will exhibit varying positions on the image receptor during tomographic movement. Note that not only are the

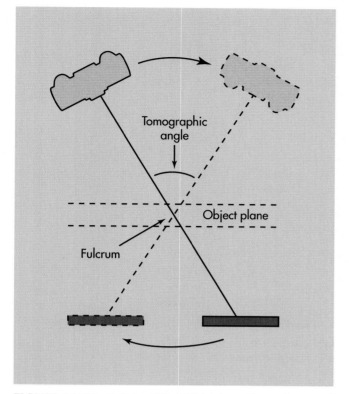

FIGURE 15-25 Relationship of fulcrum, object plane, and tomographic angle.

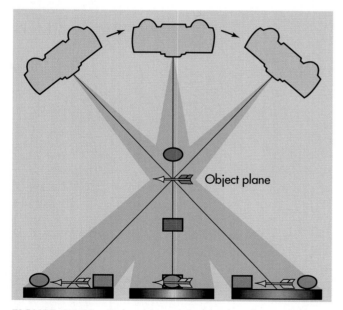

FIGURE 15-26 Only objects lying in the object plane are properly imaged. Objects above and below this plane are blurred because they are imaged across the film.

images of the ball and the box blurring because they are moving across the image receptor, but each is moving in an opposite direction.

Consequently, the ball and the box will be blurred. The larger the tomographic angle, the more blurred are the images of structures above and below the object plane.

 The farther from the object plane an anatomical structure is, the more blurred its image will be.

Objects lying outside the plane of the fulcrum will exhibit increasing motion blur with increasing distance from the object plane. The thickness of tissue that will be imaged is called the **tomographic section,** and its thickness is controlled by the **tomographic angle** (Figure 15-27).

The larger the tomographic angle, the thinner is the tomographic section.

Table 15-16 shows the approximate relationship between tomographic angle and tomographic section thickness.

When the tomographic angle is very small (for example, 0 degrees), the section thickness is the entire anatomical structure, resulting in a conventional radiograph. When the tomographic angle is 10 degrees, the section thickness is approximately 6 mm; structures lying farther than approximately 3 mm from the object plane appear blurred.

A linear anatomical structure can be imaged with less blur if the length of the structure is positioned parallel to the x-ray tube motion. This is illustrated with a tomographic test object (Figure 15-28). Conversely, Figure 15-29 shows how linear structures that lie perpendicular to the x-ray tube motion are blurred more easily.

If the tomographic angle is less than about 10 degrees, the section thickness will be quite large (see Table 15-16). This type of tomography is called zonography because a relatively large zone of tissue is imaged. Zonography is used when the subject contrast is so low that thin-section tomography would result in a poor image. Zonography finds greatest application in chest and renal examination, in which tomographic angles of 5 to 10 degrees usually are used.

Panoramic tomography was first developed for a fast dental survey but finds increasing diagnostic application of the curved bony structures of the head, such as the mandible. For this procedure, the x-ray tube and the image receptor move around the head, as shown in Figure 15-30. The x-ray beam is collimated to a slit as shown. The image receptor is likewise slit-collimated. During the examination, the image receptor translates behind the slit collimator, so it is exposed for several seconds along its length. Figure 15-31 is a clinical example.

The principal advantage of tomography is its improved radiographic contrast. Through blurring of overlying and underlying tissues, the subject contrast of tissue of the tomographic section is enhanced.

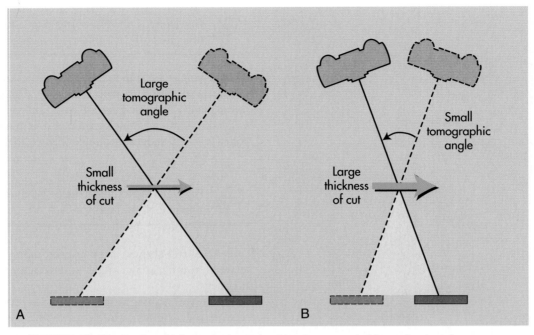

FIGURE 15-27   Section thickness is determined by the tomographic angle. **A**, A large tomographic angle results in a thin section. **B**, A small tomographic angle results in a thick section.

TABLE 15-16	Approximate Values for Section Thickness During Linear Tomography as a Function of Tomographic Angle
Tomographic Angle (degrees)	**Section Thickness (mm)**
0	Infinity
2	31
4	16
6	11
10	6
20	3
35	2
50	1

The principal disadvantage of tomography is increased patient dose. The x-ray tube is on during the entire period of tube travel, which can last several seconds. A single nephrotomographic exposure (examination of the kidneys), for example, can result in a patient dose of 1000 mrad (10 mGy$_t$).

Furthermore, most tomographic examinations require several exposures to ensure that the tomographic section of interest is imaged. A 16-film tomographic examination can result in a patient dose of several rad (mGy$_t$).

 During tomography, parallel grids must be used, and the grid lines must be oriented in the same direction as the tube movement.

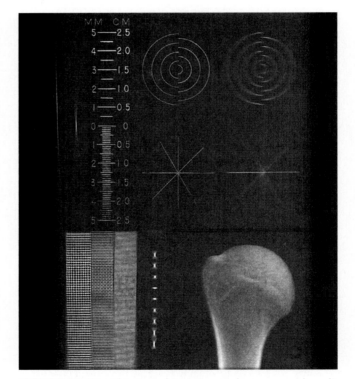

FIGURE 15-28   This test object image shows properly calibrated elevation and increased blur of objects perpendicular to the motion of the x-ray tube. (Courtesy Sharon Glaze, Baylor College of Medicine.)

Grids are used during tomography for the same reason that they are used during radiography. For linear tomography, this usually means that the grid will be positioned with its grid lines parallel to the length of the table.

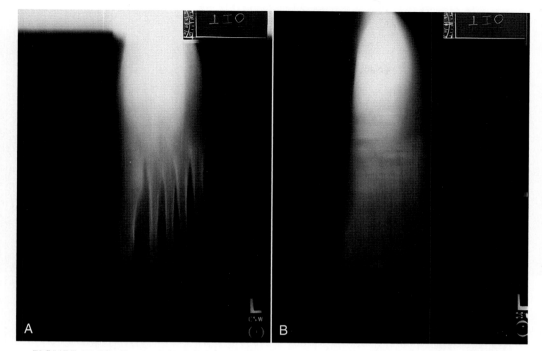

FIGURE 15-29 Foot tomographs obtained with x-ray tube motion. **A**, Parallel to the body axis. **B**, Perpendicular to the body axis. (Courtesy Rees Stuteville, Oregon Institute of Technology.)

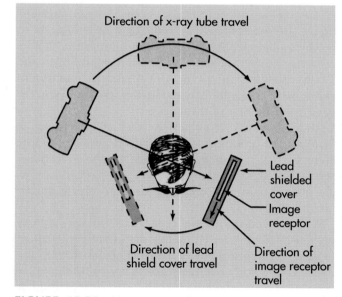

FIGURE 15-30 X-ray source–image receptor motion for panoramic tomography.

MAGNIFICATION RADIOGRAPHY

Magnification radiography is a technique that is used principally by vascular radiologists and neuroradiologists and frequently in mammography. Magnification radiography enhances the visualization of small vessels. Conventional radiography strives to minimize the OID. Magnification radiography deliberately increases the OID.

To obtain a magnified radiograph, the OID is increased, while the SID is held constant (Figure 15-32). The degree of magnification is given by the **magnification factor** (**MF**) as follows:

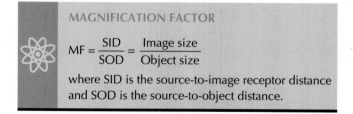

MAGNIFICATION FACTOR

$$MF = \frac{SID}{SOD} = \frac{Image\ size}{Object\ size}$$

where SID is the source-to-image receptor distance and SOD is the source-to-object distance.

Question: A magnified radiograph of the sella turcica is taken at 100 cm SID, with the object positioned 25 cm from the image receptor. If the image of the sella turcica measures 16 mm, what is its actual size?

Answer:
$$MF = \frac{100}{(100 - 25)} = 1.33$$

$$\frac{Image\ size}{Object\ size} = MF$$

$$Object\ size = \frac{Image\ size}{MF} = \frac{16}{1.33} = 12.0\ mm$$

A small focal spot must be used for magnification radiography to help reduce the loss of image detail. The focal-spot blur that results from an unnecessarily large focal spot can destroy the diagnostic value of the magnified radiograph.

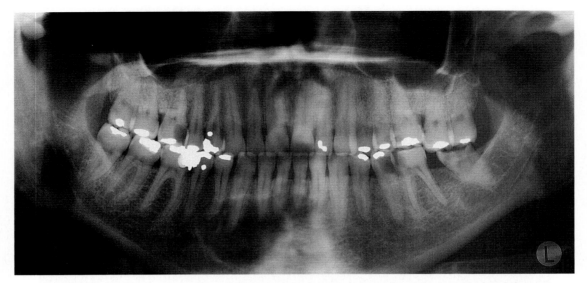

FIGURE 15-31   Panoramic tomogram showing restorations and a right mandibular defect. (Courtesy Kenneth Abramovitch, University of Texas Dental Branch.)

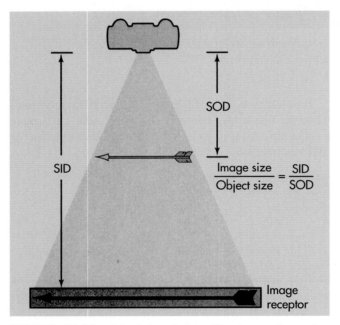

FIGURE 15-32   Principle of magnification radiography. The magnification factor is equal to the ratio of image size to object size.

Usually, grids are not needed for magnified radiography. The large OID results in a significant air-gap, so that much of the scatter radiation misses the image receptor. The larger the OID, the greater is the amount of scatter radiation that reaches the image receptor.

The principal disadvantage of magnification radiography, similar to so many specialized techniques, is increased patient dose. To obtain a magnification factor of 2, one must position the patient halfway between the x-ray tube and the image receptor. Recall that radiation intensity is related to the square of the distance, which suggests a fourfold increase in patient dose. In reality,

most magnification radiographs result in only three times the normal patient dose because grids are not used.

SUMMARY

Radiographic exposure factors (voltage, mAs, and distance) are manipulated by radiologic technologists to produce high-quality radiographs. Exposure factors influence radiographic quantity (number of x-rays) and quality (penetrability of the x-rays). Proper selection of exposure factors optimizes the spatial resolution and the contrast resolution of the image.

Radiographic technique is the combination of factors used to expose an anatomical part to produce a high-quality radiograph. Radiographic technique is characterized by the following: (1) patient factors, (2) image-quality factors, and (3) exposure technique factors.

Patient factors include anatomical thickness, body composition, and any pathology that is present. Radiographers recognize sthenic, asthenic, hyposthenic, and hypersthenic body habitus types as a way to determine body composition and thus to select proper radiographic technique. Pathology in the body may be destructive and therefore radiolucent, which requires a reduction in technique, or constructive and therefore radiopaque, which requires an increase in technique.

Image-quality factors include OD, contrast, image detail, and distortion. OD, blackening of the radiograph, is defined as the log of the incident light over the transmitted light. Contrast is the difference in OD between adjacent anatomical structures.

High kVp produces low-contrast images, whereas low kVp produces high-contrast images. Image detail is the sharpness of the image on the radiograph. To produce the sharpest image detail, use the smallest focal spot, the longest SID, and the least OID. Distortion refers to misrepresentation of object size or shape on the radiograph.

The principal radiographic exposure factors are kVp, mAs, and SID. The two technique charts used most commonly by radiographers to produce consistently high-quality radiographs are the fixed-kVp chart and the high-kVp chart. The high-kVp chart is used for barium studies and chest radiographs with kVp from 120 to 135 kVp. The fixed-kVp chart uses approximately 60 kVp for extremity radiography and approximately 80 kVp for examinations of the trunk of the body.

Even with AEC, radiographic exposure charts are required. APR uses microprocessor technology to program the technique chart into the control unit. The radiographer selects an anatomical display of the part, and the microprocessor selects the appropriate kVp and mAs settings automatically.

Although CT and MRI have replaced many plain-film conventional tomographic examinations, tomography of the chest and kidneys still is performed frequently. The emphasis is generally on linear techniques with thin 1-cm tomographic sections.

The tomographic object plane contains the fulcrum—the imaginary pivot point from which the tube and the image receptor move. The tomographic angle is the angle of movement that determines tomographic section thickness. The principal advantage of tomography is its improved radiographic contrast.

Magnification radiography is a technique that is used mainly for mammography, neurovascular, and interventional radiography.

CHALLENGE QUESTIONS

1. Define or otherwise identify the following:
   a. Kilovolt peak (kVp)
   b. Milliampere-second (mAs)
   c. Beam penetrability
   d. Fifteen percent rule
   e. Source-to-image receptor distance (SID)
   f. Inherent filtration
   g. Body habitus
   h. Image detail
   i. Image quality factors
   j. Distortion

2. Discuss how an increase in kVp changes x-ray quantity, x-ray quality, and contrast scale.
3. List and discuss the four exposure technique factors. How does each affect OD?
4. What is normally the shortest radiographic exposure time on single-phase, three-phase, and high-frequency imaging systems?
5. Describe how a change in SID from 100 cm to 180 cm should be accompanied by a change in mA and exposure time.
6. Why does an x-ray tube have two focal-spot sizes?
7. A radiographic technique calls for 82 kVp at 400mA, 200 ms, and an SID of 90 cm. What is the mAs?
8. Discuss the components of total x-ray beam filtration.
9. A radiographic technique calls for 800 mA at 50 ms. What is the mAs setting?
10. The normal lateral chest technique is 120 kVp, 100 mA, 15 ms. To reduce motion blur, the radiologic technologist shortens exposure time to 5 ms. What is the new mA?
11. Explain the following statement: Changing the mA does not change the kinetic energy of electrons flowing across the x-ray tube.
12. Why is it important to keep exposure time as short as possible?
13. Identify the range of optical densities that are too light, too dark, and within the useful range.
14. An examination requires 78 kVp/150 mAs at 100 cm SID. If the distance is changed to 180 cm, what should be the new mAs setting?
15. Describe the two focal spots available in x-ray tubes. Explain how each is used typically.
16. When a change in OD is required, what exposure technique factors should be changed, and why?
17. Explain how high-voltage generation influences x-ray beam quantity and quality.
18. How does body habitus affect the selection of technical factors?
19. What is the principal advantage of exposure with a large focal spot compared with a small focal spot?
20. Define contrast. Give examples of tissues with high contrast and with low contrast.

The answers to the Challenge Questions can be found by logging on to our website at http://evolve.elsevier.com.

16

Image Quality

OBJECTIVES

At the completion of this chapter, the student should be able to do the following:

1. Define radiographic quality, resolution, noise, and speed
2. Interpret the shape of the characteristic curve
3. Identify the toe, shoulder, and straight-line portion of the characteristic curve
4. Distinguish the geometric factors that affect image quality
5. Analyze the subject factors that affect image quality
6. Examine the tools and techniques available to create high-quality images

OUTLINE

Definitions
    Radiographic Quality
    Resolution
    Noise
    Speed
Film Factors
    Characteristic Curve
    Optical Density
    Film Processing
Geometric Factors
    Magnification
    Distortion
    Focal-Spot Blur
    Heel Effect
Subject Factors
    Subject Contrast
    Motion Blur
Tools for Improved Radiographic Quality
    Patient Positioning
    Image Receptors
    Selection of Technique Factors

MAGE QUALITY is the exactness of representation of the patient's anatomy on an image. High-quality images are required so that radiologists can make accurate diagnoses. To produce high-quality images, radiographers apply knowledge of the three major interrelated categories of radiographic quality: film factors, geometric factors, and subject factors. Each of these factors influences the quality of a radiographic image, and each is under the control of the radiologic technologist. The selection of radiographic technique factors is discussed in this chapter.

DEFINITIONS
Radiographic Quality

The term **radiographic quality (image quality)** refers to the fidelity with which the anatomical structure that is being examined is imaged on the radiograph. A radiograph that faithfully reproduces structure and tissues is identified as a **high-quality radiograph.**

The quality of a radiograph is not easy to define, and it cannot be measured precisely. A number of factors affect radiographic quality, but no precise, universally accepted measures by which to judge it have been identified. The most important characteristics of radiographic quality are **spatial resolution, contrast resolution, noise,** and **artifacts.** Artifacts are discussed in Chapter 17.

Resolution

Resolution is the ability to image two separate objects and visually distinguish one from the other. **Spatial resolution** refers to the ability to image small objects that have high subject contrast, such as a bone–soft tissue interface, a breast microcalcification, or a calcified lung nodule. Conventional radiography has excellent spatial resolution. The measure of spatial resolution is discussed more completely in Chapter 28.

 Spatial resolution improves as screen blur decreases, motion blur decreases, and geometric blur decreases.

Contrast resolution is the ability to distinguish anatomical structures of similar subject contrast such as liver–spleen and gray matter–white matter. The actual size of objects that can be imaged is always smaller under conditions of high contrast than under conditions of low contrast.

The less precise terms **detail** and **recorded detail** sometimes are used instead of **spatial resolution** and **contrast resolution.** These terms refer to the degree of sharpness of structural lines on a radiograph. **Visibility of detail** refers to the ability to visualize recorded detail when image contrast and optical density (OD) are optimized.

Noise

Noise is a term that is borrowed from electrical engineering. The flutter, hum, and whistle heard from an audio system constitute **audio noise** that is inherent in the design of the system. The "snow" on television screens, especially in weak signal areas, is **video noise,** and it too is inherent in the system.

Radiographic noise is the random fluctuation in the OD of the image.

Radiographic noise also is inherent in the imaging system (Figure 16-1). A number of factors contribute to radiographic noise, including some that are under the control of the

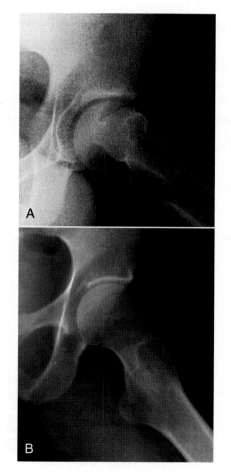

FIGURE 16-1 A, This hip radiograph demonstrates the mottled, grainy appearance associated with quantum mottle that results from the use of a low number of x-rays to produce the image. **B,** In comparison, an optimal hip image shows greater recorded detail. (Courtesy Tim Gienapp, Apollo College.)

radiologic technologist. Lower noise results in a better radiographic image because it improves contrast resolution.

Radiographic noise has four components: film graininess, structure mottle, quantum mottle, and scatter radiation. We discussed the principal source of radiographic noise—scatter radiation—in Chapters 14 and 15.

Film graininess refers to the distribution in size and space of silver halide grains in the emulsion. Structure mottle is similar to film graininess but refers to the phosphor of the radiographic intensifying screen. Film graininess and structure mottle are inherent in the image receptor. They are not under the control of the radiologic technologist, and they contribute very little to radiographic noise, with the exception of mammography.

Quantum mottle is somewhat under the control of the radiologic technologist and is a principal contributor to radiographic noise in many radiographic imaging procedures. Quantum mottle refers to the random nature by which x-rays interact with the image receptor.

If an image is produced with just a few x-rays, the quantum mottle will be higher than if the image is formed from a large number of x-rays. The use of very fast intensifying screens results in increased quantum mottle.

 The use of high-mAs, low-kVp settings and of slower image receptors reduces quantum mottle.

Quantum mottle is similar to the sowing of grass seed. If very little seed is broadcast, the resulting grass will be thin, with only a few blades. Likewise, when fewer x-rays are "cast" at the image receptor, the resulting image appears mottled or blotchy. On the other hand, if a lot of seed is cast, the resulting grass will be thick and smooth. In the same way, when more x-rays interact with the image receptor, the image appears smooth, like a lush lawn.

Speed

Two of the characteristics of radiographic quality, resolution and noise, are intimately connected with a third characteristic—**speed.** Although the speed of the image receptor is not apparent on the radiographic image, it very much influences resolution and noise. In fact, a variation in any one of these characteristics alters the other two (Figure 16-2). In general, the following rules apply:

RADIOGRAPHIC QUALITY RULES

1. Fast image receptors have high noise and low spatial resolution and contrast resolution.
2. High spatial resolution and contrast resolution require low noise and slow image receptors.
3. Low noise accompanies slow image receptors with high spatial resolution and contrast resolution.

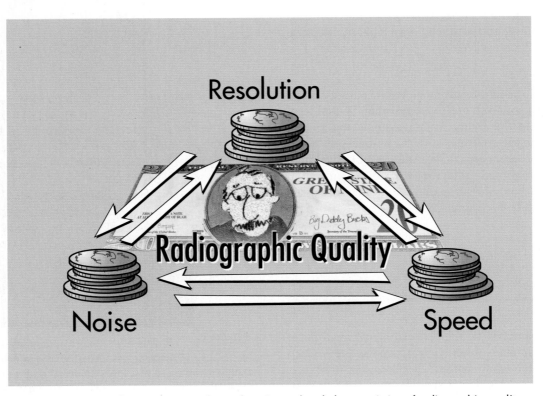

FIGURE 16-2 Resolution, noise, and speed are interrelated characteristics of radiographic quality.

The radiologic technologist is provided with all the physical tools required to produce high-quality radiographs. The skillful radiologic technologist properly manipulates these tools according to each specific clinical situation.

In general, the quality of a radiograph is directly related to an understanding of the basic principles of x-ray physics and the factors that affect radiographic quality. Figure 16-3 is an organizational chart of the principal factors that affect radiographic quality, most of which are under the control of the radiologic technologist. Each is considered in detail in this chapter.

FILM FACTORS

Unexposed x-ray film that has been processed appears quite lucent, like frosted window glass. It easily transmits light but not images. On the other hand, exposed,

processed x-ray film can be quite opaque. Properly exposed film appears with various shades of gray, and heavily exposed film appears black.

The study of the relationship between the intensity of exposure of the film and the blackness after processing is called *sensitometry*. Knowledge of the sensitometric aspects of radiographic film is essential for maintaining adequate quality control.

Characteristic Curve

The two principal measurements involved in sensitometry are the exposure to the film and the percentage of light transmitted through the processed film. Such measurements are used to describe the relationship between **OD** and radiation exposure. This relationship is called a **characteristic curve,** or sometimes the H & D curve after Hurter and Driffield, who first described this relationship.

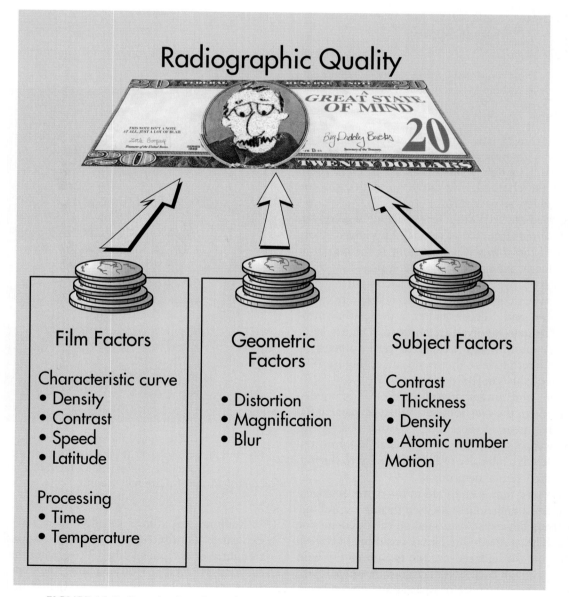

FIGURE 16-3 Organization chart of principal factors that may affect radiographic quality.

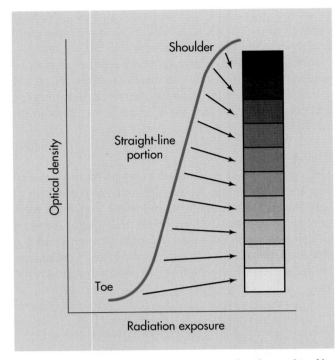

FIGURE 16-4 The characteristic curve of radiographic film is the graphic relationship between optical density (OD) and radiation exposure.

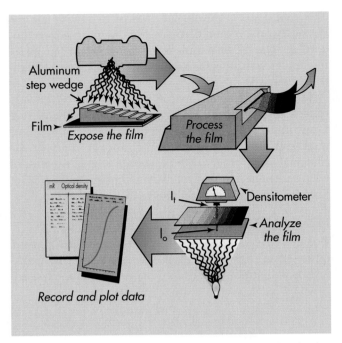

FIGURE 16-5 Steps involved in the construction of a characteristic curve.

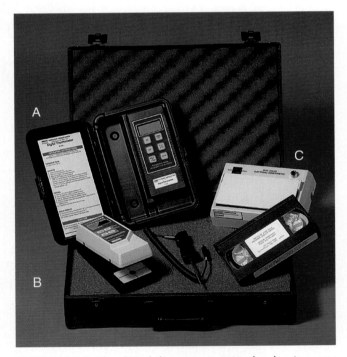

FIGURE 16-6 The digital thermometer (**A**), the densitometer (**B**), and the sensitometer (**C**) are the tools necessary for fabricating a characteristic curve and for providing routine quality control. (Courtesy Cardinal Health.)

A typical characteristic curve is shown in Figure 16-4. At low and high exposure levels, large variations in exposure result in only a small change in OD. These portions of the characteristic curve are called the **toe** and the **shoulder,** respectively.

At intermediate exposure levels, small changes in exposure result in large changes in OD. This intermediate region, called the *straight-line portion,* is the region in which a properly exposed radiograph appears.

Two pieces of apparatus are needed to construct a characteristic curve: an optical step wedge, sometimes called a *sensitometer,* and a densitometer, a device that measures OD. The steps involved are outlined in Figure 16-5, where an aluminum step wedge, or penetrometer, is shown as an alternative to the sensitometer. Figure 16-6 shows these quality control devices.

First, the film under investigation is exposed—flashed—through the sensitometer. When processed, the film will have areas of increasing OD that correspond to optical wedge steps. The sensitometer is fabricated so that the relative intensity of light exposure to the film under each step can be determined.

The processed film is analyzed in the densitometer, a device that has a light source focused through a pinhole. A light-sensing device is positioned on the opposite side of the film. The radiographic film is positioned between the pinhole and the light sensor, and the amount of light transmitted through each step of the radiographic image is measured. These data are recorded and analyzed and, when plotted, result in a characteristic curve.

Radiographic film is sensitive over a wide range of exposures. Film-screen, for example, responds to radiation intensities from less than 1 to greater than 1000 mR (0.01 to 10 mGy$_a$). Consequently, the exposure values for a characteristic curve are presented in logarithmic fashion.

Furthermore, it is not the absolute exposure that is of interest but rather the change in OD over each exposure interval. Therefore, log relative exposure (LRE) is used as the scale along the x-axis.

Figure 16-7 shows the exposure in mR, the LRE, and the relative mAs for a representative film-screen combination. The LRE scale usually is presented in increments of 0.3 because the log of 2, doubling the exposure, is 0.3. Doubling the exposure can be achieved by doubling the mAs, as the x-axis scale in Figure 16-7 shows.

 An increase in LRE of 0.3 results from doubling the radiation exposure.

Optical Density

It is not enough to say that OD is the degree of blackening of a radiograph, or that a clear area of the radiograph represents low OD and a black area represents high OD. OD has a precise numeric value that can be calculated if the level of light incident on a processed film (I_o) and the level of light transmitted through that film (I_t) are measured. The OD is defined as follows:

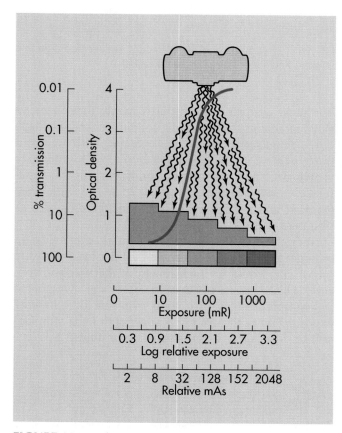

FIGURE 16-7 Relationship among log relative exposure (LRE) and relative milliampere-seconds for typical film-screen combination. Relationship between percentage transmission and optical density (OD) is shown along the y-axis.

OPTICAL DENSITY

$$OD = \log_{10} \frac{I_o}{I_t}$$

Question: The lung field of a chest radiograph transmits only 0.15% of incident light as determined with a densitometer. What is the OD?

Answer: $0.15\% = 0.0015$

$$OD = \log_{10} \frac{1}{0.0015}$$
$$= \log_{10} 666.7$$
$$= 2.8$$

OD is a logarithmic function. Logarithms allow a wide range of values to be expressed by small numbers. Radiographic film contains ODs that range from near 0 to 4. These ODs correspond to clear and black, respectively. An OD of 4 actually means that only 1 in 10,000 light photons (10^4) is capable of penetrating the x-ray film. Table 16-1 shows the range of light transmission as it corresponds to various levels of OD.

Question: The OD of a region of a lung field is 2.5. What percentage of visible light is transmitted through that region of the image?

Answer: Reference to Table 16-1 shows that an OD = 2.5 is equal to 2 of every 625 light photons that are being transmitted, or 0.32%.

Table 16-1	Relationship of the Optical Density of Radiographic Film to Light Transmission Through the Film	
Percent of Light Transmitted ($I_t/I_o \times 100$)	**Fraction of Light Transmitted (I_t/I_o)**	**Optical Density ($\log I_o/I_t$)**
100	1	0
50	1/2	0.3
32	8/25	0.5
25	1/4	0.6
12.5	1/8	0.9
10	1/10	1
5	1/20	1.3
3.2	4/25	1.5
2.5	1/30	1.6
1.25	1/80	1.9
1	1/100	2
0.5	1/200	2.3
0.32	2/625	2.5
0.125	1/800	2.9
0.1	1/1000	3
0.05	1/2000	3.3
0.032	1/3125	3.5
0.01	1/10,000	4

High-quality glass has an OD of zero, which means that all light incident on such glass is transmitted. Unexposed radiographic film allows no more than approximately 80% of incident light photons to be transmitted. Most unexposed and processed radiographic film has an OD in the range of 0.1 to 0.3, corresponding to 79% and 50% transmission, respectively.

These ODs of unexposed film are due to **base density** and **fog density** (Figure 16-8). Base density is the OD that is inherent in the base of the film. It is due to the composition of the base and the tint added to the base to make the radiograph more pleasing to the eye. Base density has a value of approximately 0.1.

Fog density has been previously described as the development of silver grains that contain no useful information. Fog density results from inadvertent exposure of film during storage, undesirable chemical contamination, improper processing, and a number of other influences. Fog density on a processed radiograph should not exceed 0.1.

 Higher fog density reduces the contrast of the radiographic image.

Question: The light incident on the radiograph of a long bone has a relative value of 1500. If the light transmitted through radiopaque bony structures has an intensity of 480 (relatively white), and the light transmitted through radiolucent soft tissue has an intensity of 2 (relatively black), what are the approximate respective ODs? Refer to Table 16-1 if necessary.

Answer: $OD = \log_{10} \dfrac{I_o}{I_t}$

a. For bone:

$OD = \log_{10} \dfrac{1500}{480} = 0.5$

b. For soft tissue:

$OD = \log_{10} \dfrac{1500}{2} = 2.9$

The useful range of OD is approximately 0.25 to 2.5. Most radiographs, however, show image patterns in the range of 0.5 to 1.25 OD. Attention to this part of the characteristic curve is essential. However, very low OD may be too light to contain an image, whereas very high OD requires a hot light to view the image.

 Base plus fog OD has a range of approximately 0.1 to 0.3.

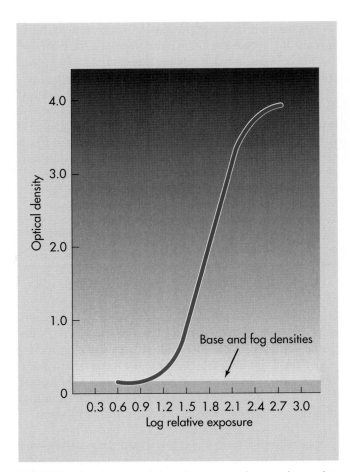

FIGURE 16-8 Base and fog densities reduce radiographic contrast and should be as low as possible.

The most useful range of OD is highly dependent on viewbox illumination, viewing conditions, and the shape of the characteristic curve. For example, with high-contrast mammography image receptors, high-luminance viewboxes, and good viewing conditions, the most useful OD range is approximately 0.25 to 2.5 with gross features, and as high as 3.5 with fine features such as skin lines.

Reciprocity Law. One would think that the OD on a radiograph would depend strictly on the total exposure (mAs) and would be independent of the time of exposure. This, in fact, is the reciprocity law. Whether a radiograph is made with short exposure time or long exposure time, the reciprocity law states that the OD will be the same if the mAs value is constant.

 The reciprocity law states that the OD on a radiograph is proportional only to the total energy imparted to the radiographic film.

The reciprocity law holds for direct exposure with x-rays, but it does not hold for exposure of film by visible light from radiographic intensifying screens.

Consequently, **the reciprocity law fails for screen-film exposures** at exposure times less than approximately 10 ms or longer than approximately 2 s.

OD is somewhat less at such short or long exposure times than exposure times within that range, even though radiation exposure is the same. The reciprocity law is important for special procedures that require very short or very long exposure times, such as angiointerventional radiography and mammography, respectively. For these few situations, increasing the mAs setting may be required if automatic exposure control does not compensate for reciprocity law failure.

Contrast. When a high-quality radiograph is placed on an illuminator, the differences in OD are obvious in the image. Such OD variations are called **radiographic contrast**. A radiograph that has marked differences in OD is a high-contrast radiograph. On the other hand, if the OD differences are small and are not distinct, the radiograph is of low contrast. Figure 16-9 illustrates the difference between high contrast and low contrast with a photograph.

Radiographic contrast is the product of two separate factors:

- **Image receptor contrast** is inherent in the screen-film combination and is influenced somewhat by processing of the film.
- **Subject contrast** is determined by the size, shape, and x-ray–attenuating characteristics of the anatomy that is being examined and the energy (kVp) of the x-ray beam.

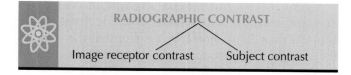

RADIOGRAPHIC CONTRAST

Image receptor contrast   Subject contrast

Radiographic contrast can be greatly affected by changes in image receptor contrast or subject contrast. In the clinical setting, it is usually best to standardize the image receptor contrast and alter the subject contrast according to the needs of the examination. Subject contrast is discussed in greater detail later.

Image receptor contrast is inherent in the type of film and radiographic intensifying screen that is being used. However, it can be influenced by two other factors: the range of ODs and the film processing technique.

Film selection usually is limited and is determined somewhat by the intensifying screen used. Film-screen images always have higher contrast compared with direct exposure images.

The best control the radiologic technologist can exercise involves exposing the image receptor properly so that the ODs lie within the diagnostically useful range of 0.25 to 2.5, and a bit higher in mammography. When exposure of the image receptor results in

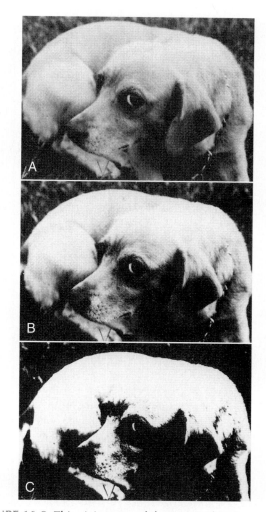

FIGURE 16-9 This vicious guard dog is posed to demonstrate differences in contrast. **A,** Low contrast. **B,** Moderate contrast. **C,** High contrast. (Courtesy Butterscotch.)

an OD outside this range, contrast is lost because the image is in the toe or the shoulder of the characteristic curve (Figure 16-10).

Standardized film processing techniques are absolutely necessary for consistent film contrast and good radiographic quality. Deviation from the manufacturer's recommendations results in reduced contrast.

 Film contrast is related to the slope of the straight-line portion of the characteristic curve.

The characteristic curve of an image receptor allows one to judge at a glance the relative degree of contrast. If the slope or steepness of the straight-line portion of the characteristic curve had a value of 1, then it would be angled at 45 degrees. An increase of 1 unit along the LRE axis would result in an increase of 1 unit along the OD axis. The contrast would be 1.

An image receptor that has a contrast of 1 has very low contrast. Image receptors with a contrast higher than 1

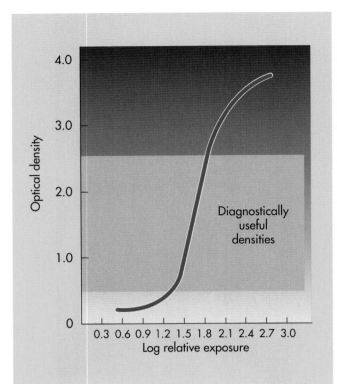

FIGURE 16-10 If exposure of the film results in optical densities (OD) that lie in the toe or shoulder region, where the slope of the curve is less, contrast is reduced.

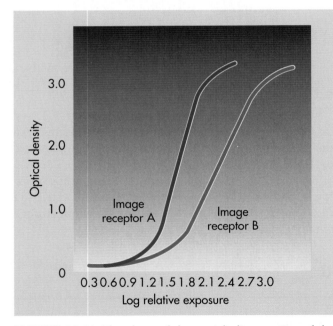

FIGURE 16-11 The slope of the straight-line portion of the characteristic curve is greater for image receptor **A** than for image receptor **B**. Image receptor **A** has greater contrast.

amplify the subject contrast during x-ray examination. An image receptor with a contrast of 3, for instance, would show large OD differences over a small range of x-ray exposure.

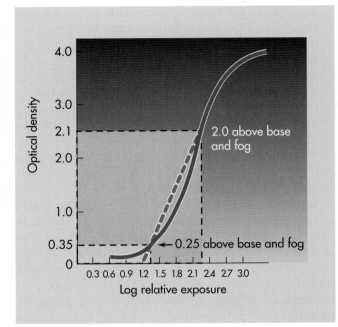

FIGURE 16-12 Average gradient is the slope of the line drawn between the points on the characteristic curve that correspond to optical density (OD) levels 0.25 and 2.0 above base and fog densities.

In general, it is not necessary for the radiologic technologist to have a precise knowledge of image receptor contrast. However, from the appearance of the characteristic curve, the technologist should be able to distinguish high-contrast image receptors from low-contrast image receptors.

Figure 16-11 shows the characteristic curves for two different image receptors. Image receptor *A* has higher contrast than *B*, as shown by the fact that the slope of the straight-line portion of the characteristic curve is steeper for *A* than for *B*.

Several methods are used to numerically specify image receptor contrast. The one most often used is the average gradient. The average gradient is the slope of a straight line drawn between two points on the characteristic curve at ODs 0.25 and 2.0 above base and fog densities. This is the approximate useful range of OD on most radiographs.

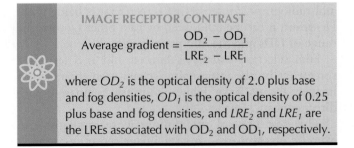

IMAGE RECEPTOR CONTRAST

$$\text{Average gradient} = \frac{OD_2 - OD_1}{LRE_2 - LRE_1}$$

where OD_2 is the optical density of 2.0 plus base and fog densities, OD_1 is the optical density of 0.25 plus base and fog densities, and LRE_2 and LRE_1 are the LREs associated with OD_2 and OD_1, respectively.

This method is diagrammed in Figure 16-12 for a film with a combined base and fog density of 0.1.

Most radiographic image receptors have an average gradient in the range of 2.5 to 3.5. Because of this, the image receptor acts as an amplifier of subject contrast. The range of the number of x-rays producing the latent image is effectively expanded, and the subject contrast is enhanced.

Question: A radiographic film has a base density of 0.06 and a fog density of 0.11. At what ODs should one evaluate the characteristic curve to determine the film contrast?

Answer: The curve should be evaluated at OD 0.25 and 2.0 above base plus fog densities. Therefore, at OD of

$OD_1 = 0.06 + 0.11 + 0.25 = 0.42$

and

$OD_2 = 0.06 + 0.11 + 2.0 = 2.17$

Image receptor contrast also may be identified by **gradient**. The gradient is the slope of the tangent *at any point* on the characteristic curve (Figure 16-13). **Toe gradient** is probably more important than average gradient for general radiography because many clinical ODs appear in the toe region of the characteristic curve. **Midgradient** or **shoulder gradient** is more important for mammography.

Question: If the ODs of 0.42 and 2.17 on the characteristic curve in the preceding example correspond to LREs of 0.95 and 1.75, what is the average gradient?

Answer: $\text{Average gradient} = \dfrac{OD2 - OD1}{LRE2 - LRE1} = \dfrac{2.17 - 0.42}{1.75 - 0.95}$

$= \dfrac{1.75}{0.8} = 2.19$

Note that the numerator in the expression for average gradient always equals 1.75.

Another way to evaluate image receptor contrast is to re-plot the data of a characteristic curve (an H & D curve) into an H & H contrast curve, as can be seen in Figure 16-14. "H & H" stands for Art Haus and Ed Hendrick, the medical physicists who first demonstrated this technique.

Speed. The ability of an image receptor to respond to a low x-ray exposure is a measure of its **sensitivity** or, more commonly, its **speed**. An exposure of less than 1 mR can be detected with a film-screen combination, whereas several mR are necessary to produce a measurable exposure with direct-exposure film.

The characteristic curve of an image receptor is also useful in identifying speed. Figure 16-15 shows the characteristic curves of two different image receptors. Because image receptor *A* requires less exposure than *B* to produce any OD, *A* is faster than *B*.

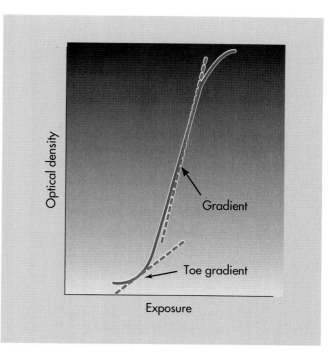

FIGURE 16-13 The gradient is the slope of the tangent at any point on the characteristic curve. Toe gradient is most important clinically.

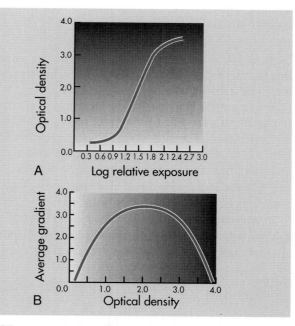

FIGURE 16-14 When the gradient of the characteristic curve (**A**) is plotted as a function of optical density, a contrast curve (**B**) results.

The characteristic curve of a fast image receptor is positioned to the left—closer to the y-axis—of that of a slow image receptor. Radiographic image receptors are identified as fast or slow according to their sensitivity to x-ray exposure.

Usually, identification of a given image receptor as so many times faster than another is sufficient for the radiologic technologist. If A were twice as fast as B, image receptor A would require only half the mAs required

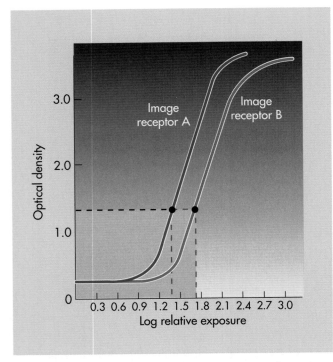

FIGURE 16-15 The speed of an image receptor is the reciprocal of the exposure, in roentgens, needed to produce an optical density (OD) of 1.0 above base plus fog. Image receptor **A** is faster than image receptor **B** (speed $A = 1/1.3 = 0.78 \ R^{-1}$; speed $B = 1/1.6 = 0.63 \ R^{-1}$).

by B to produce a given OD. Moreover, the image on image receptor A might be of poor quality because of increased radiographic noise.

When numbers are used to express speed, all are relative to 100; this is called *par speed*. Numbers higher than 100 refer to fast or high-speed image receptors. Numbers less than 100 refer to "detail" image receptors.

Do not be deceived that slower image receptors are better because they have less noise. Slower image receptors also require more patient radiation dose. A balance is required.

In sensitometry, the OD specified for determining image receptor speed is 1.0 above base plus fog density, and the speed is measured in reciprocal roentgens (1/R) as follows:

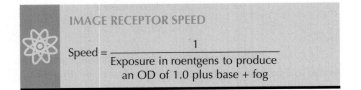

IMAGE RECEPTOR SPEED

$$Speed = \frac{1}{\text{Exposure in roentgens to produce an OD of 1.0 plus base + fog}}$$

Question: The characteristic curve of a given screen-film shows that 10 mR is needed to produce an OD of 1.0 above base plus fog density on that image receptor. What is the image receptor speed?

Answer: $Speed = \dfrac{1}{10 \ mR} = \dfrac{1}{0.01 \ R} = 100 \ R^{-1}$

Question: How much exposure is required to produce an OD of 1.0 above base plus fog density on a 600 speed image receptor?

Answer:
$$Speed = \frac{1}{exposure}$$

$$Exposure = \frac{1}{speed} = \frac{1}{600} = 0.00167 \ R$$

$$= 1.7 \ mR$$

When imaged receptors are replaced, a change in the mAs setting may be necessary to maintain the same OD. For example, if image receptor speed is doubled, the mAs must be halved. No change is required in kVp. This relationship is expressed as follows:

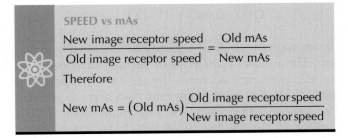

SPEED vs mAs

$$\frac{\text{New image receptor speed}}{\text{Old image receptor speed}} = \frac{\text{Old mAs}}{\text{New mAs}}$$

Therefore

$$\text{New mAs} = (\text{Old mAs}) \frac{\text{Old image receptor speed}}{\text{New image receptor speed}}$$

Question: A PA chest examination requires 120 kVp/8 mAs with a 250 speed image receptor. What radiographic technique should be used with a 400 speed image receptor?

Answer: $\text{New mAs} = (8 \ mAs)\dfrac{250}{400} = 5 \ mAs$

Therefore, the new technique is 120 kVp/5 mAs

Latitude. An additional image receptor feature easily obtained from the characteristic curve is latitude. Latitude refers to the range of exposures over which the image receptor responds with ODs in the diagnostically useful range.

Latitude also can be thought of as the margin of error in technical factors. With wider latitude, mAs can vary more and still produce a diagnostic image. Figure 16-16 shows two image receptors with different latitudes. Image receptor *B* responds to a much wider range of exposures than *A* and is said to have a wider latitude than *A*.

Latitude and contrast are inversely proportional.

Image receptors with wide latitude are said to have **long gray scale;** those with narrow latitude have **short gray scale.** When slopes of the curves in Figure 16-16 are compared, it should be clear that a high-contrast image receptor has narrow latitude, and a low-contrast image receptor has wide latitude.

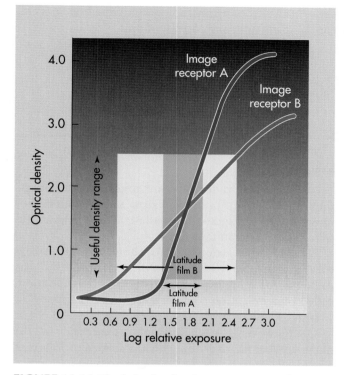

FIGURE 16-16 The latitude of an image receptor is the exposure range over which it responds with diagnostically useful optical density (OD).

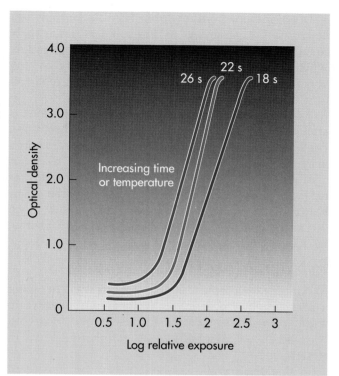

FIGURE 16-17 As development time or temperature increases, changes occur in the shape and relative position of the characteristic curve.

BOX 16-1   Factors That May Affect the Finished Radiograph

- Concentration of processing chemicals
- Degree of chemistry agitation during development
- Development time
- Development temperature

Film Processing

Proper film processing is required for optimal image receptor contrast because the degree of development has a pronounced effect on the level of fog density and on the ODs resulting from a given exposure at a given image receptor speed. Important factors that may affect the degree of development are listed in Box 16-1.

Development Time. Because development time is varied, the characteristic curve for any film changes in shape and position along the LRE axis (Figure 16-17). If characteristic curves were analyzed for contrast, speed, and fog level, each would be shown to be unique, as in Figure 16-18. Speed and fog increase with development time as it increases.

The development time recommended by the manufacturer is the time that will result in maximum contrast, at relatively high speed and with low levels of fog. When development time extends far beyond the recommended period, the image receptor contrast decreases, the relative speed increases, and the fog level increases.

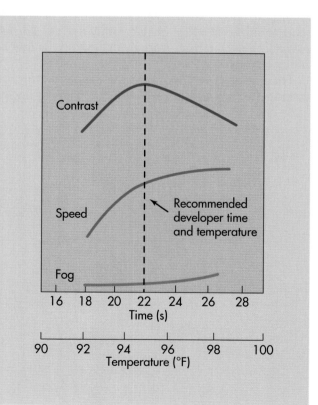

FIGURE 16-18 Analysis of characteristic curves at various development times and temperatures yields relationships for contrast, speed, and fog for 90-second automatically processed film.

Development Temperature. The relationships just described for variations in development time apply equally well to variations in development temperature. When the average gradient, speed, and fog level for any film are plotted as a function of development temperature, the results appear as in Figure 16-18.

As with time of development, maximum contrast is attained at the recommended development temperature. Fog level increases with increasing temperature, as does image receptor speed.

Within a small range, a change in time or temperature can be compensated for by a change in the other. However, a small change in time or temperature alone can result in a large change in the sensitometric characteristics of the image receptor.

GEOMETRIC FACTORS

Making a radiograph is similar in many ways to taking a photograph. Proper exposure time and intensity are required for both processes. Images are recorded both ways because x-rays and visible light photons travel in straight lines.

In that regard, an x-ray image may be considered analogous to a shadowgraph. Figure 16-19 shows the familiar shadowgraph that can be made to appear on a wall if light is shone on a properly contorted hand.

The sharpness of the shadow image on the wall is a function of a number of geometric factors. For example, the closer to the wall the hand is placed, the sharper is the shadow image. Similarly, as the light source is moved farther from the hand, the shadow becomes sharper.

These geometric conditions also apply to the production of high-quality radiographs. Three principal

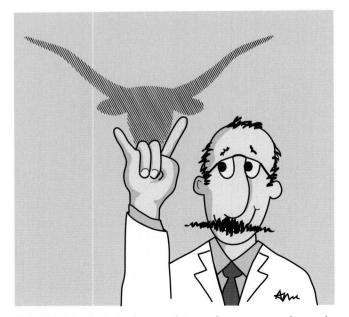

FIGURE 16-19 A shadowgraph is analogous to a radiograph. (Dedicated to Xie Nan Zhu, Guangzhou, People's Republic of China.)

geometric factors affect radiographic quality: magnification, distortion, and focal-spot blur.

> **Geometric Factors**
> - Magnification
> - Distortion
> - Focal-spot blur

Magnification

All images on the radiograph are larger than the objects they represent, a condition called **magnification.** For most medical images, the smallest magnification possible should be maintained.

During some examinations, however, magnification is desirable and is carefully planned into the radiographic examination. This type of examination, called **magnification radiography,** was discussed in Chapter 15.

Quantitatively, magnification is expressed by the magnification factor (MF), which is defined as follows:

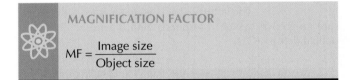

MAGNIFICATION FACTOR

$$MF = \frac{\text{Image size}}{\text{Object size}}$$

The MF depends on the geometric conditions of the examination. For most radiographs taken at a source-to-image receptor distance (SID) of 100 cm, the MF is approximately 1.1. For radiographs taken at 180 cm SID, the MF is approximately 1.05.

Question: If a heart measures 12.5 cm at its maximum width, and its image on a chest radiograph measures 14.7 cm, what is the MF?

Answer: $$MF = \frac{14.7 \text{ cm}}{12.5 \text{ cm}} = 1.176$$

Many imaging departments are changing from the traditional 100 cm SID to 120 cm SID. Such a change results in reduced magnification, improved spatial resolution, and reduced patient dose.

In the usual radiographic examination, it is not possible to determine the object size. The image size may be measured directly from the radiograph. In such situations, the MF can be determined from the ratio of SID to source-to-object distance (SOD):

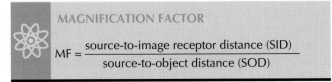

MAGNIFICATION FACTOR

$$MF = \frac{\text{source-to-image receptor distance (SID)}}{\text{source-to-object distance (SOD)}}$$

Figure 16-20 shows that this method of calculating the MF is based on the basic geometric relationship between similar triangles. If two right triangles have a common hypotenuse, the ratio of the height of one to its base will be the same as the ratio of the height of the other to its base.

This is the situation that usually is encountered in radiology. The SID is known and can be measured directly. The SOD can be estimated relatively accurately by a radiologic technologist who has a good foundation in human anatomy. The image size can be measured accurately; therefore, object size can be calculated as follows:

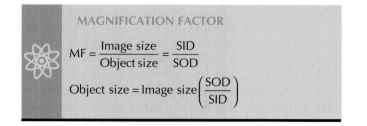

MAGNIFICATION FACTOR

$$MF = \frac{Image\ size}{Object\ size} = \frac{SID}{SOD}$$

$$Object\ size = Image\ size\left(\frac{SOD}{SID}\right)$$

Question: A renal calculus measures 1.2 cm on the radiograph. The SID is 100 cm and the SOD is estimated at 92 cm. What is the size of the calculus?

Answer:
$$Object\ size = 1.2\left(\frac{92}{100}\right) = 1.1\ cm$$

Question: A lateral view of the lumbar spine taken at 100 cm SID results in the image of a vertebral body with maximum and minimum dimensions of 6.4 cm and 4.2 cm. What is the object size if the vertebral body is 25 cm from the image receptor?

Answer:
$$MF = \frac{100}{100-25} = \frac{100}{75} = 1.33$$

Therefore, the object size is

$$\frac{6.4}{1.33} \times \frac{4.2}{1.33} = 4.81\ cm \times 33.16\ cm$$

You might ask whether these relationships hold for objects off the central ray (Figure 16-21). The MF will be the same for objects positioned off the central ray as for those lying on the central ray if the object-to-image receptor distance (OID) is the same, and if the object is essentially flat.

In summary, two factors affect image magnification: SID and OID.

MINIMIZING MAGNIFICATION

Large SID: Use as large a source-to-image receptor distance as possible.
Small OID: Place the object as close to the image receptor as possible.

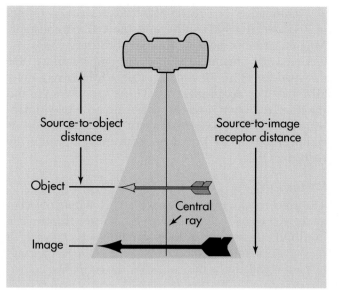

FIGURE 16-20 Magnification is the ratio of image size to object size or of source-to-image receptor distance (SID) to source-to-object distance (SOD).

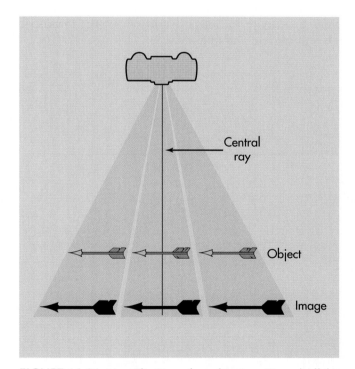

FIGURE 16-21 Magnification of an object positioned off the central ray is the same as that of an object on the central ray if the objects are in the same plane.

The SID is standard in most radiology departments at 180 cm for chest imaging, 100 cm for routine examinations, and 90 cm for some special studies, such as mobile radiography and trauma radiography.

Magnification is minimized routinely in three familiar clinical situations. Most chest radiographs are taken at 180 cm SID from the PA projection. Compared with an examination at 100 cm SID, this projection results in a larger SID/SOD ratio, and the OID is constant. Magnification is reduced because of the large SID.

Dedicated mammography imaging systems are designed for 50 to 70 cm SID. This is a relatively short SID, but it is necessary, considering the low kVp and the low radiation intensity of mammography imaging systems. Such systems have a device for vigorous compression of the breast to reduce magnification by reducing OID.

Distortion

The previous discussion assumed a very simple object—an arrow, positioned parallel to the image receptor at a fixed OID. If any one of these conditions is changed, as they all are in most medical imaging procedures, the magnification will not be the same over the entire object.

 Unequal magnification of different portions of the same object is called *shape distortion*.

Distortion can interfere with diagnosis. Three conditions contribute to image distortion: object thickness, object position, and object shape.

 DISTORTION DEPENDS ON
1. Object thickness
2. Object position
3. Object shape

Object Thickness. With a thick object, the OID changes measurably across the object. Consider, for instance, two rectangular structures of different thicknesses (Figure 16-22). Because of the change in OID across the thicker structure, the image of that structure is more distorted than the image of the thinner structure.

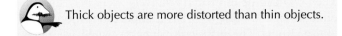 Thick objects are more distorted than thin objects.

Consider the images produced by a disc and a sphere of the same diameter (Figure 16-23). When positioned on the central axis, the images of both objects appear as circles. The image of the sphere appears less distinct because of its varying thickness, but it does appear circular.

When these objects are positioned laterally to the central ray, the disc still appears circular. The sphere appears not only less distinct but elliptical because of its thickness. This distortion resulting from object thickness is shown more dramatically in Figure 16-24 in the image of an irregular object.

These statements about discs and spheres are clinically insignificant because lateral distances off the central ray are too small. Only irregular objects, such as those shown in Figure 16-24, or the human body, show significant distortion.

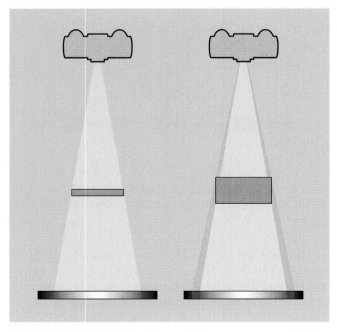

FIGURE 16-22 Thick objects result in unequal magnification and thus greater distortion compared with thin objects.

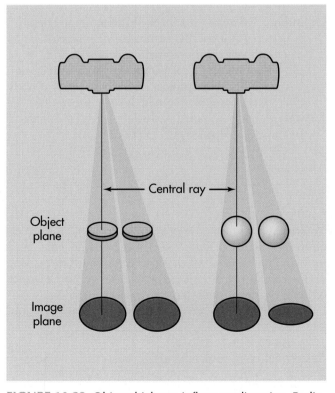

FIGURE 16-23 Object thickness influences distortion. Radiographs of a disc or sphere appear as circles if the object is on the central ray. When lateral to the central axis, the disc appears as a circle and the sphere as an ellipse.

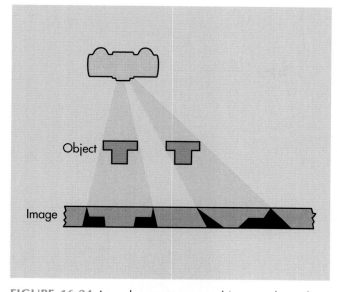

FIGURE 16-24 Irregular anatomy or objects such as these can cause considerable distortion when radiographed off the central ray.

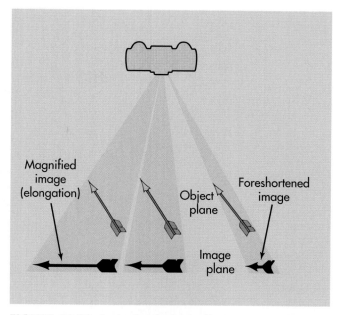

FIGURE 16-26 An inclined object that is positioned lateral to the central ray may be distorted severely by elongation or foreshortening.

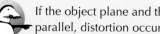 If the object plane and the image plane are not parallel, distortion occurs.

Figure 16-25, an example of gross distortion, shows that the image of an inclined object can be smaller than the object itself. In such a condition, the image is said to be **foreshortened.** The amount of foreshortening, that is, the extent of reduction in image size, increases as the angle of inclination increases.

If an inclined object is not located on the central x-ray beam, the degree of distortion is affected by the object's angle of inclination and its lateral position from the central axis. Figure 16-26 illustrates this situation and shows that the image of an inclined object can be severely foreshortened, or **elongated.**

With multiple objects positioned at various OIDs, **spatial distortion** can occur. Spatial distortion is the misrepresentation in the image of the actual spatial relationships among objects. Figure 16-27 demonstrates this condition for two arrows of the same size, one of which lies on top of the other. Because of the position of the arrows, only one image should be seen, representing the superposition of the arrows.

Unequal magnification, however, of the two objects causes arrow A to appear larger than arrow B and to be positioned more laterally. This distortion is minimal for objects lying along the central ray. As object position is shifted laterally from the central ray, spatial distortion can become more significant.

This illustrates the projection nature of x-ray images. A single image is not enough to define the three-dimensional configuration of a complex object. Therefore, most x-ray examinations are made with two or more projections.

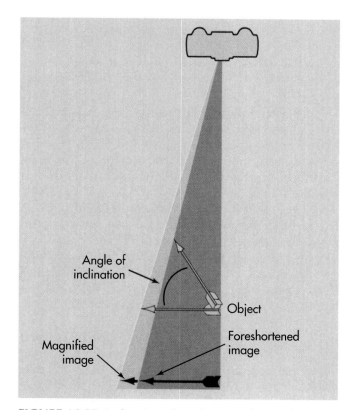

FIGURE 16-25 Inclination of an object results in a foreshortened image.

Object Position. If the object plane and the image plane are parallel, the image is not distorted. However, distortion is possible in every radiographic examination if proper patient positioning is not maintained.

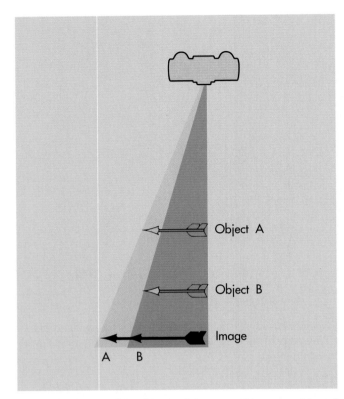

FIGURE 16-27 When objects of the same size are positioned at different distances from the image receptor, spatial distortion occurs.

Focal-Spot Blur

Thus far, our discussion of the geometric factors that affect radiographic quality has assumed that x-rays are emitted from a point source. In actual practice, there is no point source of x-radiation but, rather, a roughly rectangular source that varies in size from approximately 0.1 to 1.5 mm on a side, depending on the type of x-ray tube that is in use.

Figure 16-28 illustrates the result of using x-ray tubes with measurable effective focal spots as imaging devices. The point of the object arrow in Figure 16-28 does not appear as a point in the image plane because the x-rays used to image that point originate throughout the rectangular source.

Focal-spot blur occurs because the focal spot is not a point.

A blurred region on the radiograph over which the radiologic technologist has little control results because the effective focal spot has size. This phenomenon is called **focal-spot blur**. As illustrated, it is greater on the cathode side of the image. Focal-spot blur is undesirable.

Focal-spot blur is the most important factor for determining spatial resolution.

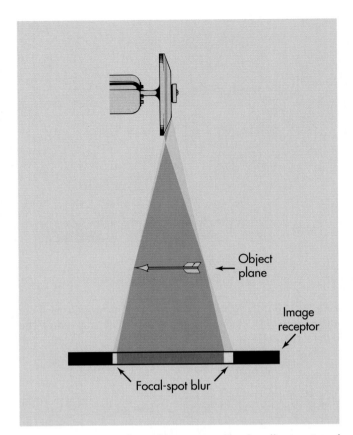

FIGURE 16-28 Focal-spot blur is caused by the effective size of the focal spot, which is larger to the cathode side of the image.

The geometric relationships that govern magnification also influence focal-spot blur. As the geometry of the source, object, and image is altered to produce greater magnification, increased focal-spot blur is produced. Consequently, these conditions should be avoided when possible.

The region of focal-spot blur can be calculated with the use of similar triangles. If an arrowhead were positioned near the x-ray tube target, the size of the focal-spot blur would be larger than that of the effective focal spot (Figure 16-29, *A*). In general, the object is much closer to the image receptor; therefore, the focal-spot blur is much smaller than the effective focal spot (Figure 16-29, *B*).

From these drawings, one can see that two similar triangles are described. Therefore, the ratio of SOD to OID is the same as the ratio of the sizes of the effective focal spot and the focal-spot blur.

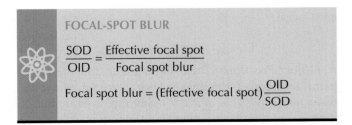

FOCAL-SPOT BLUR

$$\frac{SOD}{OID} = \frac{Effective\ focal\ spot}{Focal\ spot\ blur}$$

$$Focal\ spot\ blur = (Effective\ focal\ spot)\frac{OID}{SOD}$$

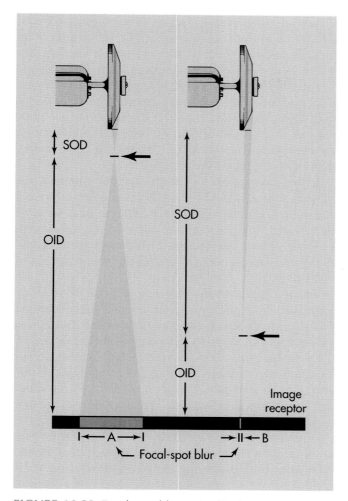

FIGURE 16-29 Focal-spot blur is small when the object-to-image receptor distance (OID) is small.

Question: An x-ray tube target with a 0.6-mm effective focal spot is used to image a calcified nodule estimated to be 8 cm from the anterior chest wall. If the radiograph is taken in a posterior-anterior projection at 180 cm SID, with a tabletop to image receptor separation of 5 cm, what will be the size of the focal-spot blur?

Answer:
$$\text{Focal spot blur} = (0.6 \text{ mm})\frac{8+5}{180-(8+5)}$$
$$= (0.6 \text{ mm})\frac{13}{167}$$
$$= (0.6 \text{ mm})(0.078)$$
$$= 0.047 \text{ mm}$$

To minimize focal-spot blur, you should use small focal spots and position the patient so that the anatomical part under examination is close to the image receptor. The SID usually is fixed but should be as large as possible. High-contrast objects that are smaller than the focal-spot blur normally cannot be imaged.

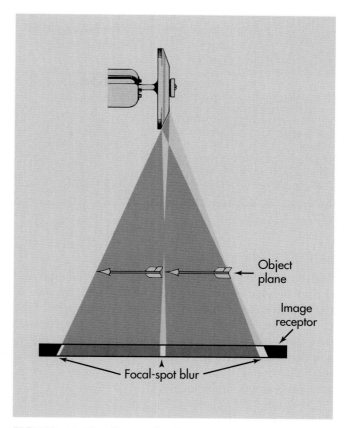

FIGURE 16-30 Effective focal spot size is largest on the cathode side; therefore, focal-spot blur is greatest on the cathode side.

Heel Effect

The heel effect, introduced in Chapter 7, is described as varying intensity across the x-ray field in the anode–cathode direction caused by attenuation of x-rays in the heel of the anode. Another characteristic of the heel effect is unrelated to x-ray intensity but affects focal-spot blur.

The size of the effective focal spot is not constant across the radiograph. An x-ray tube said to have a 1-mm focal spot has a smaller effective focal spot on the anode side and a larger effective focal spot on the cathode side (Figure 16-30).

 The focal-spot blur is small on the anode side and large on the cathode side of the image.

This variation in focal-spot size results in variation in focal-spot blur. Consequently, images toward the cathode side of a radiograph have a higher degree of blur and poorer spatial resolution than those to the anode side. This is clinically significant when x-ray tubes with small target angles are used at short SIDs. Table 16-2 lists radiographic examinations that should be performed with regard for the heel effect.

Table 16-2	Patient Positioning for Examinations That Can Take Advantage of the Heel Effect	
Examination	**Position Toward the Cathode**	**Position Toward the Anode**
PA chest	Abdomen	Neck
Abdomen	Abdomen	Pelvis
Femur	Hip	Knee
Humerus	Shoulder	Elbow
AP thoracic spine	Abdomen	Neck
AP lumbar spine	Abdomen	Pelvis

AP, Anterior-posterior.

SUBJECT FACTORS

The third general group of factors that affect radiographic quality involve the patient (Box 16-2). These factors are those associated not so much with the positioning of the patient as with the selection of a radiographic technique that properly compensates for the patient's size, shape, and tissue composition. Patient positioning is basically a requirement that is associated with the geometric factors that affect radiographic quality.

BOX 16-2 Subject Factors

- Subject contrast
- Patient thickness
- Tissue mass density
- Effective atomic number
- Object shape
- Kilovolt peak

Subject Contrast

The contrast of a radiograph viewed on an illuminator is called **radiographic contrast.** As indicated previously, radiographic contrast is a function of image receptor contrast and subject contrast. In fact, radiographic contrast is simply the product of image receptor contrast and subject contrast.

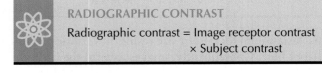

RADIOGRAPHIC CONTRAST

Radiographic contrast = Image receptor contrast × Subject contrast

Question: Screen-film with an average gradient of 3.1 is used to radiograph a long bone with subject contrast of 4.5. What is the radiographic contrast?

Answer: Radiographic contrast = (3.1)(4.5) = 13.95

Several of these subject factors were discussed in Chapter 10 in terms of their relation to the attenuation of an x-ray beam. The effect of each on subject contrast is a direct result of differences in attenuation in body tissues.

Patient Thickness. Given a standard composition, a thick body section attenuates a greater number of x-rays than does a thin body section (Figure 16-31). The same number of x-rays is incident on each section; therefore, the contrast of the incident x-ray beam is zero, that is, there is no contrast.

If the same number of x-rays left each section, the subject contrast would be 1.0. Because more x-rays are transmitted through thin body sections than through thick ones, however, subject contrast is greater than 1. The degree of subject contrast is directly proportional to the relative number of x-rays leaving those sections of the body.

Tissue Mass Density. Different sections of the body may have equal thicknesses, yet different mass densities. Tissue mass density is an important factor that affects subject contrast. Consider, for example, the radiograph of different salad ingredients (Figure 16-32). These materials have the same thickness and chemical composition. However, they have slightly different mass density from water and therefore will be imaged. The effect of mass density on subject contrast is demonstrated in Figure 16-33.

Effective Atomic Number. Another important factor that affects subject contrast is the effective atomic number of the tissue being examined. In Chapter 10, it is shown that Compton interactions are independent of atomic number, but photoelectric interactions vary in proportion to the cube of the atomic number.

The effective atomic numbers of tissues of interest are reported in Table 10-3. In the diagnostic range of x-ray energies, the photoelectric effect is of considerable importance; therefore, subject contrast is influenced greatly by the effective atomic number of the tissue that is being radiographed. When the effective atomic number of adjacent tissues is very much different, subject contrast is very high.

Subject contrast can be enhanced greatly by the use of contrast media. The high atomic numbers of iodine (Z = 53) and barium (Z = 56) result in extremely high subject contrast. Contrast media are effective because they accentuate subject contrast through enhanced photoelectric absorption.

Object Shape. The shape of the anatomical structure under investigation influences its radiographic quality, not only through its geometry but also through its contribution to subject contrast. Obviously, a structure that has a form that coincides with the x-ray beam has maximum subject contrast (Figure 16-34, *A*).

All other anatomical shapes have reduced subject contrast because of the change in thickness that they present across the x-ray beam. Figure 16-34, *B* and *C,* illustrates two shapes that result in reduced subject contrast.

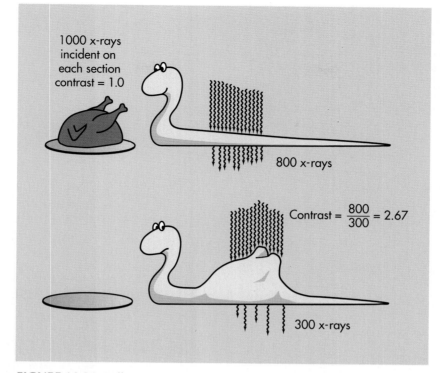

FIGURE 16-31 Different anatomical thicknesses contribute to subject contrast.

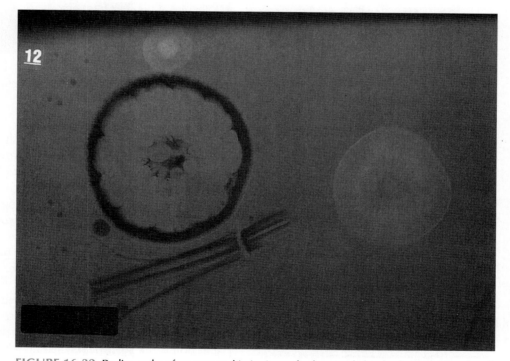

FIGURE 16-32 Radiographs of an orange, kiwi, piece of celery, and chunk of carrot show the effects of subtle differences in mass density. (Courtesy Marcy Barnes, Lexington Community College.)

This characteristic of the subject that affects subject contrast is sometimes called *absorption blur.* It reduces spatial resolution and contrast resolution of any anatomical structure, but it is most troublesome during interventional procedures in which vessels with small diameters are examined.

kVp. The radiologic technologist has no control over the four previous factors that influence subject contrast. The absolute magnitude of subject contrast, however, is greatly controlled by the kVp of operation. kVp also influences film contrast but not to the extent that it controls subject contrast.

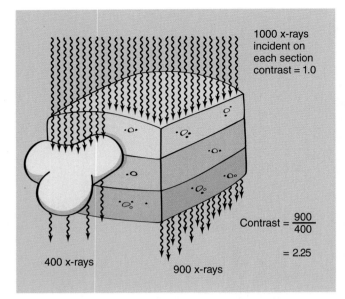

FIGURE 16-33 Variation in tissue mass density contributes to subject contrast.

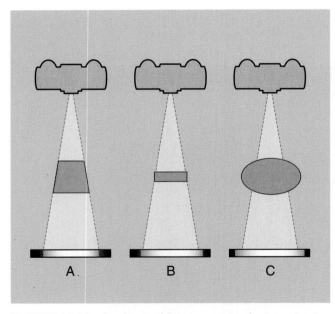

FIGURE 16-34 The shape of the structure under investigation contributes to absorption blur.

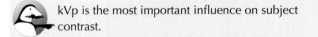

kVp is the most important influence on subject contrast.

Figure 16-35 shows a composite of a series of radiographs of an aluminum step wedge taken at kVp values ranging from 40 to 100. A low kVp results in high subject contrast, sometimes called **short gray scale contrast,** because the radiographic image appears either black or white with few shades of gray. On the other hand, high kVp results in low subject contrast or **long gray scale contrast.**

FIGURE 16-35 Radiographs of an aluminum step wedge (penetrometer) demonstrating change in contrast with varying voltage. (Courtesy Eastman Kodak Co.)

It would be easy to jump to the conclusion that low-kVp techniques are always more desirable than high-kVp techniques. However, low-kVp radiography has two major disadvantages:

1. As the kVp is lowered for any radiographic examination, the x-ray beam becomes less penetrating, requiring a higher mAs to produce an acceptable range of ODs. The result is higher patient dose. A method that can be used to estimate this increased patient dose is given in Chapter 39.
2. A radiographic technique that produces low subject contrast allows for wide latitude in exposure factors. Optimization of radiographic technique by mAs selection is not so critical when high kVp is used.

Motion Blur

Movement of the patient or the x-ray tube during exposure results in blurring of the radiographic image. This loss of radiographic quality, called **motion blur,** may result in repeated radiographs and therefore should be avoided.

Normally, motion of the x-ray tube is not a problem. In tomography, the x-ray tube is moved deliberately during exposure to blur the images of structures on either side of the plane of interest (see Chapter 15). Sometimes, the table or a restraining device is caused to move by auxiliary equipment, such as a moving grid mechanism.

 Patient motion is usually the cause of motion blur.

The radiographer can reduce motion blur by carefully instructing the patient, "Take a deep breath and hold it. Don't move."

Patient motion of two types may occur. Voluntary motion of limbs and muscles is controlled by immobilization. Involuntary motion of heart and lungs is controlled by short exposure time.

Motion blur is affected primarily by four factors. By observing the guidelines listed in Table 16-3, the radiologic technologist can reduce motion blur. Note that the last two items in this list have the same relation to motion blur as to focal-spot blur. With the use of low ripple power and high-speed image receptors, motion has been virtually eliminated as a common clinical problem.

TOOLS FOR IMPROVED RADIOGRAPHIC QUALITY

The radiologic technologist normally has the tools available to produce high-quality radiographs. Proper patient preparation, the selection of proper imaging devices, and proper radiographic technique are complex, related concepts.

For any given radiographic examination, each of these factors must be properly interpreted and applied. A small change in one may require a compensating change in another.

Patient Positioning

The importance of patient positioning should now be clear. Proper patient positioning requires that the anatomical structure under investigation be placed as close to the image receptor as is practical, and that the axis of this structure should lie in a plane that is parallel to the plane of the image receptor. The central ray should be incident on the center of the structure. Finally, the patient must be immobilized effectively to minimize motion blur.

Table 16-3	**Procedures for Reducing Motion Blur**

- Use the shortest possible exposure time.
- Restrict patient motion by providing instruction or using a restraining device.
- Use a large source-to-image receptor distance (SID).
- Use a small object-to-image receptor distance (OID).

To be able to position patients properly, the radiologic technologist must have a good knowledge of human anatomy. If multiple structures are being radiographed and are to be imaged with uniform magnification, they must be positioned at the same distance from the image receptor. The various techniques that are applied to radiographic positioning are designed to produce radiographs with minimal image distortion and maximum image resolution.

Image Receptors

Usually, a standard type of screen-film combination is used throughout a radiology department for a given examination. In general, extremity and soft tissue radiographs are taken with fine-detail screen-film combinations.

Most other radiographs use double-emulsion film with screens. The new, structured-grain x-ray films used with high-resolution intensifying screens produce exquisite images with limited patient dose.

 Principles to be considered when planning a particular examination:
1. Use of intensifying screens decreases patient dose by a factor of at least 20.
2. As the speed of the image receptor increases, radiographic noise increases and spatial resolution is decreased.
3. Low-contrast imaging procedures have wider latitude, or margin of error, in producing an acceptable radiograph.

Selection of Technique Factors

Before each examination, the radiologic technologist must select the optimum radiographic technique factors, that is, kVp, mAs, and exposure time. Many considerations determine the value of each of these factors, and they are complexly interrelated. Few generalizations are possible.

One generalization that can be made for all radiographic exposures is that the time of exposure should be as short as possible. Image quality is improved by short exposure times that cause reduced motion blur. One of the reasons why three-phase and high-frequency generators are better than single-phase generators is that shorter exposure times are possible with the former.

 Keep exposure time as short as possible.

Similar simple statements cannot be made about the selection of kVp or mA. Because time is to be kept to a minimum, the selection of kVp and mA, and the

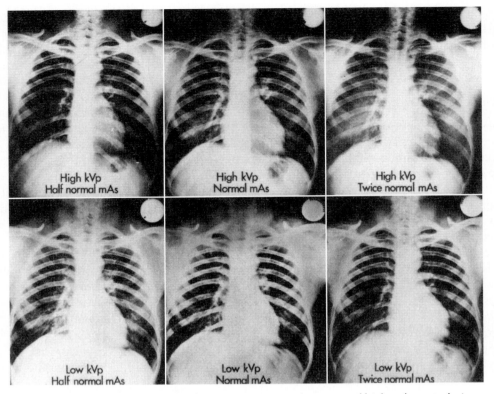

FIGURE 16-36 Chest radiographs demonstrating two advantages of high-voltage technique: greater latitude and margin for error. (Courtesy Eastman Kodak Co.)

resulting mAs value, should be considered. The radiographer should strive for optimum radiographic contrast and ODs by exposing the patient to the proper quantity and quality of x-radiation.

 The primary control of radiographic contrast is kVp.

As kVp is increased, both the quantity and quality of x-radiation are enhanced; a greater number of x-rays are transmitted through the patient, so a higher portion of the primary beam reaches the image receptor. Thus, kVp also affects OD. Among x-rays that interact with the patient, the relative number of Compton interactions increases with increasing kVp, resulting in less differential absorption and reduced subject contrast.

Furthermore, with increased kVp, the scatter radiation that reaches the image receptor is greater; therefore, radiographic noise is higher. The result of increased kVp is loss of contrast. When radiographic contrast is low, latitude is high, and the margin for error is increased.

The principal advantages of the use of high kVp include a reduction in patient dose and a wide latitude of exposures allowed in the production of a diagnostic radiograph. Figure 16-36 shows a series of chest radiographs that demonstrate increased latitude

resulting from high-kVp technique. The relative technique factors are indicated on each radiograph. To some extent, the use of grids can compensate for the loss of contrast accompanying high-kVp technique.

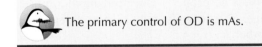 The primary control of OD is mAs.

As the mAs value is increased, the radiation quantity increases; therefore, the number of x-rays arriving at the image receptor increases, resulting in higher OD and lower radiographic noise but higher patient radiation dose.

In a secondary way, the mAs value also influences contrast. Recall that maximum contrast is attained only when the film is exposed over a range that results in OD along the straight-line portion of the characteristic curve. Too low an mAs setting results in low OD and reduced radiographic contrast because the H & D curve has flattened. Too high an mAs value results in high OD and loss of radiographic contrast for the same reason.

A number of other factors influence OD and radiographic contrast, and hence radiographic quality. Adding filtration to the x-ray tube reduces x-ray beam intensity but enhances quality. A change in SID results in a change in OD because x-ray intensity varies with

Table 16-4   Principal Factors That May Affect the Making of a Radiograph*

Increase in:	Patient Optical Dose	Radiographic Magnification	Focal Spot Blur	Motion Blur	Absorption Blur	Density	Contrast
Film speed	−	0	0	−	0	+	0
Screen speed	−	0	0	−	0	+	0
Grid ratio	+	0	0	0	0	−	+
Processing time/temperature	0	0	0	0	0	+	−
Patient thickness	+	+	+	+	+	−	−
Field size	+	0	0	0	0	+	−
Use of contrast media	0	0	0	0	0	−	+
Focal-spot size	0	0	+	0	0	0	0
SID	−	−	−	−	0	−	0
OID	0	+	+	+	0	0	+
Screen-film contact	0	0	0	0	0	0	−
Milliampere-seconds	+	0	0	0	0	+	+ or −
Time	+	0	0	+	0	+	+ or −
Voltage	+	0	0	0	0	+	−
Voltage ripple	+	0	0	+	0	+	+
Total filtration	−	0	0	0	0	−	+

SID, Source-to-image receptor distance; OID, object-to-image receptor distance.

*As the factors in the left-hand column are increased, **while all other factors remain fixed,** cross-referenced conditions are affected as shown: +, increase; −, decrease; 0, no change.

distance. Table 16-4 represents an attempt to summarize the principal factors that influence the making of a radiograph.

The continuing trend in radiographic technique is to use high kVp with a compensating reduction in mAs to produce a radiograph of satisfactory quality while reducing patient dose and the likelihood of an ordered reexamination because of an error in technique.

SUMMARY

Radiographic quality is the exactness of representation of the anatomical structure on the radiograph. Characteristics that make up radiographic quality are as follows:

- Spatial resolution, or the ability to detect small, high-contrast structures on the radiograph
- Low noise, or elimination of ODs that do not reflect anatomical structures
- Proper speed of the screen-film combination, which limits patient dose but produces a high-quality, low-noise radiograph

These characteristics and three others—film factors, geometric factors, and subject factors—combine to determine radiographic quality. Film factors involve quality control in film processing and characteristics of film.

The graph on semilogarithmic paper that presents sensitometry and densitometry data of film optical density is the characteristic curve. The characteristic curve shows film contrast, speed, and latitude.

Geometric factors that affect radiographic quality include magnification and distortion, as well as the advantageous use of object thickness, position, focal-spot blur, and the heel effect.

Subject factors that affect radiographic quality depend on the patient. A radiographer must prevent motion blur by encouraging patient cooperation. Also, by measuring patient thickness, recognizing tissue mass density, examining anatomical shape, and evaluating optimal kVp levels, a radiographer can produce a high-quality radiograph.

CHALLENGE QUESTIONS

1. Define or otherwise identify the following:
   a. Average gradient
   b. Optical density
   c. Foreshortening
   d. Focal-spot blur
   e. Opaque, radiopaque
   f. Densitometer
   g. Motion blur
   h. Spatial distortion
   i. Quantum mottle
   j. Latitude
2. What principally determines radiographic spatial resolution?

3. Describe the equipment used in sensitometry.
4. What is the importance of processor quality control in an imaging department?
5. Have the manufacturer's representative help construct a characteristic curve from the data obtained from sensitometry and densitometry of a screen-film combination used in your department.
6. The intensity of light emitted by a viewbox is 1000. The intensity of light transmitted through the film is 1. What is the optical density of the film? Will it be light, gray, or black?
7. Base and fog densities on a given radiograph are 0.35. At densities 0.25 and 2 above base and fog densities, the characteristic curve shows log relative exposure values of 1.3 and 2. What is the average gradient?
8. List factors related to film processing that may affect the finished radiograph.
9. X-ray image receptors A and B require 15 mR and 45 mR to produce an optical density of 1.0. Which is faster, and what is the speed of each?
10. What three principal geometric factors may affect radiographic quality?
11. What are standard SIDs?
12. List and explain the five factors that affect subject contrast.
13. What is the difference between foreshortening and elongation?
14. Describe the H & H contrast curve.
15. Discuss the factors that influence radiographic optical density and contrast.
16. Construct a characteristic curve for a typical screen-film combination, and carefully label the axes.
17. An x-ray examination of the heart taken at 100 cm SID shows a cardiac silhouette measuring 13 cm in width. If the OID distance is estimated at 15 cm, what is the actual width of the heart?
18. The subject contrast of a thorax is 5.3. Image receptor contrast is 3.2. What is the radiographic contrast?
19. State the reciprocity law and explain its influence on radiography.
20. How does image contrast attained with the use of a radiographic intensifying screen compare with direct exposure?

The answers to the Challenge Questions can be found by logging on to our website at http://evolve.elsevier.com.

CHAPTER

17

Image Artifacts

OBJECTIVES

At the completion of this chapter, the student should be able
to do the following:

1. Visually identify the radiographic artifacts shown in this chapter
2. List and discuss the three categories of artifacts
3. Explain the causes of exposure artifacts
4. Describe the types of artifacts caused during film processing
5. Discuss how improper handling and storage of film can cause
   artifacts

OUTLINE

Exposure Artifacts
Processing Artifacts
    Roller Marks
    Dirty Rollers
    Chemical Fog
    Wet-Pressure Sensitization
Handling and Storage Artifacts
    Light or Radiation Fog
    Kink Marks
    Static
    Hypo Retention

Artifacts can occur if the wrong film is loaded into a cassette. If high-contrast, single-emulsion mammography film is loaded into a radiographic cassette, an unexpected image results. Cassettes that have not been checked for proper screen-film contact produce smoothness in the area of poor contact that obscures detail and constitutes an artifact.

When one is trying to locate an object that has been swallowed, this is not an artifact. On the other hand, if such an object appears on an image unexpectedly, it is an artifact. Table 17-1 summarizes the exposure artifacts discussed here.

PROCESSING ARTIFACTS

Any number of artifacts can be produced during processing. Most are pressure-type artifacts caused by the transport system of the processor. Pressure-type artifacts usually sensitize the emulsion and appear as higher optical density (OD). Those that scrape or remove emulsion appear as lower OD.

> Processing artifacts are eliminated with a proper processor QC program and frequent cleaning.

Table 17-2 summarizes the processing artifacts discussed here, as well as some other common artifacts.

Roller Marks

Guide shoe marks occur when the guide shoes in the turnaround assembly of the processor are sprung or improperly positioned (Figure 17-3). If the guide shoe is used before the developer, the ridges in the guide shoes press against the film, sensitize it, and leave a characteristic mark. Guide shoe marks can be found on the leading edge or the trailing edge of the film, parallel to the direction of film travel through the processor.

Pi lines occur at 3.1416 inch (π) intervals because of dirt or a chemical stain on a roller, which sensitizes the emulsion. Because the rollers are 1 inch in diameter, 3.1416 inches represents one revolution of a roller, and the artifact appears perpendicular to the film's direction of travel through the processor. Figure 17-4 is an example of pi lines appearing on the same film.

Dirty Rollers

Dirty or warped rollers can cause **emulsion pick-off** and **gelatin buildup**, which result in **sludge** deposits on the film. These artifacts usually appear as sharp areas of increased or reduced OD. Occasionally, particles of sludge are transported through the processor and are actually dried on the film in the dryer.

Chemical Fog

Chemical fog looks like light or radiation fog and is usually a uniform dull gray. Improper or inadequate processing chemistry can result in a special type of chemical fog called a **dichroic stain.** Dichroic means two colors. The dichroic stain appears as a curtain effect on the radiograph (Figure 17-5). *Dichroic stain* is a term that is generally applied to all chemical stains.

Chemical stains on a radiograph can appear yellow, green, blue, or purple. In slow processors, the chemistry may not be squeezed properly from the film, and it either runs down the leading edge of the film or runs up the trailing edge. Both events are referred to as a **curtain effect.**

TABLE 17-1	Common Exposure Artifacts
Appearance on the Radiograph	**Cause**
Unexpected foreign object such as jewelry	Improper patient preparation
Double exposure	Reuse of cassettes already exposed
Blur	Improper patient movement, including breathing
Grid cutoff artifacts	Improper patient positioning
Obscured detail	Poor screen-film contact

TABLE 17-2	Common Processing Artifacts
Appearance on the Radiograph	**Cause**
Guide shoe marks	Improper position or springing of guide shoes in turnaround assembly
Pi lines	Dirt or chemical stains on rollers
Sharp increase or decrease in OD	Dirty or warped rollers, which can leave sludge deposits on film
Uniform dull, gray fog	Improper or inadequate processing chemistry
Dichroic stain or "curtain effect"	Improper squeezing of processing chemicals from film
Small circular patterns of increased OD	Pressure caused by irregular or dirty rollers
Yellow-brown drops on film	Oxidized developer
Milky appearance	Underreplenished fixer
Greasy appearance	Inadequate washing
Brittle appearance	Improper dryer temperature or hardener in the fixer

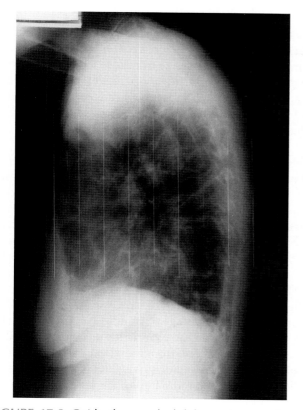

FIGURE 17-3 Guide shoe marks left by an improperly serviced turnaround assembly. (Courtesy Judy Williams, Grady Memorial Hospital, Atlanta.)

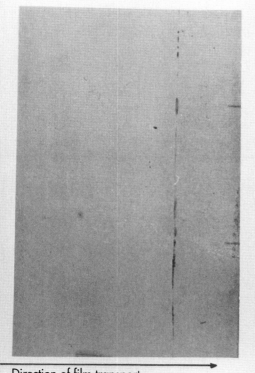

Direction of film transport →

FIGURE 17-4 Pi line artifacts due to lack of processor cleaning. (Courtesy Rita Robinson, Memorial Herman Hospital, Houston.)

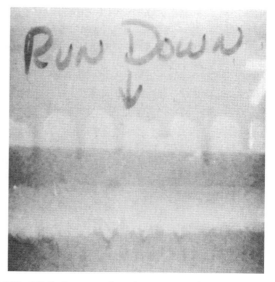

FIGURE 17-5 Excess chemistry runs down the leading edge of the film, creating a "curtain" effect. (Courtesy William McKinney, Dupont Medical Systems.)

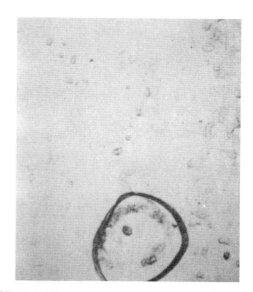

FIGURE 17-6 Wet-pressure sensitization caused by a dirty processor. (Courtesy William McKinney, Dupont Medical Systems.)

Wet-Pressure Sensitization

Wet-pressure sensitization is a common artifact that is produced in the developer tank (Figure 17-6). Irregular or dirty rollers cause pressure during development and produce small circular patterns of increased OD.

Processing artifacts in digital radiography (DR) are different from those with screen-film because the method of producing the visible image is electronic rather than chemical. Image-processing error can produce bizarre artifacts in DR. Interference with electronic components involved in processing DR images also occurs. Artifacts in DR are discussed in detail in Chapter 31.

HANDLING AND STORAGE ARTIFACTS

A number of artifacts are caused by improper film storage conditions. Image fog can result if the temperature or the humidity is too high, or if the film bin is not shielded adequately from radiation. Pressure marks can occur if the film is stacked too high. Table 17-3 summarizes the storage artifacts discussed here.

 Proper facility design helps reduce handling and storage artifacts.

Light or Radiation Fog

White-light leaks in the darkroom or within the cassette cause streaklike artifacts of increased OD. If the safelight has an improper filter, if the safelight is too bright, or if the safelight is too close to the film processing tray, the image will be fogged. Films left in the x-ray examination room during an exposure can become fogged by radiation. Radiation fog and safelight fog look alike.

Kink Marks

Characteristic artifacts can be caused by improper handling or storage either before or after processing. Rough handling before processing can cause scratches and kink marks, such as those shown in Figure 17-7. Although the kink mark may appear as a fingernail mark, it is not. It is caused by the kinking or abrupt bending of film. Both events usually appear as increased OD.

Static

Static is probably the most obvious artifact. It is caused by the buildup of electrons in the emulsion and is most noticeable during the winter or during periods of extremely low humidity. Three distinct patterns of static are crown, tree, and smudge. Tree static and smudge static are illustrated in Figure 17-8.

Hypo Retention

The yellow-brown stain that slowly appears on a radiograph after a long storage time indicates a problem with hypo retention from the fixer. With this event, not all of the residual thiosulfate from fixing was removed during washing, and silver sulfide slowly builds up and appears yellow in the stored radiograph.

TABLE 17-3	Common Handling and Storage Artifacts
Appearance on Radiographic Film	**Cause**
Fog	The temperature or humidity is too high.
	The film bin is inadequately shielded from radiation.
	The safelight is too bright, is too close to the processing tray, or has an improper filter.
	The film has been left in the x-ray room during other exposures.
Pressure or kink marks	The film is improperly or roughly handled.
	The film is stacked too high in storage (the weight causes marks).
Streaks of increased OD	The darkroom or cassette has light leaks.
Crown, tree, and smudge static	The temperature or humidity is too low.
Yellow-brown stains	Thiosulfate is left on the film because of inadequate washing.

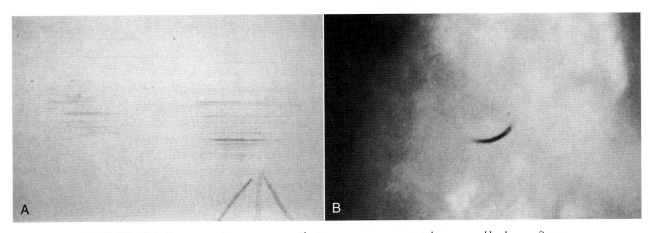

FIGURE 17-7 Preprocessing pressure artifacts can appear as scratches caused by heavy finger pressure on the feed tray, and as "fingernail" marks caused by kinking of the film. **A,** Scratches. **B,** "Fingernail" marks. (Courtesy William McKinney, Dupont Medical Systems.)

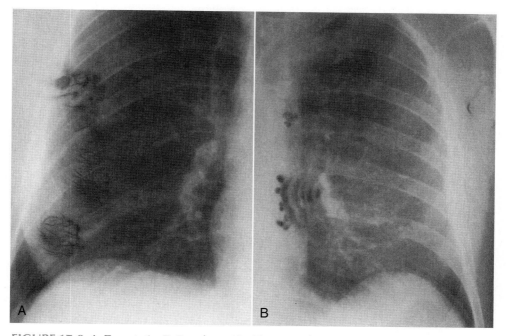

FIGURE 17-8 **A,** Tree static. **B,** Smudge static. These are the two most common types of static artifacts. (Courtesy Joel Gray, Medical Physics Consulting.)

SUMMARY

An artifact is an undesirable OD that appears on the radiograph. Artifacts occur (1) during the radiographic exposure, (2) during processing of the film, and (3) when the film is being handled and stored before or after processing.

Exposure artifacts are a result of examination technique. These include patient motion, positioning errors, wrong screen-film combinations, double exposures, and improper grid positioning.

Processing artifacts are most often pressure blemishes on the film emulsion caused by the roller transport system in the processor. They include sludge from dirty rollers, chemical fog, roller marks, and wet-pressure sensitization.

The most bothersome handling and storage artifacts are those associated with light or radiation fog, kink marks, and static.

CHALLENGE QUESTIONS

1. Define or otherwise identify the following:
   a. Exposure artifact
   b. Guide shoe marks
   c. Pick-off
   d. Pressure mark
   e. Kink mark
   f. Hypo retention
   g. Safelight
   h. Curtain effect
   i. Pi line
   j. Processing artifact

2. Why must records be kept when the QC technologist sees artifacts?
3. Describe an artifact.
4. List the four stages in diagnostic imaging during which artifacts tend to occur.
5. Give three examples of exposure artifacts.
6. How would a radiographer correct a blurred radiograph if it was the result of patient motion?
7. What is the principal reason for double exposures?
8. Name three types of processing artifacts.
9. What is a dichroic stain?
10. How do guide shoe marks occur?
11. Explain what 3.1416 inches has to do with pi lines.
12. Describe the causes of wet-pressure sensitization marks.
13. Explain three ways fog can occur on a radiograph.
14. What is the cause of a static artifact on the processed radiograph?
15. List the three types of static artifact patterns.
16. Why is it important for radiographers to be alert to film artifacts?
17. How can one best avoid processor artifacts?
18. What causes grid cutoff artifacts?
19. How do pressure-type artifacts appear?
20. What type of artifact does hypo retention cause?

The answers to the Challenge Questions can be found by logging on to our website at http://evolve.elsevier.com.

Quality Control

OBJECTIVES

At the completion of this chapter, the student should be able to do the following:

1. Define *quality assurance* and *quality control*
2. List the 10-step quality assurance model used in hospitals
3. Name the three steps of quality control
4. Describe the quality control tests and schedule for radiographic systems
5. Discuss processor quality control

OUTLINE

Quality Assurance
Quality Control
Radiographic Quality Control
    Filtration
    Collimation
    Focal-Spot Size
    kVp Calibration
    Exposure Timer Accuracy
    Exposure Linearity
    Exposure Reproducibility
    Radiographic Intensifying Screens
    Protective Apparel
    Film Illuminators
Fluoroscopy Quality Control
    Exposure Rate
    Spot-Film Exposures
    Automatic Exposure Systems
Tomography Quality Control
Processor Quality Control
    Processor Cleaning
    Processor Maintenance
    Processor Monitoring

ALL FIELDS of medicine and all hospital departments are required to develop and conduct programs that ensure the quality of patient care and management. Diagnostic imaging departments are leaders in promoting quality patient care.

This chapter discusses the properties of quality assurance and quality control, with an emphasis on radiographic imaging systems. Processor quality control is covered thoroughly in Chapter 20 ("Mammography Quality Control") and therefore is only reviewed here.

Two areas of activity are designed to ensure the best possible diagnosis at an acceptable radiation dose and with minimum cost. These areas are quality assurance (QA) and quality control (QC). There is still some confusion about the use of these terms, but responsible organizations are developing clearer definitions. Both programs rely heavily on proper record keeping.

QUALITY ASSURANCE

Health care organizations often adopt formal, structured QA models. The Joint Commission (TJC) promotes "The Ten-Step Monitoring and Evaluation Process." This QA program uses a 10-step process to resolve identified patient care problems. To ensure that a health care organization is committed to providing high-quality services and care, accrediting agencies encourage the adoption of QA models such as that recommended by TJC (Box 18-1).

Quality assurance deals with people.

A program of QA monitors proper patient scheduling, reception, and preparation, and answers the following questions: Is the scheduled examination appropriate for the patient? If so, has the patient been properly instructed before the time of the examination?

Item 8 in Box 18-1 leads to programs of continuous quality improvement (CQI); these have been implemented by many health care organizations.

QA also involves image interpretation. Did the patient's ultimate disease or condition agree with the radiologist's diagnosis? This is called **outcome analysis.**

BOX 18-1 TJC 10-Step Quality Assurance Program

1. Assign responsibility.
2. Delineate scope of care.
3. Identify aspects of care.
4. Identify outcomes that affect the aspects of care.
5. Establish limits of the scope of assessment.
6. Collect and organize data.
7. Evaluate care when outcomes are reached.
8. Take action to improve care.
9. Assess and document actions.
10. Communicate information to organization-wide quality assurance programs.

TJC, The Joint Commission.

Was the report of the diagnosis promptly prepared, distributed, and filed for subsequent evaluation? Was the clinician or patient properly informed in a timely fashion? All of these QA activities require attention from the imaging team, but they are principally the responsibility of the radiologist.

QUALITY CONTROL

Quality control (QC) is more tangible and obvious than QA. A program of QC is designed to ensure that the radiologist is provided with an optimal image produced through good equipment performance and resulting in minimal patient radiation exposure.

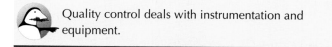

Quality control deals with instrumentation and equipment.

QC begins with the x-ray imaging systems used to produce the image and continues with the routine evaluation of image-processing facilities. QC concludes with a dedicated analysis of each image to identify deficiencies and artifacts (along with their cause) and to minimize reexamination.

Each new piece of radiologic equipment, whether it is x-ray producing or image processing, should be acceptance tested before it is applied clinically. The acceptance test must be done by someone other than the manufacturer's representative because it is designed to show that the equipment is performing within the manufacturer's specifications and is producing an acceptable patient radiation dose.

With use, the performance characteristics of all such items of equipment change and may deteriorate. Consequently, periodic monitoring of equipment performance is required. On most systems, annual monitoring is satisfactory, unless a major component such as an x-ray tube has been replaced.

TABLE 18-1	Characteristics of Various Diagnostic Imaging Systems				
Procedure	Spatial Resolution	Contrast Resolution	Temporal Resolution	Signal-to-Noise Ratio	Artifacts
Radiography	E	F	E	E	F
Mammography	E	G	G	E	F
Fluoroscopy	G	F	E	G	F
Digital R&F	G	E	G	G	G
Computed tomography	F	E	G	F	G
Magnetic resonance imaging	F	E	G	F	F
Ultrasonography	F	G	G	G	F
Nuclear medicine	F	G	F	F	F

E, Excellent; *F*, fair; *G*, good; *R&F*, radiography and fluoroscopy.

TABLE 18-2	Elements of a Quality Control Program for Radiographic Systems	
Measurement	Frequency*	Tolerance
Filtration	Annually	≥2.5 mm Al
Collimation	Semiannually	±2% SID
Focal-spot size	Annually	±50%
Calibration of kVp	Annually	±10%
Exposure timer accuracy	Annually	±5% > 10 ms ±20% ≤ 10 ms
Exposure linearity	Annually	±10%
Exposure reproducibility	Annually	±5%

*Evaluation should follow any major equipment modification.

When periodic monitoring shows that equipment is not performing as it was intended to perform, maintenance or repair is necessary. Preventive maintenance usually makes repair unnecessary.

 An acceptable QC program consists of three steps: acceptance testing, routine performance monitoring, and maintenance.

As with QA, QC requires a team effort, but QC is principally the responsibility of the medical physicist. In private offices, clinics, and hospitals, the medical physicist establishes the QC program and oversees its implementation at a frequency determined by the activity of the institution.

In a large medical center hospital where the medical physicist is a member of the professional staff, he or she performs many of the routine activities and supervises other activities. With the help of the QC technologist and radiologic engineers, the medical physicist sees that all necessary monitoring measurement and observations are performed.

In addition to ensuring patient care, a QC program in radiology is conducted for other reasons. Our litigious society demands QC records. Some insurance carriers pay for services only from facilities with an approved QC program. The Joint Commission will not place its seal of approval on facilities that do not have an ongoing QC program. Most states, through their Department of Health and with guidance from the Council of Radiation Control Program Directors (CRCPD), require QC by regulation.

The nature of a QC program is determined somewhat by the characteristics of the image produced. Table 18-1 summarizes the characteristic features of most imaging systems. Usually, the QC program focuses on the strengths of the image to ensure that those strengths are maintained.

RADIOGRAPHIC QUALITY CONTROL

Organizations such as the American College of Radiology and the American Association of Physicists in Medicine (AAPM) have developed guidelines for QC programs in radiography, as well as other imaging modalities.

Table 18-2 presents the essentials of such a program, the recommended frequency of evaluation, and the tolerance limit for each assessment. Figure 18-1 shows a medical physicist preparing dosimetry equipment for QC measurements.

Filtration

Perhaps the most important patient protection characteristic of a radiographic imaging system is filtration of the x-ray beam. State statutes require that general purpose radiographic units have a minimum total filtration of 2.5 mm Al.

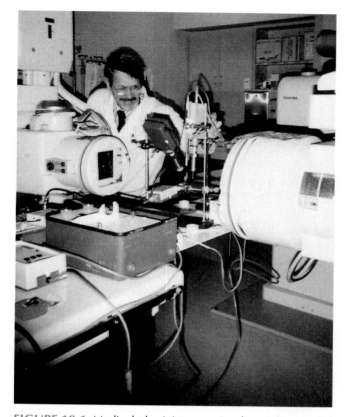

FIGURE 18-1 Medical physicist preparing for quality control (QC) measurements. (Courtesy Louis Wagner, University of Texas Medical School.)

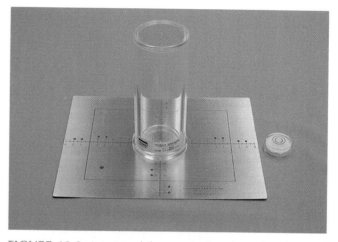

FIGURE 18-2 A test tool for monitoring the coincidence of the x-ray beam and light field. (Courtesy Cardinal Health.)

collimation can be confirmed with any of a number of test tools designed for that purpose (Figure 18-2).

 Misalignment must not exceed 2% of the source-to-image receptor distance (SID).

Most systems today are equipped with **positive beam–limiting (PBL)** collimators. These devices are automatic collimators that sense the size of the image receptor and adjust the collimating shutters to that size.

Because different sizes of image receptors must be accommodated, the PBL function must be evaluated for all possible receptor sizes. With a PBL collimator, the x-ray beam must not be larger than the image receptor, except in the override mode.

Distance and centering indicators must be accurate to within 2% and 1% of the SID, respectively. The distance indicator can be checked simply with a tape measure. The location of the focal spot usually is marked on the x-ray tube housing. Centering is checked visually for the light field, and with markers for the exposure field.

Question: The distance from the Bucky tray to the dot on the x-ray tube housing indicating focal-spot position is measured at 98.4 cm. The automatic distance indicator shows 100 cm SID. Is this acceptable?

Answer: $\dfrac{100-98.4}{100} = \dfrac{1.6}{100} = 1.6\%$, yes

Focal-Spot Size

The spatial resolution of a radiographic imaging system is determined principally by the focal-spot size of the x-ray tube. When new equipment or a replacement x-ray tube is installed, the focal-spot size must be measured (Figure 18-3).

TABLE 18-3	Minimum Half-Value Layer (HVL) Required to Ensure Adequate X-ray Beam Filtration				
Minimum HVL (mm Al)	**OPERATING kVp**				
	30	**50**	**70**	**90**	**130**
Single-phase	0.3	1.2	1.6	2.6	3.6
Three-phase/ high-frequency	0.4	1.5	2.0	3.1	4.2

It is normally not possible to measure filtration directly, so one resorts to measurement of the half-value layer (HVL) of the x-ray beam, as described in Chapter 9. The measured HVL must meet or exceed the value shown in Table 18-3 for the total filtration to be considered adequate. Filtration should be evaluated annually or at any time after a change has occurred in the x-ray tube or tube housing.

Collimation

The x-ray field must coincide with the light field of the variable-aperture light-localizing collimator. If these fields are misaligned, intended anatomy will be missed and unintended anatomy irradiated. Adequate

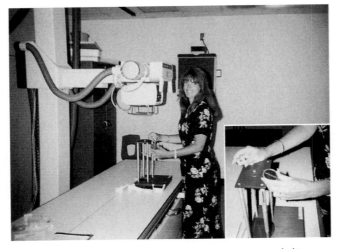

FIGURE 18-3 The pinhole camera, star pattern, and slit camera may be used to measure focal-spot size. (Courtesy Teresa Rice, Houston Community College.)

 Three tools are used for measurement of focal-spot size: the pinhole camera, the star pattern, and the slit camera.

The pinhole camera is difficult to use and requires excessive exposure time. The star pattern is easy to use but has significant limitations for focal-spot sizes less than 0.3 mm. The standard for measurement of effective focal-spot size is the slit camera.

The fabrication of an x-ray tube is an exceptionally complex process. Specification of focal-spot size depends not only on the geometry of the tube but also on the focusing of the electron beam. Consequently, vendors are permitted a substantial variance from their advertised focal-spot sizes (see Table 7-2).

Focal-spot size should be evaluated annually or whenever an x-ray tube is replaced.

An acceptable alternative to focal-spot size measurement is use of a line-pair test tool to determine limiting spatial frequency (Figure 18-4).

kVp Calibration

The radiologic technologist selects kVp for every examination. The radiologic technologist goes to exceptional lengths to determine the appropriate kVp; therefore, the x-ray generator should be properly calibrated.

A number of methods are available to evaluate the accuracy of kVp. Today, most medical physicists use one of a number of devices that are based on filtered ion chambers or filtered photodiodes (Figure 18-5). Other methods that use voltage diodes and oscilloscopes are more accurate but require an exceptional amount of time.

The kVp calibration should be evaluated annually or whenever high-voltage generator components have changed significantly. In the diagnostic range, any change

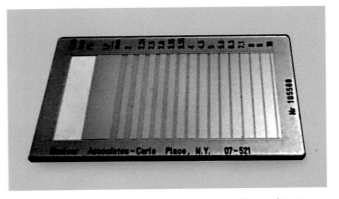

FIGURE 18-4 A line-pair test pattern. Its radiographic image measures limiting spatial resolution rather than focal-spot size.

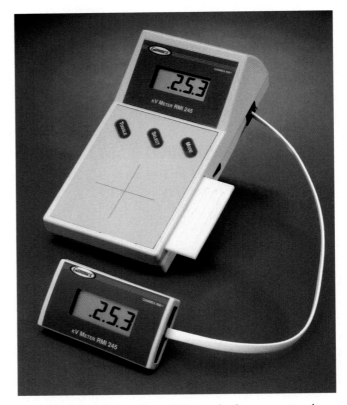

FIGURE 18-5 High-voltage (kVp) and other generator functions can be evaluated with compact test devices. (Courtesy Gammex RMI.)

in peak kilovoltage affects patient dose. A variation in kVp of approximately 4% is necessary to affect image optical density and radiographic contrast.

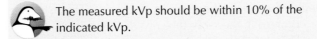 The measured kVp should be within 10% of the indicated kVp.

Exposure Timer Accuracy

Exposure time is operator selectable on most radiographic consoles. Although many radiographic systems are phototimed or controlled by mAs, exposure time is still the responsibility of the radiologic technologist. This parameter is particularly responsible for patient dose and image optical density.

Exposure timer accuracy can be assessed in several ways. Most medical physicists use one of several commercially available products that measure exposure time on the basis of irradiation time of an ion chamber or photodiode assembly (Figure 18-6).

 Exposure timer accuracy should be within 5% of the indicated time for exposure times greater than 10 ms.

The accuracy of the exposure timer should be assessed annually or more frequently if a component of the operating console or the high-voltage generator has undergone major repairs. Accuracy of 20% is acceptable for exposure times of 10 ms or less.

Automatic exposure control (AEC) also must be evaluated. These devices are designed to provide a constant optical density regardless of tissue thickness, composition, or **failure of the reciprocity law** (see Chapter 16). AEC systems are evaluated by exposing an image receptor through various thicknesses of aluminum or acrylic. Regardless of the material thickness and the absolute exposure time, the optical density of the processed image should be constant.

Insertion of a lead filter allows one to adequately assess the functioning of the backup timer. If the phototimer fails, the backup timer should terminate the exposure at 6 s or 600 mAs, whichever occurs first.

Exposure Linearity

Many combinations of mA and exposure time produce the same mAs value. The ability of a radiographic unit to produce a constant radiation output for various combinations of mA and exposure time is called **exposure linearity.**

 Exposure linearity must be within 10% for adjacent mA stations.

Exposure linearity is determined by a precision radiation dosimeter that measures radiation intensity at various combinations of mA and exposure time. Suppose, for example, that one were to choose 10 mAs for evaluation of the combinations of mA and exposure time shown in Table 18-4. Each of these combinations would be energized, and radiation intensity would be measured.

When evaluated in this fashion, the radiation output for adjacent mA stations should be within 10%. Exposure linearity should be evaluated annually or after any significant change or repair of the operating console or high-voltage generator.

This method of assessing exposure linearity is not valid if the exposure timer is inaccurate. Consequently, most would hold exposure time constant and would vary only the mA. Under these conditions, the mR/mAs value should be within 10% between adjacent mA stations.

Question: The following data are obtained to evaluate exposure linearity. Are the mA stations correctly calibrated?

Exposure Time	mA	mR
100 ms	50	29
100 ms	100	61
100 ms	200	109
100 ms	400	236

Answer:

mA	mR/mAs	% Difference
50	5.8	$\frac{6.1-5.8}{5.8} \times 100 = +5.2\%$, OK
100	6.1	$\frac{5.5-6.1}{6.1} \times 100 = -9.8\%$, OK
200	5.5	$\frac{5.9-5.5}{5.5} \times 100 = 7.3\%$, OK
400	5.9	

Exposure Reproducibility

When selecting the proper kVp, mA, and exposure time for a given examination, the radiologic technologist rightfully expects the image optical density and the contrast to be optimal. If any or all of these technique

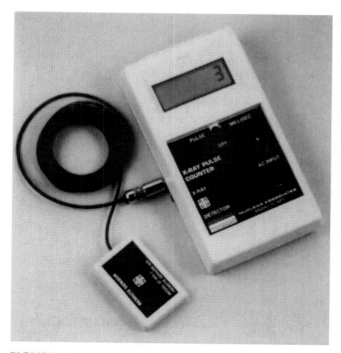

FIGURE 18-6 Device for measuring the accuracy of an exposure timer. (Courtesy Cardinal Health.)

factors are changed and then returned to the previous value, radiation exposure should be precisely the same. Radiation exposure should be **reproducible.**

> Sequential radiation exposures should be reproducible to within ±5%.

Two methods are available to evaluate exposure reproducibility; both rely on a precision radiation dosimeter. First, one can make a series of at least three exposures at the same technique factors, having changed technique controls between each exposure. If the result is not reproducible, this is usually the result of error in the kVp control. Second, one can select a combination of technique factors and hold them constant for a series of 10 exposures.

TABLE 18-4	Exposure Time and mA Combinations Equal to 10 mAs	
Exposure Time (ms)	**mA**	
1000	10	
400	25	
200	50	
100	100	
50	200	
25	400	
13	800	
10	1000	
8	1200	

Mathematical formulas can be used to determine reproducibility in both instances. These formulas basically require that output radiation intensity should not vary by more than ±5%.

Radiographic Intensifying Screens

Intensifying screens require periodic attention to minimize the appearance of artifacts. Screens should be cleaned with a soft, lint-free cloth and a cleaning solution provided by the manufacturer. The frequency of cleaning depends on the workload in the department but certainly should not occur less often than every other month.

Screen-film contact should be evaluated once or twice a year. This is done by radiographing a wire mesh pattern and analyzing the image for areas of blur (see Figures 20-14, 20-15). Should blur appear, the felt or foam pressure pad under the screen should be replaced. If this does not correct the problem, the cassette should be replaced.

Protective Apparel

All protective aprons, gloves, and gonadal shields should be radiographed or fluoroscoped annually for defects. If cracks, tears, or holes are evident, the apparel may require replacement (Figure 18-7).

Film Illuminators

Viewbox illumination should be analyzed photometrically on an annual basis. This is done with an instrument called a **photometer,** which measures light intensity at several areas of the illuminator (Figure 18-8). Intensity should be at least 1500 cd/m² and should not vary by more than ±10% over

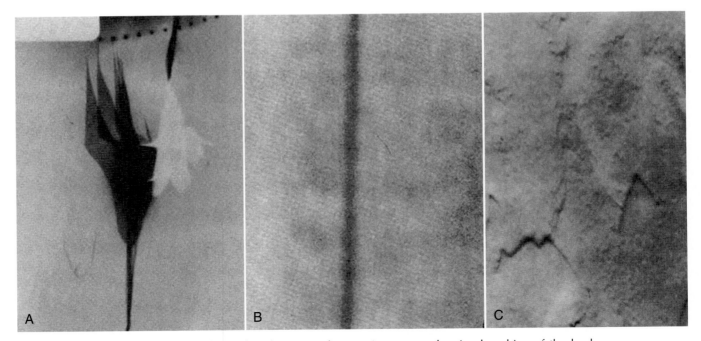

FIGURE 18-7 Radiographs of mistreated protective aprons showing bunching of the lead (**A**) from folding and tearing, a low-density area in a new apron (**B**), and cracking patterns in an apron (**C**). (Courtesy Sharon Glaze, Baylor College of Medicine.)

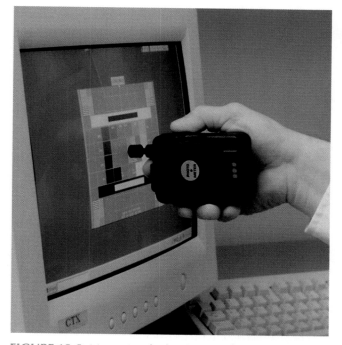

FIGURE 18-8 Measuring the luminance of a CRT screen with a photometer. (Courtesy Cardinal Health.)

TABLE 18-5	Extrance Skin Exposure With Cassette-Loaded Spot Film
kVp	**Entrance Skin Exposure (mR)**
60	450
70	270
80	170
90	150
100	130

the surface of the illuminator. If a bulb requires replacement, all bulbs in that illuminator should be replaced and matched to the type of bulb used in adjacent illuminators.

FLUOROSCOPY QUALITY CONTROL

Fluoroscopic examination can result in high patient dose. The entrance skin exposure (ESE) for an adult averages 3 to 5 R/min (30 to 50 mGy_a/min) during fluoroscopy; this can result in a skin dose of 10 rad (100 mGy_t) for many fluoroscopic examinations. For interventional procedures, a skin dose of 100 rad (1 Gy_t) is not uncommon but should be avoided if possible.

Approximate patient dose can be identified through the performance of proper QC measurements. Some measurements may be required more frequently, after significant changes have occurred in the operating console, high-voltage generator, or x-ray tube.

Exposure Rate

Federal law and most state statutes require that under normal operation, the ESE rate shall not exceed 10 R/min (100 mGy_a/min). For interventional procedures, the fluoroscope may be equipped with a high-level control, which allows an ESE up to 20 R/min (200 mGy_a/min). Unlimited exposure rates are permitted for recorded fluoroscopy, such as cineradiography.

Measurements are made with a calibrated radiation dosimeter to ensure that these levels are not exceeded. Lucite, aluminum, copper, and lead filters are used to determine the adequacy of any automatic brightness stabilization (ABS) system.

Spot-Film Exposures

Two types of spot-film devices are used; both must be evaluated for radiation exposure and proper collimation. Proper exposure of the **cassette spot film** depends on the kVp, mAs value, and sensitivity characteristics of the screen-film combination. ESEs for such a spot-film device vary widely (Table 18-5). Values reported in this table were obtained with a 10:1 grid and a 400 speed image receptor. Nongrid exposure values are approximately half of the values reported here.

> An ESE of approximately 200 mR may be assumed for a cassette spot film.

The use of photofluorospot images is routine. These images use less film, require less personnel interaction, and are produced with a lower patient dose. Photofluorospot images are recorded on film from the output phosphor of an image-intensifier tube.

In addition to the factors that affect cassette spot films, photofluorospot images depend on characteristics of the image intensifier, particularly the diameter of the input phosphor. Table 18-6 shows representative ESE for two input phosphor sizes and no grid. These are substantially lower than those attained with cassette spot films.

As the active area of the input phosphor of the image-intensifier tube is increased, patient dose is reduced in approximate proportion to the change in diameter of the input phosphor. Use of a grid during photofluorospot imaging approximately doubles the ESE.

> An ESE of approximately 100 mR may be assumed for a photofluorospot.

Question: A photofluorospot image is made at 80 kVp in the 15-cm mode without a grid, as is seen in Table 18-6. The measured ESE is 50 mR. What would be the expected ESE if the 25-cm mode were used?

Answer:
$$\frac{x}{50} = \frac{15}{25}$$

$$x = 50\left(\frac{15}{25}\right) = 30 \text{ mR}$$

Automatic Exposure Systems

All fluoroscopes are equipped with some sort of ABS or AEC. Each system functions in the manner of the phototimer of a radiographic imaging system, producing constant image brightness on the video or flat panel monitor, regardless of the thickness or composition of the anatomy. These systems tend to deteriorate or fail with use.

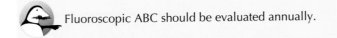

Fluoroscopic ABC should be evaluated annually.

Performance monitoring of an ABS is conducted by determining that the radiation exposure to the input phosphor of the image-intensifier tube is constant, regardless of patient thickness. With a test object in place, the image brightness on the video monitor should not change perceptibly when various thicknesses of patient-simulating material are inserted into the beam.

TABLE 18-6	Entrance Skin Exposure With Photofluorospot Imagers	
	ESE (mR)	
kVp	**15 cm II**	**25 cm II**
60	90	50
70	65	35
80	50	30
90	40	25
100	30	20

II, Image intensifier.

The input exposure rate to the image-intensifier tube is measured and should be in the range of 10 to 40 µR/s (0.1 to 0.4 µGy$_a$/s).

The test object used for ACR accreditation is shown in Figure 18-9. This test object tracks ABS versus tissue thickness and assesses spatial resolution, contrast resolution, and noise.

TOMOGRAPHY QUALITY CONTROL

In addition to the evaluations performed in the course of QC of a radiographic system, several measurements are required for those systems that can also perform conventional tomography. Precise performance standards do not exist for conventional tomography. QC measurements are designed to ensure that the characteristics evaluated remain constant.

Patient exposure should be measured for the most frequent type of tomographic examination. Table 18-7 is a sample of the results from a three-phase system and six representative tomographic examinations.

The geometric characteristics of a tomogram can be evaluated with any of a number of test objects designed for this use. Agreement between the indicated section level and the measured level should be within ±5 mm. With incrementing from one tomographic section to the next, the section level should be accurate to within ±2 mm. Constancy of ±1 mm from one QC evaluation to the next should be achieved.

Section uniformity is evaluated by imaging a hole in a lead sheet. The optical density of the image tracing of the hole should be uniform, with no perceptible variations, no gaps, and no overlaps (Figure 18-10).

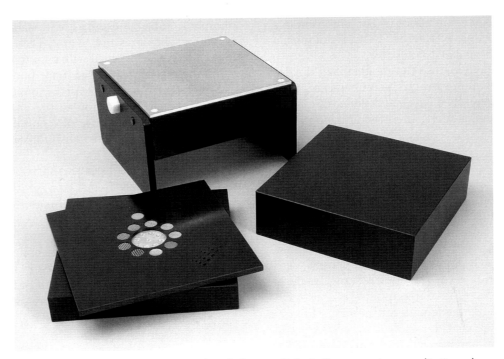

FIGURE 18-9 American College of Radiology radiologic/fluoroscopic accreditation phantom. (Courtesy American College of Radiology/CIRS.)

TABLE 18-7	Exposure Technique and Entrance Skin Exposure During Conventional Tomographic Examination	
Examination	Technique (kVp/mAs)	Entrance Skin Exposure (mR)
Temporomandibular joint	90/300	2300
Cervical spine	76/200	1300
Thoracic and lumbar spine	78/250	1700
Chest	110/8	70
Intravenous pyelogram	70/300	1800
Nephrotomogram	74/350	2200

PROCESSOR QUALITY CONTROL

QC in any activity refers to the routine and special procedures developed to ensure that the final product is of consistently high quality. QC in diagnostic radiology requires a planned continuous program of evaluation and surveillance of radiologic equipment and procedures.

When applied to automatic processing, such a program involves periodic cleaning, system maintenance, and daily monitoring. Table 18-8 lists an appropriate processor QC program.

Processor Cleaning

The first automatic processor had a dry-to-drop time of 7 minutes. Soon this was shortened to 3 minutes by what are known as *double-capacity processors*. Processing time was reduced further with the fast-access system, which is today's popular 90-second processor (Figure 18-11). Such a processor can handle up to 500 films per hour, but to do so, it requires a high concentration of processing chemistry, a high development temperature (95°F [35°C]), and a developer immersion time of 22 seconds.

The wash water temperature should be 87°F (31°C). Earlier automatic processors were supplied with hot and cold water, so the wash temperature was controlled primarily through a mixing valve. Current processors are supplied with only cold water, and temperature is maintained with a thermostatically controlled heater.

This rapid activity, carried on at high temperature with concentrated chemistry, tends to wear and corrode the mechanism of the transport system and contaminate the chemistry with processing sludge. This may lead to a deposit of sludge and debris on the rollers, which can severely affect film quality and cause artifacts if the processor is not properly cleaned at appropriate intervals.

In most facilities, cleaning is conducted weekly; records of such cleaning should be maintained. The cleaning procedure is rather simple. One removes the transport and crossover racks and cleans them and the processing tanks with appropriate fluids (Figure 18-12).

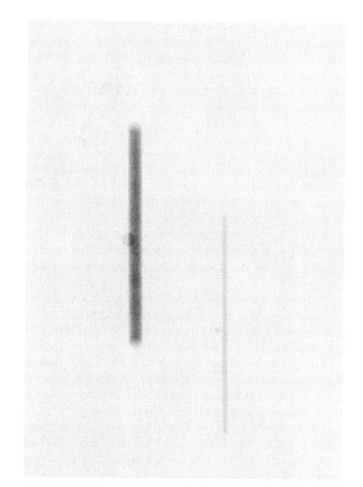

FIGURE 18-10 Images of a pinhole in a lead attenuator during linear tomography. The larger pinhole image shows modest staggering motion, resulting in varied optical density. (Courtesy Sharon Glaze, Baylor College of Medicine.)

TABLE 18-8	Quality Control Program for Radiographic Processor	
Activity	Procedure or Item	Schedule
Processor cleaning	Crossover racks	Daily
	Entire rack assembly and processing ranks	Weekly
Scheduled maintenance	Observation of belts, pulleys, and gears	Weekly
	Lubrication	Weekly or monthly
Processor monitoring	Planned parts replacement	Regularly
	Check developer temperature	Daily
	Check wash water temperature	Daily
	Check replenishment rates	Daily
	Sensitometry and densitometry	Daily

This takes no longer than a few minutes and pays great dividends in terms of reduced processor wear and consistent production of high-quality radiographs that are artifact free. When all has been reassembled, sensitometric levels must be reestablished.

Processor Maintenance

As with any electromechanical device, maintenance of the processor is essential. If equipment is not properly maintained, the processor may fail when least expected,

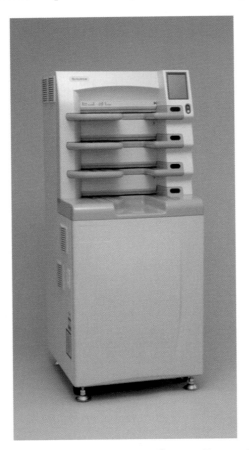

FIGURE 18-11 Automatic processor. (Courtesy Eastman Kodak.)

or when the workload is heaviest. Three types of maintenance programs should be included in the QC program for an automatic processor.

1. **Scheduled maintenance** refers to routine procedures that are performed usually weekly or monthly. Such maintenance includes observation of all moving parts for wear; adjustment of all belts, pulleys, and gears; and application of proper lubrication, to minimize wear. During processor lubrication, it is especially important to keep the lubricant off of your hands, thereby keeping it away from film and rollers and, of course, out of processor chemistry.

2. **Preventive maintenance** is a planned program of parts replacement at regular intervals. Preventive maintenance requires that a part be replaced before it fails. Such a program should avoid unexpected downtime.

3. **Nonscheduled maintenance** is, of course, the worst kind. A failure in the system that necessitates processor repair is a nonscheduled event. A proper program of scheduled maintenance and preventive maintenance keeps nonscheduled maintenance to a minimum.

Processor Monitoring

At least once per day, processor operation should be observed, and certain measurements recorded. The temperature of the developer and wash water should be noted. Developer and fixer replenishment rates should be observed and recorded.

Replenishment tanks should be checked to determine whether the floating lids are properly positioned, and whether fresh chemistry is needed. It is often appropriate to check the pH and specific gravity of developer and fixer solutions. Residual hypo should be determined.

A sensitometric strip should be passed through the processor, and fog, speed, and contrast then should be measured and recorded appropriately. Most film suppliers provide forms and assistance to establish and

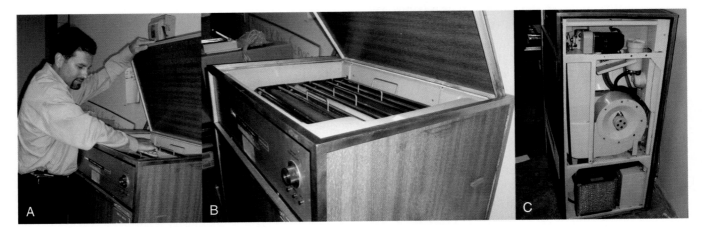

FIGURE 18-12 An automatic processor disassembled for cleaning. (Courtesy Joe Scalise, Merry X-ray Co.)

conduct a program of processor monitoring. A written record of the results of such a program is important.

The processor monitoring approach described in Chapter 20 for the dedicated mammography processor can be applied to all other processors in the health care facility.

SUMMARY

In diagnostic imaging, quality assurance (QA) involves the assessment and evaluation of patient care. Quality control (QC) is the measurement and performance evaluation of imaging equipment. Both processes ensure that the radiologist is provided with an optimal image for proper diagnosis.

The QA/QC team includes radiographers, management and secretarial personnel, the equipment manufacturer's representative, the medical physicist, radiologic engineers, and radiologists. TJC does not accredit health care facilities unless proper QA and QC programs are evident.

The three steps of QC include (1) acceptance testing, (2) routine performance evaluation, and (3) error correction. Radiographic QC evaluates filtration, collimation, focal-spot size, kVp, timers, linearity, and reproducibility.

Intensifying screens are evaluated regularly for cleanliness and screen-film contact. All lead apparel is checked for cracks, tears, and holes. Finally, viewboxes or film illuminators are examined for intensity and cleanliness.

Fluoroscopic quality control is focused on patient radiation exposure and image quality analysis.

Conventional tomography section sensitivity is evaluated regularly.

Radiographic processor QC is essential for optimal image quality. Sensitometry and densitometry are important daily functions of the QC radiographer.

CHALLENGE QUESTIONS

1. Define or otherwise identify the following:
   a. Quality assurance
   b. Required x-ray beam filtration
   c. Tomography QC
   d. Outcome analysis
   e. Minimum half-value layer
   f. CRCPD
   g. TJC 10-step program
   h. CQI
   i. Exposure linearity
   j. Quality control
2. List and explain the theory behind the TJC QA program used in hospitals.
3. Discuss the three steps of quality control for radiographic equipment.
4. Name the people on the diagnostic imaging QC team.
5. How is filtration measured in radiographic equipment?
6. Why are proper x-ray beam alignment and collimation important?
7. What are the limits for radiographic misalignment?
8. What three QC tools are used to measure focal-spot size?
9. What is the permitted variation of radiographic reproducibility?
10. What test is performed on intensifying screens and cassettes to check whether there is proper screen-film contact?
11. What products are used to clean intensifying screens?
12. How often should lead apparel be checked for protective integrity?
13. How do we ensure kVp accuracy?
14. What is the unit of luminance of a viewbox?
15. How often should an automatic processor be cleaned?
16. What is the importance of preventive maintenance for a radiographic processor?
17. A high-frequency radiographic imaging system requires how much x-ray beam filtration?
18. What is the permitted radiographic collimator misalignment?
19. When should defective protective apparel be discarded?
20. What tools are used for processor monitoring?

The answers to the Challenge Questions can be found by logging on to our website at http://evolve.elsevier.com.

PART IV

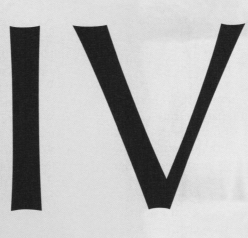

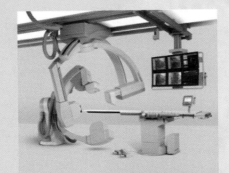

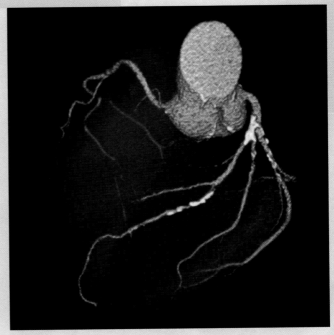

ADVANCED X-RAY IMAGING

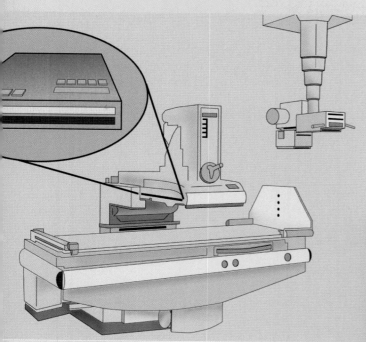

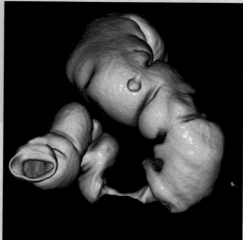

CHAPTER 10

Mammography

OBJECTIVES

At the completion of this chapter, the student should be able
to do the following:

1. Discuss the differences between soft tissue radiography and
   conventional radiography
2. Describe the anatomy of the breast
3. Identify the recommended intervals for breast self-examination and
   mammography
4. Describe the unique features of a mammographic imaging system
5. Discuss the requirement for compression in mammography
6. Describe the image receptors used and spatial resolution obtained
   in mammography
7. Explain the differences between diagnostic and screening
   mammography

OUTLINE

Soft Tissue Radiography
Basis for Mammography
   Risk of Breast Cancer
   Types of Mammography
   Breast Anatomy
The Mammographic Imaging System
   High-Voltage Generation
   Target Composition
   Focal Spot
   Filtration
   Heel Effect
   Compression
   Grids
   Automatic Exposure Control
   Magnification Mammography
Screen-Film Mammography

BREAST CANCER is the second leading cause of death from cancer in women (lung cancer is first). Each year, approximately 210,000 new cases of breast cancer are reported in the United States. One of every eight women will develop breast cancer during her life.

Early detection of breast cancer leads to more effective treatment and fewer deaths. X-ray mammography has proved to be an accurate and simple method of detecting breast cancer, but it is not simple to perform. The radiographer and support staff must have exceptional knowledge, skill, and caring.

In 1992, the U.S. government mandated regulations in the Mammography Quality Standards Act (MQSA), which set standards for image quality, radiation dose, personnel qualifications, and examination procedures.

SOFT TISSUE RADIOGRAPHY

Radiographic examination of soft tissues requires selected techniques that differ from those used in conventional radiography. These differences in technique are due to substantial differences in the anatomy that is being imaged. In conventional radiography, the subject contrast is great because of large differences in mass density and atomic number among bone, muscle, fat, and lung tissue.

In soft tissue radiography, only muscle and fat structures are imaged. These tissues have similar effective atomic numbers (see Table 10-1) and similar mass densities (see Table 10-2). Consequently, soft tissue radiographic techniques are designed to enhance differential absorption in these very similar tissues.

A prime example of soft tissue radiography is **mammography**—radiographic examination of the breast. As a distinct type of radiographic examination, mammography was first attempted in the 1920s. In the late 1950s, Robert Egan renewed interest in mammography with his demonstration of a successful technique that used low kVp, high mAs, and direct film exposure.

In the 1960s, Wolf and Ruzicka showed that **xeromammography** was superior to direct film exposure at a much lower patient dose. Detail and contrast were much improved because of characteristic **edge enhancement**—the accentuation of the interface between different tissues. This property is used frequently in the postprocessing of digital images. Xeromammography was retired by 1990 because single screen-film mammography provided better images at even lower patient radiation dose.

Mammography has undergone much change and development. It now enjoys widespread application thanks to the efforts of the American College of Radiology (ACR) volunteer accreditation program and the federally mandated Mammography Quality Standards Act (MQSA).

BASIS FOR MAMMOGRAPHY

The principal motivation for the continuing development and improvement of mammography is the high incidence of breast cancer. Breast cancer is the leading cancer among women. Unfortunately, lung cancer has passed breast cancer as the leading cause of cancer death in women because of the increasing use of tobacco.

Risk of Breast Cancer

Each year, approximately 210,000 new cases of breast cancer are reported in the United States, and this number is growing. Approximately 20% of these patients will die from this disease, but thanks to early detection, this percentage is shrinking. Several factors have been identified that increase a woman's risk of breast cancer (Box 19-1).

 One of every eight women will develop breast cancer.

Breast cancer is now a disease that is far from fatal. In 1995, the National Cancer Institute reported the first reduction in breast cancer mortality in 50 years, and this trend continues. With early mammographic diagnosis, more than 80% of patients are cured.

One important consideration in the overall efficacy of mammography is patient dose, because radiation can cause breast cancer as well as detect it. However, considerable evidence shows that the mature breast in the screening age group has very low sensitivity to radiation-induced breast cancer. Radiation carcinogenesis (the induction of cancer) is discussed in Chapter 36.

BOX 19-1   Risk Factors for Breast Cancer

- **Age:** The older you are, the higher the risk.
- **Family history:** Mother, sister with breast cancer
- **Genetics:** Presence of *BRCA1* or *BRCA2* gene
- **Breast architecture:** Dense breast tissue
- **Menstruation:** Onset before age 12
- **Menopause:** Onset after age 55
- Prolonged use of **estrogen**
- **Late age at birth of first child**, or **no children**
- **Education:** Risk increases with higher level of education.
- **Socioeconomics:** Risk increases with higher socioeconomic status.

TABLE 19-1	Recommended Intervals for Breast Examination		
	PATIENT AGE		
Examination	**<40 Years**	**40-49 Years**	**≥50 Years**
Self-examination	Monthly*	Monthly	Monthly
Physician physical examination	Annually†	Annually	Annually
X-ray mammography			
High risk	Baseline	Annually	Annually
Low risk	Baseline	Biannually	Annually

*Beginning at age 20.
†Beginning at age 35.

The dose necessary to produce breast cancer is unknown; however, the dose experienced in mammography is well known and is covered in Chapter 39. This chapter concerns the imaging technique, equipment, and procedures used in mammography.

Types of Mammography

Two different types of mammographic examination are available. **Diagnostic mammography** is performed on patients with symptoms or elevated risk factors. Two or three views of each breast may be required. **Screening mammography** is performed on asymptomatic women with the use of a two-view protocol, usually medial lateral oblique and cranial caudad, to detect an unsuspected cancer.

Screening mammography in patients 50 years or older reduces cancer mortality. Results of clinical trials show that screening of women in the 40- to 49-year age group is also beneficial in reducing mortality. Because younger women have potentially more years of life left, screening in this group results in more years of life saved.

The American Cancer Society recommends that women perform monthly breast self-examination; a health care professional teaches a woman to check her breasts regularly for lumps, thickening of the skin, or any changes in size or shape. Table 19-1 relates the recommended intervals for breast self-examination and screening mammography.

The American Cancer Society also recommends annual breast examination by a physician and a baseline mammogram. A **baseline mammogram** is the first radiographic examination of the breasts and is usually obtained before age 40. Radiologists use it for comparison with all future mammograms.

The risk of radiation-induced breast cancer resulting from x-ray mammography has been given a lot of attention. Mammography is considered very safe and effective. The ratio of benefit (lives saved) to risk (deaths caused) is estimated at 1000:1.

Breast Anatomy

The anatomy of the breast and its tissue characteristics make imaging difficult (Figure 19-1). The young breast is dense and is more difficult to image because

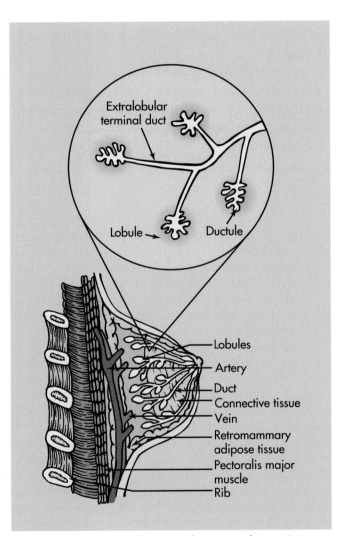

FIGURE 19-1 Breast architecture determines the requirements for x-ray imaging systems and image receptors.

of glandular tissue. The older breast is more fatty and is easier to image.

The normal breast consists of three principal tissues: fibrous, glandular, and adipose (fat). In a premenopausal woman, the fibrous and glandular tissues are structured into various ducts, glands, and connective tissues. These are surrounded by a thin layer of fat. The radiographic appearance of glandular and connective tissue is one of high optical density.

Postmenopausal breasts are characterized by a degeneration of this fibroglandular tissue and an increase in adipose tissue. Adipose tissue appears with less optical density and requires less exposure.

 The tissue most sensitive to cancer by radiation is *glandular tissue.*

If a malignancy is present, it appears as a distortion of normal ductal and connective tissue patterns. Approximately 80% of breast cancer is ductal and may have associated deposits of **microcalcifications** that appear as small grains of varying size. In terms of detecting breast cancer, microcalcifications smaller than approximately 500 μm are of interest. The incidence of breast cancer is highest in the upper lateral quadrant of the breast (Figure 19-2).

Because the mass density and atomic number of soft tissue components of the breast are so similar, conventional radiographic technique is useless. In the 70- to 100-kVp range, Compton scattering predominates with soft tissue; thus, differential absorption within soft tissues is minimal. Low kVp must be used to maximize the photoelectric effect and thereby enhance differential absorption.

Recall from Chapter 10 that x-ray absorption in tissue occurs principally by photoelectric effect and Compton effect. The degree of absorption is determined by the tissue mass density and the effective atomic number.

Absorption caused by differences in mass density is simply proportional to the mass density for photoelectric and Compton effects. Absorption caused by differences in atomic number, however, is directly proportional for Compton interactions and proportional to the cube of the atomic number for photoelectric interactions.

 At low x-ray energy, photoelectric absorption predominates over Compton scattering.

Therefore x-ray mammography requires a low-kVp technique. As kVp is reduced, however, the penetrability of the x-ray beam is reduced, which in turn requires an increase in mAs.

If the kVp is too low, an inordinately high mAs value may be required, which could be unacceptable because of the increased patient dose. Technique factors of approximately 23 to 28 kVp are used as an effective compromise between the increasing dose at low kVp and reduced image quality at high kVp.

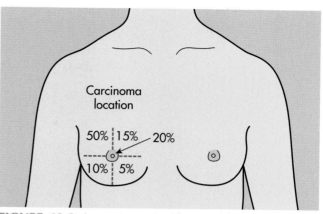

FIGURE 19-2 Approximate incidence of breast cancer by location within the breast.

THE MAMMOGRAPHIC IMAGING SYSTEM

X-ray mammography became clinically acceptable with the introduction of molybdenum as target and filter (1966) and the dedicated, single-emulsion, screen-film image receptor (1972). By 1990, grid technique, emphasis on compression, high-frequency generators, and automatic exposure control (AEC) raised mammography to the level of excellence in breast imaging.

Conventional x-ray imaging systems are unacceptable for mammography, which requires specially designed, dedicated systems. Nearly all x-ray manufacturers now produce such systems. Figure 19-3 shows two such models.

Dedicated mammographic imaging systems are designed for flexibility in patient positioning and have an integral compression device, a low ratio grid, AEC, and a microfocus x-ray tube. Desirable features of a dedicated mammography imaging system are given in Table 19-2.

High-Voltage Generation

All mammography imaging systems incorporate high-frequency generators (see Chapter 6). Such a generator accepts a single-phase input, which is rectified and capacitor-smoothed to produce a direct current (DC) voltage waveform.

This DC power is fed to an inverter circuit, which changes the power to a high frequency (typically 5 to 10 kHz) that is then capacitor-smoothed. The resulting voltage ripple in the x-ray tube is approximately 1%—essentially constant potential.

Compared with earlier single- and three-phase mammography generators, high-frequency generators are smaller and less expensive to manufacture. They provide exceptional exposure reproducibility, which contributes to improved image quality.

A maximum limit of 600 mAs is standard for preventing excessive patient radiation dose.

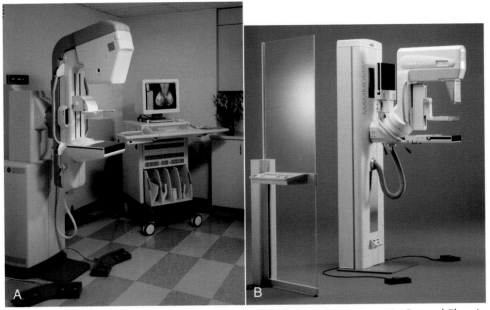

FIGURE 19-3 Representative dedicated mammography imaging systems. **A**, General Electric Senograph. **B**, Siemens Mammomat. (**A**, courtesy General Electric Medical Systems; **B**, courtesy Siemens Medical Systems.)

TABLE 19-2	**Features of a Dedicated Mammography System for Use With Screen-Film**
High-voltage	High frequency, 5-10 kHz generator
Target/filter	W/60 μm Mo
	Mo/30 μm Mo
	Mo/50 μm Rh
	Rh/50 μm Rh
KVp	20-35 kVp in 1-kVp increments
Compression	Low Z, auto adjust, and release
Grids	Ratio of 3:1 to 5:1, 30 lines/cm
Exposure control	Automatic to account for tissue thickness, composition, and reciprocity law failure
Focal spot	0.3 mm/0.1 mm (large/small)
Magnification	Up to 2
SID	50-80 cm

SID, Source-to-image receptor distance.

Target Composition

Mammographic x-ray tubes are manufactured with a tungsten (W), molybdenum (Mo), or rhodium (Rh) target. Figure 19-4 shows the x-ray emission spectrum from a tungsten target tube filtered with 0.5 mm Al operating at 30 kVp. Note that the bremsstrahlung spectrum

predominates, and that only the 12-keV characteristic x-rays from L-shell transitions are present. These L-shell x-rays all are absorbed and contribute only to patient dose—not to the image.

 Tungsten L-shell x-rays are of no value in mammography because their 12-keV energy is too low to penetrate the breast.

The x-rays most useful for enhancing differential absorption in breast tissue and for maximizing radiographic contrast are those in the range of 17 to 24 keV. The tungsten target supplies sufficient x-rays in this energy range but also an abundance of x-rays above and below this range.

Figure 19-5 shows the 26-kVp emission spectrum from a molybdenum target tube filtered with 30 μm of molybdenum; note the near absence of bremsstrahlung x-rays. The most prominent x-rays are characteristic, with energy of 17 and 19 keV resulting from K-shell interactions. Molybdenum has an atomic number of 42 compared with 74 for tungsten, and this difference is responsible for the differences in emission spectra.

The 28-kVp x-ray emission spectrum from a rhodium target filtered with rhodium appears similar to that from a molybdenum target (Figure 19-6). However, rhodium has a slightly higher atomic number (Z = 45) and therefore a slightly higher K-edge (23 keV) and more numerous bremsstrahlung x-rays.

Bremsstrahlung x-rays are produced more easily in target atoms with high Z than in target atoms with low Z.

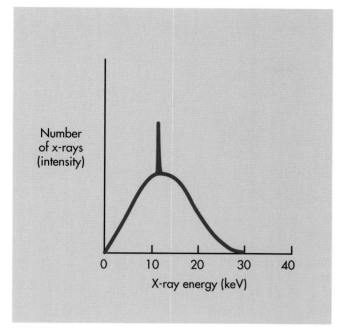

FIGURE 19-4 X-ray emission spectrum for a tungsten target x-ray tube with a 0.5-mm Al filter operated at 30 kVp.

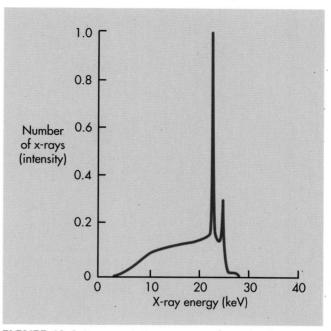

FIGURE 19-6 X-ray emission spectrum for a rhodium target x-ray tube with a 50-μm Rh filter operated at 28 kVp.

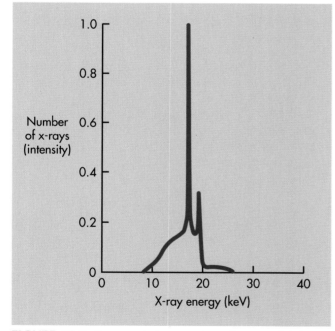

FIGURE 19-5 X-ray emission spectrum for a molybdenum target x-ray tube with a 30-μm Mo filter operated at 26 kVp.

TABLE 19-3	Mammographic Technique Chart	
Compressed Breast Thickness	**Target/Filter**	**kVp**
0-2 cm	Mo/Mo	24
3-4 cm	Mo/Mo	25, 26
5-6 cm	Mo/Rh	28
7-8 cm	Mo/Rh	32
7-8 cm	Rh/Rh*	30*

*To be used with systems that have Rh targets.

Molybdenum and rhodium K-characteristic x-rays have energy corresponding to their respective K-shell electron binding energy. This is within the range of energy that is most effective for breast imaging.

All currently manufactured breast imaging systems have target/filter combinations of Mo/Mo. Many are also equipped with Mo/Rh and Rh/Rh. Table 19-3 is an example of an appropriate mammographic technique chart.

Focal Spot

Focal-spot size is an important characteristic of mammography x-rays tubes because of the higher demands for spatial resolution. Imaging of microcalcifications requires small focal spots. Mammography x-ray tubes usually have stated focal-spot sizes—large/small of 0.3/0.1 mm.

In general, the smaller the better; however, the shape of the focal spot is also important (Figure 19-7). A circular focal spot is preferred, but rectangular shapes are common. Manufacturers shape the focal spot through clever cathode design and focusing cup voltage bias. The allowed variance is considerable for the stated nominal focal-spot size; therefore, medical physics acceptance testing of focal-spot size or spatial resolution is essential.

To obtain such small focal-spot size and adequate x-ray intensity over the entire breast, manufacturers take advantage of the line-focus principle and tilt the x-ray tube (Figure 19-8). Effective focal spots—0.3/0.1 mm—are obtained with an approximate 23-degree

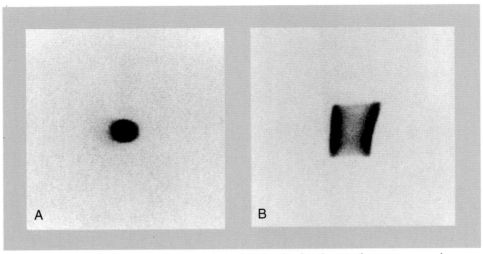

FIGURE 19-7 Pinhole camera images of **(A)** the circular focal spot of a mammography x-ray tube, and **(B)** a double banana–shaped focal spot from a general purpose x-ray tube. (Courtesy Donald Jacobson, Medical College of Wisconsin.)

anode angle and a 6-degree x-ray tube tilt. Normally, the cathode is positioned to the chest wall. This allows for easier patient positioning, as well as application of anode heel effect.

Tilting the x-ray tube to achieve an even smaller effective focal spot ensures imaging of the tissue next to the chest wall (see Figure 19-8). When the tube is tilted, the central ray parallels the chest wall, and no tissue is missed.

Filtration

At the low kVp used for mammography, it is important that the x-ray tube window not attenuate the x-ray beam significantly. Therefore, dedicated mammography x-ray tubes have either a beryllium (Z = 4) window or a very thin borosilicate glass window. Most mammography x-ray tubes have inherent filtration in the window of approximately 0.1 mm Al equivalent. Beyond the window, the proper type and thickness of x-ray beam filtration must be installed.

 Under no circumstances is total beam filtration less than 0.5 mm Al equivalent.

If a tungsten target x-ray tube is used, it should have a molybdenum or rhodium filter. The purpose of each filter is to reduce the higher-energy bremsstrahlung x-rays. Some research has suggested that 50 μm rhodium (Z = 45) is a better filter for imaging thicker and denser breasts when the x-ray tube target is tungsten. Figure 19-9 shows the emission spectrum from a tungsten target tube designed for screen-film mammography filtered by molybdenum or rhodium. The radiologic technologist selects the proper filter after determining the patient's breast characteristics.

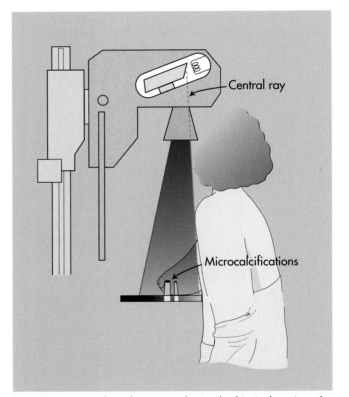

FIGURE 19-8 When the x-ray tube is tilted in its housing, the effective focal spot is small, the x-ray intensity is more uniform, and tissue against the chest is imaged.

No element can absorb its own characteristic radiation.

The use of a filter of the same element as the x-ray tube target is designed to allow the K-characteristic x-rays to expose the breast while suppressing the higher- and lower-energy bremsstrahlung x-rays. Figure 19-10

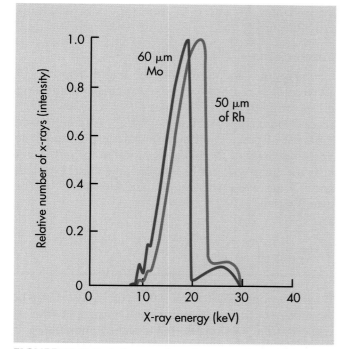

FIGURE 19-9 Emission spectrum from a tungsten target x-ray tube filtered by molybdenum and rhodium.

shows this process of selective filtration designed to shape the x-ray beam with Mo/Mo.

The unfiltered Mo beam (Figure 19-10, *A*) has a prominent characteristic x-ray emission and substantial bremsstrahlung x-ray emission. The Mo filter has its K-absorption edge at the energy of the K-characteristic x-ray emission (Figure 19-10, *B*). The combination Mo/Mo target/filter results in an emission spectrum with suppressed bremsstrahlung and prominent characteristic x-ray emission (Figure 19-10, *C*).

If an Mo target x-ray tube is used, then Mo filtration of 30 µm or Rh filtration of 50 µm is recommended. These combinations provide the Mo characteristic x-rays for imaging, along with the suppressed bremsstrahlung x-ray emission spectrum.

If an Rh target x-ray tube is used, it should be filtered with 25 µm Rh. This combination provides a slightly higher-quality x-ray beam of greater penetrability. The use of Rh as a target or filter is designed for thicker, more dense breasts. Regardless of x-ray tube target or filtration, the half-value layer is always very low.

Many x-ray tubes designed specifically for mammography have a stationary anode. Newer bi-angle and double-track anodes (one track is Mo and the other Rh) are rotating anode tubes.

Heel Effect

The heel effect is important to mammography. The conic shape of breasts should require that the radiation intensity near the chest wall must be higher than that to the nipple side to ensure near-uniform exposure of the

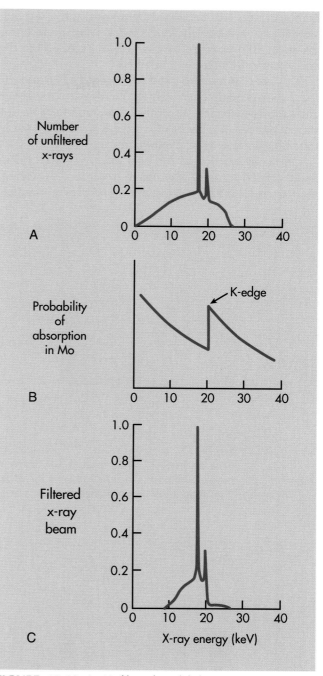

FIGURE 19-10 **A,** Unfiltered molybdenum x-ray emission spectrum. **B,** The probability of x-ray absorption in molybdenum. **C,** Bremsstrahlung x-rays are suppressed and characteristic x-ray emission becomes prominent when a molybdenum target is filtered with molybdenum.

image receptor. This is accomplished by positioning the cathode to the chest wall (Figure 19-11). However, this is not absolutely necessary because **compression** ensures imaging of a uniform thickness of tissue.

When the cathode is positioned to the chest wall, the spatial resolution of tissue near the chest wall is reduced because of the increased focal-spot blur created by the larger effective focal-spot size. However, most manufacturers of dedicated mammography imaging systems use a relatively long source-to-image receptor distance (SID) of 60 to 80 cm, with the cathode to the chest wall and the x-ray tube tilted.

This is considered the best arrangement because the focal spot is made effectively smaller, and tissue at the chest wall is imaged. It is also more comfortable for the patient because the head is always close to the x-ray tube housing during an examination.

One consequence of the heel effect is variation in focal-spot size over the image receptor. However, the use of long SID and vigorous compression makes this change in effective focal-spot size clinically insignificant.

Compression

Compression is important in many aspects of conventional radiology but is particularly important in mammography. Vigorous compression offers several advantages (Figure 19-12). A compressed breast is of greater uniform thickness; therefore, the optical density of the image is more uniform. Tissues near the chest wall are less likely to be underexposed, and tissues near the nipple are less likely to be overexposed.

> Vigorous compression must be used in x-ray mammography.

When vigorous compression is used, all tissue is brought closer to the image receptor, and focal-spot blur is reduced. Compression also reduces absorption blur and scatter radiation. All dedicated mammographic x-ray imaging systems have a built-in stiff compression device that is parallel to the surface of the image receptor. Vigorous compression of the breast is necessary to attain the best image quality.

Image quality is improved with vigorous compression, as is summarized in Table 19-4. Compression immobilizes the breast and therefore reduces motion blur. Compression spreads out the tissue and thus reduces superimposition of tissue structures.

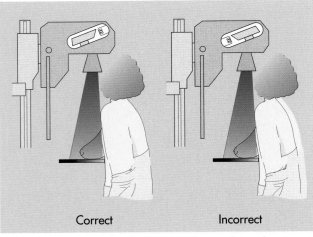

Correct   Incorrect

FIGURE 19-11 The heel effect can be used to advantage in mammography by positioning the cathode toward the chest wall to produce a more uniform optical density.

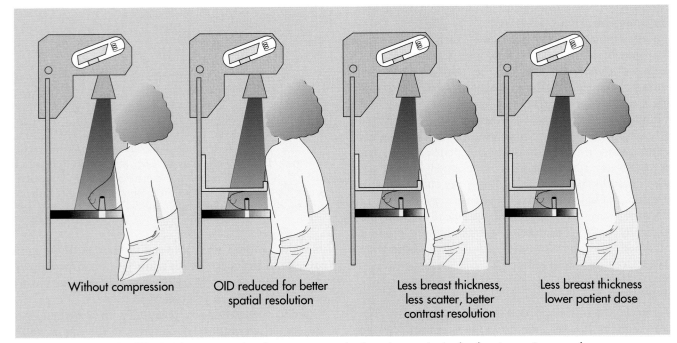

Without compression   OID reduced for better spatial resolution   Less breast thickness, less scatter, better contrast resolution   Less breast thickness lower patient dose

FIGURE 19-12 Compression in mammography has three principal advantages: improved spatial resolution, improved contrast resolution, and lower patient dose.

Table 19-4	Advantages of Vigorous Compression	
Effect	**Result**	
Immobilization of breast	Reduced motion blur	
Uniform thickness	Equal optical density on mammogram	
Reduced scatter	Improved contrast resolution radiation	
Shorter OID	Improved spatial resolution	
Thinner tissue	Reduced radiation dose	

OID, Object-to-image receptor distance.

Compression results in thinner tissue and therefore less scatter radiation and improved contrast resolution. The overall result of this improved image quality is improved ability to detect small, low-contrast lesions and high-contrast microcalcifications because of **improved spatial resolution**. Additionally, vigorous compression results in **lower patient dose.**

> Compression improves spatial resolution and contrast resolution, and reduces patient dose.

Although it may be difficult for patients to understand, compression of the breast is essential for a quality mammogram. The optimum degree of compression is unknown; however, the more vigorous the compression, the better the image and the lower the dose, but the higher the level of patient discomfort. Skilled mammographers attempt to compress the breast until it is "taut" or "just less than painful."

Grids

Grids are used routinely in mammography. Although mammographic image contrast is high because of the low kVp used, it can be improved. Most systems now have a moving grid with a ratio of 4:1 to 5:1 focused to the SID to increase image contrast. Grid frequencies of 40 lines/cm for the moving grid are typical.

Use of such grids does not compromise spatial resolution, but it does increase patient dose. The use of a 4:1 ratio grid approximately doubles the patient dose compared with nongrid contact mammography. However, the dose is acceptably low, and the improvement in contrast is significant.

A unique grid that has been developed specifically for mammography is the high-transmission cellular (HTC) grid (Figure 19-13). This grid has the clean-up characteristics of a crossed grid in that it reduces scatter radiation in two directions rather than the single direction of a parallel grid. The HTC grid has copper as grid strip material and air for the interspace, and its physical dimensions result in a 3.8:1 grid ratio.

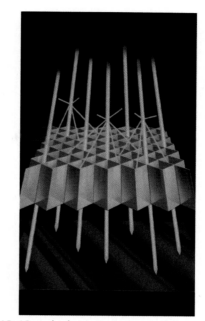

FIGURE 19-13 A high-transmission cellular grid designed specifically for mammography. (Courtesy Hologic Imaging.)

Automatic Exposure Control

Phototimers for mammography are designed to measure not only x-ray intensity at the image receptor but also x-ray quality. These phototimers are called *automatic exposure control (AEC) devices,* and they are positioned after the image receptor to minimize the object-to-image receptor distance (OID) and improve spatial resolution (Figure 19-14). Two types are used: ionization chamber and solid-state diode. Each type can have a single detector or multiple detectors, which are positioned along the chest wall/nipple axis. Some AEC devices incorporate many detectors to cover the entire breast.

The detectors are filtered differently, so the AEC can estimate the beam quality after passing through the breast. This allows assessment of breast composition and selection of proper target/filter combination. Thick, dense breasts are imaged better with Rh/Rh; thin, fatty breasts are imaged better with Mo/Mo. Such an AEC is a compensated AEC.

The AEC must be accurate to ensure reproducible images at low radiation dose. The AEC should be able to hold optical density (OD) within 0.1 OD as voltage is varied from 23 kVp to 32 kVp and for breast thickness of 2 to 8 cm, regardless of breast composition.

Magnification Mammography

Magnification techniques are used frequently in mammography, producing images up to twice the normal size. Magnification mammography requires special equipment such as microfocus tubes, adequate compression, and patient positioning devices. Effective focal-spot size should not exceed 0.1 mm.

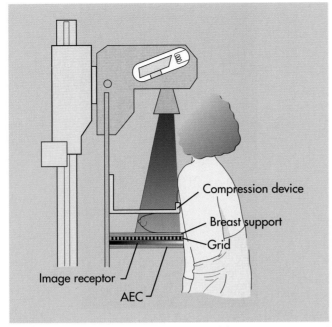

FIGURE 19-14 The relative position of the automatic exposure control (AEC) device.

Magnification mammography should not be used routinely.

Standard mammograms are adequate for most patients, so magnification mammography is usually unnecessary. The purpose of magnification mammography is to investigate small, suspicious lesions or microcalcifications seen on standard mammograms. The breast may not be completely imaged, and patient dose is approximately doubled.

SCREEN-FILM MAMMOGRAPHY

Four types of image receptors have been used for x-ray mammography: direct-exposure film, xeroradiography, screen-film, and digital detectors. Only screen-film and digital detectors are used today.

Radiographic intensifying screens and films have been designed specially for x-ray mammography. The films are single-emulsion and are matched with a single back screen. This arrangement avoids light crossover. Tabular grain emulsion has been replaced by cubic grain emulsion in most films (Figure 19-15). The result is somewhat higher contrast, especially in the toe region, which is particularly useful in mammography.

Regardless of the type of film, it must be matched for the light emission of the associated intensifying screen. Special emulsions coupled with rare Earth screen material are available.

The screen-film combination is placed in a specially designed cassette that has a low-Z front cover for low

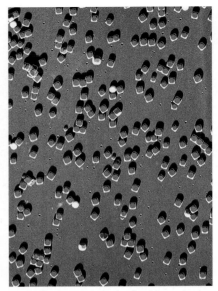

FIGURE 19-15 Photomicrograph of cubic grains in mammography film emulsions; the grains are 0.5 to 0.9 μm to produce higher contrast. (Courtesy, Michael Wilsey, Fujifilm Medical Systems.)

attenuation. It also has a low-absorbing back cover when used with an AEC. The latching/spring mechanism is designed to produce especially good screen-film contact.

The use of the radiographic intensifying screen significantly increases the speed of the imaging system, resulting in a low patient dose. The use of screens also enhances the radiographic contrast compared with that resulting from direct-exposure examination.

The emulsion surface of the film must always be next to the screen, and the film must be on the x-ray tube side of the radiographic intensifying screen.

The position of the radiographic intensifying screen and film in the cassette is important (Figure 19-16). X-rays interact primarily with the entrance surface of the screen. If the screen is between the x-ray tube and the film, screen blur is excessive. If, on the other hand, the film is between the x-ray tube and the screen, with the emulsion side to the screen, spatial resolution is better.

Processing and viewing of the mammogram are critical stages of mammography. These steps are discussed in Chapter 20, but when they are properly conducted, image receptor speeds can reach approximately 200. This results in an average glandular dose of approximately 200 mrad (2 mGy$_t$). Image receptor contrast—the average gradient—is approximately 3.5. A two-view mammogram with grid should not exceed 600 mrad (6 mGy$_t$) for a 4.5-cm-thick 50% adipose/50% glandular breast.

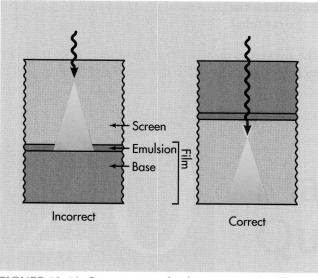

FIGURE 19-16 Correct way to load mammography film and position the cassette. Spatial resolution improves when the x-ray film is placed closest to the breast and between the x-ray tube and the radiographic intensifying screen.

SUMMARY

Breast cancer is the leading cause of death among women between 40 and 50 years of age. This is the principal reason why mammographic equipment and techniques have improved over the years, and why the Mammography Quality Standards Act was instituted.

Anatomically, the breast consists of three different tissues: fibrous tissue, glandular tissue, and adipose tissue. Premenopausal women have breasts that are composed mainly of fibrous and glandular tissue surrounded by a thin layer of fat. These breasts are dense and difficult to image. In postmenopausal women, the glandular tissue turns to fat. Because of its predominantly fatty content, the older breast is easier to image.

The mammographer must know the recommended intervals of breast self-examination, physician examination of the breasts, and mammographic examination for women of various age groups, in order to advise such patients. Diagnostic x-ray mammography often is performed every 6 months on women who have an elevated risk of breast cancer, or who have a known lesion.

Compression is an important factor in the production of high-quality mammograms.

Radiographic imaging systems are designed specially for mammographic examination. Mammographic x-ray tube targets consist of tungsten, molybdenum, or rhodium. A low kVp is used to maximize radiographic contrast of soft tissue. The x-ray beam should be filtered with 30 to 60 μm of molybdenum or rhodium to accentuate the characteristic x-ray emission.

Small focal spots should be used for imaging of microcalcifications because of the demand for increased spatial resolution. Moving grids and single-emulsion screen-film systems further increase radiographic contrast and image detail. AEC devices accommodate imaging of various sizes of breast tissue.

CHALLENGE QUESTIONS

1. Define or otherwise identify the following:
   a. Minimum filtration for mammography
   b. Mammographic SID
   c. Adipose tissue
   d. Mammographic grid ratio
   e. Molybdenum
   f. AEC
   g. Baseline mammogram
   h. Breast cancer incidence
   i. Mammographic screening projections
   j. Characteristic x-radiation
2. Describe the anatomy of the breast, including the types of tissue and structural sizes.
3. Discuss changes in image quality and patient dose in mammography as kVp is increased.
4. Graphically compare the x-ray emission of a tungsten target x-ray tube with that of a molybdenum target x-ray tube operated at 28 kVp.
5. The electron binding energies for molybdenum are K-shell, 20 keV; L-shell, 2.6 keV; and M-shell, 0.5 keV. What are the possible characteristic x-ray energies when operated at 28 kVp?
6. Discuss the influence of the heel effect on image quality in mammography.
7. Why should mammography be performed with an x-ray tube target of molybdenum or rhodium?
8. Draw the relationships among x-ray tube target, intensifying screen, film base, film emulsion, and the patient for single-emulsion screen-film mammography.
9. How is soft tissue radiography different from conventional radiography?
10. To what do the abbreviations *ACR* and *MQSA* refer?
11. What is the difference between diagnostic and screening mammography?
12. List the recommended intervals for screening x-ray mammography.
13. Explain why mammography requires a low-kVp technique.
14. List the advantages of mammographic compression.
15. Name the three materials used for mammographic x-ray tube targets.
16. What focal-spot sizes are used for mammography? Why?

MAMMOGRAPHY HAS been a screening and diagnostic tool for many years, but challenges in producing high-quality mammographic images while keeping patient radiation dose low are ongoing. A team that includes the radiologist, the medical physicist, and the mammographer works together using a quality control (QC) program to produce excellence in mammographic imaging. Each member of the team is assigned specific tasks that relate to QC. This chapter identifies these responsibilities.

QUALITY CONTROL TEAM

The American College of Radiology (ACR) and the Mammography Quality Standards Act (MQSA) have endorsed a QC program of specific duties required of the **radiologist**, the **medical physicist**, and the **mammographer** (Figure 20-1). Each of these individuals is important in ensuring the best available patient care with the least radiation exposure. This chapter discusses the responsibilities of each of these three positions but emphasizes the mammographer's duties.

Radiologist

The ultimate responsibility for mammography QC lies with the radiologist. These responsibilities often fall under the more broad area of **quality assurance (QA)**.

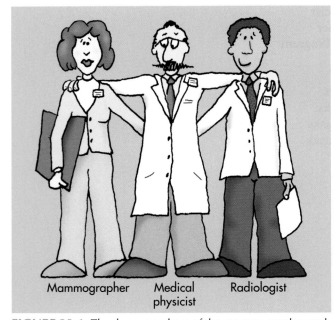

FIGURE 20-1 The three members of the mammography quality control (QC) team.

QA is an administrative program that is designed to fuse the different aspects of QC, and to ensure that all activities are carried out at the highest level. The radiologist is responsible for selecting qualified medical physicists and mammographers, and for overseeing the activities of these team members regularly.

> The radiologist's principal responsibility is supervision of the entire QA program.

Another responsibility of the radiologist involves supervising patient communication and tracking. Quality patient care is the ultimate goal of any mammography facility, and the final responsibility for this goal lies with the radiologist. The level of any QA/QC program directly reflects the radiologist's attitude and appreciation for the need for such a program. The MQSA mandates daily "clinical image evaluation" by the radiologist. Continuous quality improvement (CQI) is an extension of any QA/QC program, including administrative protocols for the continuous improvement of mammographic image quality.

Medical Physicist

The role of the medical physicist as a member of the mammography QC team is multidimensional. One such aspect is QC evaluation of the physical equipment used to produce an image of the breast. This evaluation should be performed annually or whenever a major component has been replaced. The evaluation consists of a number of measurements and tests that are summarized in Box 20-1.

The medical physicist should understand how the different technical aspects of the imaging chain affect the resulting image and therefore should be

---

BOX 20-1 Annual Quality Control Evaluation to Be Performed by the Medical Physicist

- Mammographic unit assembly inspection
- Collimation assessment
- Evaluation of spatial resolution
- kVp accuracy and reproducibility
- Beam quality assessment (half-value layer)
- Automatic exposure control performance assessment
- Automatic exposure control reproducibility
- Uniformity of screen speed
- Breast entrance exposure
- Average glandular dose
- Image-quality evaluation
- Artifact evaluation
- Radiation output intensity
- Measurement of viewing conditions

able to identify existing or potential image-quality problems. Occasionally, the medical physicist may pass information directly to the service engineer or may serve as an intermediary between the facility and the service engineer. The aim of this portion of the QC program is to ensure that equipment functions properly to provide the highest-quality images with the lowest dose to the patient.

 The medical physicist's principal responsibility is to conduct an annual performance evaluation of the imaging system.

Another role of the medical physicist is to advise the mammographer. The medical physicist should understand all tests expected of the mammographer well enough to predict likely problems or complications.

An additional responsibility is to evaluate the QC program on site at least annually. The medical physicist should review all procedures to ensure compliance with current recommendations and standards. The medical physicist should thoroughly review charts and records to check for compliance, and to ensure that they are prepared properly and contain all necessary information.

The medical physicist is an integral part of the QC team, whose full cooperation and attention is expected. This very achievable goal involves maintenance of a first-class QC program by a competent mammographer. The mammographer must call the medical physicist whenever images or the imaging system changes substantially.

Mammographer

The mammographer is extremely important to a mammography QC program. The mammographer, the most hands-on member of the QC team, is responsible for day-to-day QC and for producing and monitoring all control charts and logs for any trends that might indicate problems. In imaging facilities that use several mammographers, one should be assigned the responsibility of **QC mammographer.**

The 12 specific QC tasks for which the mammographer is responsible may be broken into categories that reflect frequency of performance. Table 20-1 outlines these tasks and estimates the time that each task requires.

QUALITY CONTROL PROGRAM

The mammographer's 12 tasks are well defined, with recommended performance standards available for each of them. To maintain a thorough and accurate QC program, the mammographer must fully understand these tasks and the reasons for recommended performance standards.

TABLE 20-1	Elements of a Mammographic QC Program	
Task	Minimum Frequency	Approximate Time to Carry Out Procedures (min)
Darkroom cleanliness	Daily	5
Processor quality control	Daily	20
Screen cleanliness	Weekly	10
Viewboxes and viewing conditions	Weekly	5
Phantom images	Weekly	30
Visual checklist	Monthly	10
Repeat analysis	Quarterly or 250 patients	60
Analysis of fixer retention in film	Quarterly	5
Conference with radiologist	Quarterly	45
Darkroom fog	Semiannually	10
Screen-film contact	Semiannually	80
Compression	Semiannually, at least	10

Total annual time required for QC: 160 hours.

Daily Tasks

Darkroom Cleanliness. The first task each day is to wipe the darkroom clean. Maintaining the cleanest possible conditions in the darkroom minimizes artifacts on mammograms (Figure 20-2). First, the floor should be damp-mopped. Next, all unnecessary items should be removed from countertops and work

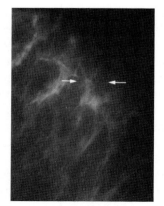

FIGURE 20-2 These specks were produced by flakes trapped between the film and the screen. (Courtesy Susan Sprinkle-Vincent, Advanced Health Education Center.)

surfaces. A clean, damp towel should be used to wipe off the processor feed tray and all countertops and work surfaces.

If a passbox is present, it should be cleaned daily as well. Hands should be kept clean to minimize fingerprints and handling artifacts. Overhead air vents and safelights should be wiped or vacuumed weekly before the other cleaning procedures are performed. Even the ceiling tiles should be cleaned to prevent flaking.

 Daily cleaning of the darkroom reduces image artifacts.

Smoking, eating, or drinking in the darkroom is prohibited. Food or drink should not be taken into the darkroom at any time. Nothing should be left on the countertop, except items used for loading and unloading cassettes, because other objects would only collect dust. No shelves should be included above the countertops in the darkroom because these also serve as sites for dust collection; such dust eventually falls onto work surfaces.

Processor QC. Before any films are processed, it should be verified that the processor chemical system is in accord with preset specifications. The first step in a processor QC program is to establish operating control levels. To begin, a new dedicated box of film should be set aside to carry out the future daily processor QC. The processor tanks and racks should be cleaned and the processor supplied with the proper developer replenisher, fixer, and developer starter fluids as specified by the manufacturer.

The developer temperature and developer and fixer replenishment rates should also be set to the levels specified by the manufacturer. A mercury thermometer should never be used. Should the thermometer break, mercury contamination could render the processor permanently useless.

Once the processor has been allowed to warm up and the developer is at the correct temperature and stable, testing may continue. In the darkroom, a sheet of control film should be exposed with a sensitometer (Figure 20-3). The sensitometric strip should always be processed in exactly the same manner. The least exposed end is fed into the processor first. The same side of the feed tray is used, with the emulsion side down. The time between exposure and processing should be similar each day.

Next, a densitometer is used to measure and record the optical density (OD) of each of the steps on the sensitometric strip. This process should be repeated each day for 5 consecutive days. The average OD is then determined for each step from the five different strips.

Once the averages have been determined, the step that has an average OD closest to 1.2 but not less than 1.2 should be identified and marked as the mid-density

(MD) step for future comparison. This is sometimes called the **speed index.**

Next, the step with an average OD closest to 2.2 and the step with an average OD closest to but not less than 0.5 should be found and marked for future comparison. The difference between these two steps is recorded as the density difference (DD), which is sometimes called the *contrast index.*

Finally, the average OD from an unexposed area of the strips is recorded as the base plus fog (B+F). The three values that have now been determined should be recorded on the center lines of the appropriate control chart. An example of a control chart is shown in Figure 20-4.

Once the control values have been established, the daily processor QC begins. At the beginning of each day, before any films are processed, a sensitometric strip should be exposed and processed according to the guidelines previously discussed. The MD, DD, and B+F are each determined from the appropriate predetermined steps and are plotted on the control charts.

The MD is determined to evaluate the constancy of image receptor speed. The DD is determined to evaluate the constancy of image contrast. These values are allowed to vary within 0.15 of the control values. If either value is out of this control limit, the point should be circled on the graph, the cause of the problem corrected, and the test repeated.

 If the value of the MD or the DD cannot be brought within the 0.15 variance of control, *no clinical images should be processed.*

If either value falls by ±0.1 outside the range of the control value, the test should be repeated. If the value continues to remain outside this range, the processor may be used for clinical processing but should be monitored closely while the problem is identified.

The B+F evaluates the level of fog in the processing chain. This value is allowed to vary within 0.03 of the control value. Anytime the value exceeds this limit, steps should be taken as described for the MD and DD values.

Weekly Tasks

Screen Cleanliness. Screens are cleaned to ensure that mammographic cassettes and intensifying screens are free of dust and dirt particles, which can resemble microcalcifications and may result in misdiagnoses. Radiographic intensifying screens should be cleaned with the use of the material and methods suggested by the screen manufacturer. If a liquid cleaner is used, screens should be allowed to air-dry while standing vertically, as shown in Figure 20-5, before the cassettes are closed or used. If compressed air is used, the air supply should be checked

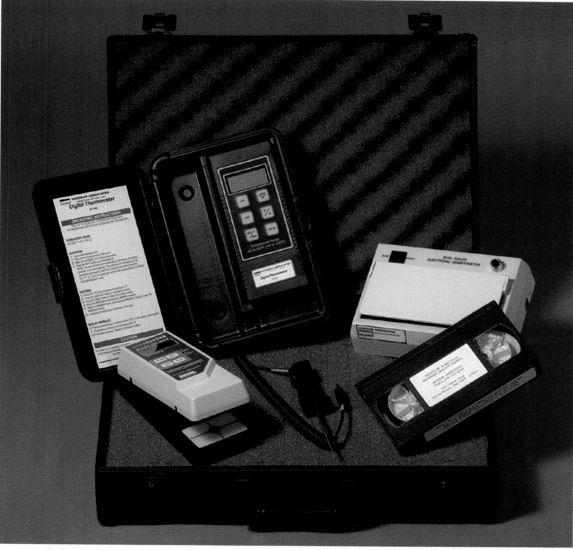

FIGURE 20-3 Processor quality control (QC) kit, including a sensitometer and a densitometer. (Courtesy Cardinal Health.)

to ensure that no moisture, oil, or other contaminants are present.

 If dust or dirt artifacts are ever noticed, the screens should be cleaned immediately.

Each screen cassette combination should be clearly labeled. Identifying information should be placed on the exterior of the cassette, as well as on a lateral border of the screen, so it will be legible on the processed film. This enables the mammographer to identify specific screens that have been found to contain artifacts.

Viewboxes and Viewing Conditions. Viewboxes and viewing conditions must be maintained at an optimal level. Viewbox surfaces should be cleaned with window cleaner and soft paper towels, ensuring that all marks have been removed.

The viewboxes should be visually inspected for uniformity of luminance and to ensure that all masking devices are functioning properly. Room illumination levels should be checked visually as well to ensure that the room is free of bright light and that the viewbox surface is free of reflections. The viewing conditions for mammographers when checking films should be the same as those for radiologists.

Any marks that are not removed easily require an appropriate cleaner that will not damage the viewbox. If the viewbox luminance appears to be nonuniform, all of the interior lamps should be replaced. Mammography viewboxes have considerably higher luminance levels than conventional viewboxes. A luminance of at least 3000 NIT (candela per square meter) is required.

All mammograms and mammography test images should be completely **masked** for viewing, so that no

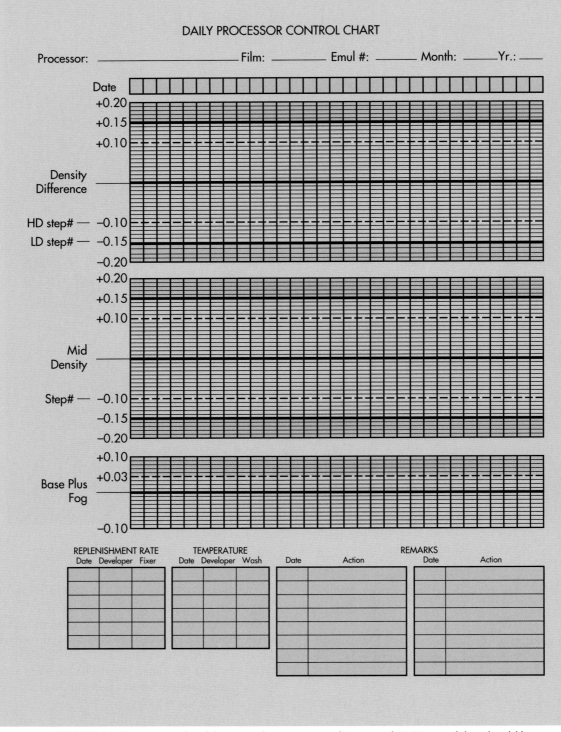

FIGURE 20-4 An example of the type of processor quality control (QC) record that should be maintained for each processor.

extraneous light from the viewbox enters the viewer's eyes. Masking can be provided simply by cutting black paper to the proper size (Figure 20-6). Commercially adjustable masks are available.

Ambient light in the area of the viewbox should be diffuse and reduced to approximately that reaching the eye through the mammogram. Sources of glare must be removed and surface reflections eliminated.

Phantom Images. Phantom images are taken to ensure optimal OD, contrast, uniformity, and image quality of the x-ray imaging system and film processor. A standard film and a cassette designated as the *control*

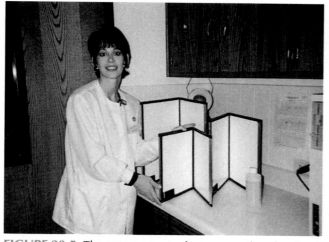

FIGURE 20-5 The proper way to dry screens after cleaning is to position them vertically. (Courtesy Linda Joppe, Rasmussen College.)

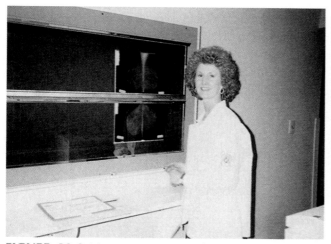

FIGURE 20-6 Mammograms must be masked for proper viewing, (Courtesy Lois Depouw, Rasmussen College.)

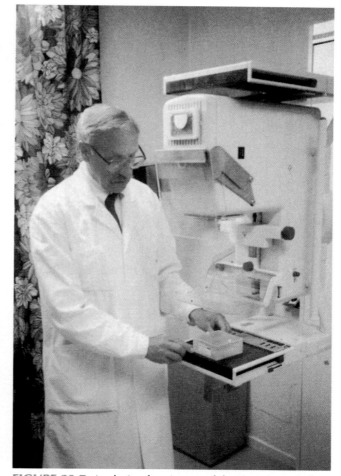

FIGURE 20-7 Analysis of an image of the American College of Radiology (ACR) mammography phantom by a medical physicist scores the detection limits of the system for fibrils, microcalcifications, and nodules. (Courtesy Art Haus, Columbus, Ohio.)

or *phantom cassette* should be used to take an image of an MQSA accreditation phantom.

The phantom should be placed on the image receptor assembly so that its edge is aligned with the chest wall edge of the image receptor, as shown in Figure 20-7. The compression device should be brought into contact with the phantom, and the automatic exposure control (AEC) sensor should be positioned in a location that will be used for all future phantom images.

The technique selected for imaging the phantom should be the same that is used clinically for a 50% adipose/50% glandular, 4.5-cm compressed breast. When the exposure is made, the time or mAs value is recorded. The film should then be processed similarly to a clinical mammogram.

A densitometer is used to determine the OD for the density disc and for the background immediately adjacent to the density disc. The time or mAs value recorded earlier, the background OD, and the DD

should be plotted on a phantom image control chart such as the one shown in Figure 20-8.

The exposure time or mAs value should stay within a range of ±15%. The background OD of the film should be approximately 1.4, with an allowed range of ±0.2. A good target value is approximately 1.6. The DD should be approximately 0.4, with an allowed range of ±0.05. However, this is defined for 28 kVp, so slightly different ODs should be expected at other kVp values.

The next step is to score the phantom image. This involves determining the number of fibers, speck groups, and masses visible in the phantom image. The ACR accreditation phantom and its image are shown in Figure 20-9. These results also should be plotted on the phantom image control chart.

Scoring of objects requires that they must always be counted from the largest object to the smallest, with each object group receiving a score of 1.0, 0.5, or zero. A fiber may be counted as 1.0 if its entire length is visible at the correct location and with the correct orientation.

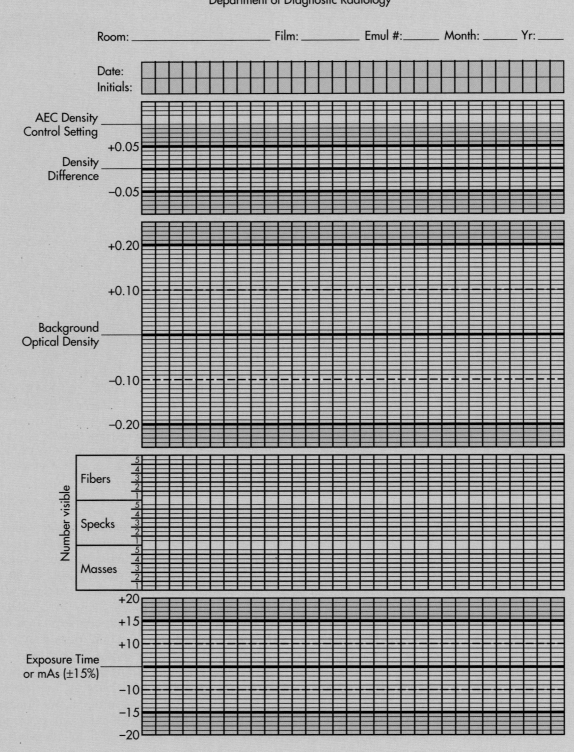

FIGURE 20-8 A phantom image control chart.

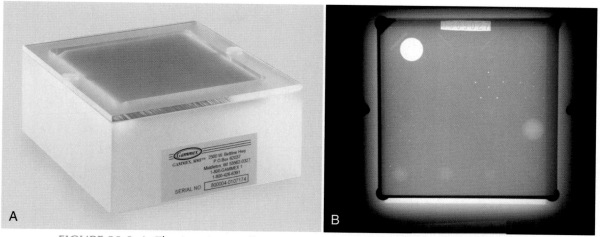

FIGURE 20-9 **A,** The American College of Radiology (ACR) accreditation phantom. **B,** Its image is shown. (Courtesy Gammex RMI.)

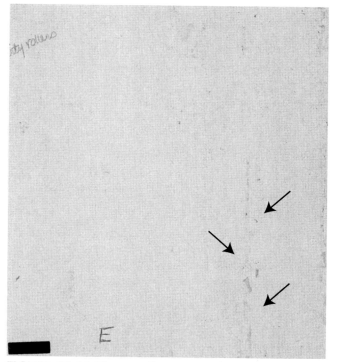

FIGURE 20-10 These really gross artifacts are caused by processor rollers that have not been cleaned. (Courtesy Cristl Thompson, El Paso Community College.)

A fiber may be given a score of 0.5 if at least half of its length is visible at the correct location and with the correct orientation. The score is zero if less than half of the fiber is visible.

A **speck group** may be counted as a full point if four or more of the six specks are visible with a magnifying glass. A score of 0.5 may be given to a speck group if at least two of the six specks are visible. If fewer than two specks in the group are visible, the score is zero.

A **mass** may be counted as a full point if a density difference is visible at the correct location with a generally

circular border. A score of 0.5 may be given to a mass if a density difference is visible at the correct location but the shape is not circular. If there is only a hint of a density difference, the score is zero.

Next, the magnifying glass is used to check the image for nonuniform areas or artifacts (Figure 20-10). If any artifacts that resemble the phantom objects are found, they should be subtracted from the score given for that object. Never subtract below the next full integer point. For example, if a score of 3.5 or 4 was given, the score cannot be subtracted below 3.

The score of phantom objects counted on subsequent phantom images for each type of object should not decrease by more than 0.5. The minimum number of objects required to pass ACR accreditation is four fibers, three speck groups, and three masses.

Phantom images should be taken after equipment installation to determine the control values of the phantom objects for future comparison. Phantom images also should be taken after the imaging equipment undergoes any maintenance.

When the phantom image results in any of the factors exceeding the control values, the cause should be investigated and corrected as soon as possible. The phantom images should always be viewed by the same person, on the same mammography viewbox, under the same viewing conditions, with the same type of magnifier that is used for mammograms, and at the same time of day.

Monthly Tasks

Visual Checklist. The visual check (1) ensures that the imaging system lights, displays, and mechanical locks, and that detents are functioning properly, and (2) confirms the optimal level of the equipment's mechanical rigidity and stability (Figure 20-11).

The mammographer should review all items on the list and should indicate the condition of each. If a particular

MAMMOGRAPHY QC VISUAL CHECKLIST

Room #:_____ Tube :_____

Month: J F M A M J J A S O N D

		J	F	M	A	M	J	J	A	S	O	N	D
C-ARM	SID indicator or marks												
	Angulation indicator												
	Locks (all)												
	Field light												
	High-tension cable/other cables												
	Smoothness of motion												
CASSETTE HOLDER	Cassette lock (small and large)												
	Compression device												
	Compression scale												
	Amount of compression: automatic manual												
	Grid												
CONTROL BOOTH	Exposure control												
	Observation window												
	Panel switches/lights/meters												
	Technique charts												
OTHER	Cones												
	Cleaning solution												
	Pass = √ Month:												
	Fail = X Date:												
	Not applicable = NA R.T.												

FIGURE 20-11 This checklist contains items that the mammographer should inspect monthly.

piece of equipment has a feature that does not appear on the checklist, this feature should be added. This helps to ensure patient safety, high-quality images, and operator convenience. If any item on the list fails visual inspection, immediate steps should be taken to remedy the problem. The checklist should be dated and initialed.

Quarterly Tasks

Repeat Analysis. This procedure is performed to determine the number and cause of repeated mammograms. Repeat analysis also identifies ways to improve efficiency, reduce costs, and reduce unnecessary patient dose. Such evaluations are valid only if patient volume results in at least 250 examinations.

To begin the analysis, all presently rejected films should be discarded, so the analysis starts at zero. A complete inventory of the remaining film supply is taken, and all rejected films are collected for the next quarter. If the workload is low, the repeat analysis is continued until 250 patient examinations have been performed. Rejected films are sorted into different categories, such as poor positioning, patient motion, too light, and the other categories shown on the reject analysis form in Figure 20-12.

MAMMOGRAPHY REPEAT ANALYSIS

From _____ To _____

Cause	Number of films	Percentage of repeats
1. Positioning		
2. Patient motion		
3. Light film		
4. Dark film		
5. Black film		
6. Static		
7. Fog		
8. Incorrect patient I.D., or double exposure		
9. Mechanical		
10. Miscellaneous		
11. Good film (no apparent problem)		
12. Clear film		
13. Wire localization		
14. Q.C.		

	Totals	
Rejects (all; 1-14)	%	
Repeats (1-11)	%	

Total film used	

FIGURE 20-12 Examination repeat analysis form.

Next, the total number of films repeated should be counted, as should the total number of films exposed. The repeat rate is computed as follows:

REPEAT ANALYSIS

$$\text{Repeat rate (\%)} = \frac{\text{number of repeated films}}{\text{total number of films}} \times 100$$

The repeat rate for each category is determined by dividing the number of repeated films in a given category by the total number of repeats. The overall repeat rate should be less than 2%, as should the rate for each category. If overall rate is high, or if a single category is higher than the others, the problem should be investigated. *All repeated films should be included in the analysis*—not only those rejected by the radiologist.

Question: A mammographic service examined 327 patients during the third calendar quarter of 2007. A total of 719 films were exposed during this period, 8 of which were repeats. What is the repeat rate?

Answer: $\text{Repeat rate} = \dfrac{8}{719} \times 100 = 1.1\%$

Analysis of Fixer Retention in Film. This task determines the amount of residual fixer in the processed film. The result is used as an indicator of archival quality.

One sheet of unexposed film is processed. Next, one drop of residual hypo test solution should be placed on the emulsion side of the film and allowed to stand for 2 minutes. The excess solution should be blotted off and the stain compared with a hypo estimator, which comes with the test solution. Use a white sheet of paper as background.

The matching number from the hypo estimator should be recorded. The comparison should be made immediately after blotting because a prolonged delay allows the spot to darken.

The hypo estimator provides an estimate of the amount of residual hypo in grams per square meter. If the comparison results in an estimate of more than 0.05 g/m^2, the test must be repeated. If elevated residual hypo is then indicated, the source of the problem should be investigated and corrected. Figure 20-13 shows the result from one such test.

Semiannual Tasks

Darkroom Fog. Darkroom fog analysis ensures that darkroom safelights and other sources of light inside and outside the darkroom do not fog mammographic films. Fog results in loss of image contrast. This test also should be performed for a new darkroom and any time safelight bulbs or filters are changed.

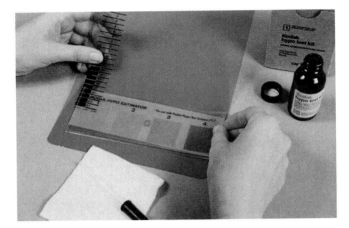

FIGURE 20-13 Analysis to determine the amount of fixer retained on the film. (Courtesy Eastman Kodak.)

Safelight filters should be checked to ensure that they are those recommended by the film manufacturer, and that they are not faded or cracked. The wattage and distance of the bulbs from work surfaces also should be checked against the recommendations of the film manufacturer.

Next, all lights should be turned off for 5 minutes; this allows the eyes to adjust to the darkness. Then the door, passbox, processor, and ceiling should be checked for light leaks. Light leaks are often visible from only one perspective, so you may have to move around the darkroom. Any leaks should be corrected before proceeding.

If fluorescent lights are present, they should be turned on for at least 2 minutes and then turned off. A piece of film should then be loaded into the phantom cassette in total darkness. Now, a phantom image should be taken as previously described. The film should be taken to the darkroom and placed emulsion side up on the countertop; one half of the image (left or right) should be covered with an opaque object. The safelights should then be turned on for 2 minutes with the half-covered film on the countertop.

After 2 minutes, the film should be processed and the OD measured very near both sides of the line separating the covered and uncovered portions of the film. The difference between the two ODs represents the amount of fog created by the safelights or by fluorescent light afterglow. This value should be recorded.

The level of this type of fog should not exceed 0.05 OD. Excessive fog levels should be investigated to find the source and take corrective action. The background OD (unfogged) of the phantom should be in the range specified previously (1.4 to 1.6).

Screen-Film Contact. Screen-film contact is evaluated to ensure that close contact is maintained between the screen and the film in each cassette. Poor screen-film contact results in image blur, again causing a loss of diagnostic information in the mammogram.

New cassettes should always be tested before they are placed into service. All cassettes and screens should be completely cleaned and allowed to air-dry for at least

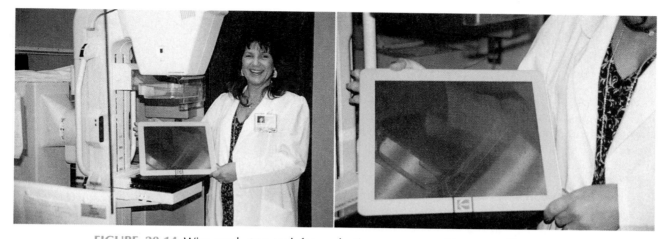

FIGURE 20-14 Wire mesh test tool for evaluating mammographic screen-film contact. (Courtesy Susan Sprinkle-Vincent, Advanced Health Education Center.)

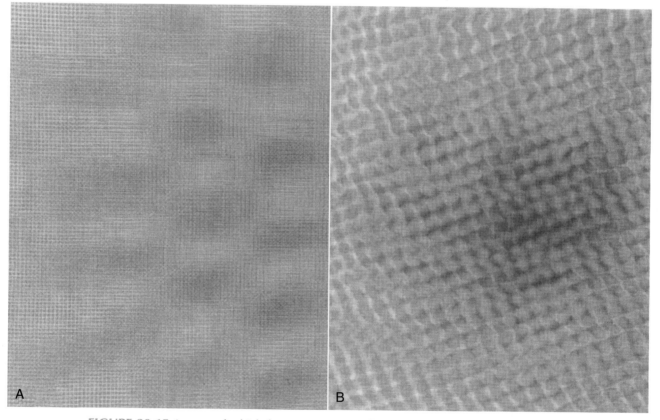

A

B

FIGURE 20-15 Images of a high-frequency wire mesh phantom showing **(A)** good and **(B)** poor screen-film contact. (Courtesy Sharon Glaze, Baylor College of Medicine.)

30 minutes before they are loaded with film for this test. After loading, the cassettes should be allowed to sit upright for 15 minutes, to allow any trapped air to escape.

The cassette to be tested should *be placed on top of the cassette holder assembly* with the test tool placed directly on top of the cassette. An appropriate test tool is made of copper wire mesh with a grid density of at least 40 wires per inch (Figure 20-14). The compression paddle should be raised as high as possible. A manual technique of approximately 26 kVp should be selected;

this results in an OD between 0.7 and 0.8 near the chest wall. Exposure time should be at least 500 ms.

A piece of acrylic should be placed between the x-ray tube and the cassette if the stated parameters cannot be met under normal circumstances. If acrylic is used, it should be placed as close as possible to the x-ray tube to reduce the scatter radiation that reaches the cassette.

The film should be processed regularly and viewed from a distance of at least 3 feet (90 cm). Dark areas on the film indicate poor screen-film contact (Figure 20-15).

Any cassettes with poor screen-film contact should be cleaned and tested again. If poor contact persists at the same spot, the problem should be investigated and the cassette removed from service until the problem has been corrected.

Compression. Observation of compression ensures that the mammographic system can provide adequate compression in the manual and power-assisted modes for an adequate amount of time. This analysis also must show that the equipment does not allow excessive compression.

To check the compression device, a towel, tennis balls, or similar cushioning material is placed on the cassette holder assembly, followed by a flat bathroom scale centered under the compression device. Another towel should be placed over the scale without covering the readout area (Figure 20-16). The compression device should be engaged automatically until it stops, the degree of compression should be recorded, and the device should then be released.

The procedure should be repeated with the manual drive, again recording the compression. Never exceed 40 pounds of compression (18 kg or 9 N) in the automatic mode. If such excess is possible, the equipment should be recalibrated, so 40 pounds of compression cannot be exceeded.

Both modes should be able to compress between 25 and 40 pounds (11 to 18 kg or 5.6 to 9 N) and to hold this compression for at least 15 seconds. If either mode fails to reach these levels, the equipment should be adjusted properly. Use of the compression paddle is the reason for a lot of patient complaints, so it is sound practice to check this device and record the results.

Firm compression is absolutely necessary for high-quality mammography. Compression reduces the thickness of tissue that the x-rays must penetrate and thus reduces scatter radiation, resulting in increased image contrast at reduced patient dose. Compression improves spatial resolution by reducing focal-spot blur and patient motion. Finally, compression serves to make the thickness of the breast more uniform, resulting in a more uniform OD and making the image easier to read.

Nonroutine Tasks

Film Crossover. When a new box of film must be opened and dedicated for processor QC, the old film must be crossed over, a very difficult and time-consuming activity. More detailed sources should be studied before this exercise is attempted.

Five strips from each of the old and new boxes of film should be exposed and processed at the same time. The OD should be read on each film for the three predetermined steps and the B+F. The five values for each of the

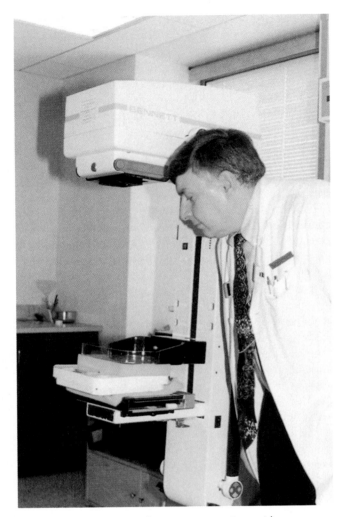

FIGURE 20-16 Testing breast compression with a conventional bathroom scale. (Courtesy Edward Nickoloff, Columbia University.)

old and the new set of films are then averaged for each of the predetermined steps.

The difference between the old and new values of MD, DD, and B+F should be determined and the control chart control values adjusted to the new values. If the B+F of the new film exceeds the B+F of the old film by more than 0.02, the cause should be investigated and remedied.

The use of strips exposed with the sensitometer longer than an hour or two before processing is unacceptable because these strips may be less sensitive to changes in the processor. The proper combination of film, processor, chemistry, developer temperature, immersion time, and replenishment rate should be used as recommended by the film manufacturer. QC also should be performed on the densitometer, sensitometer, and thermometer to maintain their proper calibrations. A log of these evaluations should be maintained.

SUMMARY

QC in mammography is part of an overall evaluation analysis and includes performance monitoring, record keeping, and evaluation of results. The three QC team members are the radiologist, who has specific duties of administration and tracking diagnostic results; the medical physicist, who examines and monitors the performance of imaging equipment; and the mammographer, who performs many tests and evaluations involving equipment, processing, and mammographic images.

The many duties and responsibilities of the QC mammographer are listed by time intervals. Daily routines include maintaining darkroom cleanliness and performing processor QC. Processor QC includes sensitometry and densitometry, as well as daily graphing of results.

Weekly routines include cleaning intensifying screens and viewbox illuminators, producing phantom images, and performing equipment checks.

Repeat analysis, based on at least 250 mammographic examinations, should occur four times a year. A repeat rate of less than 2% is required. Greater repeat rates should be investigated. Also, an archival check of film quality is performed quarterly.

Semiannually, the darkroom fog check is conducted and screen-film contact tests are performed. Finally, the compression test is done with the use of a bathroom scale under the compression paddle. Compression should never exceed 40 pounds of pressure. The automatic and manual modes should compress between 25 and 40 pounds (11 and 18 kg or 5.6 and 9 N) of compression for 15 seconds. Annually, the medical physicist evaluates the mammography imaging system.

CHALLENGE QUESTIONS

1. Define or otherwise identify the following:
   a. Quality assurance (QA)
   b. CQI
   c. Mammography phantom
   d. Density difference
   e. Repeat rate
   f. Crossover
   g. NIT
   h. Densitometer
   i. Average glandular dose
   j. MQSA
2. List two aspects of the radiologist's duties involving mammographic QC.
3. What is the most time-consuming task of the mammographic QC radiographer?
4. Which member of the QC team tracks positive diagnoses?
5. Which member of the QC team should notice a temperature error in the developer solution?
6. What do the fibrils of the ACR accreditation phantom simulate?
7. Describe how to clean radiographic intensifying screens. How often is this task performed?
8. Explain how mammographic viewboxes are different from conventional viewboxes.
9. What is masking?
10. What three objects are found in the ACR mammography phantom?
11. Describe the process of scoring phantom objects.
12. How do you check for light leaks in the darkroom?
13. What is the acceptable fog value for 2 minutes of safelight exposure of film?
14. Describe the device used to check screen-film contact.
15. What is the maximum pressure allowed for the compression device?
16. How do you ensure darkroom cleanliness?
17. What is the speed index, and how is it determined?
18. What is the minimum required luminance of a mammography viewbox?
19. When phantom images are produced, what technique should be used?
20. Show how to compute repeat rate.

The answers to the Challenge Questions can be found by logging on to our website at http://evolve.elsevier.com.

Fluoroscopy

OBJECTIVES

At the completion of this chapter, the student should be able to do the following:

1. Discuss the development of fluoroscopy
2. Explain visual physiology and its relationship to fluoroscopy
3. Describe the components of an image intensifier
4. Calculate brightness gain and identify its units
5. List the approximate kVp levels for common fluoroscopic examinations
6. Discuss the role of the television monitor and the television image in forming fluoroscopic images

OUTLINE

An Overview
Special Demands of Fluoroscopy
    Illumination
    Human Vision
Fluoroscopic Technique
Image Intensification
    Image-Intensifier Tube
    Multifield Image Intensification
Fluoroscopic Image Monitoring
    Television Monitoring
    Image Recording

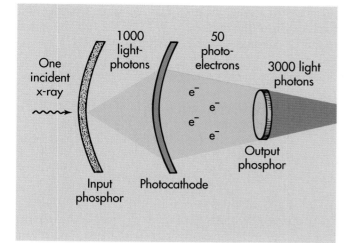

FIGURE 21-7 In an image-intensifier tube, each incident x-ray that interacts with the input phosphor results in a large number of light photons at the output phosphor. The image intensifier shown here has a flux gain of 3000.

For the image pattern to be accurate, the electron path from the photocathode to the output phosphor must be precise. The engineering aspects of maintaining proper electron travel are called **electron optics** because the pattern of electrons emitted from the large cathode end of the image-intensifier tube must be reduced to the small output phosphor.

The devices responsible for this control, called **electrostatic focusing lenses,** are located along the length of the image-intensifier tube. The electrons arrive at the output phosphor with high kinetic energy and contain the image of the input phosphor in minified form.

The interaction of these high-energy electrons with the output phosphor produces a considerable amount of light. Each photoelectron that arrives at the output phosphor produces 50 to 75 times as many light photons as were necessary to create it. The entire sequence of events from initial x-ray interaction to output image is summarized in Figure 21-7. This ratio of the number of light photons at the output phosphor to the number of x-rays at the input phosphor is the **flux gain.**

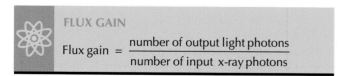

FLUX GAIN

$$\text{Flux gain} = \frac{\text{number of output light photons}}{\text{number of input x-ray photons}}$$

The increased illumination of the image is due to the multiplication of light photons at the output phosphor compared with x-rays at the input phosphor and the image minification from input phosphor to output phosphor. The ability of the image intensifier to increase the illumination level of the image is called its **brightness gain.** The brightness gain is simply the product of the **minification gain** and the **flux gain.**

BRIGHTNESS GAIN

Brightness gain = Minification gain × Flux gain

The minification gain is the ratio of the square of the diameter of the input phosphor to the square of the diameter of the output phosphor. Output phosphor size is fairly standard at 2.5 or 5 cm. Input phosphor size varies from 10 to 35 cm and is used to identify image-intensifier tubes.

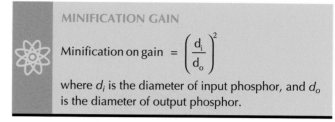

MINIFICATION GAIN

$$\text{Minification on gain} = \left(\frac{d_i}{d_o}\right)^2$$

where d_i is the diameter of input phosphor, and d_o is the diameter of output phosphor.

Question: What is the brightness gain for a 17-cm image-intensifier tube with a flux gain of 120 and a 2.5-cm output phosphor?

Answer:
$$\text{Brightness gain} = \left(\frac{17}{2.5}\right)^2 \times 120$$
$$= 46 \times 120 = 5520$$

The brightness gain of most image intensifiers is 5000 to 30,000, and it decreases with tube age and use. As an image intensifier ages, patient dose increases as a consequence of maintaining image brightness. Ultimately, the image intensifier must be replaced.

Brightness gain is now defined as the ratio of the illumination intensity at the output phosphor, measured in candela per meter squared (cd/m^2) (see Chapter 29), to the radiation intensity incident on the input phosphor, measured in milliroentgens per second (mR/s). This quantity is called the **conversion factor** and is approximately 0.01 times the brightness gain. The conversion factor is the proper quantity for expressing image intensification.

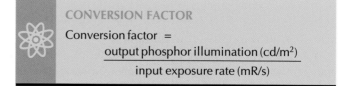

CONVERSION FACTOR

$$\text{Conversion factor} = \frac{\text{output phosphor illumination } (cd/m^2)}{\text{input exposure rate (mR/s)}}$$

Image intensifiers have conversion factors of 50 to 300. These correspond to brightness gains of 5000 to 30,000.

Figure 21-8 shows some of the modes of operation that can be accommodated with the image-intensifier tube. Fluoroscopic images are viewed on a television monitor. The spot-film camera uses 105-mm film. The cineradiography

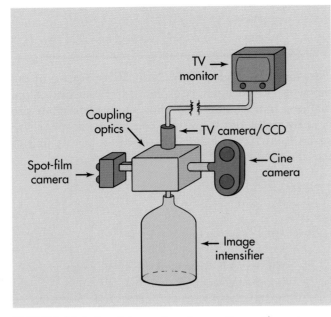

FIGURE 21-8 Possible modes of operation with an image-intensifier tube. CCD, Charge-coupled device.

camera is used almost exclusively in cardiac catheterization, but the use of digital imaging is growing.

Internal scatter radiation in the form of x-rays, electrons, and particularly light can reduce the contrast of image-intensifier tubes through a process called **veiling glare.** A veiling glare signal is produced behind a lead disc that is positioned on the input phosphor. Veiling glare is depicted in Figure 21-9. Advanced II tubes have output phosphor designs that reduce veiling glare.

Multifield Image Intensification

Most image intensifiers are of the multifield type. Multifield image intensifiers provide considerably greater flexibility in all fluoroscopic examinations and are standard components in digital fluoroscopy. Trifield tubes come in various sizes, but perhaps the most popular is 25/17/12 cm.

These numeric dimensions refer to the diameter of the input phosphor of the image-intensifier tube. The operation of a typical multifield tube is illustrated by the 25/17/12 type shown in Figure 21-10. In the 25-cm mode, photoelectrons from the entire input phosphor are accelerated to the output phosphor.

When a switch is made to the 17-cm mode, the voltage on the electrostatic focusing lenses increases; this causes the electron focal point to move farther from the output phosphor. Consequently, only electrons from the center 17-cm diameter of the input phosphor are incident on the output phosphor.

The principal result of this change in focal point is to reduce the field of view. The image now appears magnified because it still fills the entire screen on the monitor. Use of the smaller dimension of a multifield image-intensifier tube always results in a magnified

image, with a magnification factor in direct proportion to the ratio of the diameters. A 25/17/12 tube operated in the 12-cm mode produces an image that is $\frac{25}{12} = 2.1$ times larger than the image produced in the 25-cm mode.

Question: How magnified is the image of a 25/17/12 image-intensifier in the 17-cm mode compared with that produced in the 25-cm mode?

Answer: $MF = \frac{25}{17} = 1.5$ magnification

This magnified image comes at a price. In the magnified mode, the minification gain is reduced, and fewer photoelectrons are incident on the output phosphor. A dimmer image results.

To maintain the same level of brightness, the x-ray tube mA is increased by the ABC, which increases the patient dose. The increase in dose is approximately equal to the ratio of the area of the input phosphor used, or $[25^2 \div 12^2 \approx 4.4]$—the dose obtained in the wide field-of-view mode.

Question: A 23/15/10 image-intensifier tube is used in the 10-cm mode. How much higher is the patient dose in this mode compared with the 23-cm mode?

Answer: $23^2/10^2 = 5.3$ times higher!

This increase in patient dose results in better image quality. The patient dose is higher because more x-rays per unit area are required to form the image. This results in lower noise and improved **contrast resolution.**

MAGNIFICATION MODE RESULTS IN
- Better spatial resolution
- Better contrast resolution
- Higher patient dose

The portion of any image that results from the periphery of the input phosphor is inherently unfocused and suffers from **vignetting,** that is, a reduction in brightness at the periphery of the image.

Because only the central region of the input phosphor is used in the magnification mode, **spatial resolution** is also improved. In the 25-cm mode, a CsI image-intensifier tube can image approximately 0.125-mm objects (4 lp/mm); in the 10-cm mode, the resolution is approximately 0.08 mm (6 lp/mm).

The concept of spatial resolution as measured in line pairs per millimeter is discussed in Chapter 13 and more completely in Chapter 23. At this stage, it is sufficient to know that good spatial resolution is associated with a higher lp/mm value.

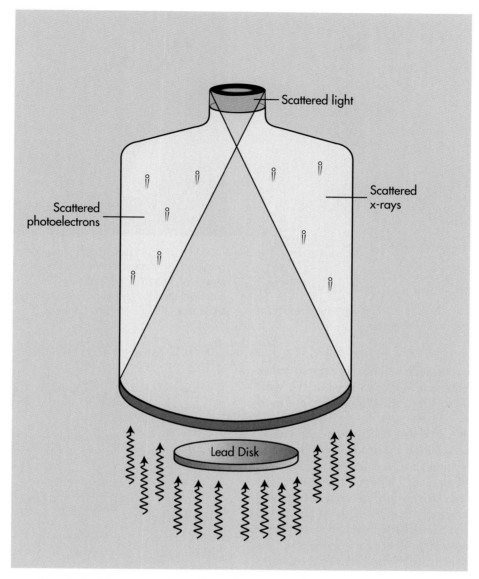

FIGURE 21-9 Veiling glare reduces the contrast of an image-intensifier tube.

FLUOROSCOPIC IMAGE MONITORING
Television Monitoring

With the **television monitoring system** of a fluoroscopic image, the output phosphor of the image-intensifier tube is coupled directly to a television camera tube. The **vidicon** (Figure 21-11) is the television camera tube that is most often used in television fluoroscopy. It has a sensitive input surface that is the same size as the output phosphor of the image-intensifier tube. The television camera tube converts the light image from the output phosphor of the image intensifier into an electrical signal that is sent to the television monitor, where it is reconstructed as an image on the television screen.

A significant advantage of television monitoring is that brightness level and contrast can be controlled electronically. With television monitoring, several observers can view the fluoroscopic image at the same time. It is even common to place monitors remote to the examination room for others to observe.

Television monitoring also allows for storage of the image in its electronic form for later playback and image manipulation.

Television Camera. Two methods are used to electronically convert the visible image on the output phosphor of the image intensifier into an electronic signal. These are the thermionic television camera tube and the solid state charge-coupled device (CCD). The CCD is discussed in Chapter 27.

The television camera consists of cylindrical housing, approximately 15 mm in diameter by 25 cm in length, that contains the heart of the television camera tube. It also contains electromagnetic coils that are used to properly steer the electron beam inside

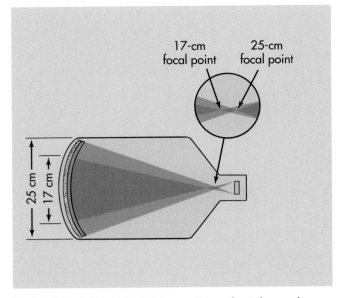

FIGURE 21-10 A 25/17/12 image-intensifier tube produces a highly magnified image in 12-cm mode.

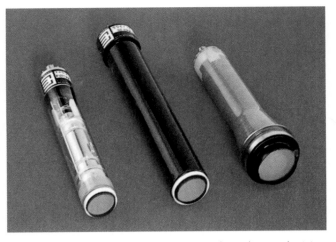

FIGURE 21-11 These three variations of a vidicon television camera tube have a diameter of approximately 2.5 cm and a length of 15 cm. The right tube uses electrostatic rather than electromagnetic electron beam deflection. (Courtesy Brad Mattinson, Philips Medical Systems.)

the tube. A number of such television camera tubes are available for television fluoroscopy, but the **vidicon** and its modified version, the **Plumbicon,** are used most often.

Figure 21-12 shows a typical vidicon. The **glass envelope** serves the same function that it does for the x-ray tube: to maintain a vacuum and provide mechanical support for the internal elements. These internal elements include the cathode, its **electron gun,** assorted **electrostatic grids,** and a **target assembly** that serves as an anode.

The electron gun is a heated filament that supplies a constant electron current by thermionic emission. The electrons are formed into an electron beam by the control grid, which also helps to accelerate the electrons to the anode.

The electron beam is further accelerated and focused by additional electrostatic grids. The size of the electron beam and its position are controlled by external electromagnetic coils known as deflection coils, focusing coils, and alignment coils.

At the anode end of the tube, the electron beam passes through a wire mesh–like structure and interacts with the target assembly. The target assembly consists of three layers that are sandwiched together. The outside layer is the **window,** the thin part of the glass envelope. Coated on the inside of the window is a thin layer of metal or graphite, called the **signal plate.** The signal plate is thin enough to transmit light yet thick enough to efficiently conduct electricity. Its name derives from the fact that it conducts the video signal out of the tube into the external video circuit.

A photoconductive layer of antimony trisulfide is applied to the inside of the signal plate. This layer, called the **target,** is swept by the electron beam. Antimony

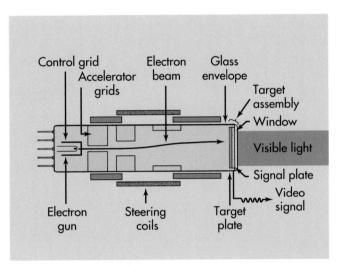

FIGURE 21-12 Vidicon television camera tube and its principal parts.

trisulfide is photoconductive because, when illuminated, it conducts electrons; when dark, it behaves as an insulator.

The mechanism of the target is complex but can be described briefly as follows. When light from the output phosphor of the image-intensifier tube strikes the window, it is transmitted through the signal plate to the target.

If the electron beam is incident on the same part of the target at the same time, some of its electrons are conducted through the target to the signal plate and from there out of the tube as the video signal. If that area of the target is dark, no video signal is produced. The magnitude of the video signal is proportional to the intensity of light (Figure 21-13).

Coupling to the Image Intensifier. Image intensifiers and television camera tubes are manufactured so that

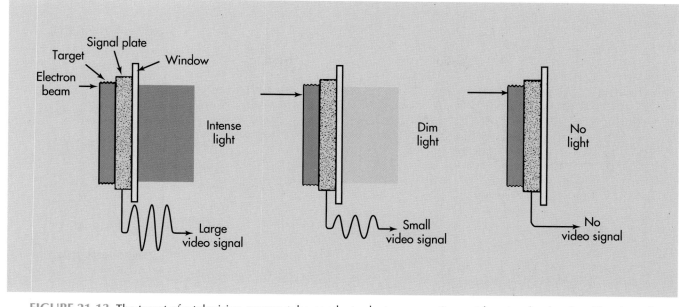

FIGURE 21-13 The target of a television camera tube conducts electrons, creating a video signal only when illuminated.

the output phosphor of the image-intensifier tube is the same diameter as the window of the television camera tube, usually 2.5 or 5 cm. Two methods are commonly used to **couple** the television camera tube to the image-intensifier tube (Figure 21-14).

The simplest method is to use a bundle of **fiber optics**. The fiber optics bundle is only a few millimeters thick and contains thousands of glass fibers per square millimeter of cross section. One advantage of this type of coupling is its compact assembly, which makes it easy to move the image-intensifier tower. This coupling is rugged and can withstand relatively rough handling.

The principal disadvantage is that it cannot accommodate the additional optics required for devices such as cine or photospot cameras.

To accept a cine or photospot camera, **lens coupling** is required. This type of coupling results in a much larger assembly that should be handled with care. It is absolutely essential that the lenses and the mirror remain precisely adjusted because malposition results in a blurred image.

The **objective lens** accepts light from the output phosphor and converts it into a parallel beam. When an image is recorded on film, this beam is interrupted by a **beam-splitting mirror** so that only a portion is transmitted to the television camera; the remainder is reflected to a film camera. Such a system allows the fluoroscopist to view the image while it is being recorded.

Usually, the beam-splitting mirror is retracted from the beam when a film camera is not in use. Both the television camera and the film camera are coupled to lenses that focus the parallel light beam onto the film and target of the respective cameras. These **camera lenses** are the most critical elements in the optical chain in terms of alignment.

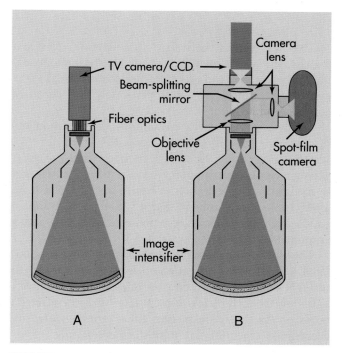

FIGURE 21-14 Television camera tubes and charge-coupled devices (CCDs) are coupled to an image-intensifier tube in two ways. **A,** Fiber optics. **B,** Lens system.

Although the lenses are shown as simple convex lenses, it should be understood that each is a compound lens system that consists of several separate lens elements.

Television Monitor. The video signal is amplified and is transmitted by cable to the television monitor, where it is transformed back into a visible image. The television monitor forms one end of a closed-circuit television system. The other end is the television camera tube or CCD.

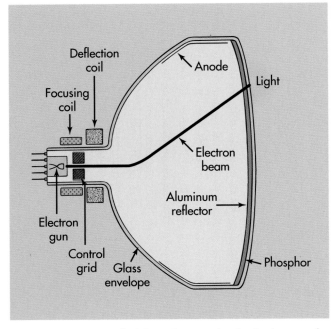

FIGURE 21-15 A television picture tube (cathode ray tube [CRT]) and its principal parts.

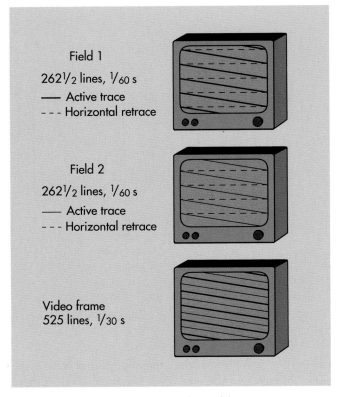

FIGURE 21-16 A video frame is formed from a raster pattern of two interlaced video fields.

Two differences between closed-circuit television fluoroscopy and a home television set are immediately obvious: no audio and no channel selection. Usually, the radiologic technologist manipulates only two controls: contrast and brightness.

The heart of the television monitor is the **television picture tube,** or the cathode ray tube (CRT) (Figure 21-15). It is similar to the television camera tube in many ways: A glass envelope, electron gun, and external coils are used to focus and steer the electron beam. It is different from a television camera tube in that it is much larger and its anode assembly consists of a fluorescent screen and a graphite lining.

The video signal received by the picture tube is **modulated,** that is, its magnitude is directly proportional to the light intensity received by the television camera tube. Different from the television camera tube, the electron beam of the television picture tube varies in intensity according to the modulation of the video signal.

The intensity of the electron beam is modulated by a **control grid,** which is attached to the electron gun. This electron beam is focused onto the output fluorescent screen by the external coils. There, the electrons interact with an output phosphor and produce a burst of light.

The phosphor is composed of linear crystals that are aligned perpendicularly to the glass envelope to reduce **lateral dispersion.** It is usually backed by a thin layer of aluminum, which transmits the electron beam but reflects the light.

Television Image. The image on the television monitor is formed in a complex way, but it can be described rather simply. It involves transforming the visible light

image of the output phosphor of the image-intensifier tube into an electrical video signal that is created by a constant electron beam in the television camera tube. The video signal then **modulates** the electron beam of the television picture tube and transforms that electron beam into a visible image at the fluorescent screen of the picture tube.

Both electron beams—the constant one of the television camera tube and the modulated one of the television picture tube—are finely focused pencil beams that are precisely and synchronously directed by the external electromagnetic coils of each tube. These beams are synchronous because they are always at the same position at the same time and move in precisely the same fashion.

The movement of these electron beams produces a **raster pattern** on the screen of a television picture tube (Figure 21-16). Although the following discussion relates to a picture tube, remember that the same electron beam pattern occurs in the camera tube.

The electron beam begins in the upper left corner of the screen and moves to the upper right corner, creating a line of varying intensity of light as it moves. This is called an **active trace.** The electron beam then is **blanked,** or turned off, and it returns to the left side of the screen as shown. This is the **horizontal retrace.**

A series of active traces then is followed by horizontal retraces until the electron beam is at the bottom of the screen. This is very similar to the action of a word processing secretary who types a line of information (the active trace): The cursor returns (the horizontal retrace) and continues this sequence to the bottom of the page. Whereas the secretary completes a page, the electron beam completes a **television field.**

The similarity stops there, however, because the secretary would continue word processing. The electron beam is blanked again and undergoes a **vertical retrace** to the top of the screen.

The electron beam now describes a second television field, which is the same as the first except that each active trace lies between two adjacent active traces of the first field. This movement of the electron beam is called **interlace,** and two interlaced television fields form a single **television frame.**

In the United States, power is supplied at 60 Hz, which results in 60 television fields per second and 30 television frames per second. This is fortunate because the flickering of home movies (shown at 16 frames per second) or old-time movies does not appear on the television image. Flickering is not detectable by the human eye at rates above approximately 20 frames per second. At a frame rate of 30 per second, each frame is 33 ms long.

> Video monitoring uses a rate of 30 frames per second.

In the television camera tube, as the electron beam reads the optical signal, the signal is erased. In the television picture tube, as the electron beam creates the television optical signal, it immediately fades, hence the term "fluorescent screen." Therefore, each new television frame represents 33 ms of new information.

Standard broadcast and closed circuit televisions are called 525-line systems because they use 525 lines of active trace per frame. Actually, only about 480 lines are used per frame because of the time required for retracing. Other special purpose systems have 875 or 1024 lines per frame and therefore have better **spatial resolution.** These high-resolution systems are particularly important for digital fluoroscopy.

In countries where power is supplied at 50 Hz, 50 television fields and thus 25 television frames are used per second. On a TV monitor, 625 lines are used per frame in two consecutive fields of 312.5 lines.

> For a 23-cm image intensifier, a 525-line TV system provides a spatial resolution of approximately 1 lp/mm; a 1024-line system provides resolution of 2 lp/mm.

The **vertical resolution** is determined by the number of scan lines. The **horizontal resolution** is determined

by **bandpass.** Bandpass is expressed in frequency (Hz) and describes the number of times per second that the electron beam can be **modulated.** A 1-MHz bandpass would indicate that the electron beam intensity could be changed a million times each second.

> The higher the bandpass, the better is the horizontal resolution.

The objective of television designers is to create a television frame that has equal horizontal and vertical resolution. Commercial television systems have a bandpass of about 3.5 MHz. Those used in fluoroscopy are approximately 4.5 MHz; 1000-line high-resolution systems have a bandpass of approximately 20 MHz.

The television monitor remains the weakest link in image-intensified fluoroscopy. A 525-line system has approximately 1-lp/mm spatial resolution, but the image intensifier is good to about 5 lp/mm. Therefore, if the superior resolution of the image intensifier is to be applied, the image must be recorded on film through an optically coupled photographic camera.

Image Recording

The conventional **cassette-loaded spot film** is one item that is used with image-intensified fluoroscopes. The spot film is positioned between the patient and the image intensifier (Figure 21-17).

During fluoroscopy, the cassette is parked in a lead-lined shroud so it is not unintentionally exposed. When a cassette spot-film exposure is desired, the radiologist must actuate a control that properly positions the cassette in the x-ray beam and changes the operation of the x-ray tube from low fluoroscopic mA to high radiographic mA. Sometimes, it takes the rotating anode a second or two to be energized to a higher speed.

The cassette-loaded spot film is masked by a series of lead diaphragms that allow several image formats. When the entire film is exposed at one time, it is called "one-on-one." When only half of the film is exposed at a time, two images result—"two-on-one." Four-on-one and six-on-one modes are also available, with the images becoming successively smaller.

Use of cassette-loaded spot film requires a higher patient dose, and the pre-exposure delay is sometimes a nuisance. Cassette-loaded spot films, however, do provide a familiar "life-sized" format for the radiologist and produce images of high quality.

The **photospot camera** is similar to a movie camera except that it exposes only one frame when activated. It receives its image from the output phosphor of the image-intensifier tube and therefore requires less patient exposure than is required by the cassette-loaded spot

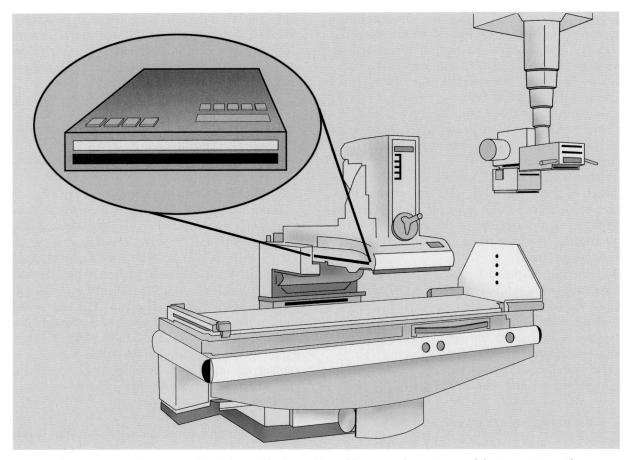

FIGURE 21-17 The cassette-loaded spot film is positioned between the patient and the image intensifier.

TABLE 21-2	**Cassette Spot Versus Photospot**	
Cassette	**Spot**	**Photospot**
Spatial resolution	8 lp/mm	5 lp/mm
Frame rate	1/s	12/s
Patient ESE	200 mR	100 mR

ESE, Entrance skin exposure.

film. The photospot camera does not require significant interruption of the fluoroscopic examination and avoids the additional heat load on the x-ray tube that is associated with cassette-loaded spot films.

The photospot camera uses film sizes of 70 and 105 mm. As a general rule, **larger film format results in better image quality but at increased patient dose.** Even with 105-mm spot films, however, the patient dose is only approximately half that used with cassette-loaded spot films.

The trend in spot filming is to use the photospot camera. The photospot camera provides adequate image quality without interruption of the fluoroscopic examination and at a rate of up to 12 images per second (Table 21-2). However, in contrast to the life-sized cassette image, the 105-mm spot film image is minified.

SUMMARY

The original fluoroscope, invented by Edison, had a zinc–cadmium sulfide screen that was placed in the x-ray beam directly above the patient. The radiologist stared directly into the screen and viewed a faint yellow-green fluoroscopic image. It was not until the 1950s that the image intensifier was developed.

In the past, fluoroscopy required radiologists to adapt their eyes to the dark before the examination was performed. Under dim viewing conditions, the human eye uses rods for vision; these have low visual acuity. The image from today's fluoroscope is bright enough to be perceived by cone vision. Cone vision provides superior visual acuity and contrast perception. When viewing the fluoroscopic image, the radiologist is able to see fine anatomic detail and differences in brightness levels of anatomic parts.

The image intensifier is a complex device that receives the image-forming x-ray beam, converts it to light, and increases the light intensity for better viewing. The input phosphor converts the x-ray beam into light. When stimulated by light, the photocathode then emits electrons and the electrons are accelerated to the output phosphor.

The following relationships define several characteristics of image-intensified fluoroscopy:

$$\text{Flux gain} = \frac{\text{number of output light photons}}{\text{number of input x-ray photons}}$$

$$\text{Minification gain} = \left(\frac{\text{diameter of input phosphor}}{\text{diameter of output phosphor}} \right)^2$$

Brightness gain is also expressed as the conversion factor:

$$\text{Conversion factor} = \frac{\text{output phosphor illumination (cd/m}^2)}{\text{input exposure rate (mR/s)}}$$

The fluoroscopy television camera is attached to the image intensifier with a lens coupling to accommodate a cine or a spot-film camera. When an image is recorded on film, a beam-splitting mirror separates the beam so that only a portion is transmitted to the television camera and the remainder is reflected to a spot-film camera.

CHALLENGE QUESTIONS

1. Define or otherwise identify the following:
   a. Photopic vision
   b. Automatic brightness control
   c. Visual acuity
   d. Flux gain
   e. Angiography
   f. Vidicon
   g. Photoemission
   h. Bucky slot cover
   i. Spot-film camera sizes
   j. Modulation
2. Draw a diagram to show the relationship between the x-ray tube, the patient table, and the image intensifier.
3. What is the difference between rod and cone vision? With which is visual acuity greater?
4. What is the approximate kVp for the following fluoroscopic examinations: barium enema, gallbladder, and upper gastrointestinal?
5. Draw a cross section of the human eye and label the cornea, lens, and retina.
6. Explain the difference between photoemission and thermionic emission.
7. Diagram the image-intensifier tube, label its principal parts, and discuss the function of each.
8. A 23-cm image intensifier has an output phosphor size of 2.5 cm and a flux gain of 75. What is its brightness gain?
9. What is vignetting?
10. Why is the television monitor considered the weakest link in image-intensified fluoroscopy?
11. What is the primary function of the fluoroscope?
12. Who invented the fluoroscope in 1896? What phosphor was used on that original fluoroscopic screen?
13. What determines the image frame rate in video fluoroscopy?
14. What limits the vertical resolution and horizontal resolution of a video monitor?
15. Does spatial resolution change when one is viewing in the magnification mode versus the normal mode?
16. What is meant by a trifield image intensifier?
17. Draw the approximate raster pattern for a conventional video monitor.
18. When the image intensifier is switched from 15-cm mode to 25-cm mode, what happens to patient dose and contrast resolution?
19. Trace the path of information-carrying elements in a fluoroscopic system from incident x-rays to video image.
20. What is the principal difference between a standard video system for fluoroscopy and a high-resolution system?

The answers to the Challenge Questions can be found by logging on to our website at http://evolve.elsevier.com.

22

Interventional Radiology

OBJECTIVES

At the completion of this chapter, the student should be able to do the following:

1. Describe the measures used to provide radiation protection for patients and personnel during interventional radiology
2. Describe the reasons why minimally invasive (percutaneous) vascular procedures often are more beneficial than traditional surgical procedures
3. Discuss the advantages that nonionic (water-soluble) contrast media offer over ionic contrast media
4. Identify the risks of arteriography
5. Describe the special equipment found in the interventional suite

OUTLINE

Types of Interventional Procedures
Basic Principles
    Arterial Access
    Guidewires
    Catheters
    Contrast Media
    Patient Preparation and Monitoring
    Risks of Arteriography
Interventional Radiology Suite
    Personnel
    Equipment

N PREVIOUS YEARS, myelography and venography were considered special procedures. Recently, the area of therapeutic angiographic intervention has undergone rapid development. We now have suites of x-ray rooms and complex equipment that have been specially designed for interventional radiology.

The following discussion concerns various interventional radiologic procedures and the special x-ray equipment necessary to perform such procedures.

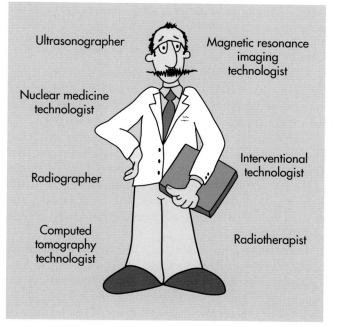

FIGURE 22-1 A radiologic technologist can specialize in many types of imaging modalities.

Isn't it interesting how advances in technology are accompanied by changes in terminology? We made radiographs with x-rays because that is how Roentgen named them. *X* is the mathematical symbol for "unknown," which is how Roentgen viewed his discovery.

As imaging technology has developed, so has our identity. First, we were called x-ray operators, then technicians, and now radiologic technologists or, more specifically, radiographers. A radiologic technologist can be a radiographer, a nuclear medicine technologist, or another imaging technologist (Figure 22-1).

In the same way that radiologic technology has been more precisely divided into disciplines, so has our imaging task. We used to do special procedures, such as pneumoencephalography, myelography, and neuroangiography. The rapid development of vascular imaging and aggressive therapeutic intervention through vessels has resulted in rooms and equipment designed especially for interventional radiologic procedures. The radiologic technologists involved are interventional radiologic technologists.

TYPES OF INTERVENTIONAL PROCEDURES

Interventional radiologic procedures began in the 1930s with **angiography**; needles and contrast media were used to enter and highlight an artery. In the early 1960s, Mason Jones pioneered **transbrachial selective coronary angiography**—entering select coronary arteries through an artery of the arm.

Also during the 1960s, transfemoral angiography— entering an artery in the thigh—of selective visceral, heart, and head arteries was developed. Melvin Judkins introduced coronary angiography, and Charles Dotter introduced visceral angiography.

Angiography refers to the opacification of vessels through injection of contrast media. **Angioplasty, thrombolysis, embolization, vascular stents,** and **biopsy** are interventional therapeutic procedures that are conducted in and through vessels. Table 22-1 lists the types

TABLE 22-1	Representative Procedures Conducted in an Interventional Radiology Suite
Imaging Procedures	**Interventional Procedures**
Angiography	Stent placement
Aortography	Embolization
Arteriography	Intravascular stent
Cardiac catheterization	Thrombolysis
Myelography	Balloon angioplasty
Venography	Atherectomy
	Electrophysiology

of imaging and interventional procedures that are likely to be conducted in an interventional radiology suite.

BASIC PRINCIPLES
Arterial Access

In 1953, Sven Ivar Seldinger described a method of arterial access in which a catheter was used. The Seldinger needle is an 18-gauge hollow needle with a stylet. Once the Seldinger needle is inserted into the femoral artery and pulsating arterial blood returns, the stylet is removed.

A guidewire then is inserted through the needle into the arterial lumen. With the guidewire in the vessel, the Seldinger needle is removed and a catheter is threaded onto the guidewire. Under fluoroscopic view, the catheter then is advanced along the guidewire.

In angiography, the common femoral artery is most often used for arterial access. The common femoral artery can be palpated by locating the pulse in the groin below the inguinal ligament, which passes between the symphysis pubis and the anterior superior iliac spine.

Guidewires

Guidewires allow the safe introduction of the catheter into the vessel. Once the catheter is in place, the guidewire allows the radiologist to position the catheter within the vascular network.

Guidewires are fabricated of stainless steel and contain an inner core wire that is tapered at the end to a soft, flexible tip. This core wire prevents loss of sections of the wire should it break. The trailing end of the guidewire is stiff and allows the guidewire to be pushed and twisted so the catheter can be positioned in the chosen vessel.

Conventional guidewires are 145 cm long. Catheters overlaying the guidewire are usually 100 cm long or less. Guidewires are categorized additionally by length to the beginning of the tapered tip, configuration of the tip, stiffness of the guidewire, and coating. They are coated with a hydrophilic material so the catheter slides over the wire more easily. This coating makes guidewires more resistant to thrombus (blood clot) and easier to irrigate while they are in the vascular system.

The J-tip for guidewires is a variation of the tip configuration that was initially designed for use in atherosclerotic vessels filled with plaque. The J-tip deflects off the edges of plaques and helps prevent subintimal dissection of the artery. The coatings on guidewires are materials that are designed to reduce friction; they include Teflon, heparin coatings, and, more recently, hydrophilic polymers. The latter type, called a **glide wire**, represents a major technologic advance in interventional radiology.

Catheters

Similar to guidewires, catheters are designed in many different shapes and sizes. Usually, catheter diameter is categorized in French (Fr) sizes, with 3 Fr equaling 1 mm in diameter. Figure 22-2 illustrates four common catheter shapes. The shaped tip of the catheter is required for selective catheterization of openings into specific arteries.

The H1 or headhunter tip designed by Vincent Hinck is used for the femoral approach to the brachiocephalic vessels. The Simmons catheter is highly curved for approach to sharply angled vessels and was also designed for cerebral angiography but was later adopted for visceral angiography. The C2 or Cobra catheter has an angled tip joined to a gentle curve and is used for introduction into celiac, renal, and mesenteric arteries.

Pigtail catheters have side holes for ejecting contrast media into a compact bolus. A catheter with side holes helps reduce a possible whiplash effect. The jet effect is minimized with the curved pigtail, which prevents injury to the vessel.

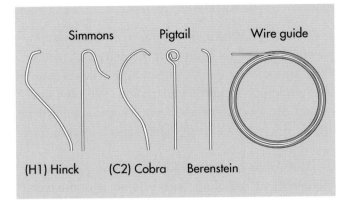

FIGURE 22-2 Typical catheter shapes.

Once the catheter is introduced into the vessel, the guidewire is removed. The catheter then must be flushed immediately to prevent clotting of blood within the catheter. Heparinized saline generally is used to flush catheters.

After catheter placement, a test injection is performed under fluoroscopy before static imaging to check that the catheter tip is not wedged and that it is in the correct vessel. Injection rates of the automatic power injector are gauged by the test flow speed.

Contrast Media

Vessels under investigation in angiography are injected with radiopaque contrast media. Initially, ionic iodine compounds were used for contrast injections; however, nonionic contrast media have largely replaced ionic agents. Because of their low concentration of ions (low osmolality), physiologic problems and adverse reactions are reduced for patients undergoing angiographic injection with nonionic contrast media.

Patient Preparation and Monitoring

Before angiography is performed, the radiologist visits the patient to establish rapport and to explain the procedure and its risks. A history and physical examination are necessary to assess the patient for allergies and other conditions so the radiologist can conclude whether a procedure is indicated and which route is optimal. Orders are written for intravenous hydration and a diet of clear liquids. The patient may be premedicated in the interventional radiologic suite to reduce anxiety.

During the procedure, monitoring by electrocardiography, automatic blood pressure measurement, and pulse oximetry is mandatory. The code or "crash" cart for life-threatening emergencies must be accessible. After the procedure has been performed, when the catheter is removed, the femoral puncture site must be manually compressed. The patient then is instructed to remain immobile for several hours after the angiographic procedure has been completed while vital signs are monitored and the puncture site inspected.

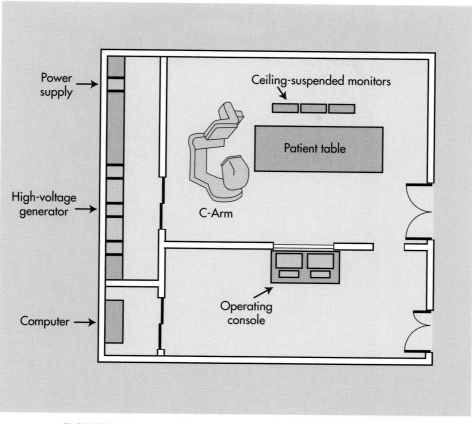

FIGURE 22-3 Typical layout for an interventional radiology suite.

Risks of Arteriography

The most common complication associated with catheter angiography is continued bleeding at the puncture site. Of course, the risk of reaction to contrast media is present, and other risk factors are related to kidney failure. Minimization of these risks requires a complete patient medical examination and the taking of surgical and allergy histories before any angiographic procedure can be done. Although uncommon, serious adverse reactions related to blood clot formation or catheter or guidewire penetrating injury can occur.

INTERVENTIONAL RADIOLOGY SUITE

Different from radiography and fluoroscopy, interventional radiology requires a suite of rooms (Figure 22-3). The procedure room itself should not be less than 20 ft along any wall and not less than 500 ft². This size is required to accommodate the quantity of equipment required and the large number of people involved in most procedures.

The procedure room usually has at least three means of access. Patient access should be available through a door wide enough to accommodate a bed. Access to the procedure room from the control room with the operating console does not usually require a door. An open passageway is adequate. Such doors interfere with movement of personnel.

The procedure room should be finished with consideration for maintaining a clean and sterile environment. The floor, walls, and all counter cabinet surfaces must be smooth and easily cleaned.

The control room should be large, perhaps 100 ft². Ideally, this room should communicate directly with the viewing areas. It also should have positive air pressure and filtered incoming air.

Personnel

A radiographer can specialize in many different fields. The radiographer who specializes in interventional radiography requires additional skills. The American Registry of Radiologic Technologists offers an examination in cardiovascular and interventional radiography. Once the examination is passed, the radiographer may add (CI) or (VI) after the RT (R).

Two or three radiographers may be present in the interventional radiography suite, as well as the interventional radiologist and a radiology nurse, who carefully monitors the patient. During procedures that require the patient to be highly medicated, an anesthesiologist also may be present.

Equipment

The x-ray apparatus for an interventional radiologic suite is generally more massive, flexible, and expensive than that required for conventional radiographic and

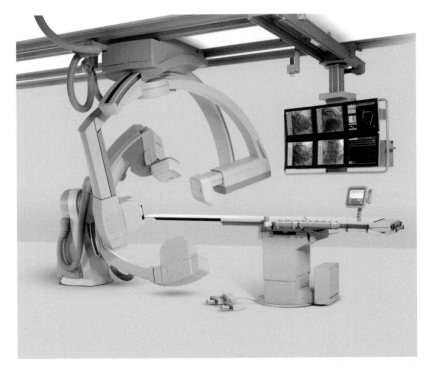

FIGURE 22-4 X-ray imaging apparatus in a typical interventional radiology suite. (Courtesy Brad Mattinson, Philips Medical Systems.)

TABLE 22-2	Specifications for a Typical Interventional X-ray Tube	
Feature	**Size**	**Why**
Focal spot	1.0 mm/0.3 mm	Large for heat load; small for magnification radiography
Disc size	15-cm diameter, 5 cm thick	To accommodate heat load
Power rating	80 kW	For rapid sequence, serial radiography
Anode heat capacity	1 MHU	To accommodate heat load

fluoroscopic imaging. Advanced radiographic and fluoroscopic equipment is required (Figure 22-4). Generally, two ceiling track–mounted radiographic x-ray tubes are required, along with an image-intensified fluoroscope mounted on a C or an L arm.

X-ray Tube. The x-ray tube used for interventional radiologic procedures has a small target angle, a large-diameter massive anode disc, and cathodes designed for magnification and serial radiography. Table 22-2 describes the specifications for such an x-ray tube.

A small focal spot of not greater than 0.3 mm is necessary for the spatial resolution requirements of small-vessel magnification radiography. Neuroangiography can be performed in contrast-filled vessels as small as 1 mm with typical selection of geometric factors and careful patient positioning.

When a source-to-image receptor distance (SID) of 100 cm and an object-to-image receptor distance (OID) of 40 cm are used, the radiographer can take advantage of the air gap to improve image contrast. A 0.3-mm focal spot results in a focal-spot blur of 0.2 mm.

Question: A left cerebral angiogram is performed with a 0.3-mm focal spot at 100 cm SID. The artery to be imaged is 20 cm from the image receptor. What is the magnification factor and the focal-spot blur?

Answer:
$$MF = \frac{100 \text{ cm SID}}{80 \text{ cm SOD}} = 1.25$$

$$FSB = 0.3\left(\frac{20 \text{ cm OID}}{80 \text{ cm SOD}}\right) = 0.075 \text{ mm}$$

Spatial resolution for this procedure can be approximated by multiplying the focal-spot blur by 2. Figure 22-5 shows geometry that results in 0.2-mm focal-spot blur images of a 1.0-mm vessel. A 0.5-mm vessel will be too blurred to be seen. Any vessel larger than 1.0 mm will be imaged.

All other essential characteristics of an interventional x-ray tube are based on required tube loading. The size and construction of the anode disc determine the anode heat capacity, which, in turn, influences the power

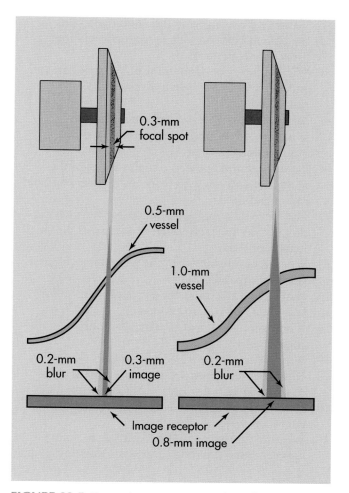

FIGURE 22-5 For a given geometry such as this one, which produces a 0.5-mm focal-spot blur, the vessels must be twice the size of the focal-spot blur.

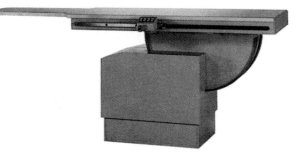

FIGURE 22-6 Typical interventional radiology patient couch with a floating, rotating, and tilting top. (Courtesy of Odelft Corporation.)

rating. An x-ray tube with a minimum 80 kW rating and 1 MHU heat capacity is required.

High-Voltage Generator. High-frequency generators are increasingly popular in all x-ray examinations, including interventional radiologic procedures. However, some interventional radiologic procedures require higher power than may be available with high-frequency generators. High-voltage generators with three-phase, 12-pulse power capable of at least 100 kW with low ripple are needed for such high power requirements.

Patient Couch. Whereas most general fluoroscopy imaging systems have a tilt table, interventional radiologic imaging systems do not. General fluoroscopy often requires head-down and head-up tilting of the patient for manipulation of contrast media. Imaging techniques such as myelography require a tilt couch; therefore, such procedures are common in general fluoroscopy.

Other imaging and interventional procedures do not require a tilt couch, but a stationary patient couch with a floating or movable tabletop is used instead

(Figure 22-6). Controls for couch positioning are located on the side of the table and are duplicated on a floor switch. The floor switch is necessary to accommodate patient positioning while a sterile field is maintained.

The patient couch may have computer-controlled **stepping** capability. This feature is necessary to allow imaging from the abdomen to the feet after a single injection of contrast medium. An additional requirement of this stepping feature is the ability to preselect the time and position of the patient couch to coincide with the image receptor.

Image Receptor. Two different types of image receptors are used in interventional radiologic procedures. The cinefluorographic camera is used during cardiac catheterization, but it is largely obsolete and has been replaced by digital image receptors. The digital image receptor begins with a television camera pickup tube or a charge-coupled device (CCD).

CCDs are photosensitive silicon chips that are rapidly replacing the television camera tube in the fluoroscopic chain. CCDs resemble computer chips and can be used anywhere that light is to be converted to a digital video image. CCDs are discussed more completely in Chapter 27.

SUMMARY

Angiography refers to the many ways of imaging contrast-filled vessels. In 1953, Sven Ivan Seldinger described a method of arterial access that uses an 18-gauge hollow needle with a stylet. Using a guidewire and a catheter, radiologists can access the vascular network without surgery. The common femoral artery is used most often for arterial access in angiography.

Catheter tip designs vary widely, and each is used for specific arteries. The contrast media used are generally nonionic; this reduces the incidence of physiologic problems and adverse reactions in patients undergoing angiographic procedures. During the procedure, the patient's vital signs must be monitored carefully. The most common risk to patients is continued bleeding at the puncture site.

The typical interventional radiologic x-ray tube is designed for magnification, high resolution, and massive heat loads. The patient couch is a floating tabletop with a stepping capability that automatically allows imaging from abdomen to feet after a single injection of contrast media.

Digital imaging generally is used for interventional procedures, with power injection of contrast media and imaging synchronized to optimize visualization of the vessel of interest.

CHALLENGE QUESTIONS

1. Define or otherwise identify the following:
   a. Angiographic contrast media
   b. Arteriography
   c. Seldinger technique
   d. Catheter
   e. Guidewire
   f. Arterial dissection
   g. Biplane imaging
   h. Tilt couch
   i. Venography
   j. Photofluorography
2. Describe cardiac catheterization.
3. What is the Seldinger method for arterial access?
4. What artery is used most often for arterial access in angiography?
5. Why is a guidewire used for arterial access of catheters?
6. List four types of catheters and the vessels for which they are designed.
7. Name two reasons why the radiologist visits the patient before an interventional radiologic procedure is performed.
8. What is the most common problem that patients encounter after an interventional radiologic procedure?
9. What are thrombolysis and embolization?
10. What is the required heating capacity of the interventional x-ray tube?
11. Name the titles and describe the duties of the team of personnel who work in the interventional radiologic suite.
12. List the focal-spot requirements for the interventional x-ray tube. For what procedure is the small focal spot used?
13. What does it mean when the patient couch has a stepping capability?
14. Name the frame rates for a cine camera.
15. List three "special procedures."
16. What is transbrachial selective coronary angiography?
17. Why are some catheters fenestrated?
18. How does osmolarity affect the action of a contrast agent?
19. What is the recommended minimum size for an interventional radiologic suite?
20. What initials may an ARRT with a specialty in interventional radiology place as a title postscript?

The answers to the Challenge Questions can be found by logging on to our website at http://evolve.elsevier.com.

Multislice Spiral Computed Tomography

OBJECTIVES

At the completion of this chapter, the student should be able
to do the following:

1. List and describe the various generations of computed tomography
   (CT) imaging systems
2. Relate the CT system components to their functions
3. Discuss image reconstruction via interpolation and back projection
4. Describe CT image characteristics of image matrix, Hounsfield unit,
   and sensitivity profile
5. Describe technique selection in CT
6. Explain the spiral imaging relationships among pitch, index, dose
   profile, and patient dose
7. Discuss image quality as it relates to spatial resolution, contrast
   resolution, noise, linearity, and uniformity
8. List the advantages and limitations of multislice spiral CT

OUTLINE

Principles of Operation
Generations of Computed
   Tomography
Imaging System Design
  Operating Console
  Computer
  Gantry
  Slip-Ring Technology
Image Characteristics
  Image Matrix
  CT Numbers
  Image Reconstruction
  Multiplanar Reformation
Image Quality
  Spatial Resolution
  Contrast Resolution
  Noise
  Linearity
  Uniformity

Multislice Spiral CT Imaging
   Principles
  Interpolation Algorithms
  Pitch
  Sensitivity Profile
Imaging Technique
  Multislice Detector Array
  Data Acquisition Rate
Computed Tomography Quality
   Control
  Noise and Uniformity
  Linearity
  Spatial Resolution
  Contrast Resolution
  Slice Thickness
  Couch Incrementation
  Laser Localizer
  Patient Dose

THE COMPUTED TOMOGRAPHY (CT) imaging system is revolutionary. No ordinary image receptor, such as film or an image-intensifier tube, is involved. A collimated x-ray beam is directed on the patient, and the attenuated image-forming x-radiation is measured by a detector whose response is transmitted to a computer.

After the signal from the detector is analyzed, the computer reconstructs the image and displays the image on a monitor. Computer reconstruction of the cross-sectional anatomy is accomplished with mathematical equations (algorithms) adapted for computer processing.

Spiral CT, which has emerged as a new and improved diagnostic tool, provides improved imaging of anatomy compromised by respiratory motion. Spiral CT is particularly good for the chest, abdomen, and pelvis, and it has the capability to perform conventional transverse imaging for regions of the body where motion is not a problem, such as the head, spine, and extremities.

This chapter introduces the physical principles of multislice spiral CT. Special imaging system design features and image characteristics are reviewed.

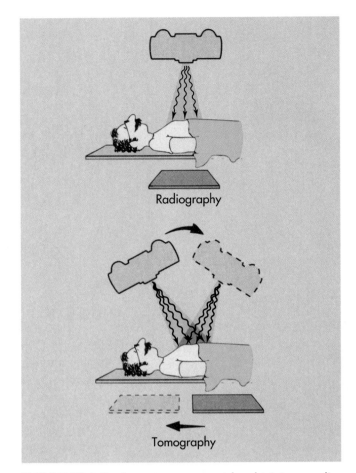

FIGURE 23-1 Equipment arrangement for obtaining a radiograph and a conventional tomograph.

The components necessary to construct a computed tomography (CT) imaging system were available to medical physicists 20 years before Godfrey Hounsfield first demonstrated the technique in 1970. Hounsfield was a physicist/engineer with EMI, Ltd., the British company most famous for recording the Beatles, and both he and his company justifiably have received high acclaim.

Alan Cormack, a Tufts University medical physicist, shared the 1979 Nobel Prize in physics with Hounsfield. Cormack had earlier developed the mathematics used to reconstruct CT images.

The CT imaging system is an invaluable radiologic diagnostic tool. Its development and introduction into radiologic practice have assumed an importance comparable with the Snook interrupterless transformer, the Coolidge hot-cathode x-ray tube, the Potter-Bucky diaphragm, and the image-intensifier tube. No other development in x-ray imaging over the past 50 years has been as significant.

PRINCIPLES OF OPERATION

When the abdomen is imaged with conventional radiographic techniques, the image is created directly on the screen-film image receptor and is low in contrast, principally because of scatter radiation. The image is

also degraded because of superposition of all the anatomic structures in the abdomen.

For better visualization of an abdominal structure, such as the kidneys, conventional tomography can be used (Figure 23-1). In nephrotomography, the renal outline is distinct because the overlying and underlying tissues are blurred. In addition, the contrast of the in-focus structures has been enhanced. Yet, the image remains rather dull and blurred.

Conventional tomography is called **axial tomography** because the plane of the image is parallel to the long axis of the body; this results in sagittal and coronal images. A CT image is a transaxial or **transverse** image that is perpendicular to the long axis of the body (Figure 23-2).

The precise method by which a CT imaging system produces a transverse image is extremely complicated, and understanding it requires strong knowledge of physics, engineering, and computer science. The basic principles, however, can be observed if one considers the simplest of CT systems, which consists of a finely collimated x-ray beam and a single detector. The x-ray source and the detector move synchronously.

When the source-detector assembly makes one sweep, or **translation,** across the patient, the internal structures

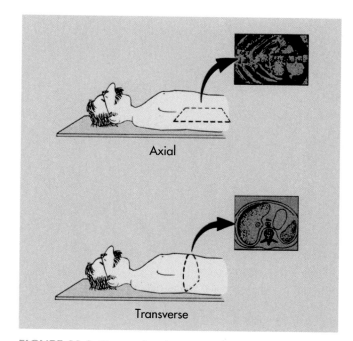

FIGURE 23-2 Conventional tomography results in an image that is parallel to the long axis of the body. Computed tomography (CT) produces a transverse image.

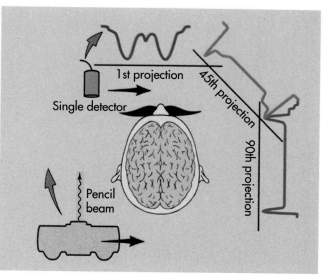

FIGURE 23-3 In its simplest form, a computed tomography (CT) imaging system consists of a finely collimated x-ray beam and a single detector, both of which move synchronously in a translate/rotate fashion. Each sweep of the source detector assembly results in a projection, which represents the attenuation pattern of the patient profile.

of the body attenuate the x-ray beam according to their mass density and effective atomic number, as was discussed in Chapter 10. The intensity of radiation detected varies according to this attenuation pattern, and an intensity profile, or **projection,** is formed (Figure 23-3).

At the end of this translation, the source detector assembly returns to its starting position, and the entire assembly **rotates** and begins a second translation. During the second translation, the detector signal again will be proportional to the x-ray beam attenuation of anatomic structures, and a second projection will be described.

If this process is repeated many times, a large number of projections are generated. These projections are not displayed visually but are stored in digital form in the computer. Computer processing of these projections involves effective superimposition of each projection to **reconstruct** an image of the anatomic structures within that slice.

Superimposition of these projections does not occur as one might imagine. The detector signal during each translation has a dynamic range of 12 bits (4096 gray levels). The value for each increment is related to the x-ray attenuation coefficient of the total path through the tissue. Through the use of simultaneous equations, a matrix of values is obtained that represents the transverse cross-sectional anatomy.

GENERATIONS OF COMPUTED TOMOGRAPHY

The previous description of a finely collimated x-ray beam and single detector assembly that translates across the patient and rotates between successive translations

is characteristic of **first-generation CT imaging systems.** The original EMI imaging system required 180 translations, which were separated from one another by a 1-degree rotation. It incorporated two detectors and split the finely collimated x-ray beam so that two contiguous slices could be imaged during each procedure. The principal drawback to these systems was that nearly 5 minutes was required to complete a single image.

 First-generation imaging system: translate/rotate, pencil beam, single detector, 5-minute imaging time.

First-generation CT imaging systems can be considered a demonstration project. They proved the feasibility of the functional marriage of the source-detector assembly, mechanical gantry motion, and the computer to produce an image.

Second-generation imaging systems were also of the translate/rotate type. These units incorporated the natural extension of the single detector to a multiple-detector assembly, while intercepting a fan-shaped rather than a pencil-shaped x-ray beam (Figure 23-4).

One disadvantage of the fan beam is the increased radiation intensity that occurs toward the edges of the beam because of body shape. This is compensated for with the use of a "bow tie" filter. These characteristic features of a first- versus a second-generation CT imaging system are shown in Figure 23-5.

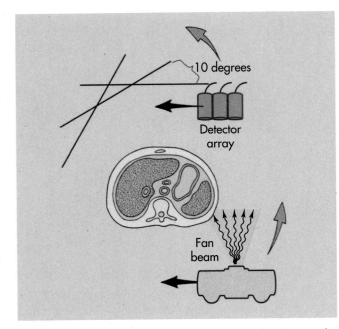

FIGURE 23-4 Second-generation computed tomography imaging systems operated in the translate/rotate mode with a multiple detector array intercepting a fan-shaped x-ray beam.

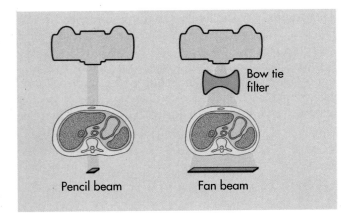

FIGURE 23-5 Profiles of two x-ray beams used in computed tomography (CT) imaging. With the fan-shaped beam of second generation, a bow-tie filter is used to equalize the radiation intensity that reaches the detector array. For first-generation CT, a pencil x-ray beam is used.

The principal advantage of the second-generation CT imaging system was speed. These imaging systems consisted of 5 to 30 detectors in the detector assembly; therefore, shorter imaging times were possible. Because of the multiple detector array, a single translation resulted in the same number of data points as several translations with a first-generation CT imaging system. Consequently, translations were separated by rotation increments of 5 degrees or more. With a 10-degree rotation increment, only 18 translations would be required for a 180-degree image acquisition.

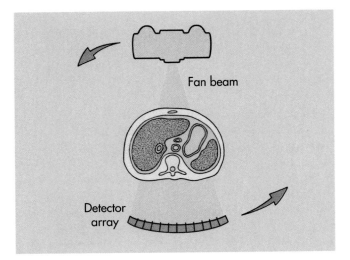

FIGURE 23-6 Third-generation computed tomography imaging systems operate in the rotate-only mode with a fan x-ray beam and a multiple detector array revolving concentrically around the patient.

Second-generation imaging system: translate/rotate, fan beam, detector array, 30-second imaging time.

The principal limitation of second-generation CT imaging systems was examination time. Because of the complex mechanical motion of translation/rotation and the enormous mass involved in the gantry, most units were designed for imaging times of 20 seconds or longer. This limitation was overcome by **third-generation CT imaging systems.** With these imaging systems, the source and the detector array are rotated about the patient (Figure 23-6). As rotate-only units, third-generation imaging systems can produce an image in less than 1 second.

The third-generation CT imaging system uses a curvilinear array that contains many detectors and a fan beam. The number of detectors and the width of the fan beam—between 30 and 60 degrees—are both substantially larger than for second-generation imaging systems. In third-generation CT imaging systems, the fan beam and the detector array view the entire patient at all times.

The curvilinear detector array produces a constant source-to-detector path length, which is an advantage for good image reconstruction. This feature of the third-generation detector assembly also allows for better x-ray beam collimation and reduces the effect of scatter radiation.

One of the principal disadvantages of third-generation CT imaging systems is the occasional appearance of ring artifacts. Should any single detector or bank of detectors malfunction, the acquired signal or lack thereof results in a ring on the reconstructed image (Figure 23-7). Software-corrected image reconstruction algorithms minimize such artifacts.

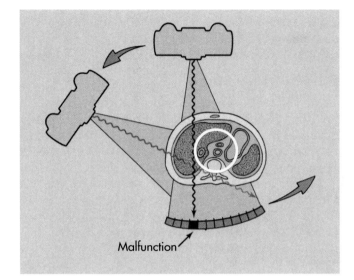

FIGURE 23-7 Ring artifacts can occur in third-generation computed tomography imaging systems because each detector views an annulus (ring) of anatomy during the examination. The malfunction of a single detector can result in the ring artifact.

 Third-generation imaging system: rotate/rotate, fan beam, detector array, subsecond imaging time, ring artifacts.

The **fourth-generation** design for CT imaging systems incorporates a rotate/stationary configuration. The x-ray source rotates, but the detector assembly does not.

Radiation detection is accomplished through a fixed circular array of detectors (Figure 23-8), which contains as many as 4000 individual elements. The x-ray beam is fan shaped with characteristics similar to those of third-generation fan beams. These units are capable of subsecond imaging times, can accommodate variable slice thickness through automatic prepatient collimation, and have the image manipulation capabilities of earlier imaging systems.

The fixed detector array of fourth-generation CT imaging systems does not result in a constant beam path from the source to all detectors, but it does allow each detector to be calibrated and its signal normalized for each image, as was possible with second-generation imaging systems. Fourth-generation imaging systems are free of ring artifacts.

 Fourth-generation imaging system: rotate/stationary, fan beam, detector array, subsecond imaging time.

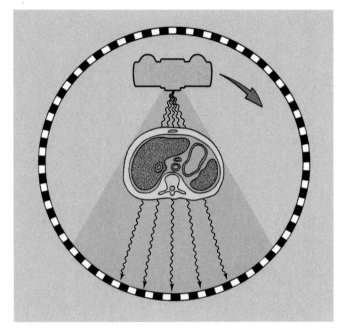

FIGURE 23-8 Fourth-generation computed tomography imaging systems operate with a rotating x-ray source and stationary detectors.

Continuing developments in CT imaging system design promise additional improvements in image quality at lower patient dose. Some incorporate novel motions of the x-ray tube or the detector array, or both. Some involve patient motion as well. None of these designs has been acclaimed as the fifth-generation design, but multislice spiral CT is the leading candidate.

Huge jumps occurred in development between the first and second generations, and even larger developments occurred between the second and third generations. The third-generation version became the de facto baseline model from which later generations were advanced.

IMAGING SYSTEM DESIGN

It is convenient to classify the components of a conventional x-ray imaging system into three major subsystems: the operating console, the generator, and the x-ray tube. It also is convenient to identify the three major components of a CT imaging system: the operating console, the computer, and the gantry (Figure 23-9). Each of these major components has several subsystems.

Operating Console

CT imaging systems can be equipped with two or three consoles. One console is used by the CT radiologic technologist to operate the imaging system. Another console may be available for a technologist to postprocess images for filming and filing. A third console may be available for the physician to view the images and manipulate image contrast, size, and general visual appearance.

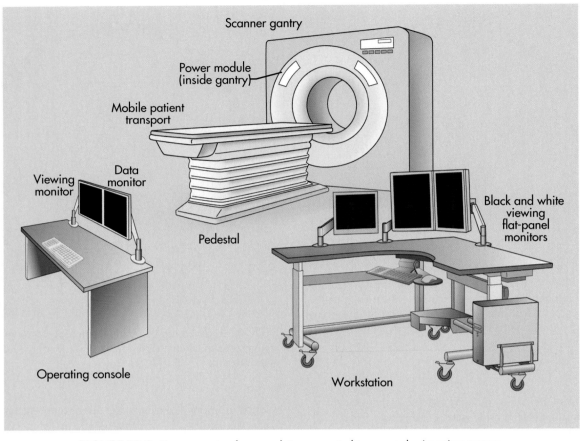

FIGURE 23-9 Components of a complete computed tomography imaging system.

The operating console contains meters and controls for selection of proper imaging technique factors, for proper mechanical movement of the gantry and the patient couch, and for the use of computer commands that allow image reconstruction and transfer. The physician's viewing console accepts the reconstructed image from the operator's console and displays it for viewing and diagnosis.

A typical operating console contains controls and monitors for the various technique factors (Figure 23-10). Operation is usually in excess of 120 kVp. The maximum mA is usually 400 mA and is modulated (varied) during imaging according to patient thickness to minimize patient dose. The thickness of the tissue slice to be imaged also can be adjusted. Nominal thicknesses are 0.5 to 5 mm. Slice thickness is selected from the console by adjustment of the automatic collimator and by selection of various rows of the detector assembly. Controls also are provided for automatic movement and for indexing of the patient support couch. This allows the operator to program for Z-axis location, tissue volume to be imaged, and spiral pitch.

The operating console usually includes two monitors. One is provided for the operator to annotate patient data on the image (e.g., hospital identification, name, patient number, age, gender) and to provide identification for each image (e.g., number, technique, couch position). The second monitor allows the operator to view the resulting image before transferring it to hard copy or to the physician's viewing console.

Physician's Work Station. This console allows the physician to call up any previous image and manipulate that image to optimize diagnostic information. The manipulative controls provide for contrast and brightness adjustments, magnification techniques, region of interest (ROI) viewing, and use of on-line computer software packages.

This software may include programs designed to generate plots of CT numbers along any preselected axis, computation of mean and standard deviations of CT values in an ROI, subtraction techniques, and planar and volumetric quantitative analysis. Reconstruction of images along coronal, sagittal, and oblique planes is also possible.

The physician's viewing console is usually remote from the CT suite and is used for postprocessing tasks for all digital images (see Chapter 29). It also can be linked to a Picture Archiving and Communication Systems (PACS) network.

Computer

The computer is a unique subsystem of the CT imaging system. Depending on the image format, as many as 250,000 equations must be solved simultaneously; thus, a large computing capacity is required.

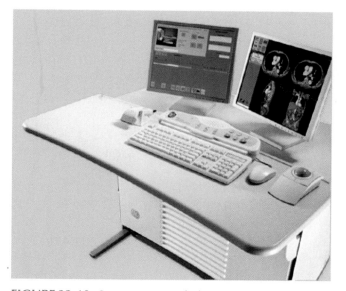

FIGURE 23-10 Operator's console for a multislice spiral computed tomography imaging system. (Courtesy Reggie Carter, General Electric Medical Systems.)

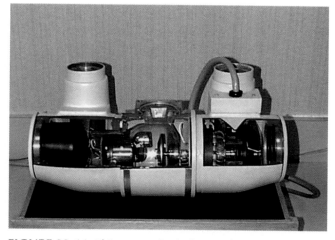

FIGURE 23-11 This x-ray tube is designed especially for spiral computed tomography. It has a 15-cm-diameter disc that is 5 cm thick with an anode heat capacity of 7 MHU. (Courtesy Randy Hood, Philips Medical Systems.)

At the heart of the computer used in CT are the microprocessor and the primary memory. These determine the time between the end of imaging and the appearance of an image—the **reconstruction time.** The efficiency of an examination is influenced greatly by reconstruction time, especially when a large number of image slices are involved.

> Reconstruction time is the time from the end of imaging to appearance of the image.

Many CT imaging systems use an **array processor** instead of a microprocessor for image reconstruction. The array processor does many calculations simultaneously and hence is significantly faster than the microprocessor.

Gantry

The gantry includes the x-ray tube, the detector array, the high-voltage generator, the patient support couch, and the mechanical support for each. These subsystems receive electronic commands from the operating console and transmit data to the computer for image production and postprocessing tasks.

X-ray Tube. X-ray tubes used in multislice spiral CT imaging have special requirements. Multislice spiral CT places a considerable thermal demand on the x-ray tube. The x-ray tube can be energized up to 60 s continuously. Although some x-ray tubes operate at relatively low tube current, for many the instantaneous power capacity must be high.

High-speed rotors are used in most for the best heat dissipation. Experience has shown that x-ray

tube failure is a principal cause of CT imaging system malfunction and is the principal limitation on sequential imaging frequency.

Focal-spot size is also important in most designs, even though the CT image is not based on principles of direct projection imaging. CT imaging systems designed for high spatial resolution imaging incorporate x-ray tubes with a small focal spot.

Multislice spiral CT x-ray tubes are very large. They have an anode heat storage capacity of 8 MHU or more. They have anode-cooling rates of approximately 1 MHU per minute because the anode disc has a larger diameter, and it is thicker, resulting in much greater mass.

The limiting characteristics are focal-spot design and heat dissipation. The small focal spot must be especially robust in design. Manufacturers design **focal-spot cooling algorithms** to predict the focal-spot thermal state and to adjust the mA setting accordingly. The x-ray tube in Figure 23-11 is designed especially for spiral CT. This x-ray tube is expected to last for at least 50,000 exposures—the approximate x-ray tube life for conventional CT.

One company has produced a revolutionary x-ray tube in which the whole insert rotates in a bath of oil during an exposure. The beam of electrons is deflected onto the anode in a process similar to that seen in a cathode ray tube (CRT). The result is that it can withstand up to 30 million heat units and cools at a rate of 5 million heat units per minute (see Figure 7-16).

Detector Array. Multislice spiral CT imaging systems have multiple detectors in an array that numbers up to tens of thousands (Figure 23-12). Previously, gas-filled detectors were used, but now, all are scintillation, solid state detectors.

Early scintillation detector arrays contained scintillation crystal–photomultiplier tube assemblies. These detectors could not be packed very tightly together, and

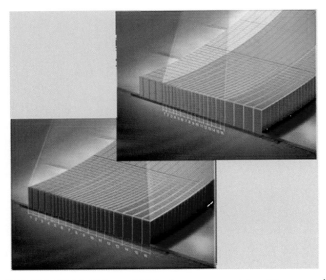

FIGURE 23-12 This multidetector array contains 64 rows of 1824 individual detectors, each 0.6 mm wide (116,736 detectors). (Courtesy Andrew Moehring, General Electric Medical Systems.)

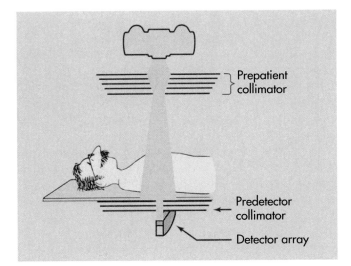

FIGURE 23-13 Multislice spiral computed tomography imaging systems incorporate both a prepatient collimator and a predetector collimator.

they required a power supply for each photomultiplier tube. Consequently, they have been replaced with scintillation crystal–photodiode assemblies.

Photodiodes convert light into an electronic signal. They are smaller and cheaper and do not require a power supply.

Sodium iodide (NaI) was the crystal used in the earliest imaging systems. This was quickly replaced by bismuth germanate ($Bi_4Ge_3O_{12}$ or BGO) and cesium iodide (CsI). Cadmium tungstate ($CdWO_4$) and special ceramics are the current crystals of choice. The concentration of scintillation detectors is an important characteristic of a CT imaging system that affects the spatial resolution of the system.

Scintillation detectors have high x-ray detection efficiency. Approximately 90% of the x-rays incident on the detector are absorbed, and this contributes to the output signal. It is now possible to pack the detectors so that the space between them is nil. Consequently, overall detection efficiency approaches 90%. The efficiency of the x-ray detector array reduces patient dose, allows faster imaging time, and improves image quality by increasing signal-to-noise ratio. Detector array design is especially critical for multisclice spiral CT.

Collimation. Collimation is required during multislice spiral CT imaging for precisely the same reasons as in conventional radiography. Proper collimation reduces patient dose by restricting the volume of tissue irradiated. Even more important is the fact that it improves image contrast by limiting scatter radiation.

In conventional radiography, only one collimator is mounted on the x-ray tube housing. In multislice spiral CT imaging, two collimators usually are used (Figure 23-13).

One collimator is mounted on the x-ray tube housing or adjacent to it. This collimator limits the area of

the patient that intercepts the useful beam, and thereby determines patient dose. This **prepatient collimator** usually consists of several sections, so a nearly parallel x-ray beam results.

> Prepatient collimation determines dose profile and patient dose.

The **predetector collimator** restricts the x-ray beam viewed by the detector array. This collimator reduces the scatter radiation incident on the detector array and, when properly coupled with the prepatient collimator, defines the slice thickness, also called the *sensitivity profile*. The predetector collimator reduces scatter radiation that reaches the detector array, thereby improving image contrast.

> The predetector collimator determines sensitivity profile and slice thickness.

High-Voltage Generator. All multislice spiral CT imaging systems operate on high-frequency power. A high-frequency generator is small because the high-voltage step-up transformer is small, so it can be mounted on the rotating gantry.

The design constraints placed on the high-voltage generator are the same as those for the x-ray tube. In a properly designed multislice spiral CT imaging system, the two should be matched to maximum capacity. Approximately 50 kW power is necessary.

Patient Positioning and the Support Couch. In addition to supporting the patient comfortably, the

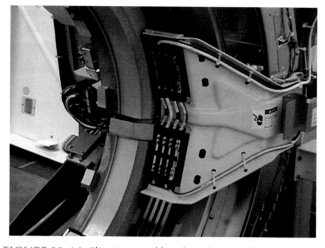

FIGURE 23-14 Slip rings and brushes electrically connect the components on the rotating gantry with the rest of the multislice spiral computed tomography imaging system. (Courtesy Terry Williams, Toshiba Medical Systems.)

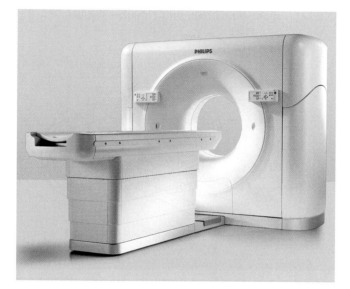

FIGURE 23-15 The gantry of this multislice spiral computed tomography imaging system contains a high-voltage generator, an x-ray tube, a detector array, and assorted control systems. (Courtesy Brad Mattinson, Philips Medical Systems.)

patient couch must be constructed of low-Z material, such as carbon fiber, so it does not interfere with x-ray beam transmission and patient imaging. It should be smoothly and accurately motor driven to allow precise patient positioning that is unaffected by the weight of the patient.

When patient couch positioning is not exact, the same tissue can be imaged twice, thus doubling the dose, or it can be missed altogether. The patient couch is indexed automatically, so the operator does not have to enter the examination room between imaging sequences. Such a feature reduces the examination time required for each patient.

Slip-Ring Technology

Slip rings are electromechanical devices that conduct electricity and electrical signals through rings and brushes from a rotating surface onto a fixed surface. One surface is a smooth ring and the other a ring with brushes that sweep the smooth ring (Figure 23-14). Spiral CT is made possible by the use of slip-ring technology, which allows the gantry to rotate continuously without interruption.

Early CT imaging was performed with a pause between gantry rotations. During the pause, the patient couch was moved and the gantry was rewound to a starting position.

In a slip-ring gantry system, power and electrical signals are transmitted through stationary rings within the gantry, thus eliminating the need for electrical cables and making continuous rotation impossible.

Slip rings make multislice spiral CT possible.

Brushes that transmit power to the gantry components glide in contact grooves on the stationary slip ring. Composite brushes made of conductive material (e.g., silver graphite alloy) are used as a sliding contact. The rings should last for the life of the imaging system. The brushes have to be replaced every year or so during preventive maintenance.

Figure 23-15 shows how compact a rotating gantry must be.

IMAGE CHARACTERISTICS

The image obtained in CT is different from that obtained in conventional radiography. It is synthetic in that it is artificially created from data received and is not a projected image. In radiography, x-rays form an image directly on the image receptor. With CT imaging systems, the x-rays form a stored electronic image that is displayed as a matrix of intensities.

Image Matrix

The CT image format consists of many cells, each assigned a number and displayed as an optical density or brightness level on the monitor. The original EMI format consisted of an 80 × 80 matrix, for a total of 6400 individual cells of information. Current imaging systems provide matrices of 512 × 512, resulting in 262,144 cells of information.

Each cell of information is a **pixel** (picture element), and the numeric information contained in each pixel is a CT number, or **Hounsfield unit (HU)**. The pixel is a two-dimensional representation of a corresponding tissue volume (Figure 23-16).

The diameter of image reconstruction is called the **field of view (FOV)**. When the FOV is increased for

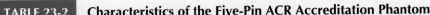

TABLE 23-2	Characteristics of the Five-Pin ACR Accreditation Phantom			
Material		Density, g/cm³	Linear Attenuation Coefficient (cm⁻¹) at 60 keV	CT Number
Polyethylene	C_2H_4	0.94	0.185	−85
Polystyrene	C_8H_8	1.05	0.196	−85
Nylon	$C_6H_{11}NO$	1.15	0.222	100
Lexan	$C_{16}H_{14}O$	1.20	0.223	115
Plexiglas	$C_5H_8O_2$	1.19	0.229	130
Water	H_2O	1.00	0.206	0

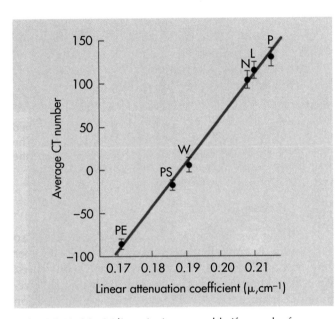

FIGURE 23-30 CT linearity is acceptable if a graph of average CT number versus the linear attenuation coefficient is a straight line that passes through 0 for water.

CT numbers along any axis of the image as a histogram or as a line graph. If all values of the histogram or line graph are within two standard deviations of the mean value ($\pm 2\sigma$), the system is said to exhibit acceptable spatial uniformity. X-ray beam hardening may cause a decrease in CT numbers so that the middle of the image appears darker than the periphery. This is the "cupping" artifact, and it can be clearly demonstrated by imaging the water bath inside a Teflon ring to simulate bone.

MULTISLICE SPIRAL CT IMAGING PRINCIPLES

Actually, the spiral motion in multislice spiral CT is not like a slinky toy; it just appears that way. Figure 23-31 shows the difference.

When the examination begins, the x-ray tube rotates continuously. While the x-ray tube is rotating, the couch moves the patient through the plane of the rotating x-ray beam. The x-ray tube is energized continuously, data are collected continuously, and an image then can

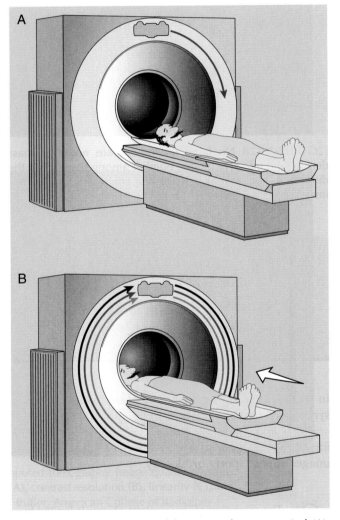

FIGURE 23-31 Movement of the x-ray tube is not spiral (A). It just appears that way because the patient moves through the plane of rotation during imaging (B).

be reconstructed at any desired z-axis position along the patient (Figure 23-32).

Interpolation Algorithms

Reconstruction of an image at any z-axis position is possible because of a mathematical process called interpolation. Figure 23-33 presents a graphic representation of interpolation and extrapolation. If one wishes

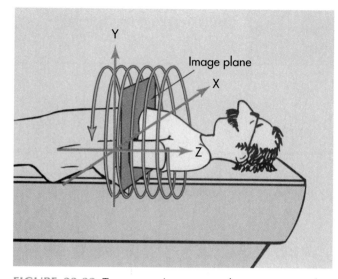

FIGURE 23-32 Transverse images can be reconstructed at any plane along the z-axis.

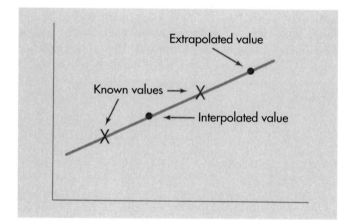

FIGURE 23-33 Interpolation estimates a value between two known values. Extrapolation estimates a value beyond known values.

to estimate a value between known values, that is interpolation; if one wishes to estimate a value beyond the range of known values, that is extrapolation.

During spiral CT, image data are received continuously, as shown by the data points in Figure 23-34, *A*. When an image is reconstructed, as in Figure 23-34, *B*, the plane of the image does not contain enough data for reconstruction. Data in that plane must be estimated by interpolation.

Data interpolation is performed by a special computer program called an **interpolation algorithm.** The first interpolation algorithms used 360-degree linear interpolation. The plane of the reconstructed image was interpolated from data acquired one revolution apart.

When these images are formatted into sagittal and coronal views, prominent blurring can occur compared with conventional CT reformatted views. The solution to the blurring problem is interpolation of values separated by 180 degrees—half a revolution of the x-ray tube.

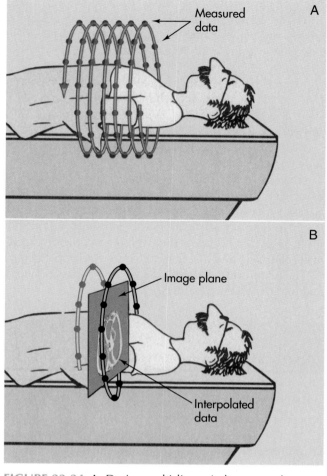

FIGURE 23-34 **A,** During multislice spiral computed tomography, image data are continuously sampled. **B,** Interpolation of data is performed to reconstruct the image in any transverse plane.

This results in improved z-axis resolution and greatly improved reformatted sagittal and coronal views.

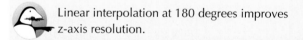

Linear interpolation at 180 degrees improves z-axis resolution.

Pitch

In addition to improved sagittal and coronal reformatted views, 180-degree interpolation algorithms allow imaging at a pitch greater than one. Spiral pitch ratio, referred to simply as **pitch,** is the relationship between patient couch movement and x-ray beam width.

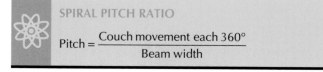

SPIRAL PITCH RATIO

$$\text{Pitch} = \frac{\text{Couch movement each } 360°}{\text{Beam width}}$$

Pitch is expressed as a ratio, such as 0.5:1, 1.0:1, 1.5:1, or 2:1. A pitch of 0.5:1 results in overlapping images and higher patient dose. A pitch of 2:1 results in extended imaging and reduced patient dose.

Question: During a 360-degree x-ray tube rotation, the patient couch moves 8 mm. Beam width is 5 mm. What is the pitch?

Answer: $\dfrac{8\,mm}{5\,mm} = 1.6:1$

Increasing pitch to above 1:1 increases the volume of tissue that can be imaged at a given time. This is one advantage of multislice spiral CT: the ability to image a larger volume of tissue in a single breath-hold. It is particularly helpful in CT angiography, radiation therapy treatment planning, and imaging of uncooperative patients.

The relationship between the volume of tissue imaged and pitch is given as follows:

VOLUME IMAGING
Tissue imaged = Beam width × Pitch × Imaging time

Table 23-3 shows this relationship for a fixed imaging time and a fixed beam width.

Question: How much tissue will be imaged if beam width is set to 8 mm, imaging time is 25 s, and pitch is 1.5:1?

Answer: Tissue imaged = 8 mm × 25 s × 1.5 = 300 mm = 30 cm

What if the gantry rotation time is not 360 degrees in 1 second? In such a situation, the volume of tissue imaged becomes as follows:

VOLUME IMAGING
$$Tissue\ imaged = \frac{Beam\ width \times Pitch \times Image\ time}{Gantry\ rotation\ time}$$

If the gantry rotation time is reduced to 0.5 seconds, Table 23-3 is changed to Table 23-4. With the availability of such fast multislice spiral CT, whole-body imaging is now possible within a single breath-hold.

TABLE 23-3   Tissue Imaged With Changing Pitch

Beam width (mm)	10	10	10	10
Imaging time (s)	30	30	30	30
Pitch	1.0:1	1.3:1	1.6:1	2.0:1
Tissue imaged (cm)	30	39	48	60

TABLE 23-4   Tissue Imaged With Changing Pitch and a Gantry Rotation Time of 0.5 s

Beam width (mm)	10	10	10
Scan time (s)	30	30	30
Gantry rotation time (s)	0.5	0.5	0.5
Pitch	1.0:1	1.5:1	2.0:1
Tissue imaged (cm)	60	90	120

Question: How much tissue will be imaged with a 5-mm beam width, a pitch of 1.6:1, and a 20-s image time at a gantry rotation time of 2 s?

Answer: $Tissue\ imaged = \dfrac{5\ mm \times 1.6 \times 20s}{2\ s}$
= 80 mm
= 8 cm

Question: One wishes to image 40 cm of tissue with a beam width of 8 mm in 25 s. If the gantry rotation time is 1.5 s, what should be the pitch?

Answer: Pitch
$= \dfrac{Tissue\ image \times Gantry\ rotation\ time}{Beam\ width \times Image\ time}$
$= \dfrac{400\ mm \times 1.5\ s}{8\ mm \times 25\ s}$
$= \dfrac{600}{200}$
$= 3.0:1$

In multislice spiral CT the entire width of the multidetector array (or at least those rows of detectors used for a particular imaging task) intercepts the collimated x-ray beam (Figure 23-35). For example, if all detectors of a 16-detector array are used, each of which is 1.25 mm in width, then when the patient couch translates 20 cm, the pitch is 1.0 because the beam width is also 20 cm (Figure 23-36).

If only the central rows of detectors are used, the x-ray beam width is collimated to 10 cm. Now, if the patient couch translates 20 cm, an extended spiral with a beam pitch of 2.0 is observed.

Question: The beam width during 64 slice spiral CT is 32 mm. If the patient couch moves 16 mm per revolution, what is the beam pitch?

Answer: $Pitch = \dfrac{Patient\ movement / 360°}{Beam\ width}$
$= 16\ mm/8\ mm$
$= 2.0:1,\ an\ extended\ spiral$

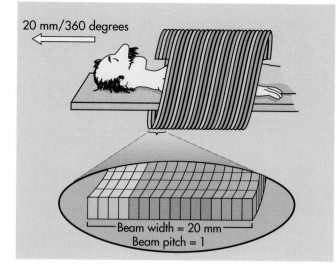

FIGURE 23-35 A 16-detector array, each array 1.25 mm wide, collimated to a 20-mm beam width results in a pitch of 1.0.

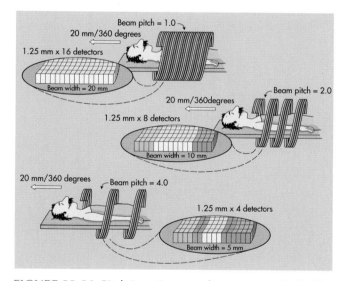

FIGURE 23-36 Pitch is patient couch movement divided by x-ray beam width.

In practice, the pitch for multislice spiral CT is usually 1.0. Because multiple slices are obtained and z-axis location and reconstruction width can be selected after imaging, overlapping images are unnecessary.

An exception is CTA, which requires a pitch of less than 1.0:1. Because of multislice capability, more slices are acquired per unit time. This results in a much larger volume of imaged tissue.

Unfortunately, when beam pitch exceeds approximately 1.0:1, the z-axis resolution is reduced because of a wide section sensitivity profile (SSP).

Sensitivity Profile

Consider the sensitivity profile of a 5-mm section obtained with a step and shoot CT imaging system (Figure 23-37). If properly collimated, it will have a **full**

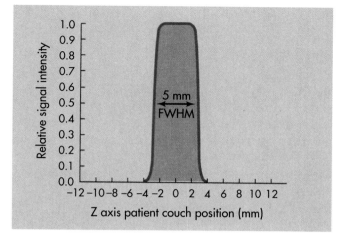

FIGURE 23-37 The section sensitivity profile (SSP) for a conventional computed tomography imaging system is nearly rectangular and is identified by its full width at half maximum (FWHM).

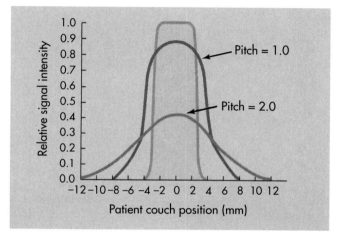

FIGURE 23-38 The section sensitivity profile for multislice spiral computed tomography widens as pitch is increased.

width at half maximum (FWHM) of 5 mm. The FWHM is the width of the sensitivity profile at one half of its maximum value.

At a multislice pitch of 1:1, the sensitivity profile is only approximately 10% wider than in conventional CT (Figure 23-38). However, at a pitch of 2:1, the sensitivity profile is approximately 40% wider.

IMAGING TECHNIQUE
Multislice Detector Array

By the end of the millennium, every CT vendor had developed and marketed multislice spiral CT imaging systems. These multislice spiral CT imaging systems have two principal distinguishing features. First, instead of a detector array, multislice spiral CT requires several parallel detector arrays that contain thousands of individual detectors (see Figure 23-12). Second, quickly energizing such a large detector array for large-volume imaging requires a very fast large-capacity computer.

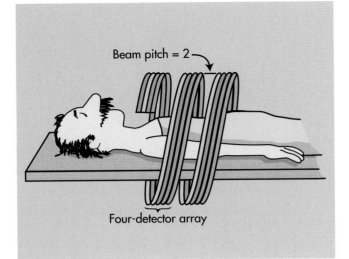

FIGURE 23-39 A four-slice spiral CT with a pitch of 2.0 covers eight times the tissue volume of single-slice spiral computed tomography.

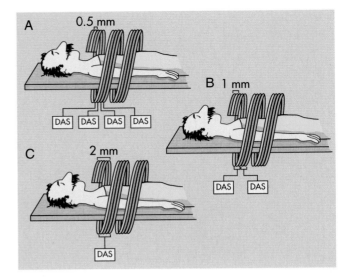

FIGURE 23-40 A four-slice spiral CT allows changes to be made in slice thickness. **A,** Four slices of 0.5 mm each. **B,** Two 0.5-slices can be combined to make two 1-mm slices. **C,** Four 0.5-mm slices can be combined to make one 2-mm slice. DAS, Data acquisition system.

After the initial demonstration of dual-slice imaging in the early 1990s, detector arrays that provide up to 320 image slices simultaneously are now available.

A simple approach to multislice spiral CT imaging is the use of four detector arrays, each of equal width. This design is shown in Figure 23-39 with a beam pitch of 2.0:1—the x-ray beam width is half the patient couch movement. The width of each detector array is 0.5 mm, resulting in four slices, each of 0.5-mm width.

The design of such a multislice CT imaging system usually allows detected signals from adjacent arrays to be combined to produce two slices of 1-mm width or one slice of 2-mm width (Figure 23-40). Wider slice imaging results in better contrast resolution at the same mA setting because the detected signal is larger.

This improvement in contrast resolution is accompanied by a slight reduction in spatial resolution due to increased voxel size. Alternatively, a larger tissue volume can be imaged with original contrast resolution at a reduced mA setting.

 Wider multislices allow imaging of greater tissue volume.

An alternate approach to four-slice imaging is shown in Figure 23-41. This design uses eight detector arrays of different widths. By combining adjacent arrays, one can obtain four 0.5-mm slices, four 1-mm slices, four 2-mm slices, or four 4-mm slices (Figure 23-42).

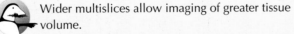 Smaller detector size results in better spatial resolution.

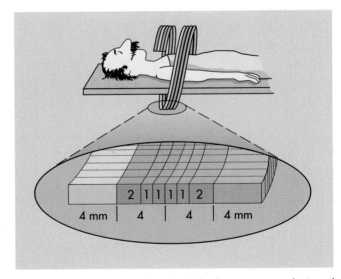

FIGURE 23-41 An asymmetric eight-detector array designed to provide four slices.

This discussion of multislice spiral CT has used four slices for simplicity as an example. In fact, multislice spiral CT has progressed from 4 to 16, to 64, and to 320 in a very short time.

A dual source multislice CT imaging system is shown in Figure 23-43. This system has two x-ray tubes and two detector arrays mounted on the revolving gantry. Imaging speed is its principal advantage; 80 ms imaging is possible.

Data Acquisition Rate

Multislice spiral CT results in acquisition of multiple slices in the same time previously required for a single slice. The slice acquisition rate (SAR) is one measure

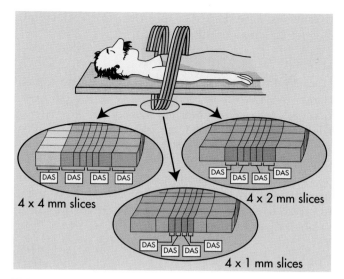

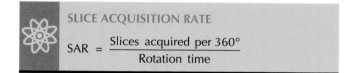

4 × 4 mm slices

4 × 2 mm slices

4 × 1 mm slices

FIGURE 23-42 The asymmetric eight-detector array allows slice thickness to be selected by switching the data acquisition system.

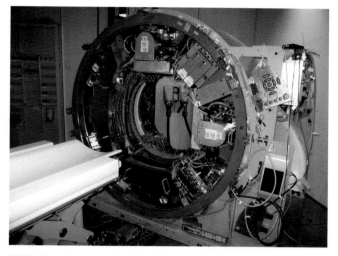

FIGURE 23-43 A dual-source multislice spiral CT imaging system. (Courtesy Jack Horwath, Siemens Medical Systems.)

of the efficiency of the multislice spiral CT imaging system.

SLICE ACQUISITION RATE

$$SAR = \frac{\text{Slices acquired per } 360°}{\text{Rotation time}}$$

Question: A 64-element multidetector array is used for 0.5-s multislice imaging. What is the SAR?

Answer:

$$SAR = \frac{\text{Slices acquired per } 360°}{\text{Rotation time}}$$

$$= \frac{64}{0.5} = 128$$

The principal advantage of multislice spiral CT is that a larger volume of tissue can be imaged. At the limit, it is now possible to image the entire body—from head to toe—in a single breath-hold. Although a volume of tissue is being imaged, this volume is represented by z-axis coverage as follows:

Z-AXIS COVERAGE (Z)

$Z = (N/R) \times W \times T \times B$

where N is the number of slices acquired, R is the rotation time, W is the slice width, T is the imaging time, and B is the pitch.

Z-AXIS COVERAGE (Z)

$Z = SAR \times W \times T \times B$

where SAR is the slice acquisition rate.

Question: A 64-slice examination is performed with a 32-mm x-ray beam width, and a 20-s examination at 0.5 s per revolution. What z-axis coverage is obtained? The patient couch translates 32 mm each revolution.

Answer: $Z = (N/R) \times W \times T \times B$
where $N = 64$,
 $R = 0.5$ s,
 $W = 0.5$ mm (64 ÷ 32 = 0.5 mm),
 $T = 20$ s, and
 $B = 1.0$.
 $Z = (64/0.5) \times 0.5 \times 20 \times 1 = 1280$ mm
 $= 128$ cm

The advantages and limitations of multislice spiral CT are summarized in Table 23-5.

COMPUTED TOMOGRAPHY QUALITY CONTROL

CT imaging systems are subject to all the misalignment, miscalibration, and malfunction difficulties of conventional x-ray imaging systems. They have the additional complexities of the multimotional gantry, the interactive console, and the associated computer.

Each of these subsystems increases the risk of drift and instability, which could result in degradation of image quality. Consequently, a dedicated quality control (QC) program is essential for each CT imaging system. Such a program includes daily, weekly, monthly, and annual monitoring, in addition to an ongoing preventive maintenance program.

Table 23-5 identifies the measurements and their required frequencies for an adequate QC program for a CT imaging system. Figure 23-44 shows a popular test object for CT measurements—the ACR CT accreditation phantom. The measurements specified for an annual performance also should be conducted for all new equipment and for all existing equipment after replacement or repair of a major component.

Noise and Uniformity

A 20-cm water bath should be imaged weekly; the average value for water should be within ±10 HU of zero. Furthermore, uniformity across the image should not vary by more than ±10 HU from center to periphery.

Nearly all CT imaging systems easily meet these performance specifications. If a system is used for quantitative CT, however, tighter specifications may be appropriate. When this assessment is performed, one should change one or more of the following: CT scan parameters, slice thickness, reconstruction diameter, or reconstruction algorithm.

Linearity

Linearity is assessed with an image of the American Association of Physicists in Medicine (AAPM) five-pin insert. Analysis of the values of the five pins should show a linear relationship between the Hounsfield unit and electron density. The coefficient of correlation for this linear relationship should be at least 0.96%, or 2 standard deviations.

This assessment should be conducted semiannually. It is particularly important for systems used for quantitative CT, which requires precise determination of the value of tissue in Hounsfield units.

TABLE 23-5	Features of Multislice Spiral Computed Tomography	
	What	**How/Why**
Advantages	No motion artifacts	Removes respiratory misregistration
	Improved lesion detection	Reconstructs at arbitrary z-axis intervals
	Reduced partial volume	Reconstructs at overlapping z-axis intervals
		Reconstructs smaller than image interval
	Optimized intravenous contrast	Data obtained during peak of enhancement
		Reduces volume of contrast agent
	Multiplanar images	Higher-quality reconstruction
	Improved patient throughput	Reduces imaging time
Limitations	Increased image noise	Bigger x-ray tubes needed
	Reduced z-axis resolution	Increases with pitch
	Increased processing time	More data, more images needed

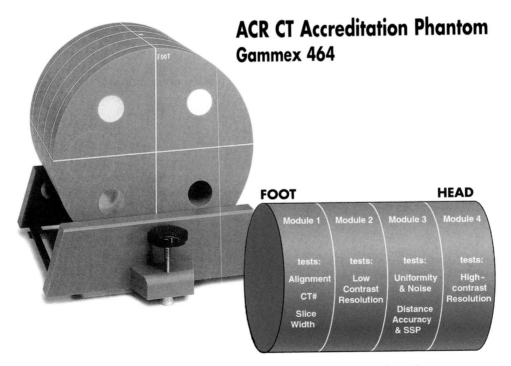

FIGURE 23-44 This CT test object is used to evaluate noise spatial resolution, contrast resolution, slice thickness, linearity, and uniformity. (Courtesy Priscilla Butler, American College of Radiology.)

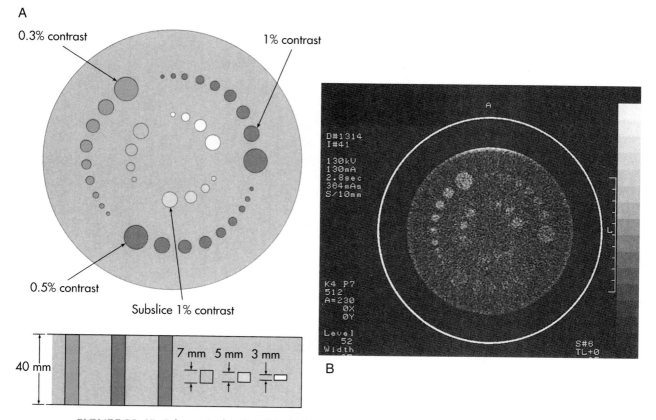

FIGURE 23-45 Schematic drawing **(A)** of a low-contrast CT test object and **(B)** its image. This test object is designed especially for multislice spiral CT. (Courtesy Josh Leavy, Phantom Laboratory.)

Spatial Resolution

Monitoring of spatial resolution is the most important component of this QC program. Constant spatial resolution ensures proper performance of the detector array, reconstruction electronics, and the mechanical components.

Spatial resolution is assessed by imaging a wire or an edge to obtain the point-spread function or the edge-response function, respectively. These functions then are mathematically transformed to obtain the modulation transfer function (MTF).

However, determining the MTF requires considerable time and attention. Most medical physicists find it acceptable to image a bar pattern or a hole pattern. Spatial resolution should be assessed semiannually and should be within the manufacturer's specifications.

Contrast Resolution

CT excels as an imaging modality because of its superior contrast resolution. The performance specifications of the various CT imaging systems differ from one manufacturer to another and from one model to another, depending on the design of the imaging system. All CT imaging systems should be capable of resolving 5-mm objects at 0.5% contrast.

Contrast resolution should be assessed semiannually. This is done with any of a number of low-contrast test objects with the built-in analytic schemes that are available on all CT imagers (Figure 23-45).

Slice Thickness

Slice thickness (sensitivity profile) is measured with the use of a specially designed test object that incorporates a ramp, a spiral, or a step wedge. This assessment should be done semiannually; the slice thickness should be within 1 mm of the intended slice thickness for a thickness of 5 mm or greater. For an intended slice thickness of less than 5 mm, the acceptable tolerance is 0.5 mm.

Couch Incrementation

With automatic maneuvering of the patient through the CT gantry, the patient must be precisely positioned. This evaluation should be done monthly. During a clinical examination with a patient-loaded couch, note the position of the couch at the beginning and at the end of the examination with the use of a tape measure and a straightedge on the couch rails. Compare this with the intended couch movement. It should be within ±2 mm.

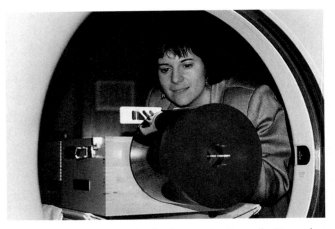

FIGURE 23-46 Medical physics evaluation of CT performance measurements using specially designed test objects. (Courtesy Cynthia McCullough, Mayo Clinic.)

Laser Localizer

Most CT imaging systems have internal and/or external laser-localizing lights for patient positioning. The accuracy of these lasers can be determined with any number of specially designed test objects. Their accuracy should be assessed at least semiannually; this is usually done at the same time as the evaluation of couch incrementation.

Patient Dose

No recommended limits are specified for patient dose during CT examination. Furthermore, dose varies considerably according to scan parameters. High-resolution imaging requires a higher dose.

When a fixed technique is used, patient dose should not vary by more than ±10% from one assessment to the next. Such an assessment should be done semiannually or should follow replacement of the x-ray tube.

Patient dose is specified as computed tomography dose index (CTDI) and can be monitored with specially designed pencil ionization chambers or thermoluminescent dosimeters. Figure 23-46 shows these measurements in progress.

SUMMARY

The multislice spiral CT imaging system does not record an image in a conventional way. The collimated x-ray beam is directed to the patient, the attenuated image-forming x-ray beam is measured by a detector array, the signal from the detector array is measured by a computer, the image is reconstructed in the computer, and, finally, the image is displayed on a television monitor or a flat-panel monitor.

Multislice spiral CT acquires transverse images, which are sections of anatomy that are perpendicular to the long axis of the body. The resultant computer image is an electronic matrix of intensities. Matrix size is usually 512 × 512 pixels. Each pixel contains numeric information called a CT number or a Hounsfield unit. The pixel is a two-dimensional representation of a corresponding tissue volume voxel.

Contrast resolution of the CT imaging system is excellent because of scatter radiation rejection due to x-ray beam collimation. The ability to image low-contrast anatomy is limited by the noise of the system. System noise is determined by the number of x-rays used by the detector array to produce the image.

Multislice spiral CT offers the following advantages over conventional step and shoot CT: (1) Motion blur is reduced, so fewer motion artifacts are noted; (2) imaging time is reduced; (3) partial volume artifact is reduced; and (4) a larger volume of tissue can be imaged.

When the examination begins, the x-ray tube rotates continuously and the patient couch moves through the plane of the rotating beam. The data collected are reconstructed at any desired z-axis position by interpolation.

Pitch is the ratio of patient couch movement to x-ray beam width. Increasing the pitch to above 1:1 increases the volume of tissue that can be imaged and at a reduced patient dose.

The need for the x-ray tube to be energized for longer periods demands higher power levels in the spiral CT x-ray tube. Solid state detector arrays with an overall detection efficiency of approximately 90% are preferred.

The volume of tissue imaged is determined by examination time, couch travel, pitch, and beam width. Improvement in z-axis spatial resolution is noted with spiral CT because no gaps in data are apparent and reconstruction images can even overlap. In addition, spiral CT excels in three-dimensional multiplanar reformation (MPR).

CHALLENGE QUESTIONS

1. Define or otherwise identify the following:
   a. Algorithm
   b. Transverse image
   c. Projection
   d. Interpolation
   e. Prepatient collimation
   f. Spatial frequency
   g. Hounsfield unit
   h. Slip ring
   i. MTF
   j. MIP
2. Name the individual who first demonstrated CT in 1970.
3. Explain the term "linear interpolation at 180 degrees."
4. What are the components in the gantry portion of the multislice spiral CT imaging system?
5. What are the special requirements of the x-ray tube as used in multislice spiral CT imaging?

6. Write the formula for the multislice spiral CT pitch.
7. What is the volume of tissue imaged with beam width thickness of 10 mm, scan time of 30 s, and pitch of 1.6:1?
8. Describe the two collimators used in CT imaging.
9. What material makes up the patient support couch?
10. Explain how slip-ring technology contributed to the development of spiral CT.
11. What is the voxel size of a CT imaging system with a 320×320 matrix size, a 20-cm reconstruction diameter, and a 0.5-cm slice thickness?
12. The volume of tissue imaged on spiral CT is determined by which technique selections?
13. Define multiplanar reformation (MPR).
14. Explain the mathematics of the multislice spiral CT image reconstruction process.

15. What type of high-voltage generator is used for multislice spiral CT?
16. A multislice spiral CT imaging system can resolve a 0.65-mm high-contrast object. What spatial frequency does this represent?
17. A 10-s multislice spiral CT examination is conducted with a 1.5:1 pitch and 5-mm beam width. How much tissue is imaged?
18. Why is multislice spiral CT pitch greater than 2:1 rarely used?
19. What determines in-plane spatial resolution?
20. What does the term *CT linearity* describe?

The answers to the Challenge Questions can be found by logging on to our website at http://evolve.elsevier.com.

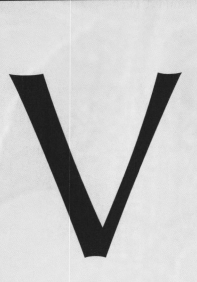

PART V

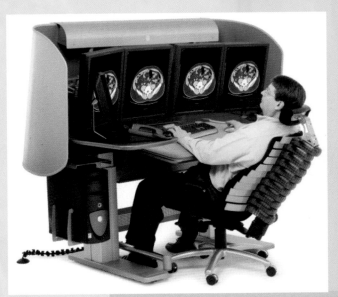

DIGITAL IMAGING

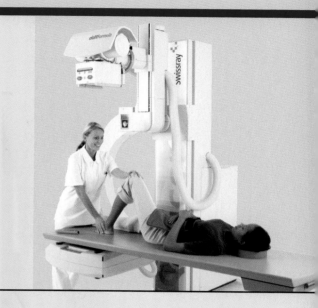

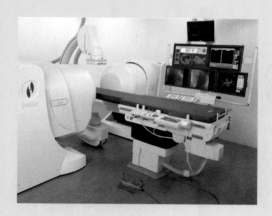

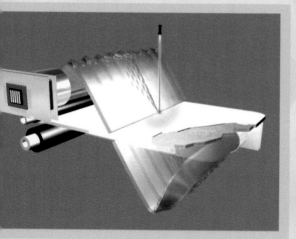

24

Computer Science

OBJECTIVES

At the completion of this chapter, the student should be able
to do the following:

1. Discuss the history of computers and the role of the transistor
2. Explain the difference betweens a microcomputer, a minicomputer, and a mainframe computer
3. List and define the components of computer hardware
4. Define "bit," "byte," and "word" as used in computer terminology
5. Contrast the two classifications of computer programs: systems software and applications programs
6. List and explain various computer languages
7. Discuss four computer processing methods

OUTLINE

History of Computers
Anatomy of a Computer
    Hardware
    Processing Methods
    Software
    Computer Languages

TODAY, THE word *computer* refers to the personal computer (PC), which is primarily responsible for the explosion in computer applications. In addition to scientific, engineering, and business applications, the computer has become evident in everyday life. For example, we know that computers are involved in video games, automatic teller machines (ATMs), and highway toll systems. Other everyday uses include supermarket checkouts, ticket reservation centers, industrial processes, touch-tone telephone systems, traffic lights, and automobile ignition systems.

Computer applications in radiology also continue to grow. The first large-scale radiology application was computed tomography (CT). Magnetic resonance imaging (MRI) and diagnostic ultrasonography use computers similarly to the way CT imaging systems do. Computers control x-ray generators and radiographic control panels, making digital fluoroscopy and digital radiography routine. Telecommunication systems have provided for the development of teleradiology—the transfer of images and patient data to remote locations for interpretation and filing. Teleradiology has changed the way human resources are allocated for these tasks.

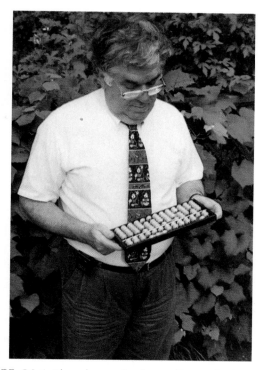

FIGURE 24-1 The abacus is the earliest calculating tool. (Courtesy Robert J. Wilson, University of Tennessee.)

HISTORY OF COMPUTERS

The earliest calculating tool, the abacus (Figure 24-1), was invented thousands of years ago in China and is still used in some parts of Asia. In the 17th century, two mathematicians, Blaise Pascal and Gottfried Leibniz, built mechanical calculators using pegged wheels that could perform the four basic arithmetic functions of addition, subtraction, multiplication, and division.

In 1842, Charles Babbage designed an analytical engine that performed general calculations automatically. Herman Hollerith designed a tabulating machine to record census data in 1890. The tabulating machine stored information as holes on cards that were interpreted by machines with electrical sensors. Hollerith's company later grew to become IBM.

In 1939, John Atansoff and Clifford Berry designed and built the first electronic digital computer.

In December 1943, the British built the first fully operational working computer, called Colossus, which was designed to crack encrypted German military codes. Colossus was very successful, but because of its military significance, it was given the highest of all security classifications and its existence was known only to relatively few people. That classification remained until 1976, which is why it is hardly ever acknowledged.

The first general purpose modern computer was developed in 1944 at Harvard University. Originally called the Automatic Sequence Controlled Calculator (ASCC), it is now known simply as the Mark I. It was an electromechanical device that was exceedingly slow and was prone to malfunction.

The first general purpose **electronic computer** was developed in 1946 at the University of Pennsylvania by J. Presper Eckert and John Mauchly at a cost of $500,000. This computer, called ENIAC (Electronic Numerical Integrator And Calculator), contained more than 18,000 vacuum tubes that failed at an average rate of 1 every 7 minutes (Figure 24-2). Neither the Mark I nor the ENIAC had instructions stored in a memory device.

In 1948, scientists led by William Shockley at the Bell Telephone Laboratories developed the transistor. A transistor is an electronic switch that alternately allows or does not allow electronic signals to pass. It made possible the development of the "stored program" computer and thus the continuing explosion in computer science.

The transistor allowed Eckert and Mauchly of the Sperry-Rand Corporation to develop **UNIVAC** (**UNIV**ersal **A**utomatic **C**omputer), which appeared in 1951 as the first commercially successful general purpose, stored-program electronic digital computer.

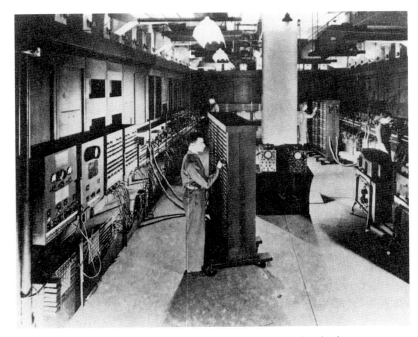

FIGURE 24-2 The ENIAC (Electronic Numerical Integrator And Calculator) computer occupied an entire room. It was completed in 1946 and is recognized as the first all-electronic, general purpose digital computer. (Courtesy Sperry-Rand Corporation.)

Computers have undergone four generations of development distinguished by the technology of their electronic devices. First-generation computers were vacuum tube devices (1939 to 1958). Second-generation computers, which became generally available in about 1958, were based on individually packaged transistors.

Third-generation computers used integrated circuits (ICs), which consist of many transistors and other electronic elements fused onto a chip—a tiny piece of semiconductor material, usually silicon. These were introduced in 1964. The microprocessor was developed in 1971 by Ted Hoff of Intel Corporation.

The fourth generation of computers, which first appeared in 1975, was an extension of the third generation and incorporated large-scale integration (LSI); this has now been replaced by very large-scale integration (VLSI), which places millions of circuit elements on a chip that measures less than 1 cm (Figure 24-3).

> The word *computer* refers to any general purpose, stored-program electronic digital computer.

The word *computer* today identifies the personal computer (PC) to most of us (Figure 24-4). This device is made of both electronic and electromechanical components. *General purpose* identifies a computer as able to solve a variety of problems. This is different from special purpose computers, which are designed for a particular singular task, such as control of an assembly line robot or an automobile ignition switch.

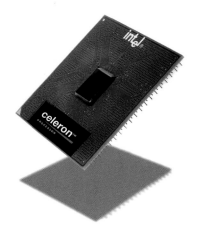

FIGURE 24-3 This Celeron microprocessor incorporates more than 1 million transistors on a chip of silicon that measures less than 1 cm on a side. (Courtesy Intel.)

All modern computers are stored-program computers because they have instructions (programs) and data stored in their memory. Stored-program computers are laid out so that the sequence of steps to be followed during any calculation is preestablished. *Electronic* implies that the computer is powered by electrical (transmits power) and electronic (transmits information) devices, rather than by a mechanical device.

Today, digital computers have replaced analog computers and the word *digital* is almost synonymous with computer. A timeline showing the evolution of computers shows how rapidly this technology is advancing (Figure 24-5).

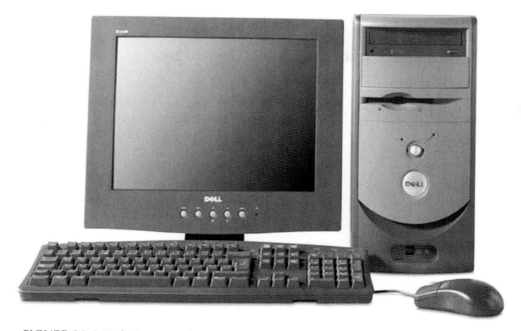

FIGURE 24-4 Today's personal computer has exceptional speed, capacity, and flexibility, and is used for numerous applications in radiology. (Courtesy Dell Computer Corporation.)

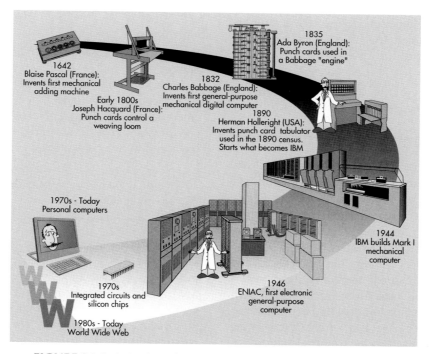

FIGURE 24-5 A timeline showing the evolution of today's computer.

 Analog refers to a continuously varying quantity; a *digital* system uses only two values that vary discretely through coding.

The difference between analog and digital is illustrated in Figure 24-6, which shows two types of watches. An analog watch is mechanical and has hands that move continuously around a dial face. A digital watch contains a computer chip and indicates time with numbers.

Analog and digital meters are used in many commercial and scientific applications. Digital meters are easier to read and can be more precise.

Computers are distinguished from calculators by their functionality. Most calculators can handle only arithmetic

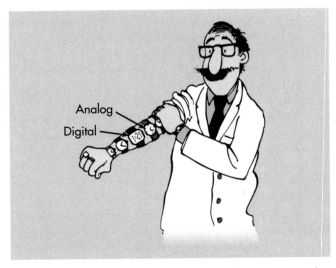

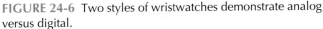

FIGURE 24-6 Two styles of wristwatches demonstrate analog versus digital.

functions, whereas computers can handle arithmetic and **logic functions:** "do," "if," "then," and "else." However, new technology has brought us advanced calculators with graphing and limited programming capabilities. Now, calculators can execute logic functions, solve equations, draw lines, and transmit data to or from other calculators or computers through cords or wireless.

 Logic functions evaluate an intermediate result and perform subsequent computations based on that result.

Computers also are often classified according to size, processing speed, and storage capacity. Distinguishing these types has become more difficult as technology improves, but they are defined as the following categories: supercomputers, mainframe computers, workstations, microcomputers, and microcontrollers.

Supercomputers are the fastest and highest-capacity computers, containing hundreds to thousands of microprocessors. They often are used for research in fields such as weather forecasting, oil exploration, and mathematics.

Mainframe computers are fast, mid-size to large, large-capacity systems that also have multiple microprocessors. They can support a few hundred to thousands of users and are found in airlines, banks, universities, and government offices.

Workstations, which were introduced in the early 1980s, are powerful desktop systems. They often are connected to larger computer systems for the purpose of transferring and sharing data and information. Workstations are used in computed radiography (CR), digital radiography (DR), and Picture Archiving and Communication System (PACS) networks for postprocessing and reporting of images.

Microcomputers, best known as PCs, also include electronic organizers and personal data assistants (PDAs), such as palmtop and hand-held systems.

Microcontrollers are tiny computers installed in "smart" appliances like microwave ovens and video games.

A radiographic operating console is controlled by a microcomputer that can analyze and control many characteristics of an examination. For example, when body part, patient size, and image receptor are selected, the microcomputer logically selects the proper radiographic technique.

ANATOMY OF A COMPUTER

A computer has two principal parts—hardware and software—each of which has several components. The **hardware** is everything about the computer that is visible—the nuts, bolts, and chips of the system that form the central processing unit (CPU) and the various input/output devices. Hardware usually is categorized according to which operation it performs. Operations include input processing, memory, storage, output, and communications.

The **software** is invisible. It consists of the computer programs that tell the hardware what to do and how to store and manipulate data.

Hardware

Input. Input hardware includes keyboards, pointing devices, and source data entry devices. A keyboard includes standard typewriter keys that are used to enter words and numbers and function keys that enter specific commands. Digital fluoroscopy (see Chapter 27) uses function keys for masking, reregistration, and time-interval difference imaging.

 Input hardware converts data into a form that the computer can use.

A **mouse** is a pointing device that the user rolls on a desktop or mouse pad to direct a pointer on the computer's display screen. High-end systems often use an optical mouse, which does not roll. The pointer is a symbol—often an arrow—that selects items from lists and menus or positions the cursor on the screen. The **cursor** indicates the insertion point on the screen where data may be entered.

A **trackball** is a variant of the mouse that usually is found in laptop computers. A **joystick** is a pointing device that is used primarily in video games and computer-aided design systems. Special joysticks are also available for people with certain disabilities.

Touchpads are small, rectangular devices that allow the user to control the cursor with a finger. A light pen connects by a wire to a computer display and, when pressed to the screen, identifies that screen position to the computer.

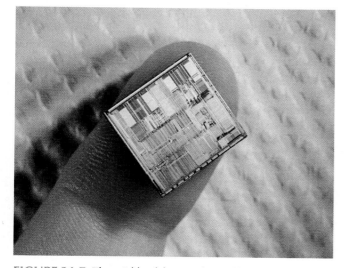

FIGURE 24-7 The width of the conductive lines in this microprocessor chip is 1.5 µm. (Courtesy Intel.)

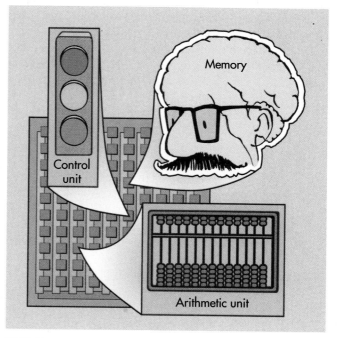

FIGURE 24-8 The central processing unit (CPU) contains a control unit, an arithmetic unit, and sometimes memory.

Pen-based systems use a penlike instrument to input handwriting and marks into a computer. Pen-based systems are used in hospitals to enter comments into patient records.

Source data entry devices include scanners, fax machines, imaging systems, audio and video devices, electronic cameras, voice-recognition systems, sensors, and biologic input devices. **Scanners** translate images of text, drawings, or photographs into a digital format recognizable by the computer. **Barcode readers,** which translate the vertical black-and-white–striped codes on retail products into digital form, are a type of scanner.

An **audio input device** translates analog sound into digital format. Similarly, video images, such as those from a VCR or camcorder, are digitized by a special video card that can be installed in a computer. Digital cameras and video recorders capture images in digital format that can easily be transferred to the computer for immediate access.

Voice-recognition systems add a microphone and an audio sound card to a computer and can convert speech into digital format. Radiologists use these systems to produce rapid diagnostic reports and to send findings to remote locations by teleradiology.

Sensors collect data directly from the environment and transmit them to a computer. Sensors are used to detect things like wind speed or temperature.

Human biology input devices detect specific movements and characteristics of the human body. Security systems that identify a person through a fingerprint or a retinal vascular pattern are examples of these devices.

Processing Methods

In large computers, the processing hardware is the central processing unit (CPU). In microcomputers, this is often referred to as the *microprocessor*. Figure 24-7 is a

photomicrograph of the Pentium microprocessor manufactured by the Intel Corporation. The Pentium processor is designed for large, high-performance, multiuser or multitasking systems.

 The electronic circuitry that does the actual computations and the memory that supports this together are called the *processor*.

A computer's processor (CPU) consists of a **control unit** and an **arithmetic/logic unit (ALU)**. These two components and all other components are connected by an electrical conductor called a **bus** (Figure 24-8). The control unit tells the computer how to carry out software instructions, which direct the hardware to perform a task. The control unit directs data to the ALU or to memory. It also controls data transfer between main memory and the input and output hardware (Figure 24-9).

The speed of these tasks is determined by an internal system clock. The faster the clock, the faster is the processing. Microcomputer processing speeds usually are defined in megahertz (MHz), where 1 MHz equals 1 million cycles per second. Today's microcomputers commonly run at up to several gigahertz (GHz; 1 GHz = 1000 MHz).

Workstations, microcomputers, and mainframes measure processing speed as MIPS (millions of instructions per second). Speeds can range from 100 MIPS in a workstation to 1200 MIPS (1.2 BIPS [billions of instructions per second]) in a mainframe. Supercomputer processing is measured in flops (floating-point

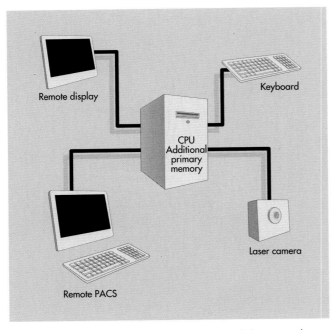

FIGURE 24-9 The control unit is a part of the central processing unit that is directly connected with additional primary memory and various input/output devices.

operations per second) and is represented as megaflops (mflops), gigaflops, and teraflops, which correspond to millions, billions, and trillions of flops, respectively.

The ALU performs arithmetic or logic calculations, temporarily holds the results until they can be transferred to memory, and controls the speed of these operations. The speed of the ALU is controlled by the system clock.

Memory. Computer memory is distinguished from storage by its function. Memory is more active, whereas storage is more archival. This active storage is referred to as memory, primary storage, internal memory, or random access memory (RAM). *Random access* means data can be stored or accessed at random from anywhere in main memory in approximately equal amounts of time, regardless of where the data are located.

RAM contents are temporary and RAM capacities vary widely in different computer systems. RAM capacity usually is expressed as megabytes (MB), gigabytes (GB), or terabytes (TB), referring to millions, billions, or trillions of characters stored.

> Main memory is the working storage of a computer.

RAM chips are manufactured with the use of CMOS (complementary metal-oxide semiconductor) technology. These chips are arranged as single-line memory modules (SIMMS).

There are two types of RAM: dynamic RAM (DRAM) and static RAM (SRAM). DRAM chips are more widely used, although SRAM chips are faster. SRAM retains its memory even if power to the computer is lost, but it is more expensive than DRAM and requires more space and power.

Special high-speed circuitry areas called *registers* are found in the control unit and the ALU. Registers are contained in the processor that hold information that will be used immediately. Main memory is located outside the processor and holds material that will be used "a little bit later."

Read-only memory (ROM) contains information supplied by the manufacturer, called *firmware,* that cannot be written on or erased. One ROM chip contains instructions that tell the processor what to do when the system is first turned on and the "bootstrap program" is initiated. Another ROM chip helps the processor transfer information between the screen, the printer, and other peripheral devices to ensure that all units are working correctly. These instructions are called ROM BIOS (basic input/output system). ROM is also one of the factors involved in making a "clone" PC; for instance, to be a true Dell clone, a computer must have the same ROM BIOS as a Dell computer.

Three variations of ROM chips are used in special situations; PROM, EPROM, and EEPROM. PROM (programmable read-only memory) chips are blank chips that a user, with special equipment, can write programs to. Once the program is written, it cannot be erased.

EPROM (erasable programmable read-only memory) chips are like PROM chips except that the contents are erasable with the use of a special device that exposes the chip to ultraviolet light. EEPROM (electronically erasable programmable read-only memory) can be reprogrammed with the use of special electron impulses.

The motherboard or system board is the main circuit board in a system unit. This board contains the microprocessor, any coprocessor chips, RAM chips, ROM chips, other types of memory, and expansion slots, which allow additional circuit boards to be added. All main memory is addressed, that is, each memory location is designated by a unique label in which a character of data or part of an instruction is stored during processing. Each address is similar to a post office address that allows the computer to access data at specific places in memory without disturbing the rest of the memory.

A sequence of memory locations may contain steps of a computer program or a string of data. The control unit keeps track of where current program instructions are stored, which allows the computer to read or write data to other memory locations, then return to the current address for the next instruction. All data processed by a computer pass through main memory. The most efficient computers, therefore, have enough main memory to store all data and programs needed for processing.

Usually, secondary memory is required in the form of diskettes and hard disc drives. Secondary memory functions similarly to a filing cabinet—you store information there until you need to retrieve it.

Once the appropriate file has been retrieved, it is copied into primary memory, where the user works on it. An old version of the file remains in secondary memory while the copy of the file is being edited/updated. When the user is finished with the file, it is taken out of primary memory and is returned to secondary memory (the filing cabinet), where the updated file replaces the old file.

The word *file* is used to refer to a collection of data or information that is treated as a unit by the computer. Each computer file has a unique name, and PC-based file names have extension names added after a period. For example, .DOC is added by a word processing program to files that contain word processing documents (e.g., REPORT.DOC).

Common file types are program files, which contain software instructions; data files, which contain data—not programs; image files, which contain digital images; audio files, which contain digitized sound; and video files, which contain digitized video images.

Storage. To understand storage hardware, it is necessary to understand the terms used to measure the capacity of storage devices. A **bit** describes the smallest unit of measure, a binary digit 0 or 1. Bits are combined into groups of 8 bits, called a **byte.**

A byte represents one character, digit, or other value. A kilobyte represents 1024 bytes. A megabyte (MB) is approximately 1 million bytes and often reflects capacities of microcomputers. A gigabyte (GB) is approximately 1 billion bytes and is used to measure the capacity of microcomputer hard disc drives and the main memory of mainframes and some supercomputers. A **terabyte** (TB) is approximately 1 thousand billion bytes.

> Storage is an archival form of memory.

The most common types of secondary storage devices are tape, diskette, hard disc, optical disc, and flash drive. Magnetic tape used to be a common storage medium for large computer systems but is now used primarily on large systems for backup and archiving of historical records, such as patient images. The "floppy disc" is also history. The compact disc (CD) is today's common transferable storage device.

CD-R (compact disc–recordable) is a CD format that allows users with CD-R drives to write data, only once, onto a specialized disc that can then be read by a standard CD-ROM drive. An example of this technology is the Photo CD system, developed by Eastman Kodak, which allows photographs taken with a 35-millimeter camera to be stored digitally on an optical disc.

Erasable optical discs, called CDE or CD-RW, allow users to erase data and use the disc over and over again.

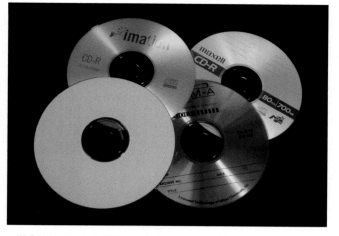

FIGURE 24-10 CDs come in various sizes and capacities.

These drives are much more durable than magnetic hard drives and they are widely used. Another technology, the DVD-ROM (digital versatile disc–read-only memory), is an optically readable digital disc that can store up to 20 GB of data. The DVD provides better audio and video quality and, in computers, can provide record and rewrite capabilities.

The CD stores data and programs as magnetized spots on a round, flat piece of mylar plastic. The CD is removable from the computer and transferable (Figure 24-10).

The most common CD is nearly 5 inches in diameter; however, smaller CDs are also available. Data are recorded on a CD in rings called *tracks,* which are invisible, closed concentric rings. The number of tracks on a CD is called TPI, or tracks per inch. The higher the TPI, the more data a CD can hold.

Each track is divided into sectors, which are invisible sections used by the computer for storage reference. The number of sectors on a CD varies according to the recording density, which refers to the number of bits per inch that can be written to the CD. CDs also are defined by their capacity, which ranges to several GB. A **CD drive** is the device that holds, spins, reads data from, and writes data to a CD.

A flash drive, sometimes called a jump drive or jump stick, is the newest of the small portable memory devices (Figure 24-11). The jump drive has a capacity of several GB; it connects through a USB port and transfers data rapidly.

In contrast to CDs, hard discs are thin, rigid glass or metal platters. Each side of the platter is coated with a recording material that can be magnetized. Hard discs are tightly sealed in a hard disc drive and data can be recorded on both sides of the disc platters. In microcomputers, hard disc drives usually are built into the system and are not removable.

Compared with CDs and flashdrives, hard discs can have thousands of tracks per inch and up to 64 sectors.

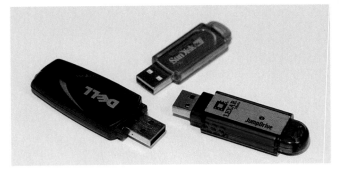

FIGURE 24-11 A jump drive is a small, solid state device that is capable of storing in excess of 1 GB of data.

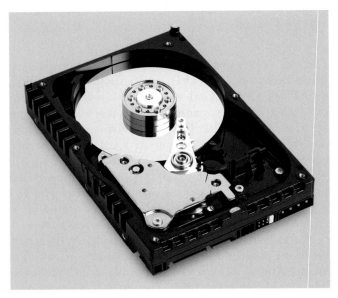

FIGURE 24-12 This disc drive reads all formats of optical compact discs and reads, erases, writes, and rewrites to a 650-MB optical cartridge.

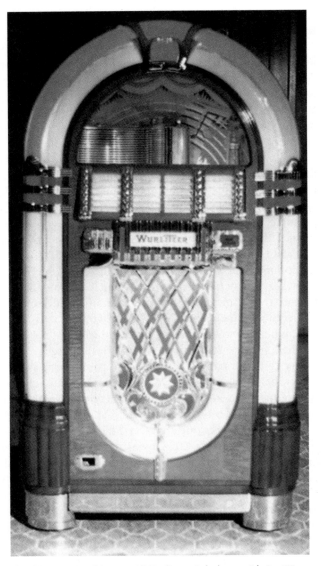

FIGURE 24-13 This 1946 Wurlitzer jukebox with its 78-rpm platters serves as a model for the optical disc jukebox of the Picture Archiving and Communication System (PACS) network. (Courtesy Raymond Wilenzek, New Orleans.)

Storage systems that use several hard discs use the cylinder method to locate data (Figure 24-12). Hard discs have greater capacity and speed than diskettes.

Microcomputer hard disc drives typically can hold up to 1 TB. Hard discs often are used in radiologic imaging procedures. The hard disc technology for large computer systems is allowing users to access large databases of information through organizations such as CompuServe and America Online. Secondary storage devices for large computers consist of removable packs of fixed disc drives.

A removable hard disc system is composed of 6 to 20 hard discs that are aligned one above the other in a sealed hard disc unit. The capacity of these units extends to many terabytes. Fixed disc drives are high-speed, high-capacity disc drives that are sealed in their own cabinets. A mainframe computer might have up to 100 of these drives attached to it.

A RAID (redundant array of inexpensive discs) system consists of two or more disc drives in a single cabinet that collectively act as a single storage system. RAID systems have greater reliability because if one disc drive fails, others can take over.

Optical discs, also called *laser discs*, are removable discs that data are written to and read from with the use of laser technology. A small laser is used to make "pits" in the disc and later to read them.

The most familiar form of optical disc is the compact disc (CD), which is used in the music industry. A single CD-ROM (compact disc–read-only memory) typically can hold 650 MB of data. CD-ROM drives used to handle only one disc at a time, but now, multidisc drives called *jukeboxes* can handle up to 100 discs. In an all-digital radiology department, the optical disc jukebox would replace the film file room (Figure 24-13).

Output. Common output devices are display screens and printers. Other devices include plotters, multifunction devices, and audio output devices.

The output device that people use most often is the display screen or monitor. The cathode ray tube (CRT) is a vacuum tube that is used as a display screen in a computer or video display terminal (VDT). Soft copy is the term that refers to the output seen on a display screen.

Flat panel displays (liquid crystal displays [LCDs]) are thinner and lighter and consume less power than CRTs. These displays are made of two plates of glass with a substance between them that can be activated in different ways.

> Output hardware consists of devices that translate computer information into a form that humans can understand.

A terminal is an input/output device that uses a keyboard for input and a display screen for output. Terminals can be dumb or intelligent.

A dumb terminal cannot do any processing on its own; it is used only to input data or receive data from a main or host computer. Airline clerks at ticketing and check-in counters usually are connected to the main computer system through dumb terminals.

An intelligent terminal has built-in processing capability and RAM but does not have its own storage capacity. Most radiologic applications use intelligent terminals.

A printer prints characters, symbols, or graphics on paper. This printed output often is called *hard copy.* Printers are categorized by the manner in which the print mechanism physically contacts the paper to print an image.

Impact printers such as dot matrix and high speed line printers have direct contact with the paper. Such printers have largely been replaced by nonimpact printers.

The two types of nonimpact printers used with microcomputers are laser printers and ink-jet printers. A laser printer operates similarly to a photocopying machine. Images are created with dots on a drum, are treated with a magnetically charged inklike substance called *toner,* and then are transferred from drum to paper.

Laser printers produce crisp images of text and graphics, with resolution ranging from 300 dots per inch (dpi) to 1200 dpi and in color. They can print up to 32 text-only pages per minute for a microcomputer and more than 120 pages per minute for a mainframe. Laser printers have built-in RAM chips to store output from the computer, ROM chips that store fonts, and their own small, dedicated processor.

Ink-jet printers also form images with little dots. These printers electrically charge small drops of ink that are then sprayed onto the page. Ink-jet printers are quieter and less expensive and can also print in color. Up to 20 pages per minute (ppm) for black text and 10 ppm for color images is possible with even modestly priced ink-jet printers.

Other specialized output devices serve specific functions. For example, plotters are used to create documents such as architectural drawings and maps. Multifunction devices deliver several capabilities such as printing, imaging, copying, and faxing through one unit. Specialized audio output devices provide the ability to output speechlike sounds, distinctive sounds such as beeps, and music.

Communications. Communications or telecommunications describes the transfer of data from a sender to a receiver across a distance. The practice of teleradiology involves the transfer of medical images and patient data.

Electric current, radiofrequency (RF), or light is used to transfer data through a physical medium, which may be a cable, a wire, or even the atmosphere, that is, wireless. Many communications lines are still analog; therefore, a computer needs a modem (modulate/demodulate) to convert digital information into analog. The receiving computer's modem converts analog information back into digital.

> Teleradiology is the transfer of images and patient reports to remote sites.

Transmission speed, the speed at which a modem transmits data, is measured in bits per second (bps) or kilobits per second (kbps). In addition to modems, computers require communications software. Often, this software is packaged with the modem, or it might be included as part of the system software.

Advances in technology have allowed for the development of faster and faster communication devices. Cable modems connect computers to cable TV systems that offer telecommunication services. Some cable providers are offering transmission speeds up to 1000 times faster than a basic telephone line.

Integrated services digital network (ISDN) transmits over regular phone lines up to five times faster than basic modems. Digital subscriber lines (DSLs) transmit at speeds in the middle range of the previous two technologies. DSLs also use regular phone lines.

Telecommunications in the form of teleradiology is changing the way we allocate human resources to improve the speed of interpretation, reporting, and archiving of images and other patient data.

Software

All that has been described thus far regarding the computer has been hardware. Hardware refers to the fixed, visible components of the system. The CPU, all input/output devices, and other auxiliary or peripheral devices are hardware. But these constitute only half of the computer. The other half is software.

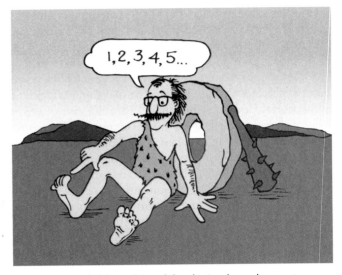

FIGURE 24-14 The origin of the decimal number system.

TABLE 24-1 Organization of Binary Number System

Decimal Number	Binary Equivalent	Binary Number
0	0	0
1	2^0	1
2	$2^1 + 0$	10
3	$2^1 + 2^0$	11
4	$2^2 + 0 + 0$	100
5	$2^2 + 0 + 2^0$	101
6	$2^2 + 2^1 + 0$	110
7	$2^2 + 2^1 + 2^0$	111
8	$2^3 + 0 + 0 + 0$	1000
9	$2^3 + 0 + 0 + 2^0$	1001
10	$2^3 + 0 + 2^1 + 0$	1010
11	$2^3 + 0 + 2^1 + 2^0$	1011
12	$2^3 + 2^2 + 0 + 0$	1100
13	$2^3 + 2^2 + 0 + 2^0$	1101
14	$2^3 + 2^2 + 2^1 + 0$	1110
15	$2^3 + 2^2 + 2^1 + 2^0$	1111
16	$2^4 + 0 + 0 + 0 + 0$	10000

 Software refers to instructions written in computer language that guide the computer through its designated operations.

TABLE 24-2 Power of Ten, Power of Two, and Binary Notation

Power of Ten	Power of Two	Binary Notation
$10^0 = 1$	$2^0 = 1$	1
$10^1 = 10$	$2^1 = 2$	10
$10^2 = 100$	$2^2 = 4$	100
$10^3 = 1000$	$2^3 = 8$	1000
$10^4 = 10,000$	$2^4 = 16$	10000
$10^5 = 100,000$	$2^5 = 32$	100000
$10^6 = 1,000,000$	$2^6 = 64$	1000000
	$2^7 = 128$	
	$2^8 = 256$	
	$2^9 = 512$	
	$2^{10} = 1024$	
	$2^{12} = 4096$	
	$2^{14} = 16,384$	
	$2^{16} = 65,536$	

Although the computer can accept and report alphabetic characters and numeric information in the decimal system, it operates in the binary system. In the decimal system, the system we normally use, 10 digits (0 to 9) are used. The word *digit* comes from the Latin for finger or toe. The origin of the decimal system is obvious (Figure 24-14).

Other number systems have been formulated to many other base values. The duodecimal system, for instance, has 12 digits. It is used to describe the months of the year and the hours in a day and night. Computers operate on the simplest number system of all—the binary number system. It has only two digits, 0 and 1.

Binary Number System. Counting in the binary number system starts with 0 to 1 and then counts over again (Table 24-1). It includes only two digits, 0 and 1, and the computer performs all operations by converting alphabetic characters, decimal values, and logic functions to binary values.

Even the computer's instructions are stored in binary form. In this way, although binary numbers may become exceedingly long, computation can be handled by properly adjusting the thousands of flip-flop circuits in the computer.

In the binary number system, 0 is 0 and 1 is 1, but there, the direct relationship with the decimal number system ends. It ends at 1 because the 1 in binary notation comes from 2^0. Recall that any number raised to the zero power is 1, therefore 2^0 is 1.

In binary notation, the decimal number 2 is equal to 2^1 plus 0. This is expressed as 10. The decimal number 3 is equal to 2^1 plus 2^0 or 11 in binary form; 4 is 2^2 plus no 2^1 plus no 2^0 or 100 in binary form. Each time it is necessary to raise 2 to an additional power to express a number, the number of binary digits increases by one.

Just as we know the meaning of the powers of 10, it is necessary to recognize the powers of 2. Power of 2 notation is used in radiologic imaging to describe image size, image dynamic range (shades of gray), and image storage capacity. Table 24-2 reviews these power notations. Note the following similarity. In both power notations, the number of 0's to the right of 1 equals the value of the exponent.

Question: Express the number 193 in binary form.
Answer: 193 falls between 2^7 and 2^8. Therefore, it is expressed as 1 followed by seven binary digits. Simply add the decimal equivalent of each binary digit from left to right:

Yes $2^7 = 1 = 128$
Yes $2^6 = 1 = 64$
Yes $2^5 = 0 = $ No 32
No $2^4 = 0 = $ No 16
No $2^3 = 0 = $ No 8
No $2^2 = 0 = $ No 4
No $2^1 = 0 = $ No 2
Yes $2^0 = 1 = 1$
————————————
11000001 = 193

Question: What is the decimal value of the binary number 100110011?
Answer: Follow the previous process by first listing the binary number and then computing each power of 2.

$1 = 2^8$ Yes $= 256$
$0 = 2^7$ No $= 0$
$0 = 2^6$ No $= 0$
$1 = 2^5$ Yes $= 32$
$1 = 2^4$ Yes $= 16$
$0 = 2^3$ No $= 0$
$0 = 2^2$ No $= 0$
$1 = 2^1$ Yes $= 2$
$1 = 2^0$ Yes $= 1$
————————————
$= 307$

Digital images are made of discrete picture elements, **pixels,** arranged in a matrix. The size of the image is described in the binary number system by power of 2 equivalents. Most images measure 256 × 256 (2^8) to 1024 × 1024 (2^{10}) for computed tomography (CT) and magnetic resonance imaging (MRI). The 1024 × 1024 matrix is used in digital fluoroscopy. Matrix sizes of 2048 × 2048 (2^{11}) and 4096 × 4096 (2^{12}) are used in digital radiography.

Bits, Bytes, and Words. In computer language, a single binary digit, 0 or 1, is called a **bit.** Depending on the microprocessor, a string of 8, 16, or 32 bits is manipulated simultaneously.

The computer uses as many bits as necessary to express a decimal digit, depending on how it is programmed. The 26 characters of the alphabet and other special characters are usually encoded by 8 bits.

> To encode is to translate from ordinary characters to computer-compatible characters—binary digits.

Bits often are grouped into bunches of eight called *bytes.* Computer capacity is expressed by the number of bytes that can be accommodated.

One kilobyte (kB) is equal to 1024 bytes. Note that *kilo* is not metric in computer use. Instead, it represents 2^{10} or 1024. The minicomputers used in radiology have capacities measured in megabytes, where 1 MB = 1 kB × 1 kB = $2^{10} × 2^{10} = 2^{20} = 1,048,576$ bytes.

Question: How many bits can be stored on a 64-kB chip?
Answer:
$$\frac{1024\ bits}{kbytes} \times 64\ kbytes \times \frac{8\ bits}{byte}$$
$$= 2^{10} \times 2^6 \times 2^3 = 2^{19} = 524,288\ bits$$

Depending on the computer configuration, two bytes usually constitute a **word.** In the case of a 16-bit microprocessor, a word would consist of 16 consecutive bits of information that are interpreted and shuffled about the computer as a unit. Sometimes half a byte is called a "nibble" and two words is a "chomp"! Each word of data in memory has its own address.

Computer Programs. The sequence of instructions developed by a software programmer is called a *computer program.* It is useful to distinguish two classifications of computer programs: systems software and application programs.

Systems software consists of programs that make it easy for the user to operate a computer to its best advantage. Computer buffs describe efficient software as "user friendly."

Application programs are those written in a higher-level language expressly to carry out some user function. Most computer programs as we know them are application programs.

> Computer programs are the software of the computer.

A computer language described as higher level is one that approaches human language and thought processes. The lowest-level computer language is machine language, that is, the only language the computer understands—binary numbers.

Systems Software. The computer program most closely related to the system hardware is the operating system. The operating system is that series of instructions that organizes the course of data through the computer to the solution of a particular problem. It makes the computer's resources available to application programs.

Commands such as "run file" to begin a sequence or "save file" to store some information in secondary memory are typical of operating system commands. MAC-OS, Windows, and Unix are popular operating systems.

This type of program usually is developed by the computer manufacturer and may be stored in ROM in the CPU. Because the CPU recognizes instructions only in binary or machine language form, formulating the operating system is perhaps the most tedious of all computer programming tasks.

Computers ultimately understand only 0's and 1's. To relieve humans from the task of writing programs in this form, other programs called *assemblers, compilers,* and *interpreters* have been written. These types of software provide a computer language that can be used to communicate between the language of the operating system and everyday language.

An assembler is a computer program that recognizes symbolic instructions such as "subtract (SUB)," "load (LD)," and "print (PT)" and translates them into the corresponding binary code. Assembly is the translation of a program written in symbolic, machine-oriented instructions into machine language instructions.

Compilers and interpreters are computer programs that translate an application program from its high-level language, such as BASIC, C++, or Pascal, into a form that is suitable for the assembler, or into a form that is accepted directly by the CPU. Interpreters make program development easier because they are interactive. Compiled programs run faster because they create a separate machine language program.

Application Programs. Computer programs that are written by the computer manufacturer, a software manufacturer, or by the users themselves to guide the computer to perform a specific task are called *application programs.* Examples are Lotus, Quicken, and Excel.

Application programs allow the user to print a mailing list, complete an income tax form, evaluate a financial statement, or reconstruct an image from an x-ray transmission pattern. They are written in one of many high-level computer languages and then are translated through an interpreter or a compiler into a corresponding machine language program that subsequently is executed by the computer.

The diagram in Figure 24-15 illustrates the flow of the software instructions from turning the computer on to completing a computation. When the computer is first turned on, nothing is in its memory except a program called a *bootstrap.* This is frozen permanently in ROM. When the computer is started, it automatically runs the bootstrap program, which is capable of transferring other necessary programs off the disc and into the computer memory.

The bootstrap program loads the operating system into primary memory, which, in turn controls all subsequent operations. A machine language application

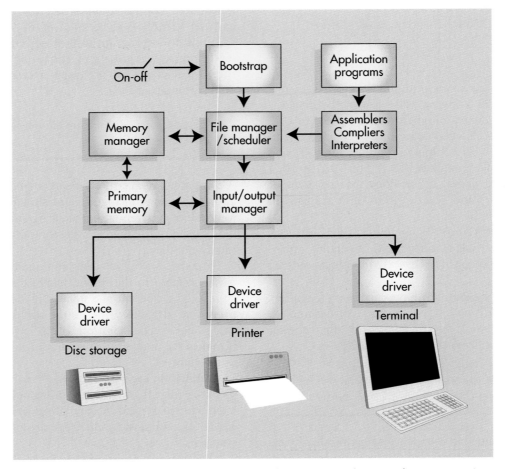

FIGURE 24-15 The sequence of software manipulations required to complete an operation.

program likewise can be copied from the disc into primary memory, where prescribed operations occur. After completion of the program, results are transferred from primary memory to an output device under the control of the operating system.

Hexadecimal Number System. The hexadecimal number system is used by assembly level applications. As you have seen, assembly language acts as a midpoint between the computer's binary system and the user's human language instructions. The set of hexadecimal numbers is 0, 1, 2, 3, 4, 5, 6, 7, 8, 9, A, B, C, D, E, and F. Each of these symbols is used to represent a binary number or, more specifically, a set of four bits. Therefore, because it takes eight bits to make a byte, a byte can be represented by two hexadecimal numbers. The set of hexadecimal numbers corresponds to the binary numbers for 0 to 15, as is shown in Table 24-3.

Computer Languages

High-level programming languages allow the programmer to write instructions in a form that approaches human language, with the use of words, symbols, and decimal numbers rather than the 1's and 0's of machine language. A brief list of the more popular programming languages is given in Table 24-4. With the use of one of these high-level languages, a set of instructions can be written that will be understood by the system software and will be executed by the computer through its operating system.

FORTRAN. The oldest language for scientific, engineering, and mathematical problems is FORTRAN (FORmula TRANslation). It was the prototype for today's algebraic languages, which are oriented toward computational procedures for solving mathematical and statistical problems.

Problems that can be expressed in terms of formulas and equations are sometimes called **algorithms.** An algorithm is a step-by-step process used to solve a problem, much in the way a recipe is used to bake a cake, except that the algorithm is more detailed, that is, it would include instructions to remove the shell from the egg. FORTRAN was developed in 1956 by IBM in conjunction with some major computer users.

BASIC. Developed at Dartmouth College in 1964 as a first language for students, BASIC (Beginners All-purpose Symbolic Instruction Code) is an algebraic programming language. It is an easy-to-learn, interpreter-based language. BASIC contains a powerful arithmetic facility, several editing features, a library of common mathematical functions, and simple input and output procedures.

TABLE 24-3	The Hexadecimal Number System	
Decimal	Binary	Hexadecimal
0	0000	0
1	0001	1
2	0010	2
3	0011	3
4	0100	4
5	0101	5
6	0110	6
7	0111	7
8	1000	8
9	1001	9
10	1010	A
11	1011	B
12	1100	C
13	1101	D
14	1110	E
15	1111	F

TABLE 24-4	Programming Languages	
Language	Date Introduced	Description
FORTRAN	1956	First successful programming language; used for solving engineering and scientific problems
COBOL	1959	Minicomputer and mainframe computer applications in business
ALGOL	1960	Especially useful in high-level mathematics
BASIC	1964	Most frequently used with microcomputers and minicomputers; science, engineering, and business applications
BCPL	1965	Development-stage language
B	1969	Development-stage language
C	1970	Combines the power of assembly language with the ease of use and portability of high-level language
Pascal	1971	High-level, general purpose language; used for teaching structured programming
ADA	1975	Based on Pascal; used by the U.S. Department of Defense
VisiCalc	1978	First electronic spreadsheet
C	1980	Response to complexity of C; incorporates object-oriented programming methods
QuickBASIC	1985	Powerful high-level language with advanced user features
Visual C	1992	Visual language programming methods; design environments
Visual BASIC	1993	Visual language programming methods; design environments; advanced user-friendly features

QuickBASIC. Microsoft developed BASIC into a powerful programming language that can be used for commercial applications and for quick, single-use programs. QuickBASIC's advanced features for editing, implementing, and decoding make it an attractive language for professional and amateur programmers.

COBOL. One high-level, procedure-oriented language designed for coding business data processing problems is COBOL (**CO**mmon **B**usiness **O**riented **L**anguage). A basic characteristic of business data processing is the existence of large files that are updated continuously. COBOL provides extensive file-handling, editing, and report-generating capabilities for the user.

Pascal. Pascal is a high-level, general purpose programming language that was developed in 1971 by Nicklaus Wirth of the Federal Institute of Technology at Zürich, Switzerland. A general purpose programming language is one that can be put to many different applications. Currently, Pascal is the most popular programming language for teaching programming concepts, in part because its syntax is relatively easy to learn and closely resembles that of the English language in usage.

C, C++. C is considered by many to be the first modern "programmer's language." It was designed, implemented, and developed by real working programmers and reflects the way they approached the job of programming. C is thought of as a middle-level language because it combines elements of high-level languages with the functionality of an assembler (low-level) language.

In response to the need to manage greater complexity, C++ was developed by Bjarne Stroustrup in 1980, who initially called it "C with Classes." C++ contains the entire C language, as well as many additions designed to support object-oriented programming (OOP).

Once a program exceeds approximately 30,000 lines of code, it becomes so complex that it is difficult to grasp as a single object. Therefore, OOP is a method of dividing up parts of the program into groups, or objects, with related data and applications, in the same way that a book is broken into chapters and subheadings to make it more readable.

Visual C++, Visual Basic. Visual programming languages are the most recent languages, and they are under continuing development. They are designed specifically for the creation of Windows applications. Although Visual C++ and Visual Basic use their original respective programming language code structures, both were developed with the same goal in mind: to create user-friendly Windows applications with minimal effort from the programmer.

In theory, the most inexperienced programmer should be able to create complex programs with visual languages. The idea is to have the programmer design the program in a design environment without ever really writing extensive code. Instead, the visual language creates the code to match the programmer's design.

Macros. Most spreadsheet and word processing applications offer built-in programming commands called *macros*. These work in the same way as commands in programming languages, and they are used to carry out user-defined functions or a series of functions in the application. One application that offers a very good library of macro commands is Excel, a spreadsheet. The user can create a command to manipulate a series of data by performing a specific series of steps.

Macros can be written or they can be designed in a fashion similar to that of visual programming. This process of designing a macro is called *recording*. The programmer turns the macro recorder on, carries out the steps he wants the macro to carry out, and stops the recorder. The macro now knows exactly what the programmer wants implemented and can run the same series of steps repeatedly.

Other program languages have been developed for other purposes. LOGO is a language that was designed for children. ADA is the official language approved by the U.S. Department of Defense for software development. It is used principally for military applications and artificial intelligence.

SUMMARY

The word *computer* is used as an abbreviation for any general purpose, stored-program electronic digital device. "General purpose" means the computer can solve problems. "Stored-program" means the computer has instructions and data stored in its memory. "Electronic" means the computer is powered by electrical and electronic devices. "Digital" means that the "data" are in discrete values.

A computer has two principal parts: the hardware and the software. The hardware is the computer's nuts and bolts. The software is the computer's programs, which tell the hardware what to do.

Hardware consists of several types of components: central processing unit (CPU), control unit, arithmetic unit, memory units, input and output devices, video terminal display, secondary memory devices, printer, and modem.

The basic parts of the software are the bits, bytes, and words. In computer language, a single binary digit, either 0 or 1, is called a *bit*. Bits grouped in bunches of eight are called *bytes*. Computer capacity is expressed in gigabytes.

Computers use a specific language to communicate commands in software systems and programs. Computers operate on the simplest number system of all—the binary system, which includes only two digits, 0 and 1. The computer performs all operations by converting alphabetic characters, decimal values, and logic functions into binary values. Other computer languages allow the programmer to write instructions in a form that approaches human language.

CHALLENGE QUESTIONS

1. Define or otherwise identify the following:
   a. Logic function
   b. Central processing unit
   c. Modem
   d. Character generator
   e. Byte
   f. Operating system
   g. Bootstrap
   h. Algorithm
   i. BASIC
   j. RAM
2. Name three operations in diagnostic imaging departments that are computerized.
3. The acronyms ASCC, ENIAC, and UNIVAC stand for what titles?
4. What is the difference between a calculator and a computer?
5. Explain the differences between the microcomputer, the minicomputer, and the mainframe computer.
6. What are the two principal parts of a computer and the distinguishing features of each?
7. List and define the several components of computer hardware.
8. Define *bit, byte,* and *word* as used in computer terminology.
9. Distinguish systems software from applications programs.
10. List several types of computer languages.
11. What is the difference between a CD and a DVD?
12. A memory chip is said to have 256 MB of capacity. What is the total bit capacity?
13. What is high-level computer language?
14. What computer language was the first modern programmers' language?
15. List and define the four computer processing methods.
16. What type of computer is used by the U.S. Census Bureau?
17. Describe a CPU. List its three principal parts and describe their functions.
18. What input/output devices are commonly used in radiology?
19. Convert the decimal number 147 into binary form.
20. Convert the binary number 110001 into decimal form.

The answers to the Challenge Questions can be found by logging on to our website at http://evolve.elsevier.com.

CHAPTER 25

Computed Radiography

OBJECTIVES

At the completion of this chapter, the student should be able
to do the following:

1. Describe several advantages of computed radiography over
   screen-film radiography
2. Identify workflow changes when computed radiography replaces
   screen-film radiography
3. Discuss the relevant features of a storage phosphor imaging plate
4. Explain the operating characteristics of a computed radiography
   reader
5. Discuss spatial resolution, contrast resolution, and noise related to
   computed radiography
6. Identify opportunities for patient radiation dose reduction with
   computed radiography

OUTLINE

The Computed Radiography Image Receptor
    Photostimulable Luminescence
    Imaging Plate
    Light Stimulation–Emission
The Computed Radiography Reader
    Mechanical Features
    Optical Features
    Computer Control
Imaging Characteristics
    Image Receptor Response Function
    Image Noise
Patient Characteristics
    Radiation Dose
    Workload

Presently, an acceleration in the conversion from screen-film radiography (analog) to digital radiography (DR) is occurring. Digital imaging began with computed tomography (CT) and magnetic resonance imaging (MRI).

DR was introduced in 1981 by Fuji with the first commercial computed radiography (CR) imaging system. After many improvements that were made over the next decade, CR became clinically acceptable and today enjoys widespread use.

Today, medical imaging is complemented by multiple forms of DR in addition to CR. At this time, CR is the mostly widely used DR modality, and although other DR systems are increasing in use, it seems there will always be a need for CR because of its unique properties.

This chapter discusses CR, but the reader should understand that much of the information relevant to CR applies also to DR because CR is a form of DR.

Before computed radiography (CR) is discussed, a review of the workload steps associated with screen-film radiography is in order. Consider the sequence outlined in Figure 25-1.

To conduct a screen-film radiographic examination, one should first produce a paper trail of the study, then process the image with wet chemistry, and finally physically file the image after accepting that it is diagnostic. CR imaging eliminates some of these steps and can produce better medical images at lower patient dose.

COMPUTED RADIOGRAPHY (CR) TERMS

- PSL = photostimulable luminescence
- PSP = photostimulable phosphor
- SPS = storage phosphor screen
- IP = imaging plate
- SP = storage phosphor
- PMT = photomultiplier tube
- PD = photodiode

THE COMPUTED RADIOGRAPHY IMAGE RECEPTOR

Many similarities have been observed between screen-film imaging and CR imaging. Both modalities use as the image receptor an x-ray sensitive plate that is encased in a protective cassette. The two techniques can be used interchangeably with any x-ray imaging system. Both carry a latent image, albeit in a different form, that must be made visible via processing.

Here, however, the similarities stop. In screen-film radiography, the radiographic intensifying screen is a scintillator that emits light in response to an x-ray interaction. In CR, the response to x-ray interaction is seen as trapped electrons in a higher-energy metastable state.

Photostimulable Luminescence

Some materials such as barium fluorohalide with europium (BaFBr:Eu or BaFI:Eu) emit some light promptly, in the way that a scintillator does following x-ray exposure. However, they also emit light some time later when exposed to a different light source. Such a process is called *photostimulable luminescence (PSL)*.

The europium (Eu) is present in only very small amounts. It is an **activator** and is responsible for the storage property of the PSL. The activator is similar to the sensitivity center of a film emulsion because without it, there would be no latent image.

In the same way that the photographic effect is not fully understood and continues to be studied, so too the physics of PSL is not fully understood.

The atoms of barium fluorobromide have atomic numbers of 56, 9, and 35, respectively, with K-shell electron binding energies of 37, 5, and 12 keV. Many Compton and photoelectric x-ray interactions occur with outer-shell electrons, sending them into an excited, metastable state (Figure 25-2). When these electrons return to the ground state, visible light is emitted (Figure 25-3).

Over time, these metastable electrons return to the ground state on their own. However, this return to the ground state can be accelerated or stimulated by exposing the phosphor to intense infrared light from a laser—hence the term **photostimulable luminescence** from a photostimulable phosphor (PSP).

The PSP, barium fluorohalide is fashioned similarly to a radiographic intensifying screen, as is shown in Figure 25-4. Because the latent image occurs in the form of metastable electrons, such screens are called **storage phosphor screens (SPSs)**.

The SPS appears white because the small PSP particles (3 to 10 mm) scatter light excessively. Such a scattering is called **turbid**. PSP particles are randomly positioned throughout a **binder**.

SPSs are mechanically stable, electrostatically protected, and fashioned to optimize the intensity of stimulated light. Some SPSs incorporate phosphors

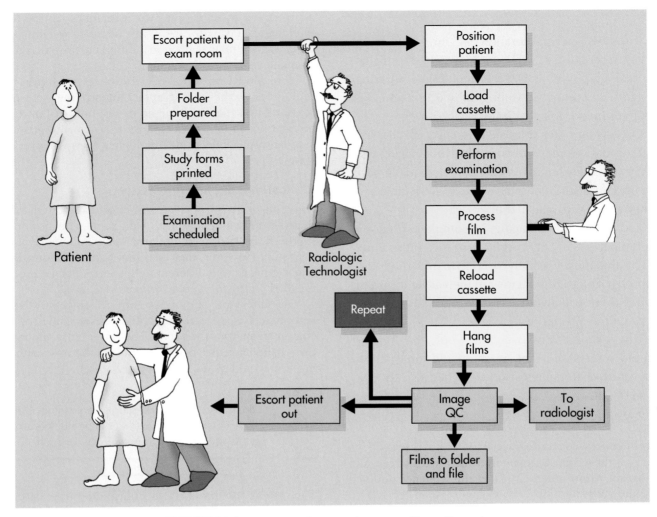

FIGURE 25-1 Sequence of activity for screen-film radiography.

grown as linear filaments (Figure 25-5) that enhance the absorption of x-rays and limit the spread of stimulated emission.

Imaging Plate

The PSP screen is housed in a rugged cassette and appears similar to a screen-film cassette (Figure 25-6). In this form as an image receptor, the PSP screen-film cassette is called an **imaging plate (IP).**

The IP is handled in the same manner as a screen-film cassette; in fact, this is a principal advantage of CR. CR can be substituted for screen-film radiography and used with any x-ray imaging system. The PSP screen of the IP is not loaded and unloaded in a dark room. Rather, it is handled in the manner of a screen-film daylight loader.

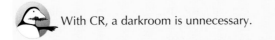 With CR, a darkroom is unnecessary.

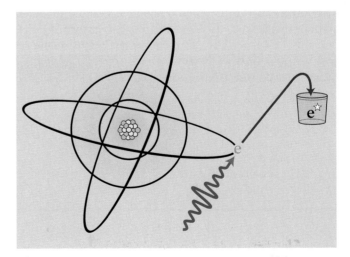

FIGURE 25-2 X-ray interaction with a photostimulable phosphor results in excitation of electrons into a metastable state.

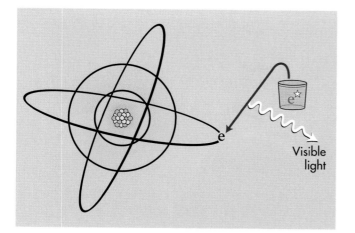

FIGURE 25-3 When metastable electrons return to their ground state, visible light is emitted.

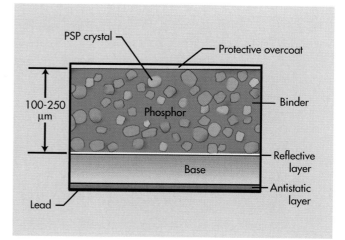

FIGURE 25-4 Cross section of a photostimulable phosphor (PSP) screen.

The IP has lead backing that reduces backscatter x-rays. This improves the contrast resolution of the image receptor.

Light Stimulation–Emission

Thermoluminescent dosimetry (TLD) and optically stimulated luminescence (OSL) are the main radiation detectors used for occupational radiation monitoring (see Chapter 40). Light is emitted when a TLD crystal is heated. Light is emitted when an OSL crystal is illuminated. PSL is similar to OSL.

The sequence of events engaged in producing a PSL signal begins as shown in Figure 25-7. When an x-ray beam exposes a PSP, the energy transfer results in excitation of electrons into a metastable state. Approximately 50% of these electrons return to their ground state immediately, resulting in **prompt emission** of light, with wavelength λe.

The remaining metastable electrons return to the ground state over time. This causes the latent image to fade and requires that the IP must be read soon after exposure. CR signal loss is objectionable after approximately 8 hours.

The next step in CR imaging is stimulation (Figure 25-8). The finely focused beam of infrared light with wavelength λs and beam diameter of 50 to 100 nm is directed at the PSP. As laser beam intensity increases, so does the intensity of the emitted signal.

> The diameter of the laser beam affects the spatial resolution of the CR imaging system.

Note that as the laser beam penetrates, it spreads. The amount of spread increases with PSP thickness.

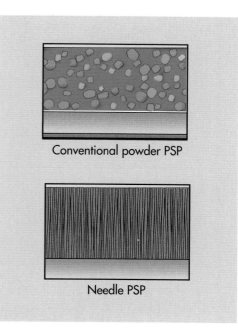

FIGURE 25-5 Some storage phosphor screens (SPSs) incorporate phosphors grown as linear filaments that increase the absorption of x-rays and limit the spread of stimulated emission.

Figure 25-9 illustrates the third step in this imaging process—detect (read) the stimulated emission. The laser beam with wavelength λs causes metastable electrons to return to the ground state with the emission of a shorter-wavelength light λe in the blue region of the visible spectrum. Through this process, the latent image is made visible.

Some signal is lost as the result of (1) scattering of the emitted light, and (2) the collection efficiency of the photodetector. Photomultiplier tubes (PMTs) and photodiodes (PDs) are the light detectors of choice for CR.

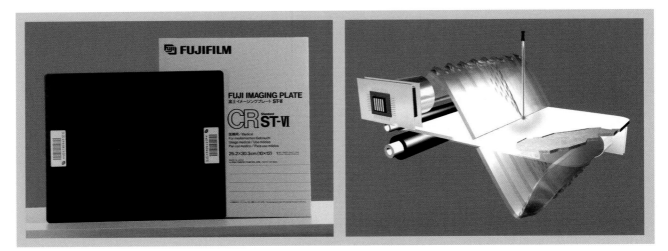

FIGURE 25-6 A Fuji computed radiography imaging plate. (Courtesy Michael Wilsey, Fuji Medical Systems.)

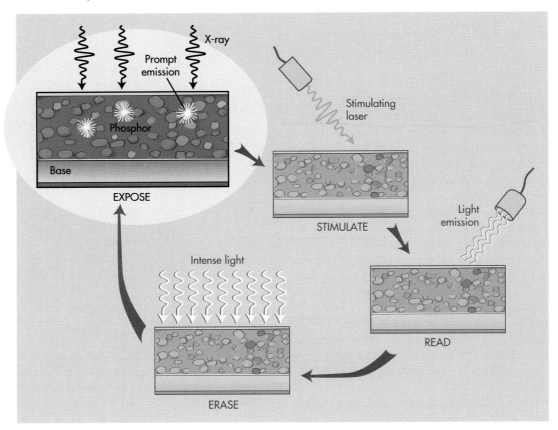

FIGURE 25-7 *Exposure:* The first of a sequence of events that results in an x-ray–induced image-forming signal.

The final stage in PSL signal production is shown in Figure 25-10. The stimulation cycle of PSL signal acquisition does not completely transition all metastable electrons to the ground state. Some excited electrons remain.

If residual latent image remained, ghosting could appear on subsequent use of the IP. Any residual latent image is removed by flooding the phosphor with very intense white light from a bank of specially designed fluorescent lamps.

The stimulation portion of PSP processing would result in no latent image if the laser beam were made to dwell longer at each position on the PSP, but this would require an unacceptable processing time.

 Imaging plates should be used soon after the erase cycle has been completed.

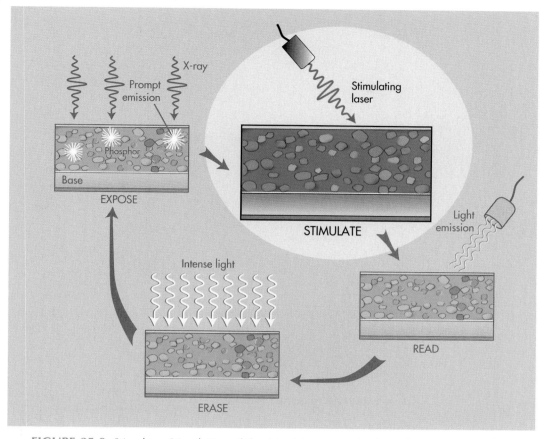

FIGURE 25-8 *Stimulate:* Stimulation of the latent image results from the interaction of an infrared laser beam with the photostimulable phosphor (PSP).

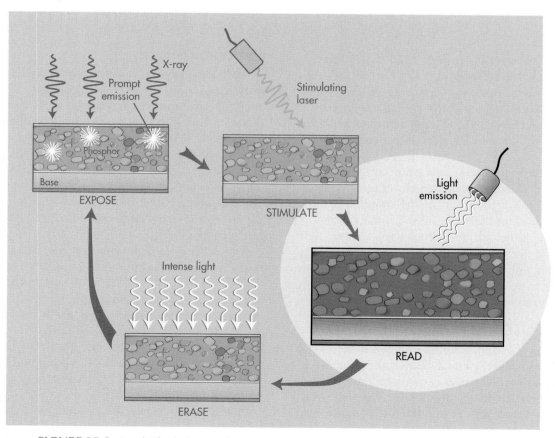

FIGURE 25-9 *Read:* The light signal emitted after stimulation is detected and measured.

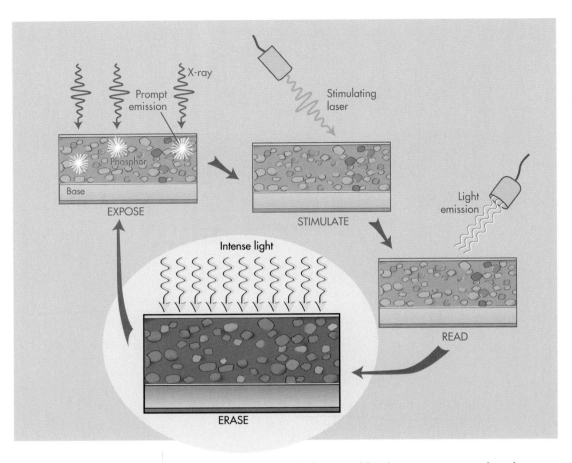

FIGURE 25-10 *Erase:* Prior to reuse, any residual metastable electrons are moved to the ground state by an intense light.

The PSP is sufficiently sensitive that it can become fogged by background radiation.

The laser light used to stimulate the PSP has a wavelength λs and is monochromatic, as can be seen in Figure 25-11. A HeNe gas laser used to be the stimulating source of choice, but this has been largely replaced by a solid state laser.

The resulting emission, λe, has a polychromatic emission spectrum. The emitted light intensity is many orders of magnitude lower than that of the stimulating light; this poses additional challenges to the entire process.

Solid state lasers produce longer-wavelength light and therefore are less likely to interfere with emitted light. Even so, optical filters are necessary to allow only emitted light to reach the photodetector while blocking the intense stimulated light.

THE COMPUTED RADIOGRAPHY READER

A commercial computed radiography reader, as is shown in Figure 25-12, could be mistaken for a day-light film processor. However, a daylight film processor is based on wet chemistry processing. The CR reader represents the marriage of mechanical, optical, and computer modules.

Mechanical Features

When the CR cassette is inserted into the CR reader, the IP is removed and is fitted to a precision drive mechanism. This drive mechanism moves the IP constantly, yet slowly ("**slow scan**") along the long axis of the IP. Small fluctuations in velocity can result in banding artifacts, so the motor drive must be absolutely constant.

While the IP is being transported in the slow scan direction, a deflection device such as a rotating polygon (shown in Figure 25-13) or an oscillating mirror deflects the laser beam back and forth across the IP. This is the **fast scan** mode.

These drive mechanisms are coupled so the laser beam is blanked during retrace, similar to the situation described in Chapter 21 for a video monitor. The error tolerance for this mechanism is fractions of a pixel. Image edges from a CR reader that is out of tolerance appear "wavy."

Another method is for the cassette to be placed in the reader vertically with the IP withdrawn downward. As this occurs, the cassette is scanned by a horizontal laser.

The IP barely leaves the cassette, so it is not subject to roller damage. Furthermore, the scan is nearly always

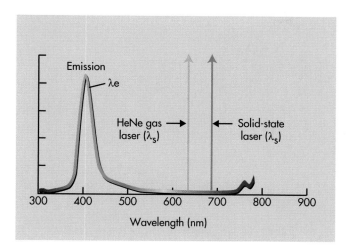

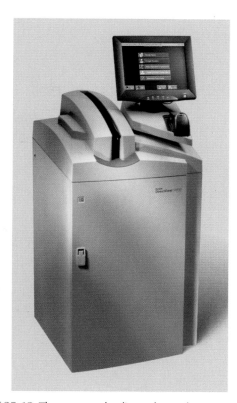

FIGURE 25-11 The laser light used to stimulate the photo-stimulable phosphor is monochromatic. Resultant emitted light is polychromatic.

FIGURE 25-12 The computed radiography reader is a compact mechanico, optico, computer assemble. (Courtesy Eastman Kodak Co.)

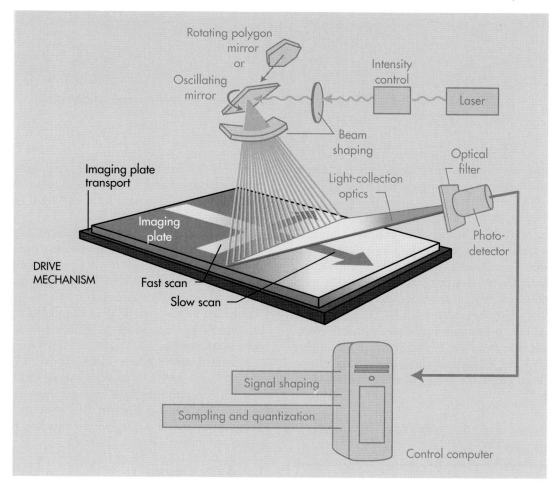

FIGURE 25-13 The drive mechanisms of the computed radiography (CR) reader move the imaging plate (IP) slowly along its long axis, while an oscillating beam deflection mirror causes the stimulating laser beam to sweep rapidly across the IP.

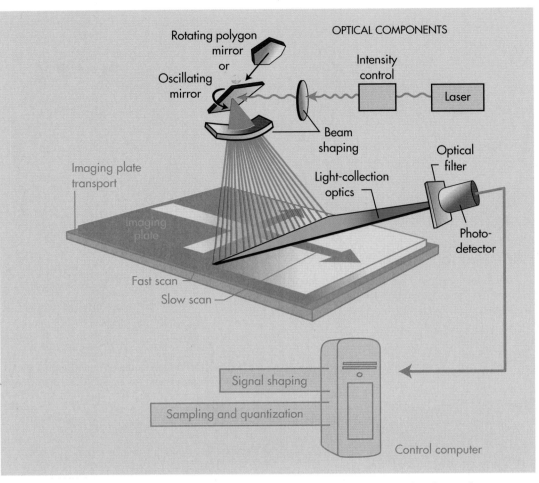

FIGURE 25-14 The optical components and optical path of a computed radiography (CR) reader are highlighted.

located at right angles to the direction of any grid lines; in this way, aliasing artifacts are reduced.

Optical Features

The challenge to the CR reader is to precisely interrogate each metastable electron of the latent image in a precise fashion. Components of the optical subsystem include the laser, beam-shaping optics, light-collecting optics, optical filters, and a photodetector. These components are shown in Figure 25-14.

The laser is the source of stimulating light; however, it spreads as it travels to the rotating/oscillating reflector. This light beam is focused onto the reflector by a lens system that keeps the beam diameter small—less than 100 μm.

> Laser beam size is critical for ensuring high spatial resolution.

As the laser beam is deflected across the IP, it changes size and shape. Special beam-shaping optics keeps constant the beam size, shape, speed, and intensity.

Ralph Schaetzing describes a flashlight exercise to explain what is needed for beam shaping. Shine a flashlight perpendicularly on a wall, and what do you see? A circle of light.

Now, move the beam along the wall slowly but with constant velocity, and what do you see? The beam becomes distorted, moves faster, and is less intense. These types of changes in a CR reader are corrected with the use of beam-shaping optics.

Emitted light from the IP is channeled into a funnel-like fiber optic collection assembly and is directed at the photodetector, PMT, PD, or charge-coupled device (CCD). Before photodetection occurs, the light is filtered, so that none of the long-wavelength stimulation light reaches the photodetector and swamps emitted light. In this case, emitted light is the signal and stimulating light the noise; therefore, proper filtering improves the signal-to-noise ratio.

Computer Control

The output of the photodetector is a time-varying analog signal that is transmitted to a computer system that has multiple functions (Figure 25-15).

The time-varying analog signal from the photodetector is processed for amplitude, scale, and compression. This shapes the signal before the final image is formed. Then, the analog signal is digitized, with attention paid to proper **sampling** (time between samples) and **quantization** (the value of each sample).

> Sampling and quantization are the process of analog-to-digital conversion (ADC).

The **image buffer** is usually a hard disc. This is the place where a completed image can be stored temporarily until it is transferred to a workstation for interpretation or to an archival computer.

The computer of the CR reader is in control of the slow scan and the fast scan. This control works off the computer clock in gigahertz (GHz).

IMAGING CHARACTERISTICS

Medical imaging with CR is not much different from that with screen-film imaging. A cassette is exposed with an existing x-ray imaging system to form a latent image.

The cassette is inserted into an automatic processor (reader) and the latent image is made manifest.

Here the similarity ends. The four principal characteristics of any medical image consist of spatial resolution, contrast resolution, noise, and artifacts. Such characteristics are different for all DR, including CR from screen-film imaging. These are discussed in greater depth in Chapters 28 through 31.

Image Receptor Response Function

The shape of the characteristic curve for screen-film imaging was described in detail in Chapter 16. It is presented again in Figure 25-16, along with the "characteristic curve" for a CR image receptor. In CR and DR, it is not really a characteristic curve but rather an **image receptor response function.**

Figure 25-16 suggests several differences between CR and screen-film image receptors. The response of screen-film extends through an optical density (OD) range from 0 to 3 because OD is a logarithmic function that represents three orders of magnitude, or 1000.

However, the screen-film image can display only approximately 30 shades of gray on a viewbox. That is

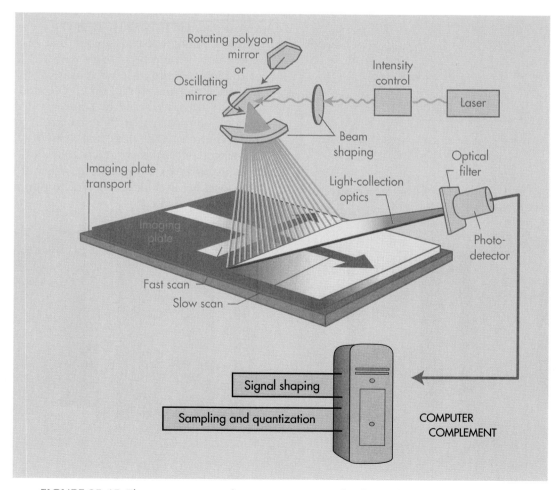

FIGURE 25-15 The computer complement to a computed radiography (CR) reader provides signal amplification, signal compression, scanning control, analog-to-digital conversion, and image buffering.

why radiographic technique is so critical in screen-film imaging. Most screen-film imaging techniques aim for radiation exposure on the toe side of the characteristic curve.

CR imaging is characterized by extremely wide latitude. Four decades of radiation exposure results in 10,000 gray levels, each of which can be evaluated visually by postprocessing.

Proper radiographic technique and exposure are essential for screen-film radiography. Overexposure and underexposure result in unacceptable images (Figure 25-17).

With CR, radiographic technique is not so critical because contrast does not change over four decades of radiation exposure. Figure 25-18 shows the appearance of CR images acquired through the same radiographic technique range as those used for Figure 25-17.

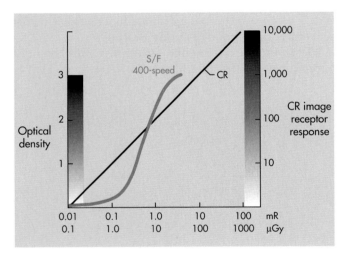

FIGURE 25-16 The image receptor response for computed radiography (CR) is shown with the characteristic curve of a screen-film image receptor.

 A 14-bit CR image has 16,384 gray levels.

Image Noise

The principal source of noise on a radiographic image is scatter radiation; this is the same whether screen-film or CR image receptors are used. Box 25-1 reviews sources of noise in screen-film radiography.

Image noise associated with CR includes all sources listed in Box 25-1, plus those provided in Box 25-2. Each of the three subsystems of CR contributes noise to the image.

Fortunately, CR noise sources are bothersome only at very low image receptor radiation exposure. Newer CR systems promise lower noise levels and therefore additional patient radiation dose reduction.

PATIENT CHARACTERISTICS
Radiation Dose

Consider the lower left quadrant of Figure 25-16, as shown in Figure 25-19. At image receptor radiation exposure less than approximately 0.5 mR (5μGy), CR is a faster image receptor when compared with a 400-speed screen-film system; therefore, lower patient exposure should be possible with CR.

Lower radiographic technique that results in lower patient dose should be possible with CR if it were not for the image noise at low exposure. This will be discussed again in Chapter 28 for all DR modalities.

At this time, it should be emphasized that the conventional approach that "kVp controls contrast" and "mAs controls OD" does not hold for CR. Because CR image contrast is constant, regardless of radiation exposure, images can be made at higher kVp and lower mAs, resulting in additional reduction in patient radiation dose.

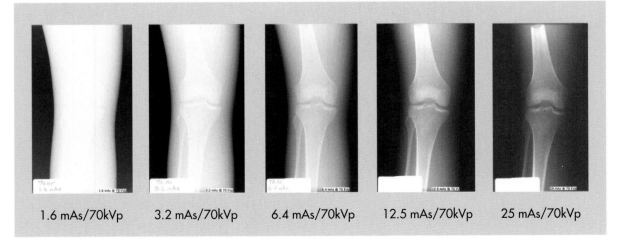

| 1.6 mAs/70kVp | 3.2 mAs/70kVp | 6.4 mAs/70kVp | 12.5 mAs/70kVp | 25 mAs/70kVp |

FIGURE 25-17 Improper radiographic technique with a screen-film image receptor results in an unacceptable image. (Courtesy Betsy Shields, Presbyterian Hospital, Charlotte, North Carolina.)

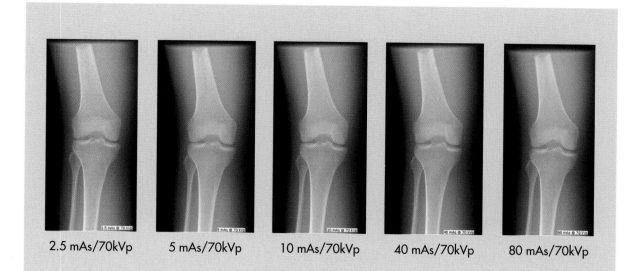

| 2.5 mAs/70kVp | 5 mAs/70kVp | 10 mAs/70kVp | 40 mAs/70kVp | 80 mAs/70kVp |

FIGURE 25-18 Computed radiography (CR) images obtained through the same radiographic technique used in Figure 25-17. (Courtesy Betsy Shields, Presbyterian Hospital, Charlotte, North Carolina.)

BOX 25-1 Sources of Image Noise in Screen-Film Radiography

- Quantum noise
  - X-ray quanta absorbed
  - X-ray quanta scattered
- Latent image fading
- Image receptor noise
- Phosphor structure
- Phosphor particle size
- Phosphor particle size distribution
- Overcoat/reflection/backing layers

BOX 25-2 Sources of Image Noise in Computed Radiography

MECHANICAL DEFECTS
- Slow scan driver
- Fast scan driver

OPTICAL DEFECTS
- Laser intensity control
- Scatter of stimulating beam
- Light quanta emitted by screen
- Light quanta collected

COMPUTER DEFECTS
- Electronic noise
- Inadequate sampling
- Inadequate quantization

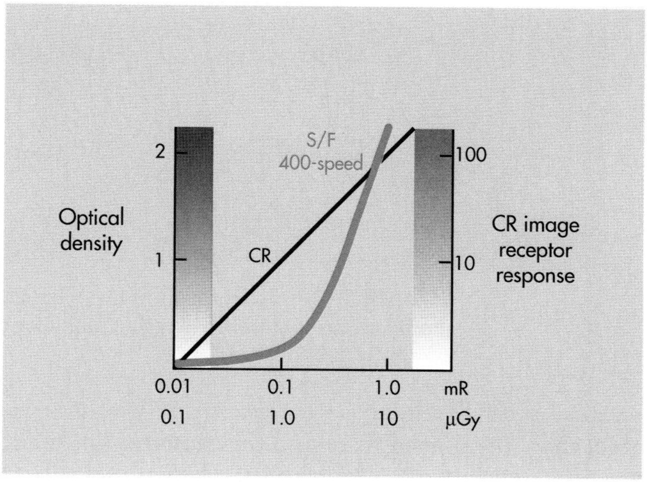

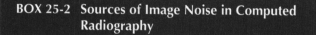

FIGURE 25-19 This region of the image receptor response curve suggests that significant patient radiation dose reduction may be possible with computed radiography (CR).

Workload

The transition from screen-film radiography to CR brings several significant changes. Fewer repeat examinations should be needed because of the wide exposure latitude. Contrast resolution will be improved and patient dose may be reduced.

 CR should be performed at lower techniques than screen-film radiography.

The radiographer will notice one less step in the workload described in Figure 25-1 (Figure 25-20).

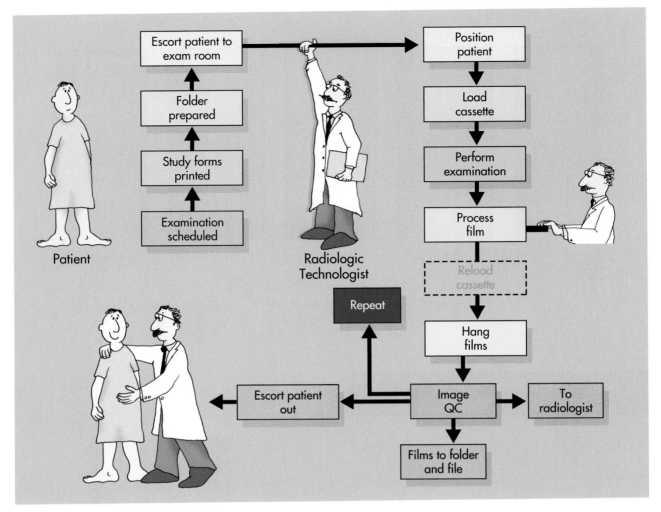

FIGURE 25-20 The transition from screen-film radiography to computed radiography (CR) removes one step from the radiography workload process.

Because the CR reader is automatic and the IP reusable, there is no need to reload the cassette. But wait, it gets much better, as you will read about in subsequent chapters.

SUMMARY

The first applications of digital radiography appeared in the early 1980s as computed radiography (CR). CR is based on the phenomenon of photostimulable luminescence (PSL).

X-rays interact with a storage phosphor screen (SPS) and form a latent image by exciting electrons to a higher-energy metastable state. In the CR reader, the latent image is made visible by releasing the metastable electrons with a stimulating laser light beam.

On returning to the ground state, electrons emit shorter-wavelength light in proportion to the intensity of the x-ray beam. The emitted light signal is digitized and reconstructed into a medical image.

The value of each CR pixel describes a linear characteristic curve over four decades of radiation exposure and a 10,000 grayscale. This wide latitude can result in reduced patient dose and improved contrast resolution. A useful rule of thumb is that current "average" screen-film exposure factors represent the absolute maximum factors for the body part in CR.

CHALLENGE QUESTIONS

1. Define or otherwise identify the following:
    a. Imaging plate
    b. Activator
    c. λs and λe
    d. Metastable electron
    e. Polychromatic
    f. Fast scan
    g. Prompt emission
    h. Storage phosphor
    i. Turbid
    j. Photodiode

2. What workload steps are omitted when one is converting from screen-film radiography to computed radiography?

3. Identify three photostimulable phosphors.

4. How is the latent image formed in computed radiography?

5. What causes a photostimulable phosphor to appear turbid?

6. How do we reduce backscatter radiation in computed radiography, and why?

7. What is the approximate color of stimulating light and emitted light?

8. What is the purpose of an optical filter positioned before the photodetector?

9. What is the difference between fast scan and slow scan?

10. What is the difference between an analog signal and a digital signal?

11. What is the difference between sampling and quantization?

12. What is the purpose of a buffer?

13. Why is beam shaping required for the laser beam?

14. What are the three subsystems of a CR reader?

15. How is ghosting due to residual latent image reduced?

16. What is the approximate difference in wavelength between prompt emission and stimulated emission?

17. How differently should one handle a computed radiography imaging plate compared with a screen-film cassette?

18. How is the latent image made visible in computed radiography?

19. What is the purpose of europium (Eu) in a photostimulable phosphor?

20. Diagram the various layers of a CR imaging plate.

The answers to the Challenge Questions can be found by logging on to our website at http://evolve.elsevier.com.

26

Digital Radiography

OBJECTIVES

At the completion of this chapter, the student should be able
to do the following:

1. Identify five digital radiographic modes in addition to computed
   radiography
2. Define the difference between direct digital radiography and indirect
   digital radiography
3. Describe the capture, coupling, and collection stages of each type of
   digital radiographic imaging system
4. Discuss the use of silicon, selenium, cesium iodide, and gadolinium
   oxysulfide in digital radiography

OUTLINE

Scanned Projection Radiography
Charge-Coupled Device
Cesium Iodide/Charge-Coupled Device
Cesium Iodide/Amorphous Silicon
Amorphous Selenium
Digital Mammography

The acceleration to all-digital imaging continues because it provides several significant advantages over screen-film radiography.

Screen-film radiographic images require chemical processing, time that can delay completion of the examination. Once an image has been obtained on film, little can be done to enhance the information content.

When the examination is complete, images are available in the form of hard copy film that must be catalogued, transported, and stored for future review. Furthermore, such images can be viewed only in a single place at one time.

These and other limitations are eliminated or reduced with the use of digital radiography (DR). This chapter describes various approaches to DR. Subsequent chapters present information on the digital image, the soft copy read of the digital image, and quality control measures for the digital image.

Because of its widespread application, computed radiography was discussed thoroughly in Chapter 25. This chapter discusses alternate approaches to DR.

Several approaches may be used to produce digital radiographs, and it is not yet clear whether one of these approaches ultimately will prevail. Furthermore, the vocabulary applied to digital radiography (DR) is not yet standard or universally accepted. The characterization and organization of DR as discussed in this book are depicted in Figure 26-1.

> Digital radiography is more efficient in time, space, and personnel than screen-film radiography.

Ehsan Samei has reported a clever approach to describing and identifying the various DR imaging systems—capture element, coupling element, and collection element.

The **capture element** is that in which the x-ray is captured. In computed radiography (CR), the capture element is the photostimulable phosphor. In the other DR modes, the capture element may be cesium iodide (CsI), gadolinium oxysulfide (GdOS), or amorphous selenium (a-Se).

The **coupling element** is that which transfers the x-ray–generated signal to the collection element. The coupling element may be a lens or fiber optic assembly, a contact layer, or a-Se.

The **collection element** may be a photodiode, a charge-coupled device (CCD), or a thin-film transistor (TFT). The photodiode and the CCD are light-sensitive devices that collect light photons. The TFT is a charge-sensitive device that collects electrons.

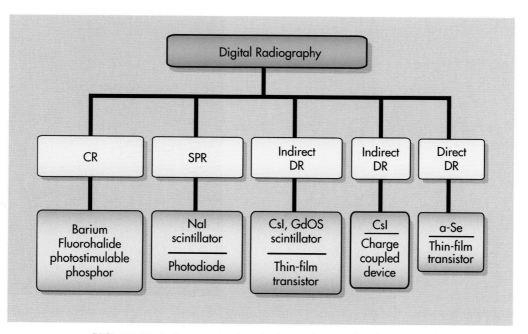

FIGURE 26-1 An organizational scheme for digital radiography.

SCANNED PROJECTION RADIOGRAPHY

Shortly after the introduction of third-generation computed tomography (CT), scanned projection radiography (SPR) was developed by CT vendors to facilitate patient positioning (Figure 26-2). It remains in use with virtually all current multislice spiral CT imaging systems.

CT vendors give this process various trademarked names, but SPR is similar for all. The patient is positioned on the CT couch and then is driven through the gantry while the x-ray tube is energized. The x-ray tube and the detector array do not rotate but are stationary, and the result is a digital radiograph (Figure 26-3).

During the 1980s and the early 1990s, SPR was developed for dedicated chest DR (Figure 26-4). The principal advantage of SPR was collimation to a fan x-ray with associated scatter radiation rejection and improvement in image contrast.

In SPR, the x-ray beam is collimated to a fan by pre-patient collimators. Postpatient image-forming x-rays likewise are collimated to a fan that corresponds to the detector array—a scintillation phosphor, usually cesium iodide (CsI)—and is married to a linear array of CCDs through a fiber optic light path.

This development was not very successful because chest anatomy has high subject contrast, so scatter radiation rejection is not all that important. Furthermore, the scanning motion required several seconds, resulting in motion blur.

At the present time, SPR is re-emerging with some modification as a promising adjunct to digital mammography tomosynthesis (DMT). The purpose of all forms of tomography is to improve image contrast, and that is the goal of DMT.

Every technical characteristic of mammography—low kVp, compression, radiographic grid—is designed to improve the image contrast of this soft tissue anatomy. First, a discussion of the CCD is provided because this device is involved in several approaches to digital radiography.

CHARGE-COUPLED DEVICE

The CCD was developed in the 1970s as a highly light-sensitive device for military use. It has since that time found major application in astronomy and digital photography.

The CCD, which is the light-sensing element for most digital cameras, has three principal advantageous imaging characteristics: sensitivity, dynamic range, and size. The CCD is a silicon-based semiconductor and is shown as an image receptor in Figure 26-5.

Sensitivity is the ability of the CCD to detect and respond to very low levels of visible light. This sensitivity is important for photographing the heavens through a telescope and for low patient radiation dose in digital imaging.

Dynamic range is the ability of the CCD to respond to a wide range of light intensity, from very dim to very bright. The dynamic range relative to that of a 400 speed screen-film radiographic image receptor is shown in Figure 26-6.

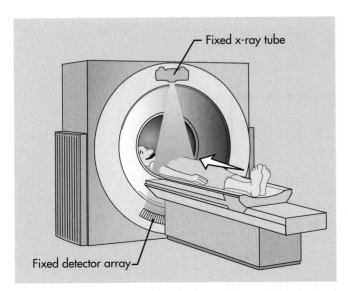

FIGURE 26-2 A scanned projection radiograph is obtained in computed tomography by maintaining the energized x-ray tube/detector array fixed while the patient is translated through the gantry.

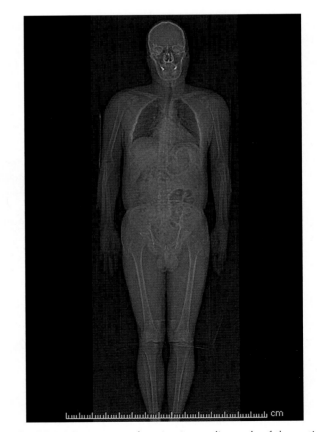

FIGURE 26-3 A scanned projection radiograph of the entire trunk of the body obtained in computed tomography. (Courtesy Colin Bray, Baylor College of Medicine.)

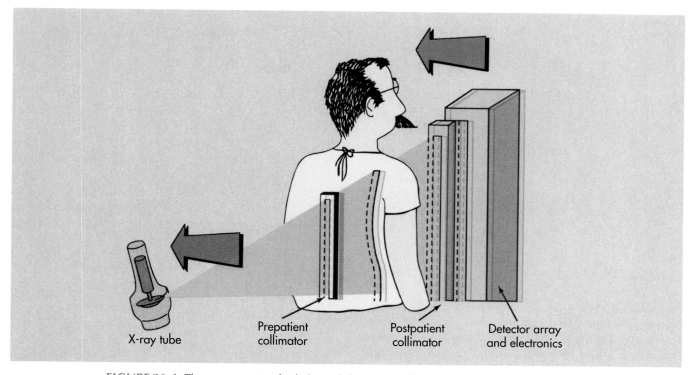

FIGURE 26-4 The components of a dedicated chest scanned projection radiography. (Courtesy Gary Barnes, University of Alabama, Birmingham.)

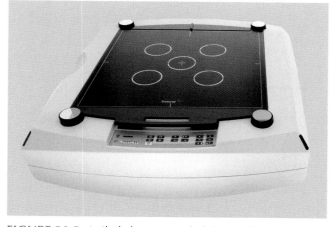

FIGURE 26-5 A tiled charge-coupled device (CCD) designed for digital radiography (DR) imaging. (Courtesy Bob Millar, Swissray.)

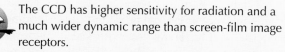

The CCD has higher sensitivity for radiation and a much wider dynamic range than screen-film image receptors.

Note that the CCD radiation response is linear, but the screen-film image receptor has the characteristic H & D (Hurter & Driffield) curve response. Although the screen-film image receptor has three decades of radiation response—optical density (OD) from 0 to 3—only approximately 30 shades of gray are perceivable by the human eye. We attempt to produce radiographs low

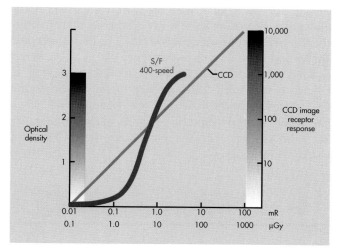

FIGURE 26-6 The radiation response of a charge-coupled device (CCD) compared with that of a 400 speed screen-film image receptor.

on the linear portion of the H & D curve to maximize image contrast.

With the use of a CCD image contrast is unrelated to image receptor x-ray exposure. Furthermore, each of the four decades of radiation response—0 to 10,000—can be visualized by image postprocessing.

Also, it should be noted that at very low x-ray exposure, the response of a CCD system is greater than that of screen-film. This should result in lower patient dose during DR.

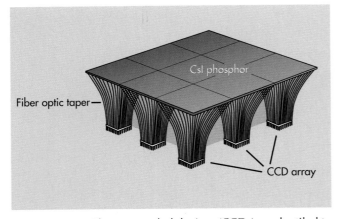

FIGURE 26-7 Charge-coupled devices (CCDs) can be tiled to receive the light from an area x-ray beam as it interacts with a scintillation phosphor such as cesium iodide (CsI).

A CCD is very small, and this makes it highly adaptable to DR in its various forms. The CCD itself measures approximately 1 to 2 cm, but the pixel size is an exceptional 100 × 100 μm!

CESIUM IODIDE/CHARGE-COUPLED DEVICE

One successful approach to DR is shown in Figure 26-7. This use of tiled CCDs receiving light from a scintillator allows the use of an area x-ray beam, so that, in contrast to SPR, exposure time is short. The image receptor shown in Figure 26-5 is of this type.

The scintillation light from a CsI phosphor is efficiently transmitted through fiber optic bundles to the CCD array. The result is high x-ray capture efficiency and good spatial resolution—up to 5 lp/mm. Figure 26-8 shows a versatile imaging system that is based on CsI/CCD technology.

 CsI/CCD is an indirect DR process by which x-rays are converted first to light then to electric signal.

The assembly of multiple CCDs for the purpose of viewing an area x-ray beam presents the challenge to create a seamless image at the edge of each CCD. This is accomplished by interpolation of pixel values at each tile interface.

CESIUM IODIDE/AMORPHOUS SILICON

An early application of DR involved the use of CsI to capture the x-ray, as in Figure 26-9, as well as transmission of the resulting scintillation light to a collection element. The collection element is silicon-sandwiched as a TFT. Silicon is a semiconductor that usually is grown as a crystal. When identified as amorphous silicon (a-silicon), the silicon is not crystalline but is a fluid that can be painted onto a supporting surface.

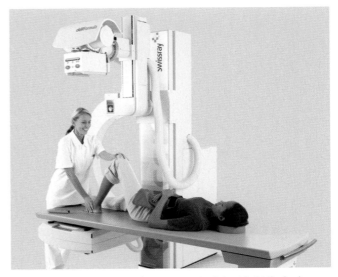

FIGURE 26-8 A versatile cesium iodide (CsI)/tiled charge-coupled device (CCD); digital radiographic imaging system. (Courtesy Bob Millar, Swissray.)

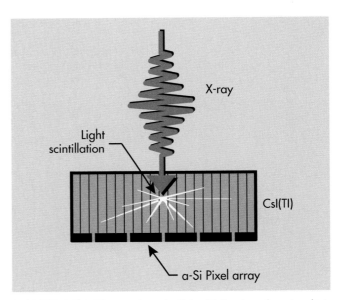

FIGURE 26-9 The cesium iodide (CsI) phosphor in digital radiography image receptors is available in the form of filaments to improve x-ray absorption and reduce light dispersion.

CsI has a high photoelectric capture because the atomic number of cesium is 55 and that of iodine is 53. Therefore, x-ray interaction with CsI is high, resulting in low patient radiation dose. The DR image receptor is fabricated into individual pixels, as shown in Figure 26-10. Each pixel has a light-sensitive face of a-Si, with a capacitor and a TFT embedded.

 CsI/a-Si is an indirect DR process by which x-rays are converted first to light then to electric signal.

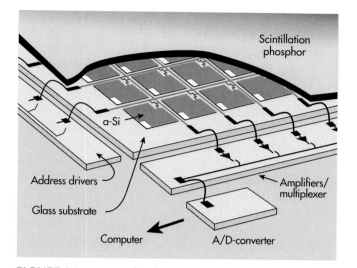

FIGURE 26-10 Digital radiographic images can be produced from the cesium iodide (CsI) phosphor light detected by the active matrix array (AMA) of silicon photodiodes.

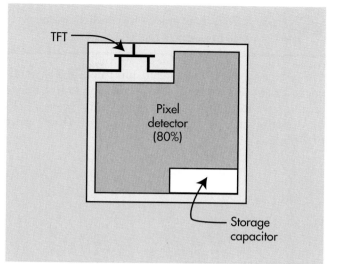

FIGURE 26-12 The fill factor is that portion of the pixel element that is occupied by the sensitive image receptor.

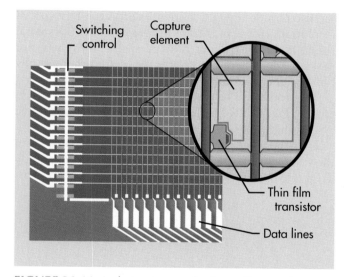

FIGURE 26-11 A photomicrograph of an active matrix array–thin-film transistor (AMA-TFT) digital radiography (DR) image receptor with a single pixel highlighted.

Figure 26-11 is a micrograph of an a-Si array that shows contacts for the switch control address drivers and the data lines. An exploded view of a single pixel shows that a large portion of the face of the pixel is covered by electronic components and wires that are not sensitive to the light emitted by the CsI phosphor.

The geometry of each individual pixel is very important, as illustrated in Figure 26-12. Because a portion of the pixel face is occupied by conductors, capacitors, and the TFT, it is not totally sensitive to the incident image-forming x-ray beam.

The percentage of the pixel face that is sensitive to x-rays is the **fill factor**. The fill factor is approximately 80%; therefore, 20% of the x-ray beam does not contribute to the image.

This represents one of the dilemmas for DR. As pixel size is reduced, spatial resolution improves but at the expense of the patient radiation dose. With smaller pixels, the fill factor is reduced and x-ray intensity must be increased to maintain adequate signal strength.

CsI has been used for years as the capture element of an image-intensifier tube. Similarly, GdOS has been widely used as the capture element of most rare Earth radiographic intensifying screens.

What has been described for the CsI/a-Si image receptor can be repeated for the GdOS/a-Si image receptor. In screen-film radiographic imaging, GdOS thickness determines speed at the image receptor.

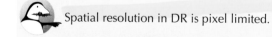

Spatial resolution in DR is pixel limited.

As GdOS screen-film speed was increased, spatial resolution was reduced because of light dispersion in the GdOS. Such is not the case with DR. Increasing thickness of GdOS in a DR image receptor increases the speed of the system, with no compromise in spatial resolution.

AMORPHOUS SELENIUM

The final DR modality is identified by some as **direct DR** because no scintillation phosphor is involved. The image-forming x-ray beam interacts directly with amorphous selenium (a-Se), producing a charged pair as shown in Figure 26-13. The a-Se is both the capture element and the coupling element.

a-Se is a direct DR process by which x-rays are converted to electric signal.

The a-Se is approximately 200 μm thick and is sandwiched between charged electrodes. The entire image receptor would appear as that shown in Figure 26-10 for CsI/a-Si and described as an active matrix array of TFTs.

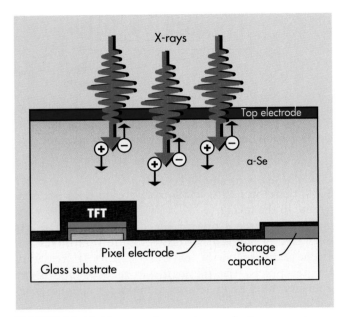

FIGURE 26-13 The use of amorphous selenium as an image receptor capture element eliminates the need for a scintillation phosphor.

X-rays incident on the a-Se create electron hole pairs through direct ionization of selenium. The created charge is collected by a storage capacitor and remains there until the signal is read by the switching action of the TFT.

DIGITAL MAMMOGRAPHY

Digital radiography received a large boost in the late 1990s with the application of DR to mammography, called digital mammography (DM). One might think that DR should have better spatial resolution than screen-film mammography because of the situation illustrated in Figure 26-14.

Light from a radiographic intensifying screen spreads and exposes a rather large area of the film. The result is limited spatial resolution. The signal emitted during CR also spreads, limiting spatial resolution. The curves shown in Figure 26-14, called *line spread functions*, indicate the relative degree of spatial resolution.

According to the description provided for Figure 26-14, the use of a-Se for DR should result in the best spatial resolution. However, such is not the case because spatial resolution in DR is limited by pixel size, with the result that no DR system can match screen-film radiography for spatial resolution.

This topic will be revisited in greater depth in Chapter 29. Figure 26-15 shows a digital mammographic system that is based on a-Se technology.

Digital mammography got a significant boost from the results of the Digital Mammography Imaging Study Trial (DMIST), which were released in late 2005. This

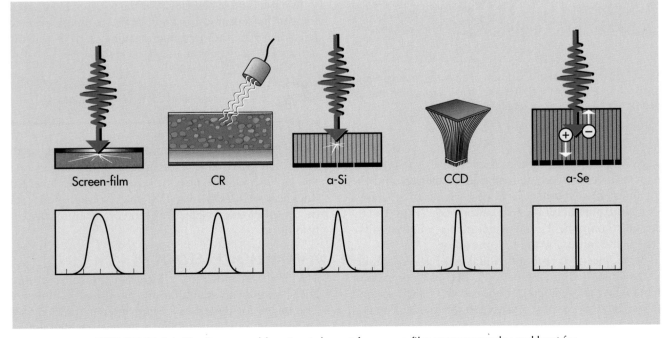

FIGURE 26-14 The line spread function is largest for screen-film mammography and least for amorphous selenium (a-Se) digital mammography.

investigation involved the imaging of nearly 50,000 women with screen-film mammography and DM interpreted from a properly designed viewing station (Figure 26-16).

The stated intention of DMIST was to determine whether digital mammography was as good as screen-film mammography. The suspicion was that it was not, because the spatial resolution of DM (5 lp/mm) was much lower than that of screen-film mammography (15 lp/mm).

On the basis of radiologists' interpretation, results showed that not only was digital mammography equal to screen-film mammography for all patients, it was better for imaging dense, glandular breast tissue. This finding suggests that contrast resolution is more important than spatial resolution for mammography and possibly for all medical imaging. This is discussed further in Chapter 28.

> Contrast resolution is more important than spatial resolution for soft tissue radiography.

Digital mammography tomosynthesis (DMT) is a recent advanced application of DM. With DMT, an area x-ray beam interacts with the digital mammographic image receptor, producing a digital mammogram. This digital mammogram is repeated several times at different angles, as shown in Figure 26-17.

Each image is available in digital form and can be reconstructed as a three-dimensional matrix of values, each representing a voxel. This is not different from CT but occurs at substantially lower patient radiation doses. With these digital data available, a tomographic section can be reconstructed with enhanced image contrast at acceptable patient radiation dose (Figure 26-18).

Figure 26-19 is a further rendition of the radiographic workflow for DR. Several additional steps are unnecessary.

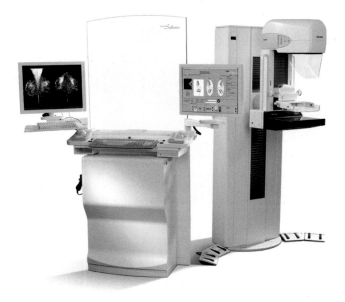

FIGURE 26-15 A digital mammographic imaging system based on amorphous selenium (a-Se) technology. (Courtesy Hologic.)

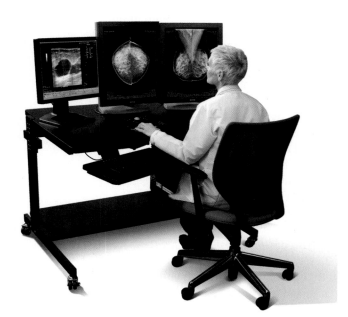

FIGURE 26-16 Secur View

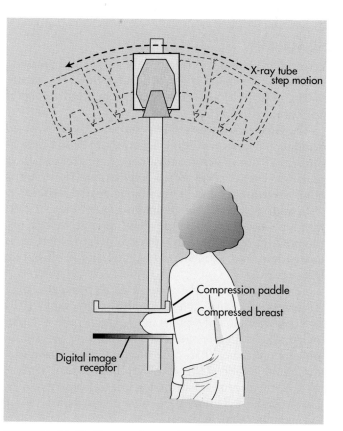

FIGURE 26-17 The projection/reconstruction scheme for digital mammography tomosynthesis.

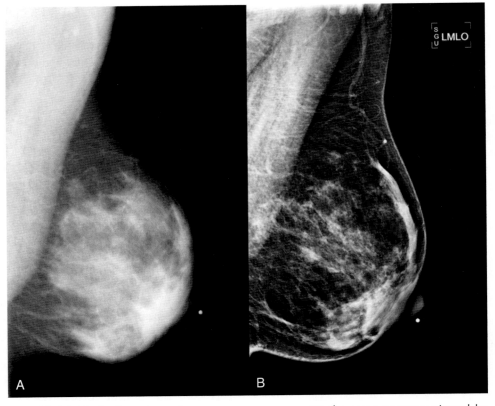

FIGURE 26-18 **A,** One view of a mammogram versus **(B)** the same anatomy viewed by digital mammography tomosynthesis.

SUMMARY

Screen-film radiology has been the medical imaging process of choice for 100 years. Now, however, we are in the midst of a rapid transfer of technology to digital radiography (DR).

The earliest DR was a spin-off from CT and involved a collimated fan x-ray beam. Scanned projection radiography (SPR) provides the advantage of scatter radiation reduction due to x-ray beam collimation. The result is better contrast resolution but limited spatial resolution.

Spatial resolution is limited to pixel size in DR; this fact has held back the development of DR until recently. It is now clear that contrast resolution is more important in medical imaging, and in this area, DR prevails.

Currently, four methods are used to produce a digital projection radiograph. Computed radiography (CR) uses photostimulable phosphor to generate a latent image. The visible image results when the photostimulable luminescence (PSL) is scanned with a laser beam.

Cesium iodide (CsI) scintillation phosphor can be used as the capture element for image-forming x-rays. This signal is channeled to a charge-coupled device through fiber optic channels.

Gadolinium oxysulfide (GdOS) or CsI is used to capture x-rays. The light from these scintillators is conducted to an active matrix array (AMA) of thin-film transistors (TFTs), whose sensitive element is amorphous silicon (a-Si).

Finally, amorphous selenium is used as a capture element for x-rays in an alternate DR method.

A recent mammographic investigation (Digital Mammography Imaging Study Trial [DMIST]) has shown DR to be superior to screen-film mammography.

CHALLENGE QUESTIONS

1. Define or otherwise identify the following:
   a. SPR
   b. Amorphous
   c. Spatial resolution
   d. Fan x-ray beam
   e. Charge-coupled device
   f. Scintillation phosphor
   g. DMIST
   h. Spatial frequency
   i. Dynamic range
   j. Tomosynthesis
2. Describe some applications for use of a CCD in addition to medical imaging.
3. What are the two principal phosphors used in DR?
4. What was the result of the DMIST investigation?

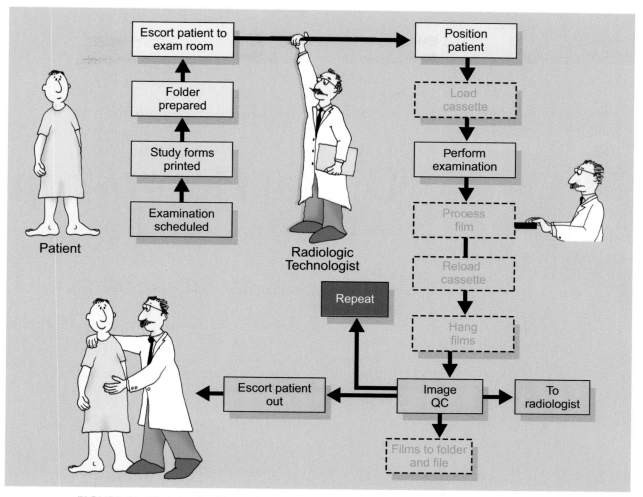

FIGURE 26-19 Several additional steps are eliminated when progressing from screen-film radiography through CR to DR.

5. By what four methods can a digital radiograph be produced?
6. Why is interest in digital mammography tomosynthesis ongoing?
7. How does pixel size in CCD DR compare with that in other forms of DR?
8. Why is fill factor important?
9. How is the tiled CCD mosaic made to appear as a single image?
10. How does the image line spread function change for the four types of DR?
11. What properties make GdOS a good DR image receptor?
12. What is the principal advantage of SPR over tiled CCDs for use in DR?
13. What is the meaning of "sensitivity" in DR?

14. Describe the role of an AMA-TFT assembly.
15. Two conducting leads are present for each digital pixel. What are they, and what do they do?
16. How does DMT show promise for improved breast cancer detection?
17. What are the respective atomic numbers for the x-ray capture elements of the various DR systems?
18. What are the consequences of producing flat panel digital image receptors with smaller pixels?
19. What is meant by "limited spatial resolution"?
20. What are the capture, couple, and collection stages for amorphous selenium (a-Se)–based DR?

The answers to the Challenge Questions can be found by logging on to our website at http://evolve.elsevier.com.

Digital Fluoroscopy

OBJECTIVES

At the completion of this chapter, the student should be able
to do the following:

1. Describe the parts of a digital fluoroscopy system and explain their
   functions
2. Compute pixel size in digital fluoroscopy
3. Describe the use of a CCD instead of a TV camera tube
4. Outline the procedures for temporal subtraction and energy
   subtraction

OUTLINE

Digital Fluoroscopy Imaging System
Image Capture
  Charge-Coupled Device
  Flat Panel Image Receptor
Image Display
  Video System
  Flat Panel Image Display
Digital Subtraction Angiography
  Image Formation
  Roadmapping
  Patient Dose

CONVENTIONAL FLUOROSCOPY produces a shadowgraph-type image on a receptor that is directly produced from the transmitted x-ray beam. Image-intensifier tubes serve as the fluoroscopic image receptor. These tubes usually are coupled electronically to a television monitor for remote viewing, as described in Chapter 21. Figure 27-1 diagrams the components used in conventional fluoroscopy.

Digital fluoroscopy (DF) is a digital x-ray imaging system that produces dynamic images obtained with an area x-ray beam. The difference between conventional fluoroscopy and DF is the nature of the image and the manner in which it is digitized.

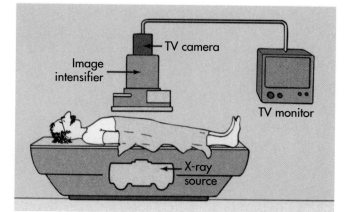

FIGURE 27-1 The imaging chain in conventional fluoroscopy.

Question: What is the pixel size of a 1000-line DF system operating in the 5-inch mode?

Answer: Five inches equals 127 mm (5 × 25.4 mm/inch). Therefore, the size of each pixel is
$$\frac{127 \text{mm}}{1024} = 0.124 \text{mm}$$

The medical physics groups at the University of Wisconsin and the University of Arizona independently initiated studies of digital fluoroscopy (DF) in the early 1970s. These studies have been continued by the research and development groups of most x-ray imaging system manufacturers.

The early approach was to use fluoroscopic equipment while placing a computer between the television camera pickup tube and the television monitor. The video signal from the television camera was routed through the computer, manipulated in various ways, and transmitted to a television monitor in a form ready for viewing.

 Advantages of DF over conventional fluoroscopy include the speed of image acquisition and postprocessing to enhance image contrast.

The initial investigators of DF demonstrated that nearly instantaneous, high-contrast subtraction images could be obtained after intravenous injection of contrast media. Although the intravenous route is still widely used, intra-arterial injections are also used with DF.

A 1024 × 1024 image matrix sometimes is described as a 1000-line system. In DF, the spatial resolution is determined both by the image matrix and by the size of the image intensifier. Spatial resolution is limited by pixel size.

DIGITAL FLUOROSCOPY IMAGING SYSTEM

A DF examination is conducted in much the same manner as a conventional fluoroscopic study. To the casual observer, the equipment is the same, but such is not the case (Figure 27-2). A computer has been added, as have multiple monitors and a more complex operating console (Figure 27-3).

Figure 27-4 shows a representative operating console of a dedicated DF imaging system. It contains alphanumeric and special function keys in the right module for entering patient data and communicating with the computer. The right portion of the console contains additional special function keys for data acquisition and image display.

The module on the right also contains computer-interactive video controls and a pad for cursor and region-of-interest (ROI) manipulation. Other systems use a trackball, a joystick, or a mouse instead of the pad. At least two monitors are used. Here the right monitors are used to edit patient and examination data and to annotate final images. The left monitors display subtracted images.

During DF, the under-table x-ray tube actually operates in the radiographic mode. Tube current is measured in hundreds of mA instead of less than 5 mA, as in image-intensifying fluoroscopy.

This is not a problem, however. If the tube were energized continuously, it would fail because of thermal overloading, and the patient dose would be exceedingly high. Images from DF are obtained by pulsing the x-ray beam in a manner called *pulse-progressive fluoroscopy*, as is shown in Figure 27-5.

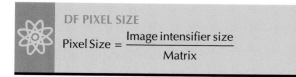

DF PIXEL SIZE

$$\text{Pixel Size} = \frac{\text{Image intensifier size}}{\text{Matrix}}$$

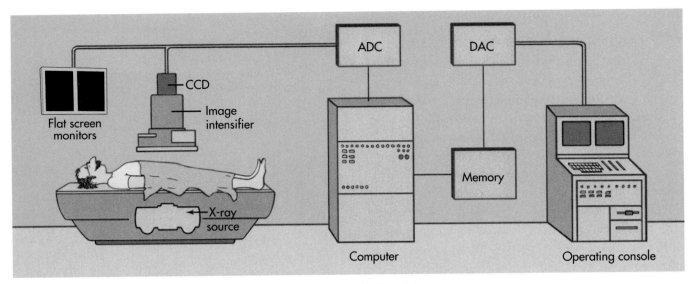

FIGURE 27-2 The components of a digital fluoroscopy system.

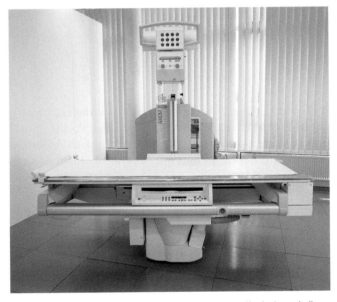

FIGURE 27-3 An installed remotely controlled digital fluoroscopic system with over-table tube and under-table image receptor. (Courtesy Siemens Medical Solutions USA.)

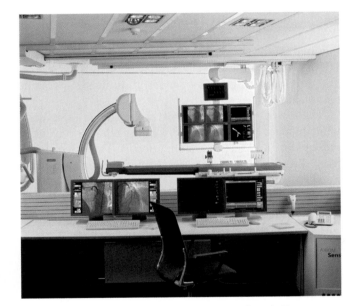

FIGURE 27-4 Operating console for a digital fluoroscopy system. (Courtesy Siemens Medical Solutions USA.)

 During DF, the x-ray tube operates in the radiographic mode.

Image acquisition rates of 1 per second to 10 per second are common in many examinations. Because 33 ms is required to produce a single video frame, x-ray exposures longer than this can result in unnecessary patient doses. This is a theoretical limit, however, and longer exposures may be necessary to ensure low noise and good image quality.

If a flat panel is the fluoroscopic image receptor instead of an II tube, x-ray exposure time can be continuously varied for even greater patient dose reduction. Each time the flat panel is exposed, it is read immediately and the image projected until the next image is acquired.

Consequently, the x-ray generator must be capable of switching on and off very rapidly. The time required for the x-ray tube to be switched on and reach selected levels of kVp and mA is called the **interrogation time.** The time required for the x-ray tube to be switched off is the **extinction time** (see Figure 27-5). DF systems must incorporate high-frequency generators with interrogation and extinction times of less than 1 ms.

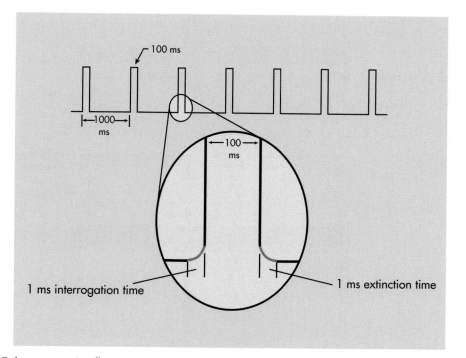

FIGURE 27-5 Pulse-progressive fluoroscopy involves terms such as *duty cycle, interrogation time,* and *extinction time.*

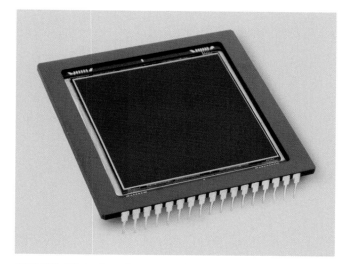

FIGURE 27-6 This charge-coupled device consists of 14-μm pixels arrayed in a 2048 × 2048 matrix; it views the light output of an image-intensifier tube. (Courtesy Apogee Instruments Inc.)

The fraction of time that the x-ray tube is energized is called the duty cycle. Figure 27-5 shows that the x-ray tube is energized for 100 ms every second. This represents a 10% **duty cycle**. This feature of pulse-progressive DF can result in significant patient radiation dose reduction.

IMAGE CAPTURE
Charge-Coupled Device

A major change from conventional fluoroscopy to DF is the use of a charge-coupled device (CCD) instead of a TV camera pickup tube, as is shown in Figure 27-2.

The charge-coupled device (CCD) was developed in the 1970s for military applications, especially in night vision scopes. Today, CCDs are used in the home camcorder, commercial television, security surveillance, and astronomy (Figure 27-6).

The demands of medical imaging are much more rigorous than in these other applications. That is why the application of the CCD in fluoroscopy is a recent development.

The sensitive component of a CCD is a layer of crystalline silicon (Figure 27-7). When this silicon is illuminated, electrical charge is generated, which is then sampled, pixel by pixel, and manipulated to produce a digital image.

The CCD is mounted on the output phosphor of the image-intensifier tube and is coupled through fiber optics or a lens system (Figure 27-8). In fact, such coupling is far more complex than that shown in Figure 27-8. A commercial CCD coupling housing is shown in Figure 27-9.

Note the device in Figure 27-9 that is labeled "ABS sensor." With a lens-coupled CCD, a sample of light is measured and is used to drive the automatic brightness stabilization (ABS) system. When the CCD is coupled to the image intensifier, the entire CCD signal is sampled and drives the ABS system.

The principal advantage of CCDs in most applications, such as a camcorder, is their small size and ruggedness. The principal advantages of their use for medical imaging are listed in Box 27-1.

The spatial resolution of a CCD is determined by its physical size and pixel count. Systems that incorporate a 1024 matrix can produce images with 10 lp/mm

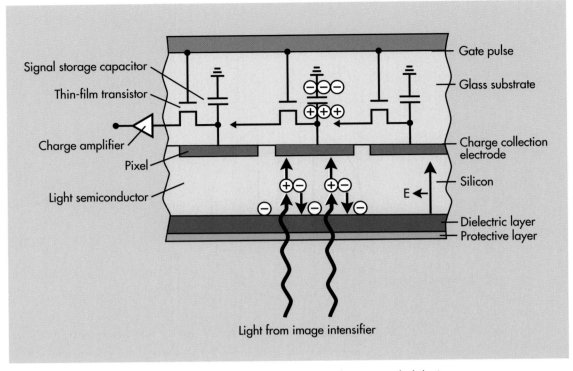

FIGURE 27-7 Cross-sectional view of a charge-coupled device.

spatial resolution. Television camera tubes can show spatial distortion in what is described as "pin cushion" or "barrel" artifact. No such distortion occurs with a CCD.

The CCD has greater sensitivity to light (detective quantum efficiency [DQE]) and a lower level of electronic noise than a television camera tube. The result is a higher signal-to-noise ratio (SNR) and better contrast resolution. These characteristics also result in substantially lower patient dose.

The response of the CCD to light is very stable. Warm-up of the CCD is not required. Neither image lag nor blooming is present. It has essentially an unlimited lifetime and requires no maintenance.

Perhaps the single most important feature of CCD imaging is its linear response (Figure 27-10). The linear response feature is particularly helpful for subtraction imaging and results in improved dynamic range and better contrast resolution.

 DF with CCD results in wider dynamic range and better contrast resolution than conventional fluoroscopy.

Flat Panel Image Receptor

The next improvement in this type of DF imaging is developing quickly: flat panel image receptors (FPIRs) composed of cesium iodide (CsI)/amorphous silicin (a-Si) pixel detectors, as described in Chapter 26 for

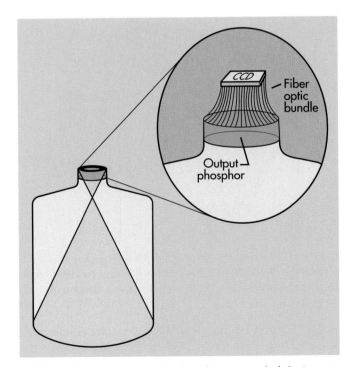

FIGURE 27-8 Manner in which a charge-coupled device can be coupled to the image-intensifier tube.

digital radiography. Faster than the time it takes for all television camera tubes to be replaced by CCDs, CCDs will begin to be replaced by FPIRs.

An installed FPIR fluoroscopic system is shown in Figure 27-11. Several features are immediately obvious.

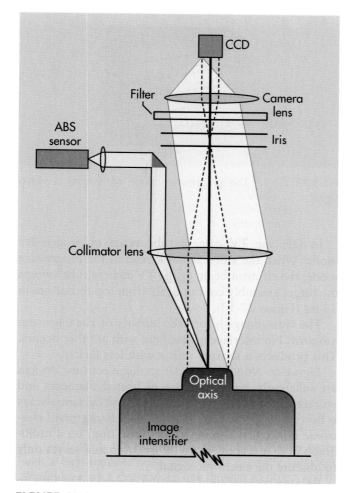

FIGURE 27-9 An example of a lens-coupling system for a charge-coupled device (CCD) to an image intensifier.

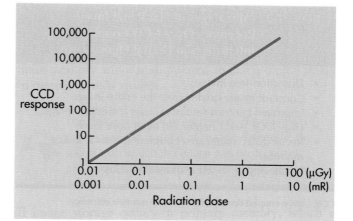

FIGURE 27-10 The response to light of a charge-coupled device is linear and can be electronically manipulated.

BOX 27-1 Advantages of Charge-Coupled Devices for Medical Imaging

- High spatial resolution
- High signal-to-noise ratio
- High detective quantum efficiency (DQE)
- No warm-up required
- No lag or blooming
- No spatial distortion
- No maintenance
- Unlimited life
- Unaffected by magnetic fields
- Linear response
- Lower patient dose

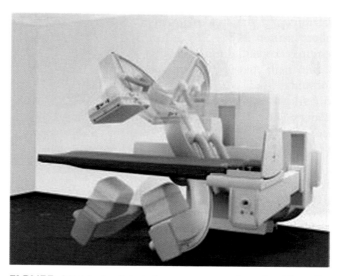

FIGURE 27-11 A digital fluoroscope equipped with a flat panel image receptor. (Courtesy Siemens Medical Solutions USA.)

The FPIR is much smaller and lighter and is manipulated more easily than an image intensifier. The FPIR imaging suite provides easier patient manipulation and radiologist/technologist movement, and there are no radiographic cassettes.

However, ease of use is not the principal reason why FPIR will prevail as the digital fluoroscope of the future.

Box 27-2 lists some advantages of FPIR over image-intensified fluoroscopy.

The image intensifier is limited by nonuniform spatial resolution and contrast resolution from the center to the periphery of the circular image. Veiling glare and pincushion distortion increase with age on an image intensifier. The response of an FPIR is uniform over the entire receptor and does not degrade with age.

The image captured by an FPIR is square or rectangular, similar to the associated flat panel monitors (see Chapter 29).

In contrast to an image-intensifier tube, the FPIR is insensitive to external magnetic fields. This has made possible a new area of interventional radiography: image-guided catheter navigation (Figure 27-12).

A special catheter with a magnetic tip is introduced into the patient vasculature. This catheter is manipulated remotely through tortuous vessels by two large steering

Table 27-2	Approximate Patient Dose in a Representative Fluoroscopic Examination	
	PATIENT DOSE	
Imaging Mode	**Conventional**	**Digital**
5 minutes' fluoroscopy	20 rad (200 mGy)	10 rad (100 mGy)
3 spot films— normal mode	0.6 rad (6 mGy)	0.2 rad (2 mGy)
3 spot films— mag 1 mode	1.0 rad (10 mGy)	0.3 rad (3 mGy)
Total dose	21.6 rad (216 mGy)	10.5 rad (105 mGy)

compares a representative fluoroscopic study performed conventionally versus one performed digitally.

Digital spot images are so easy to acquire that it is possible to make more exposures than are necessary. If the fluoroscopist gets carried away, patient dose savings will disappear.

SUMMARY

Digital fluoroscopy (DF) has added a computer, at least two monitors, and a complex control panel to conventional fluoroscopy equipment. The minicomputers in DF control the image matrix size, the system dynamic range, and the image acquisition rate. Eight to 30 images per second can be acquired with DF, depending on the image matrix mode.

Subtraction is the process of removing or masking all unnecessary anatomy from an image and enhancing only the anatomy of interest. With DF, subtraction is accomplished by temporal or energy subtraction.

Digital image processing can be used in diagnostic imaging departments for the Picture Archiving and Communication System (PACS). The file room can be replaced by a magnetic or optical memory device about the size of a desk. Teleradiology is the remote transmission of digital images to workstations in other areas of the hospital or offsite.

CHALLENGE QUESTIONS

1. Define or otherwise identify the following:
   a. Digital subtraction angiography
   b. Registration
   c. Interrogation time
   d. Hybrid subtraction
   e. CCD
   f. FPIR
   g. Progressive video scan
   h. Duty cycle
   i. ABS
   j. Flat panel display

2. What are the principal advantages of DF over conventional fluoroscopy?
3. Describe the sequence of image acquisition in mask-mode fluoroscopy.
4. Describe the differences between a video system operating in the interlace mode and one operating in the progressive mode.
5. Why are all electronic devices inherently noisy?
6. Describe the process of energy subtraction.
7. What determines the spatial resolution of a DF system?
8. A DF system is operated in a 512 × 512 image mode with a 23-cm image intensifier. What is the size of each pixel?
9. The dynamic range of some DF systems is described as 12 bits deep. What does this mean?
10. What principally determines spatial resolution in digital fluoroscopy?
11. How is automatic brightness stabilization implemented with FPIR fluoroscopy?
12. What is the pixel size of a 1000-line video system when the DF image intensifier is operated in the 12-cm mode?
13. How does a fluoroscopic image captured by FPIR differ from that captured with an II-CCD?
14. What additional equipment is required to progress from conventional fluoroscopy to DF?
15. Discuss the patient dose implications associated with DF compared with conventional fluoroscopy.
16. What is image-guided catheter navigation?
17. What x-ray energy (keV) would result in greatest contrast in digital subtraction angiography when an iodinated contrast agent is used (E_B = 33 keV)?
18. What are some advantages associated with the use of a CCD instead of a TV camera tube?
19. How can misregistration artifacts be corrected?
20. Why is signal-to-noise ratio important in DF?

The answers to the Challenge Questions can be found by logging on to our website at http://evolve.elsevier.com.

CHAPTER 28

The Digital Image

OBJECTIVES

At the completion of this chapter, the student should be able to do the following:

1. Distinguish between spatial resolution and contrast resolution
2. Identify the use and units of spatial frequency
3. Interpret a modulation transfer function curve
4. Discuss how postprocessing allows the visualization of a wide dynamic range
5. Describe the features of a contrast-detail curve
6. Discuss the characteristics of digital imaging that should result in lower patient radiation dose

OUTLINE

Spatial Resolution
    Spatial Frequency
    Modulation Transfer Function
Contrast Resolution
    Dynamic Range
    Postprocessing
    Signal-to-Noise Ratio
Contrast-Detail Curve
Patient Dose Considerations
    Image Receptor Response
    Detective Quantum Efficiency

CONVENTIONAL RADIOGRAPHIC imaging systems have worked well for over a century, providing increasingly better diagnostic images. However, conventional radiology has limitations.

Screen-film radiographic images require processing time that can delay the completion of the examination. Once an image is obtained, very little can be done to enhance the information content. When the examination is complete, images are available in the form of hard copy film that must be catalogued, transported, and stored for future review. Furthermore, such images can be viewed only in a single geographic location at a time.

Another and perhaps more severe limitation is the noise inherent in these images. Radiography uses a large area beam of x-rays. The Compton-scattered portion of the image-forming x-ray beam increases with increasing field size. This increases the noise of the radiographic image and severely degrades contrast resolution.

Medical images are obtained to help in the diagnosis of diseases or defects in anatomy. Each medical image has two principal characteristics: spatial resolution and contrast resolution. Additional image properties such as noise, artifacts, and archival quality are noted, but spatial resolution and contrast resolution are most important.

SPATIAL RESOLUTION

Spatial resolution (resolution in space) is the ability of an imaging system to resolve and render on the image a small high-contrast object. Figure 28-1 shows black dots of diminishing size on a white background.

The black on light tan is high contrast. If the dots were shades of gray, they would not exhibit high contrast, but rather low contrast.

The dots range in size from 10 mm down to 50 μm. Most people can see objects as small as 200 μm; therefore, the spatial resolution of the eye is described as 200 μm. If the dots were not high contrast, the spatial resolution of the eye would require larger dots.

Spatial resolution is usually described as the size of an object that can be viewed. In medical imaging, spatial resolution is described by the quantity "spatial frequency." Spatial frequency was introduced in Chapter 25 and is discussed further here because it is an important characteristic that is used to describe medical images and medical imaging systems.

Spatial Frequency

The fundamental concept of spatial frequency does not refer to size but to the **line pair**. A line pair is a black line on a white background, as is shown in Figure 28-2. One line pair consists of the line and an interspace of the same width as the line. Six line-pair patterns are shown, with each line and each interspace representing the size of the dots in Figure 28-1.

 Spatial frequency is expressed in line pair per millimeter (lp/mm).

Spatial frequency relates the number of line pairs in a given length, expressed as centimeters or millimeters. The unit of spatial frequency as used in medical imaging describes line pair per millimeter (lp/mm). Figure 28-3 shows the spatial frequency of the six sets of line pairs.

Question: A digital radiographic imaging system has a spatial resolution of 3.5 lp/mm. How small an object can it resolve?

Answer: 3.5 lp/mm = 7 objects in 1 mm, or 7/mm. Therefore, the reciprocal is the answer, or 1/7 mm = 0.143 mm = 143 μm

Clearly, as the spatial frequency becomes larger, the objects become smaller. Higher spatial frequency indicates better spatial resolution.

Question: A screen-film mammography imaging system operating in the magnification mode can image high-contrast microcalcifications as small as 50 μm. What spatial frequency does this represent?

Answer: It takes two 50-μm objects to form a single line pair. Therefore, 1 lp = 100 μm, or 1 lp/100 μm = 1 lp/0.1 mm = 10 lp/mm.

The concept of spatial frequency is demonstrated in Figure 28-4 by the dress of three entrepreneurs. The undertaker's plain black suit has a spatial frequency of zero. No change is seen from one part of the suit to another.

The banker's pinstripe suit has zero vertical spatial frequency but high horizontal spatial frequency. The used car salesman's coat has high spatial frequency in all directions.

Anatomy also can be described as having spatial frequency. Large soft tissues such as liver, kidney, and brain have low spatial frequency and therefore are easy to image. Bone trabeculae, breast microcalcifications, and contrast-filled vessels are high-frequency objects, and therefore, they are more difficult to image.

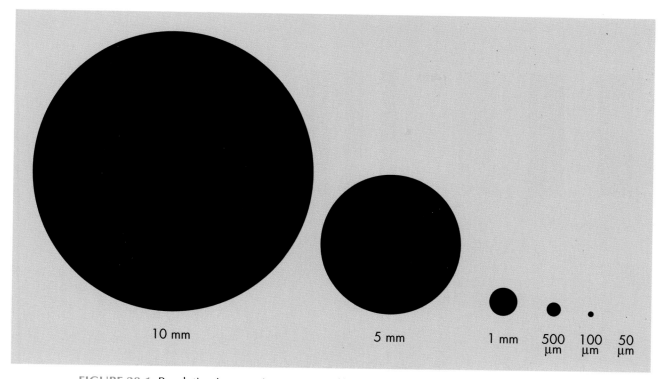

FIGURE 28-1 Resolution in space is a measure of how small an object one can see on an image.

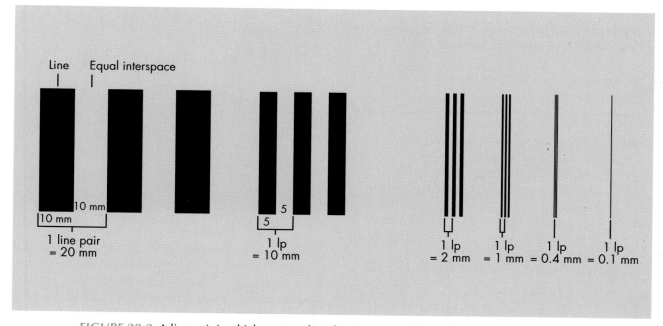

FIGURE 28-2 A line pair is a high-contrast line that is separated by an interspace of equal width.

An imaging system with higher spatial frequency has better spatial resolution.

Table 28-1 presents the approximate spatial resolution for various medical imaging systems. Sometimes, the spatial resolution for nuclear medicine, computed tomography, and magnetic resonance imaging is stated in terms of lp/cm instead of lp/mm.

Question: The image from a nuclear medicine gamma camera can resolve just 1/4 inch. What spatial frequency does this represent?

Answer: 1/4 in × 25.4 mm/in = 6.35 mm
It takes two 6.35-mm objects to form a line pair, hence 12.7 mm/lp.
The reciprocal is 1 lp/12.7 mm
= 0.08 lp/mm = 0.8 lp/cm.

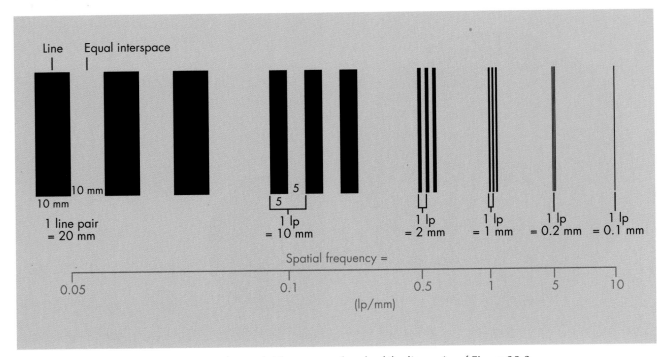

FIGURE 28-3 The spatial frequency of each of the line pairs of Figure 28-2.

The spatial resolution of projection radiography is determined by the geometry of the system, especially focal-spot size. Mammography is best because of its small focal spot—0.1 mm—for magnification.

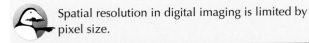 Spatial resolution in digital imaging is limited by pixel size.

Question: What is the spatial resolution of a 512 × 512 computed tomography (CT) image that has a field of view of 30 cm? What spatial frequency does that represent?

Answer: 512 pixels/30 cm = 512 pixels/300 mm
300 mm/512 pixels = 0.59 mm/pixel

Two pixels are required to form a line pair; therefore

$$2 \times 0.59 \text{ mm} = 1.2 \text{ mm/lp}$$
$$1 \text{ lp}/1.2 \text{ mm} = 0.83 \text{ lp/mm} = 8.3 \text{ lp/cm}.$$

Spatial resolution in all of the digital imaging modalities is limited by the size of the pixel. No digital imaging system can image an object smaller than one pixel. This CT imaging system is limited to a spatial resolution of 0.59 mm. or 8.3 lp/p/cm.

Modulation Transfer Function

Modulation transfer function (MTF) is a term borrowed from radio electronics that has been applied to the description of the ability of an imaging system to render objects of different sizes onto an image. Objects with

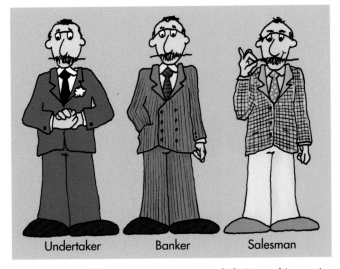

FIGURE 28-4 Three entrepreneurs and their working attire demonstrate the concept of spatial frequency.

high spatial frequency are more difficult to image than those with low spatial frequency. This is just another way of saying that small objects are harder to image.

Regardless of the size of the object, the object is considered to be high contrast, black on white, for the purpose of MTF evaluation. The ideal imaging system is one that produces an image that appears exactly as the object. Such a system would have an MTF equal to one.

 Modulation transfer function can be viewed as the ratio of image to object as a function of spatial frequency.

An ideal imaging system does not exist. The line pairs of Figure 28-1 become more blurred with increasing spatial frequency. The amount of blurring can be represented by the reduced amplitude of the representative frequency, as is shown in Figure 28-5.

Quality control test objects and tools have been designed to measure the amount of blurring as a function of spatial frequency. Figure 28-6 shows two bar pattern test tools with spatial frequencies up to 20 lp/mm. Such

tools used with a microdensitometer can measure the modulation of each spatial frequency pattern and can use those data to construct an MTF curve.

When the modulation of the bar pattern is plotted against spatial frequency, as is done in Figure 28-7, an MTF curve results. When an imaging system is evaluated through this method, the 10% MTF often is identified as the system spatial resolution.

 Imaging system spatial resolution is spatial frequency at 10% MTF.

The curve in Figure 28-7 is representative of screen-film radiography. At low spatial frequencies (large objects), good reproduction is noted on the image. However, as the spatial frequency of the object increases (the objects get smaller), the faithful reproduction of the object on the image gets worse. This MTF curve shows a limiting spatial resolution of approximately 8 lp/mm.

At low spatial frequencies, the contrast of the object is preserved, but at high spatial frequencies, contrast

TABLE 28-1	Approximate Spatial Resolution for Various Medical Imaging Systems	
Gamma camera	0.1 lp/mm
Magnetic resonance imaging	1.5 lp/mm
Computed tomography	1.5 lp/mm
Diagnostic ultrasound	2 lp/mm
Fluoroscopy	3 lp/mm
Digital radiography	4 lp/mm
Computed radiography	6 lp/mm
Radiography	8 lp/mm
Mammography	15 lp/mm

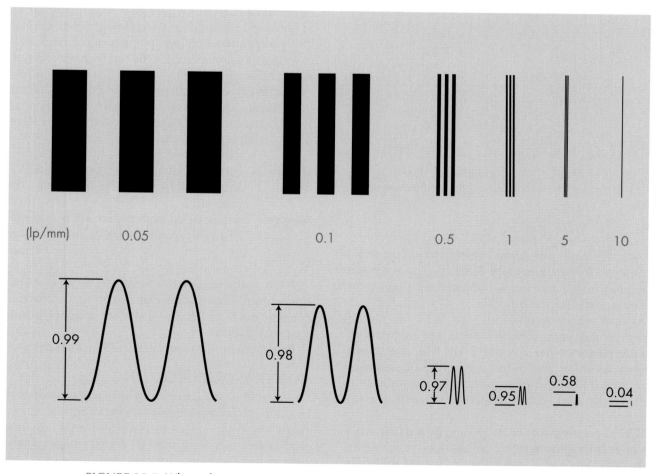

FIGURE 28-5 When a line pair pattern is imaged, the higher spatial frequencies become blurred, resulting in reduced modulation.

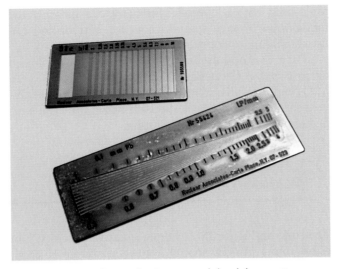

FIGURE 28-6 These plastic-encased lead bar patterns are imaged to construct a modulation transfer function (MTF). (Courtesy Fluke Biomedical.)

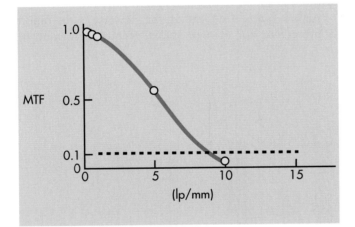

FIGURE 28-7 A plot of the modulation data from Figure 28-5 results in a modulation transfer function (MTF) curve.

is lost; this limits the spatial resolution of the imaging system. Inspect Figure 28-8, where a radiographic screen-film imaging system is compared with a mammographic screen-film system.

At low spatial frequencies, the MTF for radiography should be higher than that for mammography because two screens are used. The use of two screens amplifies the contrast of large objects with little blur. However, this is not the case because of the low kVp and tissue compression used for mammography.

With increasing spatial frequency, image blur worsens in radiography. Image blur worsens in mammography also, but not as quickly as in radiography. The use of a single screen in mammography allows better visualization of smaller objects.

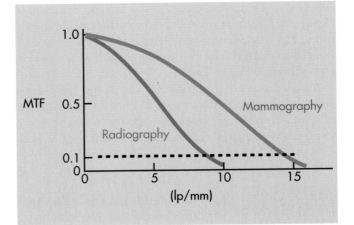

FIGURE 28-8 Screen-film mammography has a higher modulation transfer function (MTF) at low spatial frequencies and higher spatial frequencies than screen-film radiography.

As Figure 28-8 shows, radiography has a limiting spatial resolution of approximately 8 lp/mm, but that for mammography is approximately 15 lp/mm. The single screen and smaller focal spot result in better spatial resolution with mammography.

Figure 28-9 shows two photographic representations of the MTF curves of Figure 28-8 to give a better sense of how a change in MTF affects image rendition. Figure 28-9, *A* represents radiography whereas Figure 28-9, *B* represents mammography with better spatial resolution and contrast resolution.

The MTF curve that represents digital radiography (DR) (Figure 28-10) has the distinctive feature of a cutoff spatial frequency. No DR imaging system can resolve an object smaller than the pixel size.

Question: Figure 28-10 indicates a cutoff spatial frequency of 4 lp/mm for DR. What is the pixel size?

Answer: 4 lp/mm = 8 objects/mm = 8 pixels/mm
Therefore, pixel size is 1/8 mm = 0.125 mm = 125 μm.

Note also that DR has higher MTF at low spatial frequencies. This is due principally to the expanded dynamic range of DR and its higher detective quantum efficiency (DQE).

Both of these characteristics are discussed here.

CONTRAST RESOLUTION

One hundred percent contrast is black and white. The lettering on this page shows very high contrast. Contrast resolution is the ability to distinguish many shades of gray from black to white. All digital imaging systems have better contrast resolution than screen-film imaging. The principal descriptor for contrast resolution is grayscale, also called *dynamic range*.

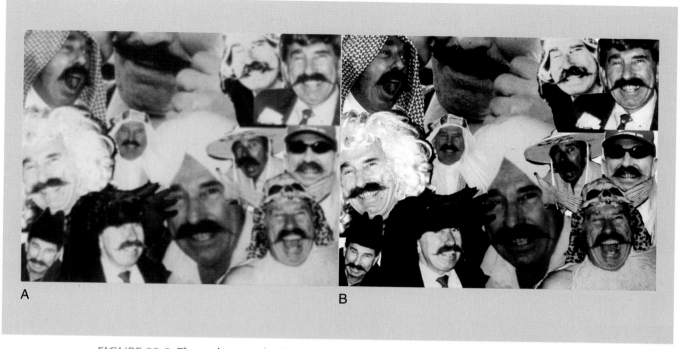

FIGURE 28-9 These photographs illustrate differences in image appearance associated with the modulation transfer function (MTF) curves of **(A)** radiography and **(B)** mammography.

Dynamic Range

The dynamic range of a screen-film radiograph is essentially three orders of magnitude, from an optical density (OD) of near 0 to 3.0 (Figure 28-11). This represents a dynamic range of 1000, but the viewer can visualize only about 30 shades of gray.

The grayscale can be made more visible with the use of specific radiographic techniques designed to increase image latitude; however, still no more than 30 shades of gray will be viewed because of the limitations of the human visual system.

> Dynamic range is the number of gray shades that an imaging system can reproduce.

The dynamic range of digital imaging systems is identified by the bit capacity of each pixel. Computed tomography and magnetic resonance imaging systems generally have a 12-bit dynamic range ($2^{12} = 4096$ shades of gray). DR may have a 14-bit dynamic range ($2^{14} = 16,384$ shades of gray). Because contrast resolution is so important in mammography, such digital systems have a 16-bit dynamic range ($2^{16} = 65,536$ shades of gray). Table 28-2 summarizes the dynamic range of various imaging systems.

Over the range of exposures used for screen-film imaging, the response of a digital imaging system is four to five orders of magnitude (Figure 28-12). Still, the human visual system is not able to visualize such a grayscale. With the postprocessing exercise of window

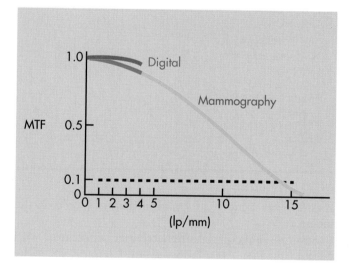

FIGURE 28-10 The modulation transfer function (MTF) curve for any digital radiographic imaging system is characterized by a cutoff frequency determined by pixel size. In this illustration the cutoff frequency is 41 lp/mm, which indicates a 125-µm pixel size,

and level, each grayscale can be visualized—not just 30 or so.

Postprocessing

A principal advantage of digital imaging is the ability to preprocess and postprocess the image for the purpose of extracting even more information. With screen-film radiographic images, what you see is what you get. One

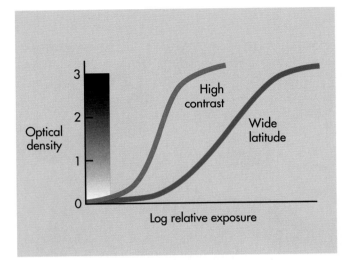

FIGURE 28-11 The contrast of a radiographic image can be somewhat controlled, but the visual range remains at approximately 30 shades of gray.

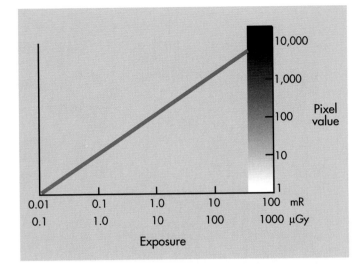

FIGURE 28-12 Digital imaging systems have a dynamic range greater than four orders of magnitude.

Table 28-2	Dynamic Range of Digital Medical Imaging Systems	
	DYNAMIC RANGE	
Imaging System	**Bit Depth**	**Shades of Gray**
Diagnostic ultrasound	2^8	256
Nuclear medicine	2^{10}	1024
Computed tomography	2^{12}	4096
Magnetic resonance imaging	2^{12}	4985
Digital radiography	2^{14}	16,384
Digital mammography	2^{16}	65,536

cannot extract more information than is visible on the image.

Several image-processing activities associated with digital imaging are discussed in Chapter 29. One postprocessing activity—window and level—is discussed here because it makes possible visualization of the entire dynamic range of the grayscale.

Consider the grayscale presented in Figure 28-13, which represents a 14-bit dynamic range. The 16,384 distinct values for the grayscale are far more than we can visualize.

The range from white to black has been arbitrarily divided into 10 gray levels. Place a pencil over one of the dividers and see if you can distinguish the adjacent gray levels from one another. For most people, approximately 30 gray levels is about the limit of contrast resolution.

With use of the window and level postprocessing tool, any region of this 16,384 grayscale can be expanded into

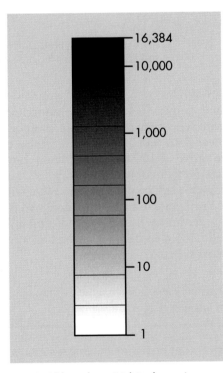

FIGURE 28-13 Although a 14-bit dynamic range contains 16,384 shades of gray, we can see only about 30 of them.

a white-to-black grayscale, as is shown in Figure 28-14. This postprocessing tool is especially helpful when soft tissue images are evaluated.

Postprocessing allows visualization of all shades of gray.

The breast consists of essentially totally soft tissue and therefore is difficult to image. The subject contrast

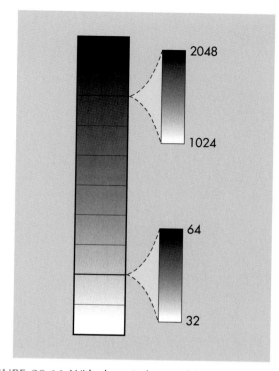

FIGURE 28-14 With the window and level postprocessing tool, any region and range of the 16,384 can be rendered as 30 shades of gray.

is poor; this requires that low kVp must be used to accentuate photoelectric interaction.

Figure 28-15, *A,* shows a screen-film mammogram of good quality. Figure 28-15, *B,* is a digital mammogram of the same breast that shows somewhat better contrast. Figure 28-15, *C* and *D* are digital mammograms of the same breast that show even better contrast because of window and level postprocessing.

In early 2006, results of the Digital Mammography Imaging Screening Trial (DMIST) were reported. This study was commissioned by the American College of Radiology Imaging Network (ACRIN) and the National Institutes of Health (NIH). A total of 50,000 women were imaged with screen-film mammography and digital mammography, and results show that for the younger, denser breast, digital mammography was better.

For older, less dense breasts, digital mammography was equal to screen-film mammography. This suggests that contrast resolution is more important than spatial resolution when soft tissue is imaged.

Signal-to-Noise Ratio

The signal in a radiographic image is that portion of the image-forming x-rays that represents anatomy. In all radiographic imaging, the number of such x-rays is huge. The signal represents the difference between those x-rays transmitted to the image receptor and those absorbed photoelectrically, as is seen in Figure 28-16.

Other sources of noise in addition to scatter radiation may be associated with the image receptor, regardless of whether it is the screen-film or digital type. The signal-to-noise ratio (SNR) is important to any medical image. Noise limits contrast resolution; therefore, practitioners strive for as high an SNR as possible, in keeping with ALARA (As Low As Reasonably Achievable).

> Image noise limits contrast resolution.

In general, as the mAs is increased, the SNR also is increased, although at the expense of increased patient dose. This is a dilemma that is faced in digital imaging, as is discussed later in this chapter.

Another way to increase SNR is seen in digital subtraction angiography (DSA). Suppose a single DSA image has an SNR of 1:1, this represents a signal value of 1 and a noise value of 1. If two sequential DSA images are integrated, that is, added to each other, the signal is doubled, but the noise is increased only by the square root of two, or 1.414. Therefore, the SNR is 2/1.414 = 1.414.

Signal increases in proportion to the number of images integrated; noise increases in proportion to the square root of the number of images.

When four DSA frames are integrated, the signal is increased four times. The noise is increased by the square root of four or two. Therefore, SNR = 4/2 = 2 after four-image integration.

CONTRAST-DETAIL CURVE

Another method for evaluating the spatial resolution and contrast resolution of an imaging system is the contrast-detail curve. This method involves information similar to an MTF curve, but most find it easier to interpret.

Quality control test tools such as that shown in Figure 28-17 simplify the construction of a contrast-detail curve for any imaging system. Such tools have rows of holes of varying sizes that are fashioned into a plastic or aluminum sheet. Each row is associated with a column of holes of the same size that are drilled to a different depth. A similar test tool is shown in Figure 28-18, *A.* Its image is shown in Figure 28-18, *B* where the result is a pattern on the image of holes of varying size and contrast *(arrow).*

Upon close inspection of the image of Figure 28-18, *B* one can carve out a curve of those holes that are visible. The result is a curve that appears as in Figure 28-19. This contrast-detail curve is a plot of the just perceptible visualization of size as a function of object contrast.

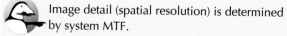

> Image detail (spatial resolution) is determined by system MTF.

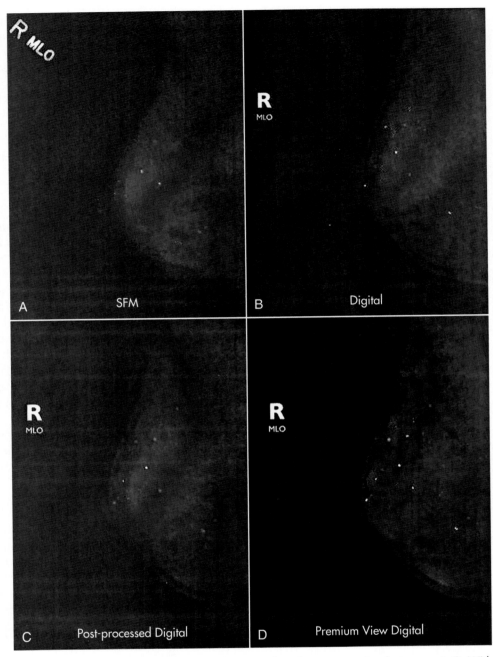

FIGURE 28-15 A, With screen-film mammography what you see is what you get. **B,** With digital mammography contrast is enhanced. **C** and **D,** By postprocessing the digital image, contrast can be further enhanced. (Courtesy Ed Hendrick, Northwestern University.)

The contrast-detail curve shows that when object contrast is high, small objects can be imaged. When object contrast is low, large objects are required for visualization on an image.

The left side of the contrast-detail curve, that related to high-contrast objects, is said to be limited by the MTF of the imaging system. Spatial resolution is determined by the MTF of the imaging system.

The right side of the curve, which relates to low-contrast objects, is said to be noise limited. Noise reduces contrast resolution.

An example of the use of a contrast-detail curve is shown in Figure 28-20, which compares two digital radiographic imaging systems that have different pixel sizes. The system with the smaller pixel size will have better spatial resolution, but the contrast resolution of both will be the same if the same imaging technique is used.

If the mAs is increased during digital radiography, spatial resolution remains the same but contrast resolution is improved at the higher mAs. This is shown in Figure 28-21; it may seem strange that the higher

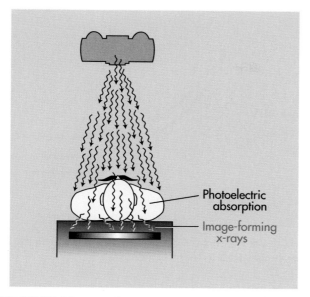

FIGURE 28-16 Image-forming x-rays are those that are transmitted through the patient unattenuated (signal) and those that are Compton scattered (noise).

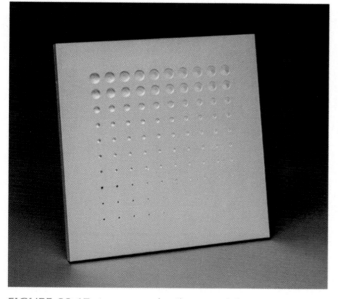

FIGURE 28-17 A contrast-detail test tool for constructing a contrast-detail curve. (Courtesy Fluke Biomedical.)

mAs image results in a lower curve. The lower curve represents better contrast resolution because tissue with lower subject contrast can be imaged.

Contrast resolution is limited by noise or SNR.

The object of the contrast-detail curve is to better understand that which influences spatial resolution—MTF—and that which influences contrast resolution—

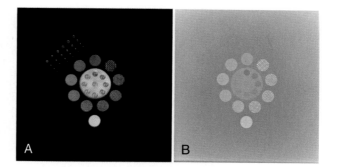

FIGURE 28-18 A contrast-detail tool (**A**) and its image (**B**) allows construction of a contrast-detail curve. (**A** courtesy American College of Radiology; **B** courtesy David Albers, Rice University.)

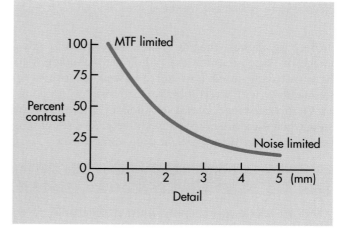

FIGURE 28-19 The contrast-detail curve is a plot of minimum visual size as a function of contrast.

SNR—for various imaging systems. It is an instructive method of understanding how technique factors and imaging system factors influence spatial resolution and contrast resolution.

Figure 28-22 shows the relative contrast-detail curves for various medical imaging systems. Note that mammography has the best spatial resolution, principally because of focal-spot size.

Magnetic resonance imaging (MRI) has the best contrast resolution because of the range of the tissue values of proton density, TI relaxation time, and T2 relaxation time. Computed tomography, however, has the best contrast resolution of all x-ray imaging systems because of x-ray beam collimation and the resultant reduction in scatter radiation.

PATIENT DOSE CONSIDERATIONS

With acceleration to all-digital imaging, practitioners have the opportunity to reduce patient dose by 20% to 50%, depending on the examination. However, quite the opposite has occurred—something that many call "dose creep."

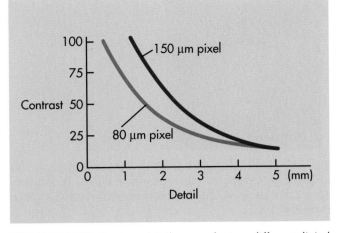

FIGURE 28-20 Contrast-detail curves for two different digital imaging systems with different pixel sizes.

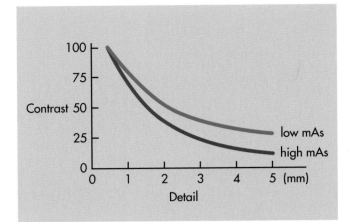

FIGURE 28-21 Contrast-detail curves for a single digital imaging system operated at different mAs.

Because digital imaging can always yield a good image, it is possible for the radiologic technologist to be unwittingly lured into not adjusting exposures as frequently as with screen-film, for example, by not changing factors between a lateral view and an anteroposterior view when these are taken consecutively. As a result, it is possible for the overall patient dose to increase.

BOX 28-1 Dose Reduction With Digital Radiography

- Exposures should not be repeated in digital radiography (DR) because of brightness or contrast concerns.
- DR systems cannot compensate for excessive noise caused by quantum mottle.
- Overexposed images do not have to be repeated and should not become a habit.

Patient dose reduction should be possible because of the manner in which the digital image receptor responds to x-rays and because of a property of the digital image receptor known as *detective quantum efficiency,* which was introduced earlier.

Image Receptor Response

Consider again the responses of a screen-film image receptor and a digital image receptor, as shown in Figure 28-23. These curves relate to the contrast resolution of the respective imaging system; they do not represent spatial resolution. Recall that spatial resolution in screen-film radiography is determined principally by focal-spot size, but spatial resolution in digital imaging is determined by pixel size.

 Spatial resolution in screen-film radiography is determined principally by focal spot size.

Because digital image receptor response is linearly related to radiation dose, image contrast does not change with dose. One cannot overexpose or underexpose a digital image.

Therefore a digital image should never require repeating because of exposure factors. The exposure factor–related repeat rate for screen-film radiography ranges to approximately 5%, and this translates directly to a dose reduction for digital imaging patients.

Figure 28-23 shows the range for a properly exposed 400 speed screen-film radiograph. When overexposed or underexposed image contrast is reduced. Such is not the case for digital imaging, and this affords a considerable opportunity for dose reduction.

Contrast resolution is preserved in digital imaging, regardless of dose.

The screen-film radiographs of a foot phantom shown in Figure 28-24 are labeled with the technique used for each. Screen-film radiographs are overexposed or underexposed easily; however, this is not the case with digital images.

Figure 28-25 shows the same foot phantom imaged digitally at the same techniques of Figure 28-24. The respective radiation exposure values are shown to emphasize the possible patient radiation dose reduction with digital imaging.

Radiographic technique for screen-film imaging requires (1) that an appropriate kVp should be selected on the basis of the anatomy that is being imaged, and (2) that the proper mAs should be selected to produce proper OD on the finished image. For screen-film imaging, kVp controls contrast, and mAs controls OD.

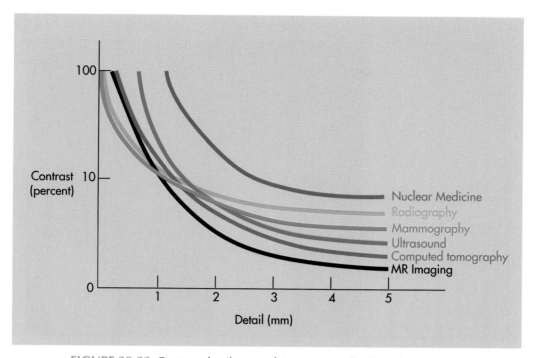

FIGURE 28-22 Contrast-detail curves for various medical imaging systems.

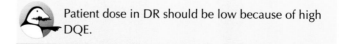

Technique creep should replace dose creep.

Digital imaging techniques must be approached differently. Instead of "dose creep," "technique creep" should be used with each of the various digital imaging systems. The result will be patient dose reduction.

Because digital image contrast is unrelated to dose, kVp becomes less important. When digital examination of specific anatomy is conducted, the kVp should start to be increased, and an accompanying reduction in mAs should be noted with successive examinations. The result will be adequate contrast resolution, constant spatial resolution, and reduced patient dose.

The patient dose reduction that is possible is limited. Figure 28-26 is an additional rendering of the image receptor response curves of Figure 28-23, except here, the region for digital image receptor exposure is highlighted.

The problem with very low technique for digital imaging is low SNR. Noise can predominate and compromise the interpretation of soft tissue anatomy.

Detective Quantum Efficiency

The probability that an x-ray will interact with an image receptor is determined by the thickness of the capture layer and its atomic composition. The descriptor used for medical imaging is detective quantum efficiency (DQE). DQE is related to the absorption coefficient and to the spatial frequency of the signal.

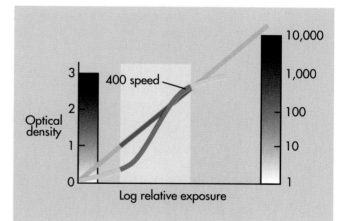

FIGURE 28-23 Response of a screen-film and a digital image receptor.

Patient dose in DR should be low because of high DQE.

For present purposes, DQE can be regarded as the absorption coefficient; it is highly x-ray energy dependent. Table 28-3 presents the atomic number for various elements used in digital and screen-film image receptors and the K-shell absorption edge for the most responsive element.

Lanthanum oxysulfide (LaOS) and gadolinium oxysulfide (GdOS) are the two principal image capture elements used in radiographic screens. Barium fluorobromide (BaFBr), cesium iodide (CsI), and

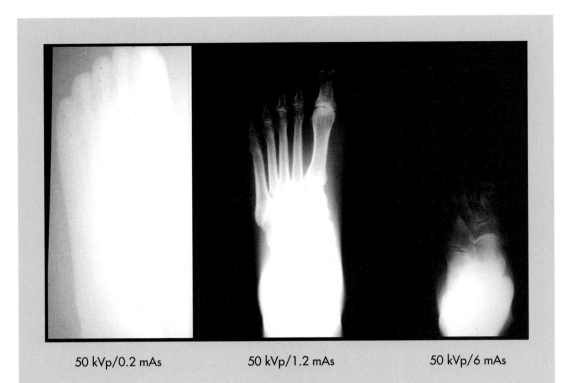

50 kVp/0.2 mAs   50 kVp/1.2 mAs   50 kVp/6 mAs

FIGURE 28-24 Screen-film radiographs of a foot phantom showing overexposure and underexposure because of wide-ranging technique. (Courtesy Anthony Siebert, University of California, Davis, California.)

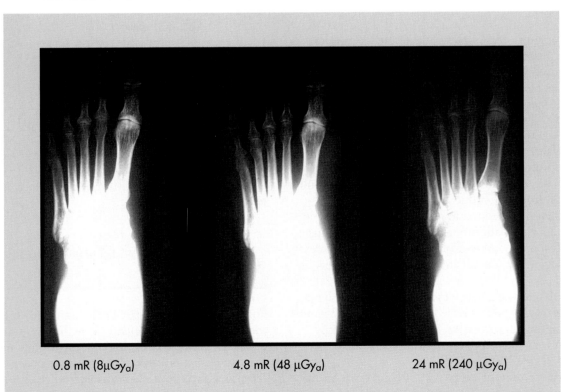

0.8 mR (8μGy$_a$)   4.8 mR (48 μGy$_a$)   24 mR (240 μGy$_a$)

FIGURE 28-25 Digital images of a foot phantom using the same radiographic techniques as in Figure 28-24 show the maintenance of contrast over a wide range of patient dose. (Courtesy Anthony Siebert, University of California, Davis, California.)

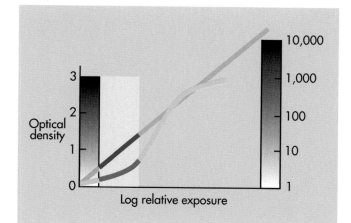

FIGURE 28-26 At very low exposure of a digital image receptor, spatial resolution and contrast are maintained but image noise may be troublesome.

TABLE 28-3	Atomic Number and K-Shell Binding Energy for Various Image Receptors		
Image Receptor	Capture Element	Atomic Number	K-Shell Binding Energy
GdOS	Gd	64	55 keV
LaOS	La	57	39 keV
BaFBr	Ba	56	37 keV
CsI	Cs	55	35 keV
	I	53	33 keV
a-Se	Se	34	12 keV

a-Se, Amorphous selenium; *BaFBr*, barium fluorobromide; *CsI*, cesium iodide; *GdOS*, gadolinium oxysulfite; *LaOS*, lanthanum oxysulfide.

amorphous selenium (a-Se) are used with digital image receptors. The value of DQE for each of these capture elements is strongly dependent on x-ray energy, as is shown in Figure 28-27.

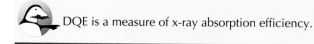

DQE is a measure of x-ray absorption efficiency.

Figure 28-28, a simplification of Figure 28-27, combines the various DQE values for screen-film, computed radiography (CR), and DR image receptors with a 90-kVp x-ray emission spectrum. Note that the DQE for DR is higher than that for CR or screen-film. CR has a slightly higher DQE than screen-film.

The relative value of DQE for various image receptors means that fewer x-rays are required by the higher DQE

receptors to produce an image; this translates into lower patient dose. The additional feature shown in Figure 28-28 is that most x-rays have energy that matches the K-shell binding energy; this relates to greater x-ray absorption at that energy.

The scatter x-ray beam has lower energy than the primary x-ray beam.

One final feature of this analysis of DQE and patient radiation dose relates to the x-ray beam incident on the image receptor. When the 90-kVp x-ray beam interacts with the patient, most of the x-rays are scattered and are reduced in energy as shown in Figure 28-28. This results in even greater absorption of image-forming x-rays.

This analysis of image receptor response and DQE shows that both characteristics of digital image receptors suggest that patient dose should be less with digital imaging than with screen-film imaging. Coupled with a new approach to radiographic technique that is based on increased kVp and reduced mAs, digital imaging will result in reduced patient radiation dose.

SUMMARY

The digital medical image is limited by one deficiency when compared with screen-film radiography—spatial resolution. Spatial resolution, the ability to image small high-contrast objects, is limited by pixel size in digital imaging.

However, digital imaging has several important advantages over screen-film imaging. Digital images are obtained faster than screen-film images because wet chemistry processing is unnecessary. Digital images can be viewed simultaneously by multiple observers in multiple locations. Digital images can be transferred and archived electronically, thereby saving imaging retrieval time and film file storage space.

It is even more important to note that digital images have a wider dynamic range, and this results in better contrast resolution. With postprocessing, thousands of gray levels can be visualized, allowing extraction of more information from each image. The modulation transfer function curve and the contrast-detail curve represent the favorable characteristics of a digital image.

Perhaps the principal favorable characteristic of digital imaging is the opportunity for patient radiation dose reduction. This occurs because of the linear manner in which the image receptor responds to x-rays, and because of the greater detective quantum efficiency of the digital image receptor.

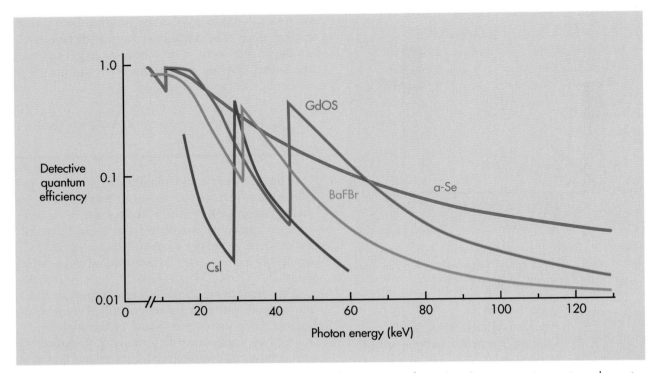

FIGURE 28-27 Detective quantum efficiency as a function of x-ray energy for various image receptor capture elements.

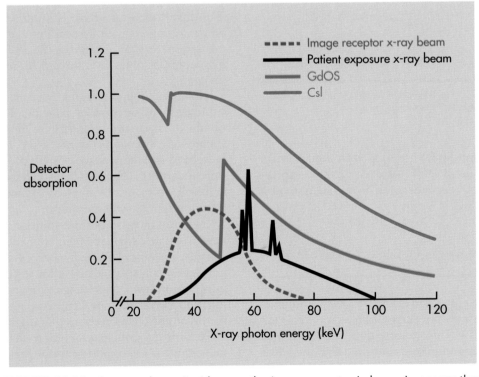

FIGURE 28-28 The x-ray beam incident on the image receptor is lower in energy than the beam incident on the patient and better matches the x-ray absorption of capture elements.

CHALLENGE QUESTIONS

1. Define or otherwise identify the following:
   a. Spatial frequency
   b. Detective quantum efficiency
   c. Contrast resolution
   d. Modulation transfer function
   e. K-shell binding energy
   f. Bar pattern test tool
   g. Contrast detail curve
   h. Dynamic range
   i. DMIST
   j. Postprocessing
2. What is the spatial frequency of a 100-μm high-contrast object?
3. The best a magnetic resonance imaging system can do is approximately 2 lp/cm. What is this limit in lp/mm?
4. The limiting spatial resolution for computed radiography is approximately 6 lp/mm. What size object does this represent?
5. What tissues would be considered low spatial frequency structures?
6. What tissues would be considered high spatial frequency structures?
7. What medical imaging system has the best spatial resolution? Why?
8. What medical imaging system has the best contrast resolution? Why?
9. What units are found along the vertical and horizontal axes of an MTF curve?
10. What units are found along the vertical and horizontal axes of a contrast-detail curve?
11. How is image blur related to object spatial frequency?
12. What value of MTF is generally considered the limiting spatial resolution of an imaging system?
13. Why does a digital imaging system have a cutoff spatial frequency?
14. Compare the dynamic range of the human visual system with those of screen-film radiography and digital imaging.
15. A 12-bit dynamic range has how many shades of gray?
16. What were the principal findings of the DMIST, and what are their implications for medical imaging?
17. How does image integration in DSA improve signal-to-noise in the image?
18. Describe the quality control test tool designed to produce a contrast-detail curve.
19. Which—spatial resolution or contrast resolution—is more influenced by image noise?
20. Discuss "dose creep" and "technique creep."

The answers to the Challenge Questions can be found by logging on to our website at http://evolve.elsevier.com.

CHAPTER 29

Viewing the Digital Image

OBJECTIVES

At the completion of this chapter, the student should be able
to do the following:

1. Identify quantities and units used in photometry
2. Explain the variation in luminous intensity of digital display devices
3. Describe differences in hard copy and soft copy and in the interpretation of each
4. Discuss the features of an AMLCD
5. Describe the features of preprocessing and postprocessing
6. Identify application of the Picture Archiving and Communication System

OUTLINE

Photometric Quantities
    Response of the Eye
    Photometric Units
    Cosine Law
Hard Copy–Soft Copy
Active Matrix Liquid Crystal Display
    Display Characteristics
    Image Luminance
    Ambient Light
Preprocessing the Digital Image
Postprocessing the Digital Image
Picture Archiving and Communication System
    Network
    Storage System

TO THIS point in medical imaging, understanding the physical concepts and associated quantities of energy and radiation has been necessary. The adoption of digital imaging and the "soft read" of images on a digital display device requires an understanding of an additional area of physics—photometry.

Photometry is the science of the response of the human eye to light. Refer to the discussion in Chapter 21 for an overview of human vision and a brief description of the anatomy of the eye.

PHOTOMETRIC QUANTITIES

A description of human visual response is exceptionally complex and involves psychology, physiology, and physics, among other disciplines. The first attempt to quantify human vision was made in 1924 by the newly formed Commission Internationale de l'Éclairage (CIE) and included a definition of light intensity, the candle, the footcandle, and candle power.

Response of the Eye

The CIE recognized the difference between photopic bright light vision with cones and scotopic dim light vision with rods. This resulted in the standard CIE photopic and scotopic response curves shown in Figure 29-1. Bright vision is best at 555 nm, and dim vision is best at 505 nm.

Photometric Units

Now the radiologic technologist must have some familiarity with all units used to express photometric quantities. The basic unit of photometry is scaled to the maximum photopic eye response at 555 nm and is the **lumen**.

> The basic photometric unit is the lumen.

Luminous flux, the fundamental quantity of photometry, is expressed in lumens (lm). Luminous flux describes the total intensity of light from a source. Household lamps are rated by the power they consume in watts. An equally important value found on each lamp package is its luminous flux in lumens.

Illuminance describes the intensity of light incident on a surface. One lumen of luminous flux incident on a single square foot is a footcandle (fc). This English unit, the fc, is still in wide use. The metric equivalent is 1 lumen per square meter, which is 1 lux (lx) (1 footcandle = 10.8 lux).

Luminance intensity is a property of the source of light, such as a viewbox or a digital display device. Luminance intensity is the luminous flux that is emitted into the entire viewing area; it is measured in lumens per steradian or **candela.**

Luminance is a quantity that is similar to luminance intensity. Luminance is another measure of the brightness of a source such as a digital display device expressed as units of candela per meter squared or **nit.**

Table 29-1 summarizes these photometric quantities and their associated units.

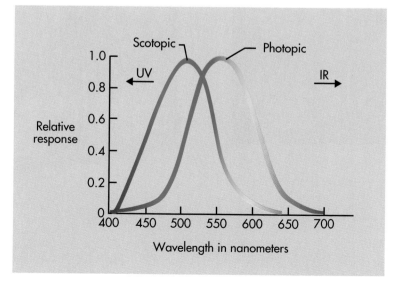

FIGURE 29-1 Photometric response curves for human vision.

Table 29-2 shows the range of illuminance for several familiar situations. Most indoor work and play areas are illuminated to 100 to 200 footcandles.

Cosine Law

Two fundamental laws are associated with photometry. Luminous intensity decreases in proportion to the inverse square of the distance from the source. This is the famous **inverse square law** (see Chapter 4).

TABLE 29-1	Photometric Quantities and Units	
Quantity	Units	Abbreviation
Luminous flux	Lumen	lm
Illuminance	Lumen/ft²	fc
	Lumen/m²	lx
Luminous intensity	Lumen/steradian	cd
Luminance	Candela/m²	nit

TABLE 29-2	Illuminance in Modern Lighting Scene Illuminance (fc)
Digital image reading room	1
Twilight	5
Corridor	20
Waiting room	30
Laboratory	100
Tennis court	200
Cloudy day	1000
Surgery	3000
Sunny day	10,000

The **cosine law** is important when one is describing the luminous intensity of a digital display device. When a monitor is viewed straight on, the luminous intensity is maximum. When a monitor is viewed from an angle, the contrast and the luminous intensity, as seen in Figure 29-2, are reduced.

> The best viewing of a digital display device is straight on.

This reduced projected surface area follows a mathematical function called a *cosine*. Luminous intensity falls off rapidly as one views a digital display device at larger angles from perpendicular.

HARD COPY–SOFT COPY

Until the mid 1990s, essentially all medical images were "hard copy," that is, the images were presented to the radiologist on film. The image was interpreted from the film, which was positioned on a lighted viewbox.

Computed tomography (1974) and magnetic resonance imaging (1980) represent the first widespread digital medical images. However, until recently, even these digital images were interpreted from film placed on a lighted viewbox.

Now, essentially all digital images are read or interpreted from presentation on a digital display device. The knowledge required of a radiologic technologist regarding the viewing of a film image on a viewbox is

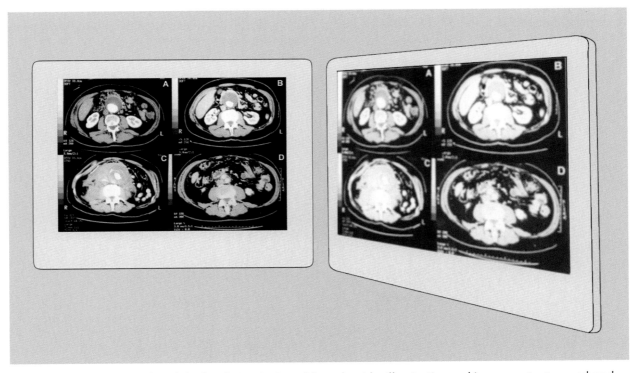

FIGURE 29-2 When a digital display device is viewed from the side, illumination and image contrast are reduced.

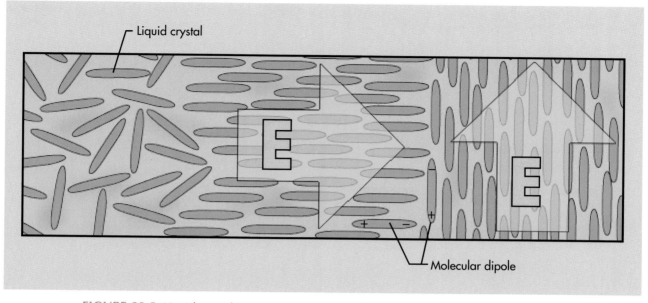

FIGURE 29-3 Liquid crystals are randomly oriented in the natural state and are structured under the influence of an external electric field.

rather simple. The knowledge required for soft copy viewing on a digital display device is not only different but difficult.

Soft copy viewing is performed on a digital cathode ray tube (CRT) or an active matrix liquid crystal display (AMLCD). The essentials of CRT imaging were discussed in Chapter 21.

This chapter concentrates on the AMLCD as the principal soft copy digital display device.

ACTIVE MATRIX LIQUID CRYSTAL DISPLAY

We all know that matter takes the form of gas, liquid, or solid. A liquid crystal is a material state between that of a liquid and a solid.

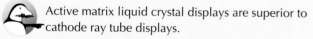

Active matrix liquid crystal displays are superior to cathode ray tube displays.

A liquid crystal has the property of a highly ordered molecular structure—a crystal—and the property of viscosity—a fluid. Liquid crystal materials are linear organic molecules (Figure 29-3) that are electrically charged, forming a natural molecular dipole. Consequently, the liquid crystals can be aligned through the action of an external electric field.

Display Characteristics

AMLCDs are fashioned pixel by pixel. The AMLCD has a very intense white backlight that illuminates each pixel. Each pixel contains light-polarizing filters and films to control the intensity and color of light transmitted through the pixel.

The differences between color and monochrome AMLCDs involve the design of the filters and films. Color AMLCDs have red-green-blue filters within each pixel fashioned into subpixels, each with one of these three filters.

Medical flat panel digital display devices are monochrome AMLCDs. Figure 29-4 illustrates the design and operation of a single pixel. Blacklight illuminates the pixel and is blocked or transmitted by the orientation of the liquid crystals.

The pixel consists of two glass plate substrates that are separated by embedded spherical glass beads of a few microns in diameter that act as spacers. Additionally, bus lines—conductors—control each pixel with a thin-film transistor (TFT).

Spatial resolution improves with the use of higher-megapixel digital display devices.

Medical flat panel digital display devices are identified by the number of pixels in the AMLCD. A 1-megapixel display will have a 1000 × 1000-pixel arrangement. A high-resolution monitor will have a 5-megapixel display, or a 2000 × 2500-pixel arrangement. Table 29-3 reports the matrix array for popular medical flat panel digital display devices.

Image Luminance

The AMLCD is a very inefficient device. Only approximately 10% of the backlight is transmitted through a monochrome monitor, and half of that through a color monitor. This inefficiency is due in part to light absorption in the filters and polarizers. Because a

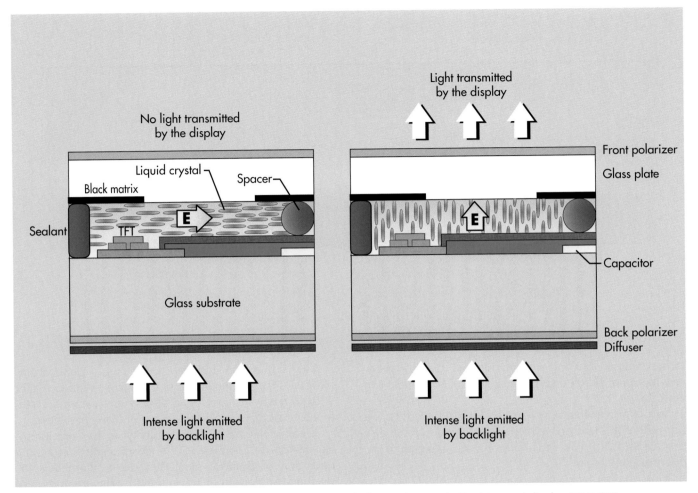

FIGURE 29-4 Cross-sectional rendering of one pixel of an active matrix liquid crystal display (AMLCD).

substantial portion of each pixel is blocked by the TFT and the bus lines, efficiency is reduced still further.

The portion of the pixel face that is available to transmit light is the "aperture ratio." Aperture ratios of 50% to 80% are characteristic of medical AMLCDs.

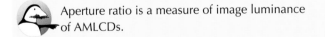 Aperture ratio is a measure of image luminance of AMLCDs.

The term "active" in AMLCD refers to the ability to control individually each pixel of the digital display device. This differs from the nature of reading a digital image receptor line by line, which is called a "passive" read. The TFT is required for the active read.

Some of the principal differences between digital CRT displays and AMLCDs are shown in Table 29-4. AMLCDs are rapidly replacing CRTs because most of these characteristics favor the AMLCD.

AMLCDs have better grayscale definition than CRTs. AMLCDs are not limited by veiling glare or reflections in the glass faceplate; thus better contrast resolution is attained. The intrinsic noise of an AMLCD is less

TABLE 29-3	Standard Sizes of Medical Flat Panel Digital Display Devices
Description of Size	**Matrix Array**
1 MP	1000 × 1000 pixels
2 MP	1200 × 1800 pixels
3 MP	1500 × 2000 pixels
5 MP	2000 × 2500 pixels

MP, Megapixel.

than that of a CRT; this also results in better contrast resolution.

Ambient Light

AMLCDs are designed to better reduce the influence of ambient light on image contrast. The principal disadvantage of an AMLCD is the angular dependence of viewing. Figure 29-5 shows that the image contrast falls sharply as viewing angle increases.

This characteristic of flat panel digital display devices has led to considerable ergonomic design of digital workstations. Ergonomics is the act of matching a worker to the work environment for maximum efficiency.

TABLE 29-4	Principal Differences Between CRT and AMLCD Digital Display Devices	
CRT	**AMLCD**	
Light emitting	Light modulating	
Curved face	Flat face	
Scanning electron beam	Active matrix address	
Veiling glare distortion	Pixel cross-talk distortion	
Spot pixel	Square pixel	
Phosphor nonuniformity	LC nonuniformity	

AMLCD, Active matrix liquid crystal display; *CRT,* cathode ray tube; *LC,* liquid crystal.

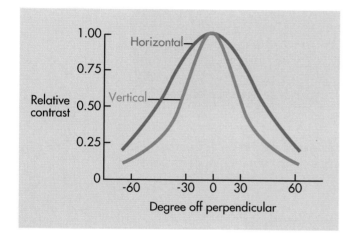

FIGURE 29-5 Loss of image contrast as a function of off-perpendicular viewing of an active matrix liquid crystal display (AMLCD).

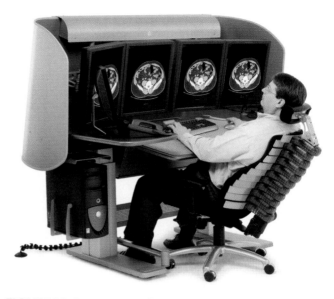

FIGURE 29-6 Ergonomically designed digital image workstation. (Courtesy Anthro Corporation.)

TABLE 29-5	Digital Image Preprocessing
Problem	**Solution**
Defective pixel	Interpolate adjacent pixel signals
Image lag	Offset correction
Line noise	Correct from dark reference zone

Figure 29-6 shows an example of an ergonomically designed digital image workstation. Levels of ambient light at the workstation must be reduced to near darkness for best viewing.

PREPROCESSING THE DIGITAL IMAGE

A principal advantage of digital imaging over screen-film imaging is the ability to manipulate the image before display—preprocessing—and after display—postprocessing. Preimage processing and postimage processing alter image appearance, usually for the purpose of improving image contrast.

 Preprocessing of digital images is largely automatic.

Preprocessing actions are outlined in Table 29-5. Preprocessing is designed to produce artifact-free digital images. In this regard, preprocessing implements electronic calibration to reduce pixel-to-pixel, row-to-row, and column-to-column response differences. The processes of pixel interpolation, lag correction, and noise correction are automatically applied with most systems.

Offset images and **gain images** are automatic calibration images designed to make the response of the image receptor uniform. Gain images are generated every few months, and offset images are generated many times each day.

These preprocessing calibration techniques are identified as **flatfielding** and are shown in Figure 29-7. Averaging techniques also are employed to reduce noise and improve contrast.

Digital image receptors and display devices have millions of pixels; therefore, it is reasonable to expect some individual pixels to be defective and to respond differently or not at all. Such defects are corrected by **signal interpolation.** The response of pixels surrounding the defective pixel is averaged, and that value is assigned to the defective pixel.

Each type of digital image receptor generates an electronic latent image that may not be made visible completely. What remains is **image lag,** and this can be troublesome when one is switching from high-dose to low-dose techniques, such as switching from digital subtraction angiography (DSA) to fluoroscopy. The solution is application of an **offset voltage** before the next image is acquired.

Some voltage variations may be seen along the buses that drive each pixel. This defect, called **line noise,** can cause linear artifacts to appear on the final image. The

FIGURE 29-7 **A,** Exposure to a raw x-ray beam shows the heel effect on the image. **B,** Flatfielding corrects this defect and makes the image receptor response uniform. (Courtesy Anthony Siebert, University of California Davis.)

solution is to apply a voltage correction from a row or a column of pixels in a dark, unirradiated area of the image receptor.

POSTPROCESSING THE DIGITAL IMAGE

Postprocessing is where digital imaging shines. In contrast to preprocessing, which is largely automatic, postprocessing requires intervention by the radiologic technologist and the radiologist. Postprocessing refers to anything that can be done to a digital image after it is acquired by the imaging system.

> Postprocessing of digital images requires operator manipulation.

Postprocessing of the digital image is performed to optimize the appearance of the image for the purpose of better detecting pathology. Table 29-6 lists the more useful postprocessing functions.

Annotation is the process of adding text to an image. In addition to patient identification, annotation is often helpful in informing the clinician about anatomy and diagnosis.

Digital images have dynamic ranges up to 16-bit, 65,536-gray levels. Yet, the human visual system can visualize only approximately 30 shades of gray. By **window and level** adjustment, the radiologic technologist can make all 65,536 shades of gray visible.

TABLE 29-6	Digital Image Postprocessing
Process	**Results**
Annotation	Label the image
Window and level	Expand the digital grayscale to visible
Magnification	Improve visualization and spatial resolution
Image flip	Reorient image presentation
Image inversion	Make white-black and black-white
Subtraction (DSA)	Improve image contrast
Pixel shift	Reregister an image to correct for patient motion
Region-of-interest	Determine average pixel value for use in quantitative imaging

DSA, Digital subtraction angiography.

This amplification of image contrast may be the most important feature of digital imaging.

The larger matrix size digital display devices have better spatial resolution because they have smaller pixels. This allows, among other properties, **magnification** of a region of an image to render the smallest detail visible. Magnification in digital imaging is similar to using a magnifying glass with a film image.

At times, multiple digital images must be flipped horizontally or vertically. This process, called **image flip,** is used to bring images into standard viewing order.

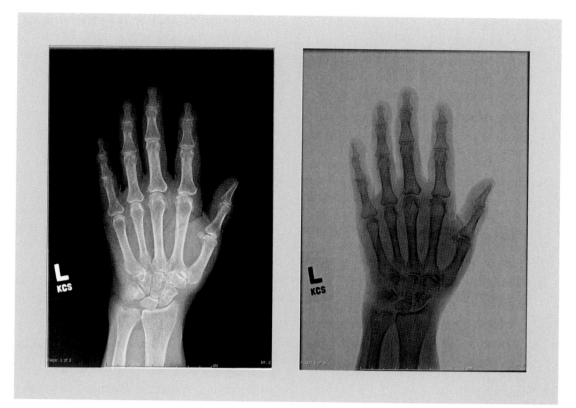

FIGURE 29-8 Digital image inversion is sometimes helpful in making disease more visible, as in this case of a digital hand image. (Courtesy Colin Bray, Baylor College of Medicine.)

Most digital images are viewed through the contrast rendition of screen-film images: Bone is white and soft tissue is black. However, sometimes, pathology can be made more visible with **image inversion,** which results in a black appearance of bone and a white appearance of soft tissue (Figure 29-8).

Image subtraction, as used in DSA, was discussed in Chapter 27. Subtraction of digital radiographic images obtained months apart—temporal subtraction—is used to amplify changes in anatomy or disease. The purpose of image subtraction is to enhance contrast.

Misregistration of a subtraction image occurs when the patient moves during serial image acquisition. This can be corrected by reregistering the image through a technique called **pixel shift.**

Greater use is being made of quantitative imaging, that is, use of the numeric value of pixels to help in diagnosis. This requires identifying a **region-of-interest (ROI)** and computing the mean pixel value for that ROI. This is an area of digital imaging that has been identified as quantitative radiology; it is finding application in bone mineral assay, calcified lung nodule detection, and renal stone identification.

Edge enhancement is effective for fractures and small, high-contrast tissues. **Highlighting** can be effective in identifying diffuse, nonfocal disease. **Pan, scroll, and zoom** allows for careful visualization of precise regions of an image.

PICTURE ARCHIVING AND COMMUNICATION SYSTEM

Radiology is adopting digital imaging very rapidly. Estimates of the present level of digitally acquired images range up to 70%.

These digital images come from every area of medical imaging—nuclear medicine, diagnostic ultrasonography, radiography, fluoroscopy, computed tomography, and magnetic resonance imaging. Screen-film radiographs can be digitized with the use of a device such as that shown in Figure 29-9. Such film digitizers are based on laser beam technology.

A Picture Archiving and Communication System (PACS), when fully implemented, allows not only the acquisition but also the interpretation and storage of each medical image in digital form without resorting to film (hard copy). The projected efficiencies of time and cost are enormous.

> PACS improves image interpretation, processing, viewing, storage, and recall.

The four principal components of a PACS are the image acquisition system, the display system, the network, and the storage system. Chapter 26 presented

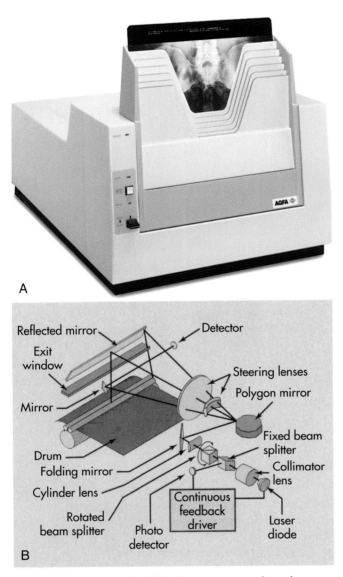

FIGURE 29-9 **A,** A thin film digitizer uses a laser beam to convert an analog radiograph into a digital image. **B,** The printing to film is similar to that of a laser printer. (**A** courtesy Agfa; **B** courtesy Imation.)

digital image acquisition, and the earlier sections of this chapter have discussed the digital display system.

Network

To be truly effective, each of these image-processing modes must be quick and easy to use. This requires that each workstation must be microprocessor controlled and must interact with each imaging system and the central computer. To provide for such interaction, a network is required.

Computer scientists use the term *network* to describe the manner in which many computers can be connected to interact with one another. In a business office, for instance, each secretary might have a microprocessor-based workstation, which is interfaced with a central office computer, so

that information can be transferred from one workstation to another, or to and from a main computer or server.

In some countries, national networks are used for medical data. All patients have a unique identifier—a number that is exclusively theirs for life.

Any hospital at any time can enter the unique identifier and access the medical records for that patient. At the moment, this is primarily limited to text, but as PACS networks expand, the system will include images.

In radiology, in addition to secretarial workstations, the network may consist of various types of devices that allow storage, retrieval, and viewing of images, PACS workstations, remote PACS workstations, a departmental mainframe, and a hospital mainframe (Figure 29-10). Each of these devices is called a **client** of the network.

> Clients are interconnected, usually by cable in a building, by telephone or cable television lines among buildings, and by microwave or satellite transmission to remote facilities.

Teleradiology is the process of remote transmission and viewing of images. To ensure adaptability between different imaging systems, the American College of Radiology (ACR), in cooperation with the National Electrical Manufacturers Association (NEMA), has produced a standard imaging and interface format called DICOM—Digital Imaging and Communications in Medicine.

The network begins at the digital imaging system, where data are acquired. Images reconstructed from data are processed at the console of the imaging system or are transmitted to a PACS workstation for processing.

At any time, such images can be transferred to other clients within or outside the hospital. Instead of running films up to surgery for viewing on a viewbox, one simply transfers the image electronically to the PACS workstation in surgery.

When a radiologist is not immediately available for image interpretation, the image can be transferred to a PACS workstation in the radiologist's home. Essentially, everywhere that film used to be required, electronic images can be substituted. Time is essential when one is considering image manipulation; therefore, fast computers and networks with high bandwidth are required for this task.

These requirements are relaxed for the information management and database portion of PACS, which is the Radiology Information System (RIS). Such lower-priority RIS functions include message and mail utilities, calendar reporting, storage of text data, and financial accounting and planning.

From the RIS workstation, any number of coded diagnostic reports can be initiated and transferred to a secretarial workstation for report generation. The secretarial workstation in turn can communicate with the

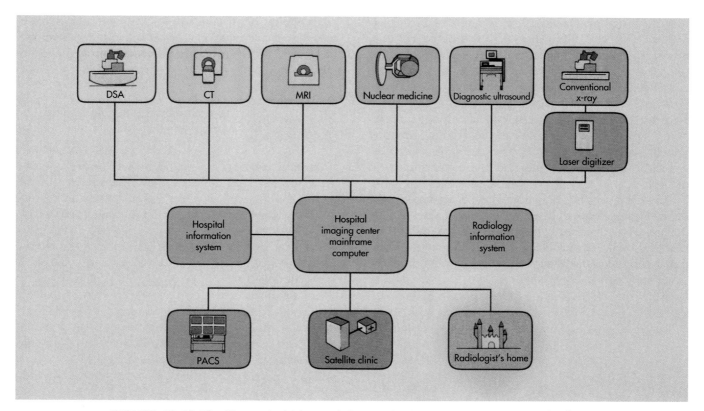

FIGURE 29-10 The Picture Archiving and Communication System (PACS) network allows interaction among the various modes of data acquisition, image processing, and image archiving.

main hospital computer for patient identification, billing, accounting, and interaction with other departments.

Such interconnection allows for the "pre-fetching" of images from the archive. The moment a patient reports to any reception desk anywhere in the facility, the process of recovering archived records commences automatically. By the time the patient reaches the examination room, all previous images and reports are available.

Similarly, a secretarial workstation at the departmental reception desk can interact with a departmental computer for scheduling of patients, technologists, and radiologists, and for analysis of departmental statistics. Finally, at the completion of an examination, PACS allows for more efficient image archiving.

Storage System

One motivation for PACS is archiving. How often are films checked out from the file room and never returned? How many films disappear from jackets? How many jackets disappear? How often are films copied for clinicians?

 Just the cost of the hospital space to accommodate a film file room may be sufficient to justify PACS.

Image storage requirements are determined by the number of images and the image data file size. Image file size is the product of the matrix size and the grayscale bit depth. The following examples should help with this understanding.

Question: How much computer capacity is required to store a magnetic resonance imaging (MRI) examination that consists of 120 images, each with image matrix size of 256 × 256 and 256 shades of gray?

Answer:

Size of Matrix		Shades of Gray
256 × 256	×	256
256 × 256	×	8 bit
65,536	×	1 byte
		= 65,536 bytes

120 × 65,536 = 7,864,320 bytes, or approximately 8 MB

Question: How much computer capacity is required to store a single chest image with a 4096 × 4096 matrix size and a 12-bit dynamic range (considered by most as minimally acceptable)?

Answer: This is a 4096 × 4096 matrix with 1024 shades of gray.

Size of Matrix	Shades of Gray
4096 × 4096	12 bit
16,777,216	1.5 byte
	= 25,165,824 bytes, or approximately 25 MB

With PACS, a film file room is replaced by a magnetic or optical memory device. The future of PACS, however, depends on the continuing development of the optical disc.

Optical discs can accommodate tens of gigabytes (GB) of data and images and, when stored in a "jukebox" (see Figure 24-13), can accommodate terabytes (TB). However, because of the dynamic range of DR and digital mammography file storage is stretched. Table 29-7 shows the file size for various medical images.

An entire hospital file room can be accommodated by a storage device the size of a desk. Electronically, images can be recalled from this archival system to any workstation in seconds. Backup image storage is accommodated offsite at a digital data storage vendor in the case that the main file is corrupted.

Furthermore, by employing PACS with digital imaging, the workflow chart is greatly reduced, as is shown in Figure 29-11. This leads to much improved imaging efficiency.

Table 29-7	Approximate Digital File Size for Various Medical Images	
Medical Image	Image Size	Examination Size
Nuclear medicine	0.25 MB	5 MB
Diagnostic ultrasound	0.25 MB	8 MB
Magnetic resonance imaging	0.25 MB	12 MB
Computed tomography	0.5 MB	20 MB
Digital radiography	5 MB	20 MB
Digital mammography	10 MB	60 MB

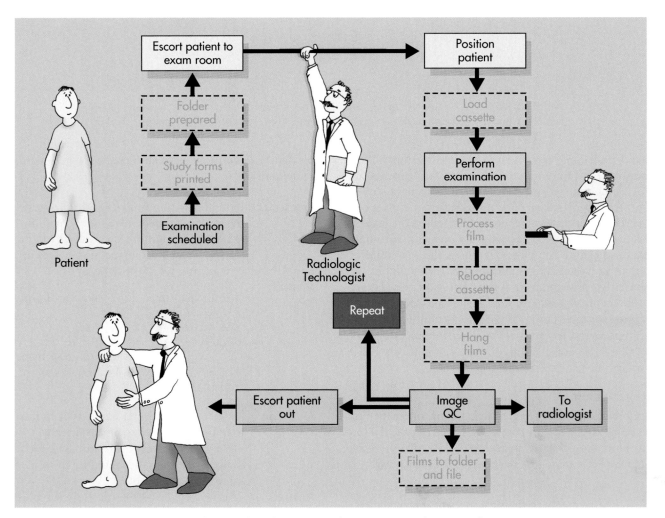

FIGURE 29-11 Combining digital images with a Picture Archiving and Communication System (PACS) network eliminates even more steps in medical imaging workflow and enhances efficiency.

SUMMARY

Viewing of digital images requires that the radiologic technologist must have an introductory knowledge of photometry. Knowledge of photometric units and concepts is essential to successful digital imaging. Photopic vision and scotopic vision are used for viewing of digital images.

The active matrix liquid crystal display (AMLCD) is the principal system for viewing soft copy digital images. The characteristics of an AMLCD affect image luminance. Ambient light is also of great consideration with the use of an AMLCD.

Preprocessing and postprocessing of the digital image are the properties that propel digital imaging to be superior to analog medical imaging.

The Picture Archiving and Communication System (PACS) is the design for integrating medical images into the health care environment. Among other characteristics, the film file room is replaced by electronic memory devices the size of a box. Teleradiology is the remote transmission of digital images.

CHALLENGE QUESTIONS

1. Define or otherwise identify the following:
   a. PACS
   b. Hard copy
   c. Lumen
   d. Ambient light
   e. Photometry
   f. Scotopic
   g. Pixel shift
   h. Network client
   i. Footcandle
   j. Interpolation
2. What is image registration, and how is it used?
3. Describe the effect of off-axis viewing of a digital display system.
4. What equipment is required to implement teleradiology?
5. What portion of medical imaging is now digital?
6. What photometric quantity best describes image brightness?
7. Describe the properties of a liquid crystal.
8. How much digital capacity is required to store a 2000 × 2500 digital mammogram with a 16-bit grayscale?
9. How is interpolation used to preprocess a digital image?
10. What is the difference between bright vision and dim vision?
11. What is the approximate illumination of an office, major league night baseball, and a sunny snow scene?
12. How is DICOM used with medical images?
13. Briefly, how does an AMLCD work?
14. What is the difference between monochrome and polychrome?
15. What are some advantages of digital display devices over a digital cathode ray tube?
16. Describe image inversion.
17. If the transmission speed of a teleradiology system is 1 MB/s, how long will it take to transmit two 3-MB chest images with a 12-bit grayscale?
18. What is the aperture ratio of a medical AMLCD?
19. What ergonomic properties are incorporated into a digital image workstation?
20. What are four major photometric quantities?

The answers to the Challenge Questions can be found by logging on to our website at http://evolve.elsevier.com.

Digital Display Quality Control

OBJECTIVES

At the completion of this chapter, the student should be able to do the following:

1. Describe various factors associated with the performance of digital display devices
2. Explain the various test patterns suggested by AAPM TG 18 on digital display device performance assessment
3. Discuss the quality control tests and schedule used for digital display devices

OUTLINE

Performance Assessment Standards
  SMPTE
  NEMA-DICOM
  DIN 2001
  VESA
  AAPM TG 18
Luminance Meter
Digital Display Device Quality Control
  Geometric Distortion
  Reflection
  Luminance Response
  Display Resolution
  Display Noise
Quality Control by the Technologist

WITH THE ADVENT of digital imaging, the scope of conventional quality assurance protocols has expanded beyond the traditional areas of medical imaging with screen-film image receptors. Quality control (QC) procedures for the support of screen-film imaging are directed to wet chemistry processors, screens, and viewboxes. Digital imaging QC is directed to the reading environment and the digital display device.

In any modern radiology reading room, reading light boxes are being replaced with digital monitors for medical image review and diagnosis. Any malfunctioning component in the display system can produce image degradation that can simulate or obscure disease. To ensure proper functioning of display devices, it is essential that a comprehensive QC program should be implemented under the supervision of a qualified medical physicist.

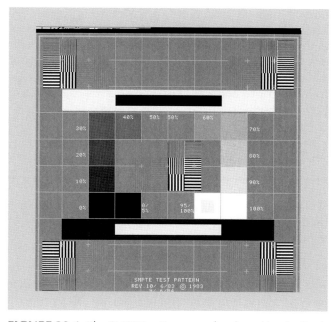

FIGURE 30-1 The SMPTE pattern was developed by the Society of Motion Picture and Television Engineers.

PERFORMANCE ASSESSMENT STANDARDS

Numerous initiatives have been developed to standardize soft copy digital display device performance standards.

SMPTE

The Society of Motion Picture and Television Engineers (SMPTE) has described the format, dimensions, and contrast characteristics of a pattern used to make measurements of the resolution of display systems. One outcome of these performance recommendations is what is commonly referred to as the "SMPTE pattern" (Figure 30-1).

Among other characteristics that the pattern provides, the most common is the observation of 5% and 95% luminance patches. This helps to point out any gross deviations in luminance adjustments.

In its standards for teleradiology, the American College of Radiology (ACR) has recommended that the SMPTE pattern should be used for quality control (QC) purposes as well. Most digital imaging equipment vendors provide the pattern in a format such that it can be displayed on the monitor for evaluation purposes.

NEMA-DICOM

The ACR and the National Electrical Manufacturers Association (NEMA) formed a committee that generated a standard for Digital Imaging and Communication that is referred to as the DICOM standard. They presented their work as a document known as the Gray Scale Display Function (GSDF). The intent of this standard was to allow medical images to be transferred according

to the DICOM standard to be displayed on any DICOM-compatible display device with a consistent grayscale appearance.

The consistent appearance was achieved in keeping with the principle of **perceptual linearization,** wherein equal changes in digital values associated with an image translate into equal changes in perceived brightness at the display. GSDF is now mandated for all digital display devices.

DIN 2001

In 2001, the German standards institution, Deutsches Institut für Normung, published a document called, "Image Quality Assurance in X-ray Diagnostics; Acceptance Testing for Image Display Devices" (DIN 2001). DIN 2001 was developed as an acceptance testing standard to address the requirements for digital display systems. It called for joint performance evaluation of the imaging modality and the digital display device.

VESA

In 1998, the Flat Panel Display Measurement standard (FPDM), version 1.0, was released by the Video Electronics Standard Association (VESA). This standard provides a set of instructions that can be used to help in the evaluation of system performance according to a compliance standard.

AAPM TG 18

To evaluate a digital display device comprehensively toward the goal of ensuring acceptable clinical performance, the American Association of Physicists in Medicine (AAPM) developed a set of test patterns and outlined related procedures in Task Group Report 18. The following sections explain the various patterns recommended by the AAPM, along with prescribed methods for use. Particular emphasis is placed on details of associated patterns that can be used by a radiologic technologist to perform checks to ensure proper system performance.

 AAPM TG 18 measurements and observations should be instituted for all digital display devices.

We begin with an introduction to the test tools that are used by medical physicists for comprehensive testing of digital display devices.

LUMINANCE METER

The luminance response of monitors and luminance uniformity measurements require the use of a properly calibrated photometer. Two types of photometers are commonly used: near-range and telescopic; these are shown in Figure 30-2.

 Photometric evaluation of digital display devices and ambient light levels is essential to digital QC.

Near-range photometers are used in close proximity to monitors; telescopic photometers are used to test from a distance of 1 m.

The response from the two types of photometers may be slightly different, depending on the contribution that is made by stray sources of light. However, the readings from both types are acceptable as long as measurements are performed in a consistent manner. Contributions from ambient light should be kept constant when either photometer is used.

The luminance meter should use a calibration method that is traceable to the National Institute of Standards and Technology (NIST) and should be able to measure luminance in the range of 0.05 to 1000 cd/m^2 with better than 5% accuracy and a precision of at least 0.01. The photometer also should comply with the Commission Internationale de l'Éclairage (CIE) standard photopic spectral response within a range of 3%.

To evaluate monitor display reflection and to assess ambient light conditions, an **illuminance meter** is used. The illuminance meter should be calibrated according to NIST standards; response to better than 5% at a 50-degree angulation should be required.

It is important to quantify the color tint of various grayscale displays to match multiple monitors that may be used at a single workstation. Colorimeters are used to measure CIE-specified color coordinates of a digital display device. These are available in near-range and telescopic styles.

DIGITAL DISPLAY DEVICE QUALITY CONTROL

To carefully evaluate the comprehensive characteristics of the digital display device, a range of tests are performed. For most of these, AAPM TG 18 patterns are used to perform qualitative and quantitative tests. For a few tests, no test patterns are required.

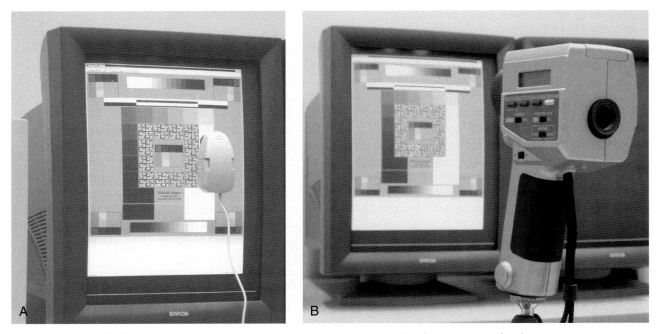

FIGURE 30-2 Examples of near-range **(A)** and telescopic **(B)** photometric and colorimetric evaluation. (Courtesy Eshan Samei, Duke University, North Carolina.)

Geometric Distortion

Geometric distortion arises from problems that cause the displayed image to be geometrically different from the original image. This can affect the relative size and shape of image features.

Visual assessment of geometric distortion can be carried out with the use of TG 18-QC and TG 18-LPV/LPH test patterns (Figure 30-3). By filling the entire screen with the test pattern, one can look for pincushion and barrel-like distortions. These types of distortions are common in cathode ray tube–based display devices. All lines in the pattern in general should appear straight.

By measuring distances in the square areas of the pattern with the help of a flexible plastic ruler, one can quantify the level of distortion in the images. Measurements are performed in various quadrants to look at variation in geometric distortion in different areas of the monitor.

With primary class devices, the acceptable level of distortion in various quadrants in either direction is 2%. The corresponding criterion for secondary class devices is 5%.

Reflection

An ideal display device has a luminance that is based on the light generated only by the device itself. In reality, the ambient light significantly contributes to the light reflected by the display device, which, in turn, depends on the display characteristics of the display device. It is important to characterize these reflection characteristics of the display monitor.

Usually, the display reflection is characterized as specular and diffuse. **Specular reflection** results in the generation of mirror images of light sources surrounding the monitor. In diffuse reflection, light is randomly scattered on the monitor.

In Figure 30-4 diffuse and specular reflections are illustrated for a color *(left)* and a monochrome *(right)* display device with the power off. Monochrome has reduced specular reflection because of an improved antireflective coating.

A simple test to assess specular reflection is to simply turn off the monitor and look for sources of illumination within a 15-degree angle of observation at an approximate distance of 30 to 50 cm. Look for images of various light sources and any high-contrast patterns from viewers' clothing or the surroundings.

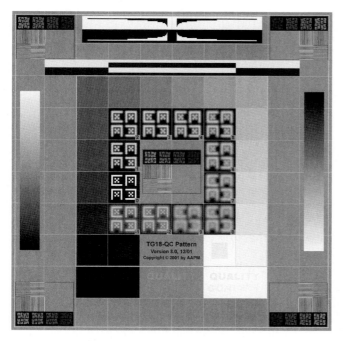

FIGURE 30-3 TG 18-QC test pattern.

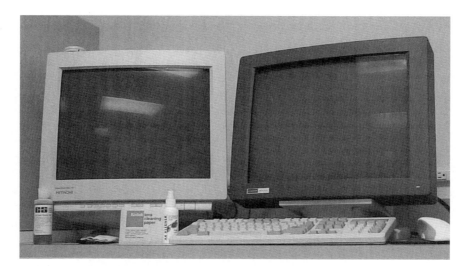

FIGURE 30-4 Diffuse and specular reflections are illustrated for a color *(left)* and a monochrome *(right)* display device with the power off. Monochrome has reduced specular reflection caused by an improved antireflective coating. (Courtesy Eshan Samei, Duke University, North Carolina.)

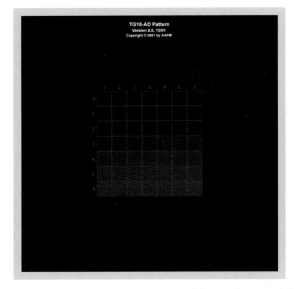

FIGURE 30-5 TG 18-AD pattern used for evaluating diffuse reflection.

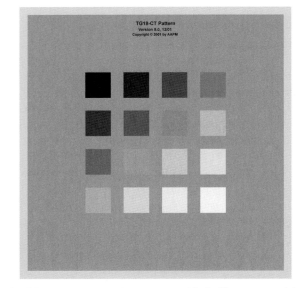

FIGURE 30-6 TG 18-CT pattern with half-16 area of half-moon targets.

The TG 18-AD pattern (Figure 30-5) consists of uniformly varying low-contrast patterns. To evaluate diffuse reflection, one has to observe the threshold of visibility for low-contrast patterns under ambient lighting conditions and in total darkness. Under both conditions, the threshold of visibility should be the same. If the ambient lighting changes the threshold, then ambient lighting should be reduced.

Luminance Response

The image acquired by a digital modality is stored as an array of pixel values. These pixel values are also gray-scale values, and they are sent to a digital display device as **presentation values or p-values.**

These p-values then are transformed into **digital driving levels,** or **DDLs,** that then are transformed into luminance values through a **look-up table,** or **LUT.** Transformation of presentation values to DDLs is performed according to the DICOM standard, which ensures that when these DDLs are displayed as luminance levels, corresponding equal changes in perceived brightness correspond to equal changes in p-values.

> Digital image data arrive at the digital display device as p-values, transformed into digital driving levels and viewed as luminance levels.

The luminance response of a digital display device refers to the relationship between displayed luminance and input values of a standardized display system. Displayed luminance consists of light produced by the display device; it varies between L_{min} and L_{max} and receives a fixed contribution from diffusely reflected ambient light—L_{amb}.

The TG 18-CT test pattern (Figure 30-6) is used to perform a qualitative evaluation of the luminance response of a digital display device. This pattern has low-contrast targets that should be visible in all 16 regions of the pattern. The pattern should be evaluated from a distance of approximately 30 cm. A common failure is to be unable to see targets in one or two of the dark regions.

With the use of an external photometer and TG 18-LN test patterns (Figure 30-7), the luminance in the test region should be recorded for the 18 DDLs. Ambient lighting conditions should be reduced to minimum levels. The maximum luminance value should be greater than 171 cd/m². Maximum luminance values should be verified against the manufacturer's quoted value.

The luminance response of a display device varies as a function of location on the display surface. In addition, the contrast behavior is a function of the viewing angle as well. The maximum variation of luminance across the display area when a uniform pattern is displayed is referred to as luminance nonuniformity. Cathode ray tube displays have luminance nonuniformity from the center to the edges and corners of the display.

TG 18-UN10 and 80 test patterns (Figure 30-8) can be used for visual evaluation of nonuniformity. By observing the patterns across the display screen, one can observe any gross variations in uniformity. No luminance variations with dimensions on the order of 1 cm or larger should be observed.

For qualitative or visual assessment of angular dependence, the TG 18-CT test pattern is used. By first observing the half-moon targets straight on-axis and then comparing them with viewing angles in which the visibility of half-moon targets is altered, one can gain

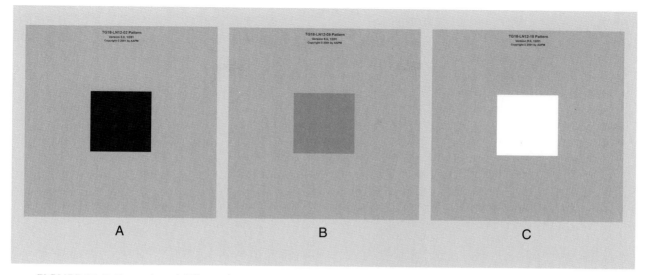

FIGURE 30-7 Examples of different luminance patches for measurement of luminance response of the system.

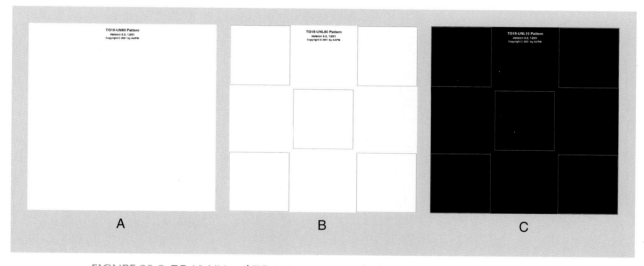

FIGURE 30-8 TG 18-UN and TG 18-UNL patterns for luminance uniformity assessment.

an understanding of viewing angle dependency of a particular display device.

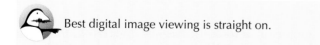
Best digital image viewing is straight on.

The viewing angle within which the monitor shows no variation in viewed patterns will define a conelike region and is the region in which the monitor should be used clinically. Established viewing angle limits may be clearly labeled on the front of the display device. For multiple LCD monitor workstations, displays should be adjusted in such a way that the displays optimally face the user.

For quantitative evaluation of luminance uniformity, one measures the luminance in different regions of TG 18-UNL10 and TG 18-UNL80 patterns with an external photometer. Luminance is measured at five different locations of the monitor.

Maximum deviation in uniformity is calculated as the percent difference between maximum and minimum luminance values relative to their average value as follows:

$$200 \times (L_{max} - L_{min})/(L_{max} + L_{min})$$

Maximum nonuniformity for an individual display device should be less than 30%.

Display Resolution

Spatial resolution is the quantitative measure of the ability of the display system to produce separable images of different points of an object with high fidelity.

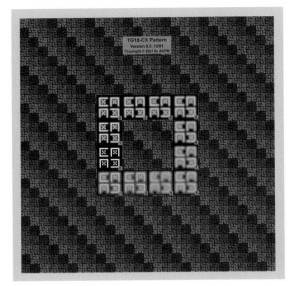

FIGURE 30-9 TG 18-CX pattern for display resolution evaluation.

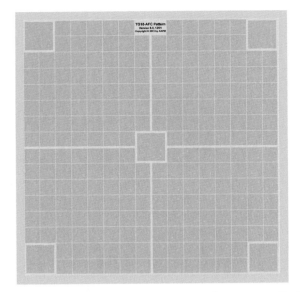

FIGURE 30-11 TG 18-AFC pattern used to assess display noise.

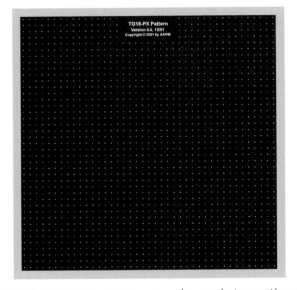

FIGURE 30-10 TG 18-PX pattern for resolution uniformity evaluation.

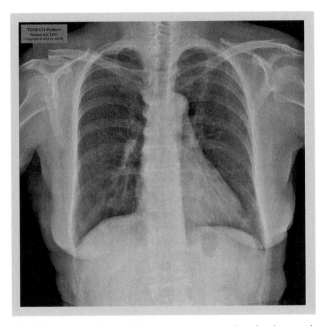

FIGURE 30-12 TG 18-CH anatomic image for display evaluation.

TG 18-CX (Figure 30-9) and TG 18-QC patterns can be used to evaluate display resolution. The CX patterns in the middle and in the corners can be evaluated with a magnifying glass and compared. The TG 18-PX (Figure 30-10) pattern can be used to evaluate resolution uniformity.

Display Noise

Noise in an image, along with image contrast and size, is an important factor in determining the visibility of an object. Any high-frequency fluctuations/patterns that interfere with detection of the true signal would be classified as noise. Noise can be quantified with the TG 18-AFC test pattern (Figure 30-11), which is based on the method used to determine just noticeable luminance difference as a function of size.

The test pattern contains a large number of regions with changing target positions. Size and contrast, however, are constant in four of the four quadrants into which the pattern is subdivided.

In addition to all the patterns that have been described here, other patterns are designed to evaluate characteristics such as veiling glare and display chromaticity. Also, some reference anatomic images, such as the digital chest image shown in Figure 30-12, are available for overall display system evaluation.

QUALITY CONTROL BY THE TECHNOLOGIST

To ensure proper operation of the digital display device, it is important to develop a continuous quality control program. This should include the following:

- Medical physicist's acceptance testing of any new digital display devices
- Routine quality control tests by the QC technologist
- Periodic review of QC program by a qualified medical physicist
- Annual and postrepair medical physics performance evaluations

> The TG 18-QC test pattern should be viewed daily.

Although a comprehensive QC program is strongly desirable, daily evaluation of monitors with the TG 18-QC test pattern is important. A quick review of the pattern should give the technologist an idea about any gross changes in system performance. For example, a change in contrast-detail "QUALITY CONTROL" letters may be indicative of a malfunctioning system; this may necessitate further testing by a medical physicist and the engineering staff.

SUMMARY

Several national scientific organizations have published protocols that are based on electronic test patterns for assessing the quality of a digital display device. Assessment requires visual interpretation of a test pattern and photometric measurement of emitted light intensity and stray light intensity.

A spatial electronic display pattern should be used for the evaluation of various digital display characteristics. The TG 18-QC test pattern should be used daily for overall display evaluation.

CHALLENGE QUESTIONS

1. Define or otherwise identify the following:
   a. SMPTE pattern
   b. Specular reflection
   c. GSDF
   d. cd/m^2
   e. Veiling glare
   f. Presentation value
   g. VESA
   h. TG 18
   i. NIST
   j. Pincushion distortion
2. Which TG 18 test pattern is used to evaluate diffuse reflection, and how does the pattern appear?
3. What type of device is used to evaluate diffuse reflection?
4. What are the time requirements on technologist QC of a digital display device?
5. Which TG 18 test pattern is used to evaluate digital display resolution, and how does the pattern appear?
6. What luminance range should be measurable?
7. What does L_{amb} represent, and what is its preferred value?
8. Which TG 18 test pattern is used to evaluate display noise, and how does it appear?
9. What is the principle of perceptual linearization?
10. When should a medical physicist perform digital display device quality control?
11. What TG 18 electronic test pattern is used to evaluate contrast resolution of a digital display device, and how does it appear?
12. What is threshold of visibility?
13. What are the standard descriptions for digital display devices?
14. What is display noise?
15. Which TG 18 electronic test pattern is used for luminance uniformity assessment, and how does it appear?

The answers to the Challenge Questions can be found by logging on to our website at http://evolve.elsevier.com.

CHAPTER 31

Digital Image Artifacts

OBJECTIVES

At the completion of this chapter, the student should be able to do the following:

1. Discuss the three types of digital imaging artifacts and how to avoid them
2. Identify the difference between for-processing images and for-presentation images
3. Describe the basis for data compression and the difference between lossless and lossy compression
4. Analyze the use of an image histogram in digital image artifacts
5. Explain how digital image artifacts occur because of improper collimation, partition, or alignment

OUTLINE

Image Receptor Artifacts
Software Artifacts
    Preprocessing
    Image Compression
Object Artifacts
    Image Histogram
    Collimation/Partition
    Alignment

AS WE LEARNED in Chapter 17, an artifact is any false visual feature on a medical image that simulates tissue or obscures tissue. Artifacts interfere with diagnosis and must be avoided. Similar to accidents, artifacts are, by definition, avoidable.

Artifacts can be controlled when the cause of the artifact is understood. In screen-film imaging, three classifications of artifacts occur—processing, exposure, and handling/storage. Likewise, in digital imaging, three classifications of artifacts can be described—image receptor, software, and object.

When digital images are printed, processing artifacts may have to be considered, as they are with screen-film images. Such considerations are not repeated here.

The three digital imaging artifact classes are shown in Figure 31-1, along with the subsets of each.

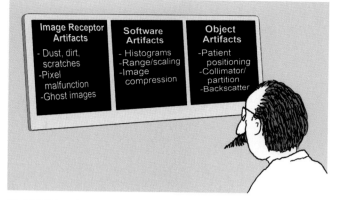

FIGURE 31-1 Digital imaging artifacts classification scheme.

IMAGE RECEPTOR ARTIFACTS

As can occur with screen-film image receptors, digital image receptors can suffer from rough handling, scratches, and dust (Figure 31-2). Artifacts produced by dust can be corrected easily with proper cleaning unless the dust is internal to the optics of a computed radiography (CR) imaging system. Figure 31-3 shows a CR image taken with an imaging plate contaminated with residual glue that could not be removed. Dust on any section of the CR optical path—mirrors and lenses—cannot be corrected by the radiologic technologist and will require professional service.

Scratches or a substantial malfunction of pixels likely will require replacement of the image receptor.

 Digital image receptors have unique artifacts associated with pixel failure.

Digital radiography (DR) and CR imaging plates (IPs) should last for thousands of exposures. There is no such thing as "radiation fatigue" on these IPs. Routine quality control (QC) should include regular documentation of imaging frequency, imaging performance, and the physical condition of each IP, to reduce artifact appearance and help prevent failure. Figure 31-4 is an example of a QC form for such regular documentation.

Environmental radiation can contribute to ghost artifacts.

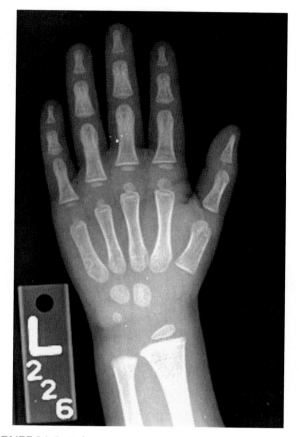

FIGURE 31-2 Debris on image receptor in digital radiography (DR) can be confused with foreign bodies. (Courtesy Charles Willis, M.D. Anderson Cancer Center.)

The appearance of ghost images (Figure 31-5) occurs because of incomplete erasure of a previous image on a computed radiography IP. Usually, such artifacts can be corrected by additional signal erasure techniques. If a computed radiography IP has not been used for 24 hours, it should be erased again before use. When a completely erased IP is processed, the resultant image should be uniform and artifact free.

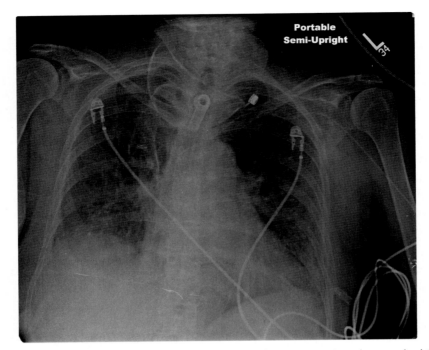

FIGURE 31-3 Residual glue on a computed radiography (CR) imaging plate resulted in this artifact, causing the plate to be removed from service. (Courtesy David Clayton, M.D. Anderson Cancer Center.)

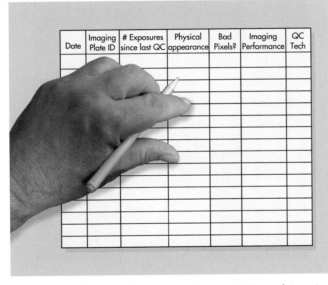

FIGURE 31-4 Form for routine documentation of imaging plate performance to help reduce artifacts.

Rough handling or faulty construction of a digital IP can result in artifacts. Figure 31-6 shows the result on the image from a damaged CR imaging plate.

SOFTWARE ARTIFACTS

Digital images are obtained as raw data sets. As such, these images are ready "for processing." For-processing images are manipulated into "for-presentation" images that the radiologic technologist can use for QC and for interpretation by the radiologist.

Preprocessing

Before an image is prepared "for processing," several manipulations of the output of an image receptor may be necessary to correct for potential artifacts. Such artifacts can occur because of dead pixels or dead rows or columns of pixels (Figure 31-7).

A single pixel or a single row or column normally will not interfere with diagnosis. However, many of these defects must be corrected. Correction algorithms specific to each type of digital image receptor employ interpolation techniques to assign digital values to each dead pixel, row, or column.

Irradiation of a digital image receptor by the raw x-ray beam may show variations over the image, producing an irregular pattern that could interfere with diagnosis (Figure 31-8, *A*). With this irregular pattern, a preprocessing manipulation known as *flatfielding* is performed, resulting in a uniform response to a uniform x-ray beam (Figure 31-8, *B*).

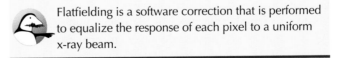

Flatfielding is a software correction that is performed to equalize the response of each pixel to a uniform x-ray beam.

CR cassettes are highly sensitive to background radiation and scatter. If a CR cassette has not been used for several days, it should be inserted into the reader for re-erasure (Figure 31-9). The practice of leaving cassettes in a supposedly "radiation safe" area in an x-ray room during an examination must be discouraged.

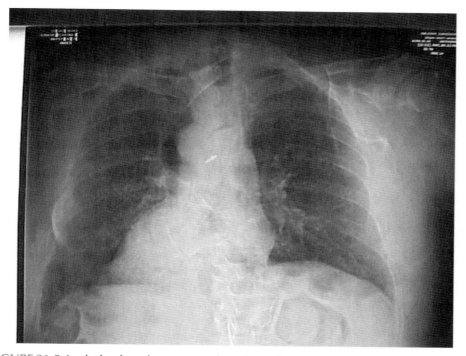

FIGURE 31-5 Look closely and you can see the pelvis at the top of this image and the bowel pattern at the bottom. This resulted because the imaging plate was not fully erased before the chest examination was performed. (Courtesy Barbara Smith Pruner, Portland Community College.)

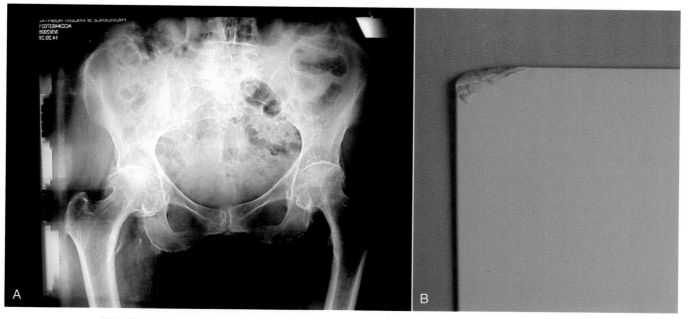

FIGURE 31-6 A, Note the white shapes on the left side, which resulted when the computed radiography (CR) imaging plate came apart. **B,** This is the CR plate, which shows corner damage and peeling. (Courtesy Barbara Smith Pruner, Portland Community College.)

Image Compression

Digital imaging becomes evermore robust in terms of the digital files generated. This would not represent a problem if it were not for increasing application of teleradiology, which requires the electronic transmission of images. Table 31-1 presents the relative file sizes per image for various digital imaging modalities.

At up to 50 MB per image on a 24 × 30-cm imaging plate (2e16 and 50-μm pixel size), a four-view

mammography study can generate 200 MB. Transmitting and archiving this amount of data is technically difficult; therefore, compression techniques are employed.

Data compression takes advantage of redundancy of data, as occurs with exposure to the raw x-ray beam when all values are the same. Such compression techniques are described as *lossless* or *lossy*.

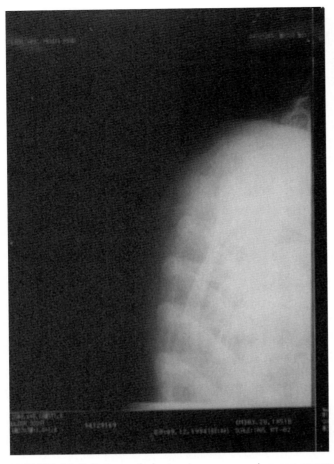

FIGURE 31-7 Failure of electronic preprocessing can cause uninterpretable images in digital radiography (DR). (Courtesy Charles Willis, M.D. Anderson Cancer Center.)

An image file that is compressed in a lossless mode is one that can be reconstructed to be exactly the same as the original image. Lossless compression reduces the data file to 10% (10:1) to 50% (2:1) of the original file. However, this is not satisfactory for large image files because transmission time and data manipulation time can still be unacceptable.

Lossy compression, which can provide compression factors of up to 100:1 or greater, can be used on images in which exact measurement or fine detail is not required, such as video recordings that are to be replayed on a standard domestic television.

 Lossless compression up to 3:1 generally is considered acceptable and helpful in digital image management.

Lossy compression is that which is something greater than an order of magnitude compression less than 10:1. Such a level of compression supports teleradiology but not computer-aided diagnosis (CAD) or image archiving. CAD systems require uncompressed for-processing images. Compressed images may cause the CAD system to miss lesions because of the compression artifact, which actually represents a lack of data.

OBJECT ARTIFACTS

Object artifacts can arise from the technologist's errors in patient positioning, x-ray beam collimation, and histogram selection. Backscatter radiation also can be troublesome because of the sensitivity of the digital image receptor.

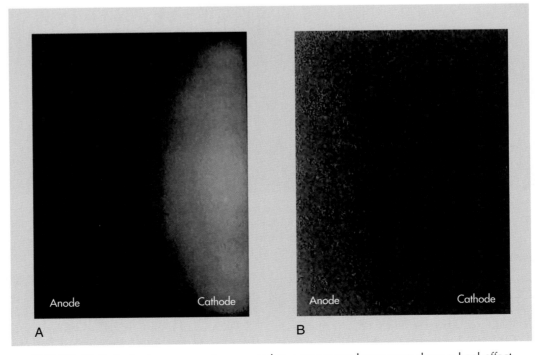

FIGURE 31-8 **A,** An image receptor exposed to a raw x-ray beam may show a heel-effect response. **B,** Flatfielding preprocessing can make the response uniform.

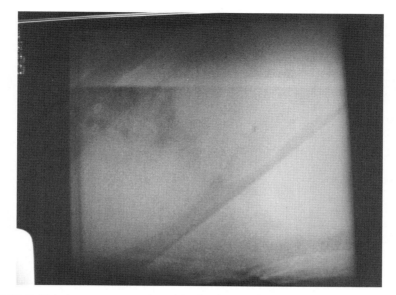

FIGURE 31-9 This image was produced by background radiation on a computed radiography (CR) plate that had not been used for days. (Courtesy Barbara Smith Pruner, Portland Community College.)

TABLE 31-1	Approximate Digital File Sizes for Various Imaging Modalities
Image Modality	**File Size per Image**
Nuclear medicine	2 MB
Magnetic resonance imaging	5 MB
Computed tomography	10 MB
Computed radiography	20 MB
Digital radiography	20 MB
Digital mammography	50 MB

If a lot of scattering material is present behind the image receptor, backscatter radiation can cause a phantom image. If this type of artifact is discovered, the back side of the image receptor should be shielded to reduce backscatter x-rays.

Image Histogram

Digital image histograms are very important for digital image production. However, they can be the source of bothersome digital image artifacts if they are not properly understood and manipulated.

All digital radiographic imaging systems have the ability to evaluate the original image data through histogram analysis. A histogram is a plot of the frequency of appearance of a given object characteristic.

A sample histogram is shown in Figure 31-10, where the height of 500 Emperor Penguins and 500 Little Blue Penguins is plotted. The average height of the Emperor Penguin is approximately 110 cm (range, 60 to 160 cm). The same value for the Little Blue Penguins is approximately 30 cm (range, 15 to 80 cm).

 A histogram is a graph of frequency of occurrence versus digital value intervals.

A histogram is a discrete plot of values rather than a continuous plot. The histogram in Figure 31-10 is a plot of the number of penguins (frequency) that have a given height as a function of that height (value interval). Because there are two penguin populations, two peaks are evident on this histogram.

Consider the simulated chest radiograph of Figure 31-11, and note where each identified part of the image would appear on a screen-film response curve—the characteristic curve. The collimated portion is white with no contrast, and the fully exposed portion is black, also with no contrast. Those two portions of every radiograph set limits on the useful portion of the image.

When the chest radiograph is digital, each region of the image (Figure 31-12, A) can be represented by the frequency distribution of the digital values of each pixel, as shown in Figure 31-12, B. The location of those image regions on the digital image receptor response curve is shown in Figure 31-12, C. The relative shape of this histogram is characteristic of all posteroanterior (PA) chest digital radiographs.

Even more important is the fact that the shape of an image histogram is characteristic of each anatomical projection. Figure 31-13 shows the characteristic shapes of image histograms of additional radiographic projections.

Most digital imaging systems have the ability to store and analyze characteristic image histograms for each radiographic projection. By storing 50 PA chest image histograms and averaging the value of each frequency interval, a representative histogram is produced for each image receptor. The histogram can be regularly updated from newer images.

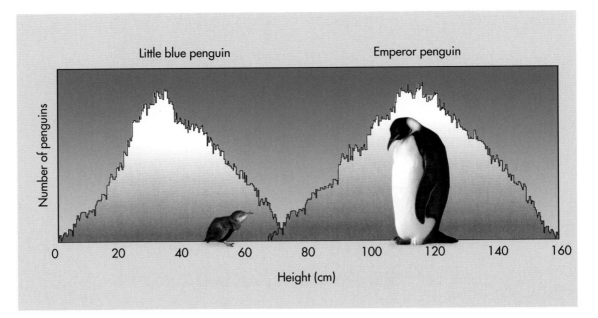

FIGURE 31-10 This histogram is a plot of the number of penguins as a function of the height of each penguin.

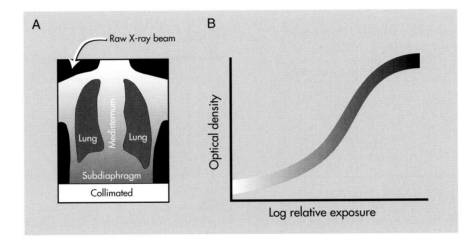

FIGURE 31-11 A, Simulated chest radiograph shows areas of lung and tissue that are unexposed (collimated) or fully exposed (raw x-ray beam). **B,** The point where each would fall on a characteristic curve.

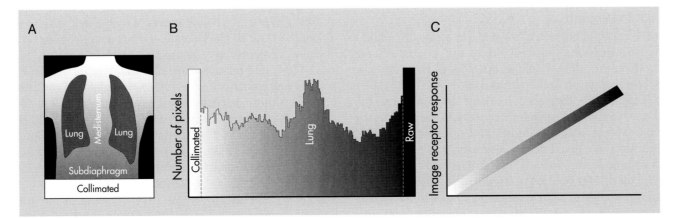

FIGURE 31-12 A, Region of a simulated digital chest radiograph, and **(B)** the corresponding image histogram. **C,** The placement of each region in **A** on the response curve of the digital image receptor.

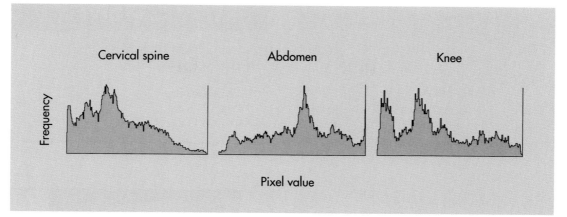

FIGURE 31-13 Characteristic histograms for cervical spine, abdomen, and knee.

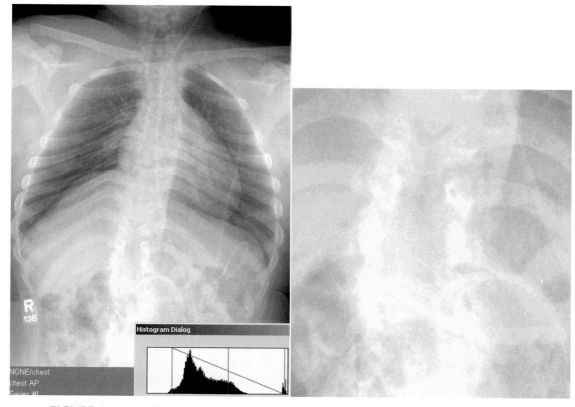

FIGURE 31-14 Underexposure in digital radiography (DR) causes loss of contrast in dense anatomy because of increased noise. (Courtesy Charles Willis, M.D. Anderson Cancer Center.)

This places an additional responsibility on the radiographer. In addition to selecting technique, the radiographer must engage the appropriate histogram before examination so as to apply the appropriate reconstruction algorithm to the final image (Figure 31-14).

Collimation/Partition

If the x-ray exposure field is not properly collimated, sized, and positioned, exposure field recognition errors may occur. These can lead to histogram analysis errors, because signal outside the exposure field is included in the histogram.

The result is very dark or very light or very noisy images (Figure 31-15).

> Automatic radiation field recognition is essential for artifact-free images.

Digital radiographic imaging plates now are available in the standard sizes shown in Box 31-1. The 14 × 17-inch image receptor is history; it has been replaced by a 35 × 43-cm image receptor.

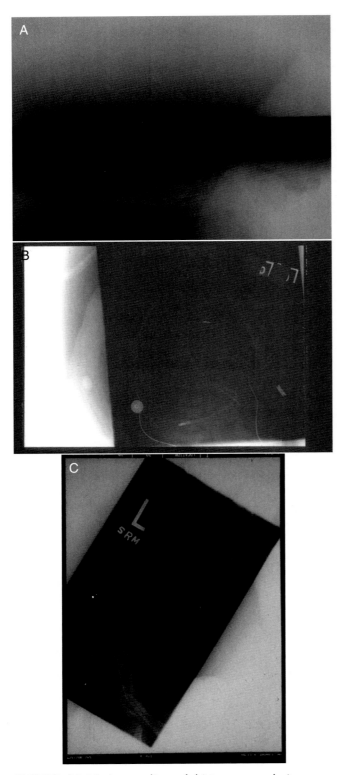

FIGURE 31-15 A sampling of histogram analysis errors. (Courtesy Barry Burns, University of North Carolina.)

CR, Computed radiography; DR, digital radiography.

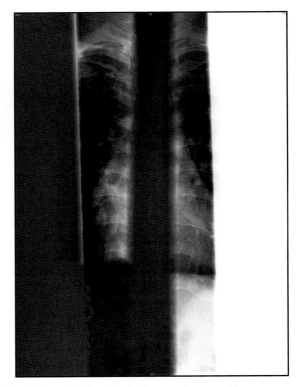

FIGURE 31-16 The blacked-out spine on this anteroposterior view was restored by engaging the automatic collimation feature. The white out on the patient's left side was fixed by postconing that area and then engaging the "collimated image." (Courtesy Dennis Bowman, Community Hospital of the Monterrey Peninsula.)

histogram can be improperly analyzed, resulting in an artifact such as that shown in Figure 31-16.

 Proper collimation and centering prevent histogram errors that can lead to artifacts.

Collimation of the projected area x-ray beam is important for patient radiation dose reduction and for improved image contrast in screen-film radiography. In DR, proper collimation has the added value of defining the image histogram. If improperly collimated, the

Digital image receptors normally can recognize even-numbered (i.e., two or four) x-ray exposure fields that are centered and cleanly collimated. Three on one and four on one are not recommended unless the unexposed portion is shielded. Figure 31-17 is a good example of reduced contrast when three on one is employed.

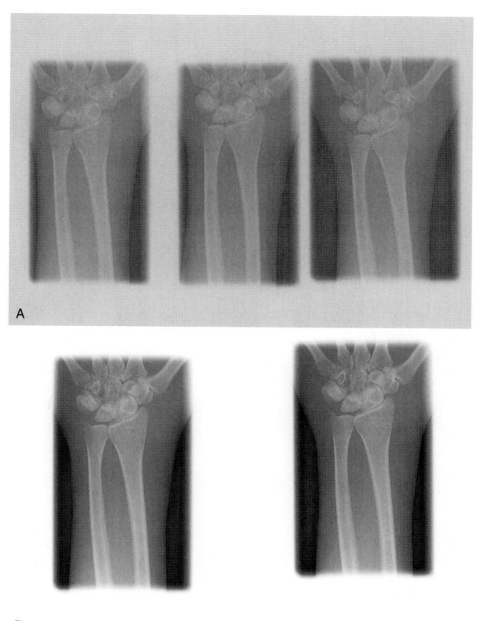

A

B

FIGURE 31-17 Loss of contrast is obvious when three on one versus two on one imaging is compared. (Courtesy Barry Burns, University of North Carolina.)

For the image histogram to be properly analyzed, each collimated field should consist of four distinct collimated margins, as seen in Figure 31-18. The use of three collimated margins usually works, but when fewer than three are used, artifacts may result.

If images are not collimated and centered, image receptor exposure will not be accurate and cannot be used for image quality evaluation.

If multiple fields are projected onto a single imaging plate, each must have clear, collimated edges and margins between each field. This process, called *partitioning*, allows two or more images to be projected on a single IP. Figure 31-19 illustrates the opposite situation.

 Partitioning of multiple digital images on a single IP results in proper separation and collimation of each image.

The cause of these collimation artifacts is vendor algorithm related. The exposure field recognition algorithm is unable to match image histograms if the fields are not clear. This algorithm is based on edge detection or area detection. Further postprocessing of each image requires digital data representative of anatomy—not twice-irradiated or unirradiated portions of the IP.

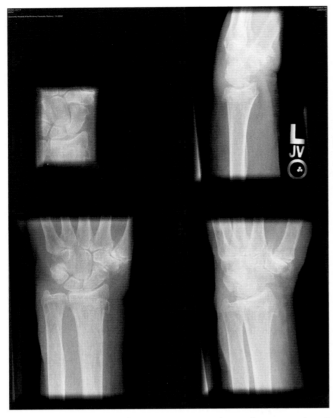

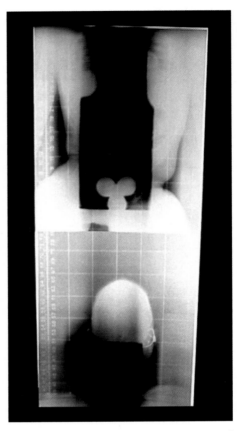

FIGURE 31-18 If all four wrist images have the same signal intensity, the radiographer changed technique appropriately. Technique was not properly adjusted for the oblique view in the lower right region. (Courtesy Dennis Bowman, Community Hospital of the Monterrey Peninsula.)

FIGURE 31-19 Two computed radiography (CR) plates used for spine imaging were placed into the processor in the wrong order. (Courtesy Barbara Smith Pruner, Portland Community College.)

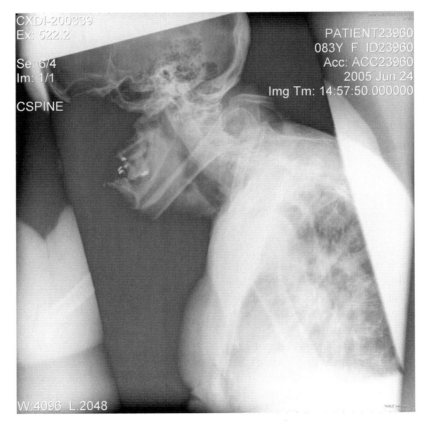

FIGURE 31-20 Improperly collimated multiple fields not aligned with the imaging plate (IP) edge result in overexposure and the artifact seen here. (Courtesy David Clayton, M.D. Anderson Cancer Center.)

Alignment

Alignment of the exposure field on the IP is important in the same way and for the same reason as collimation. When an image field, such as that shown in Figure 31-20, is not oriented with the size and dimensions of the IP, image artifacts can appear.

⊙

CHALLENGE QUESTIONS

1. Define or otherwise identify the following:
   a. Histogram
   b. Artifact
   c. Partition
   d. IP
   e. Compression
   f. CAD
   g. Frequency distribution
   h. For presentation
   i. Flatfielding
   j. Radiation fatigue
2. What are the three general classifications of digital image artifacts?
3. What is the for-processing image, and how is it manipulated?
4. What does it mean when a single digital image is not properly aligned with the IP? Diagram such a situation.
5. What is the appearance of the radiation response curve for a digital image receptor?
6. Which digital imaging modality generates the largest image file, and approximately how large is it?
7. What is the difference between lossless and lossy compression?
8. Diagram improper margins of three digital images on a single IP.
9. How many distinct margins should appear on a digital radiograph?
10. Why is backscatter radiation important in digital radiography?
11. What are the units on each axis of a digital image histogram?
12. What type of algorithm is used to correct for malfunctioning pixels?
13. Why is data compression often required for digital images?
14. What do the two outlying peaks on a digital image histogram represent?
15. What is the life expectancy of a CR imaging plate?
16. Relate the tissues of a digital radiography to position on the radiation response curve.
17. Why is it important for the radiologic technologist to select the proper imaging protocol for each digital imaging examination?
18. How does the heel effect appear on a digital image receptor?
19. Excessive compression can result in what form of image artifact?
20. Is an image histogram updated from time to time? If so, why?

The answers to the Challenge Questions can be found by logging on to our website at http://evolve.elsevier.com.

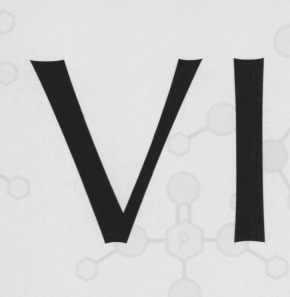

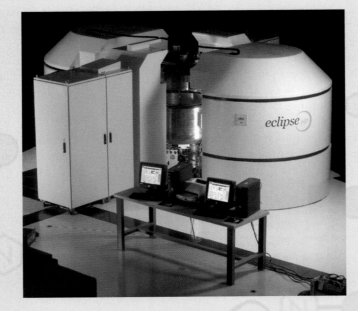

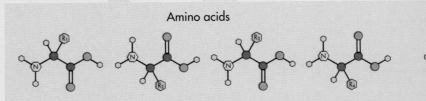

PART VI

Amino acids

○ Oxygen   ● Carbon   Ⓝ Nitrogen   Ⓡ Various side chains   ○ Hydrogen

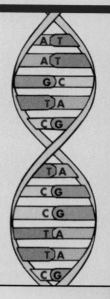

RADIOBIOLOGY

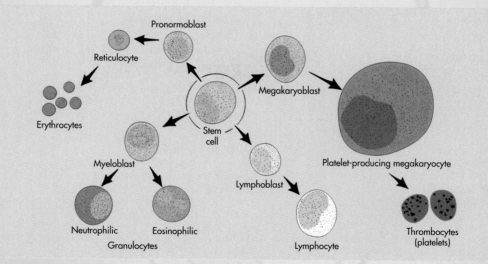

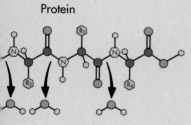

Protein

Human Biology

OBJECTIVES

At the completion of this chapter, the student should be able
to do the following:

1. Discuss the cell theory of human biology
2. List and describe the molecular composition of the human body
3. Explain the parts and function of the human cell
4. Describe the processes of mitosis and meiosis
5. Evaluate the radiosensitivity of tissues and organs

OUTLINE

Human Radiation Response
Composition of the Body
Cell Theory
    Molecular Composition
The Human Cell
    Cell Function
    Cell Proliferation
    Mitosis
    Meiosis
Tissues and Organs

T IS KNOWN beyond the shadow of a doubt that x-rays are harmful. If sufficiently intense, x-rays can cause skin burns, cataracts, cancer, leukemia, and other harmful effects. What is not known for certain is the degree of effect, if any, after exposure to diagnostic levels of x-radiation.

The benefits derived from diagnostic applications of x-rays are enormous. It is the job of the radiologic technologist, the radiologist, and the medical physicist to produce high-quality x-ray images with minimal radiation exposure. This approach results in the greatest benefit with the lowest risk to patients and radiation workers. This is the practice known as *ALARA*—"as low as reasonably achievable."

This chapter examines the concepts of human biology and discusses the known radiosensitivity of tissues, organs, and cells.

HUMAN RADIATION RESPONSE

The effect of x-rays on humans is the result of interactions at the atomic level (see Chapter 10). These atomic interactions take the form of ionization or excitation of orbital electrons and result in the deposition of energy in tissue.

Deposited energy can produce a molecular change, the consequences of which can be measurable if the molecule involved is critical. Figure 32-1 summarizes the sequence of events between radiation exposure and resultant human injury.

When an atom is ionized, its chemical binding properties change. If the atom is a constituent of a large molecule, ionization may result in breakage of the molecule or relocation of the atom within the molecule. The abnormal molecule may in time function improperly or cease to function, which can result in serious impairment or death of the cell.

At each stage in the sequence, it is possible to repair radiation damage and recover.

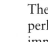

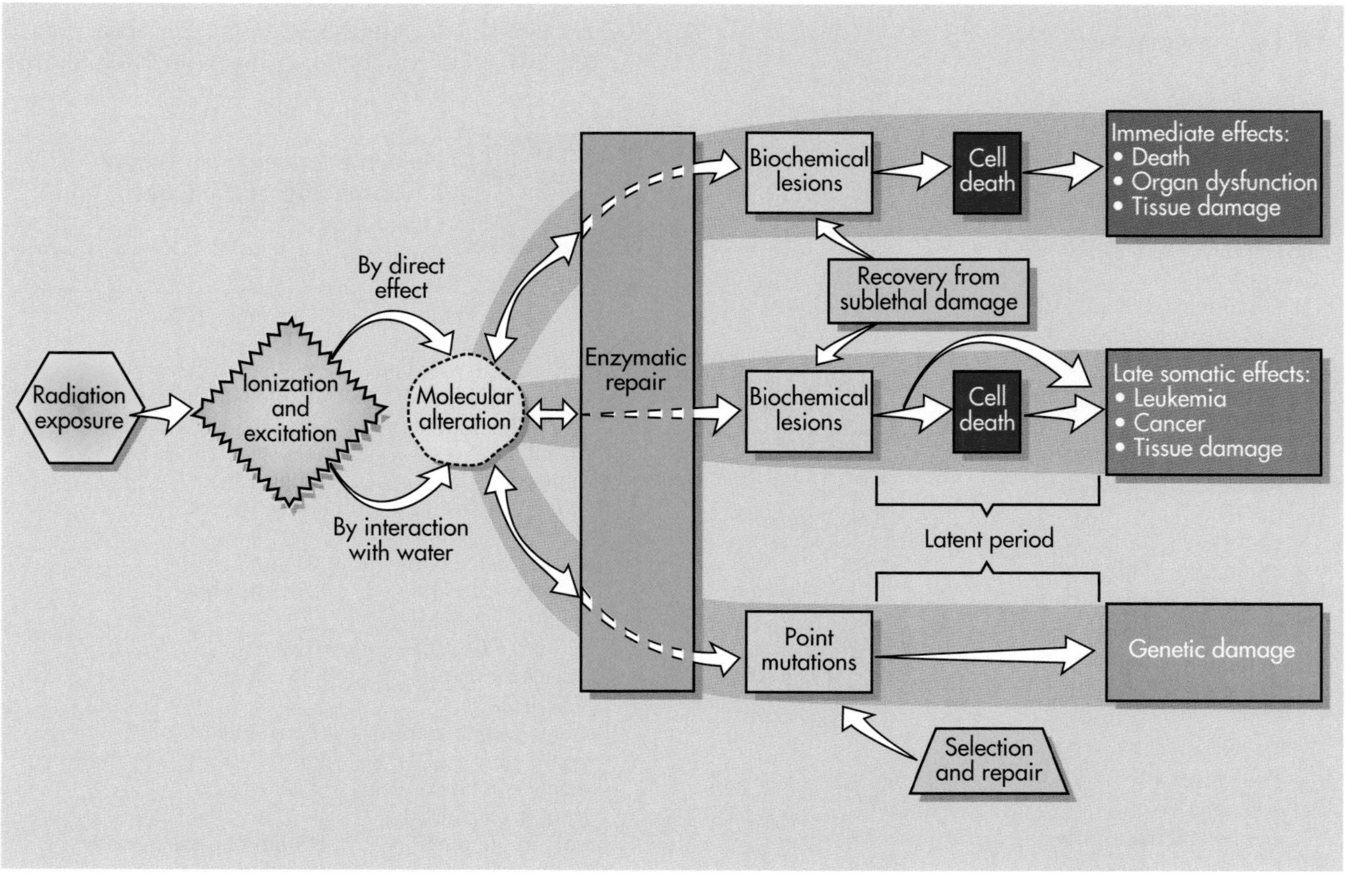

FIGURE 32-1 The sequence of events after radiation exposure of humans can lead to several radiation responses. At nearly every step, mechanisms for recovery and repair are available.

This process is reversible. Ionized atoms can become neutral again by attracting a free electron. Molecules can be mended by repair enzymes. Cell and tissues can regenerate and recover from radiation injury.

If the radiation response occurs within minutes or days after the radiation exposure, it is classified as an **early effect of radiation.** On the other hand, if the human injury is not observed for months or years, it is called a **late effect of radiation.**

A general classification scheme of possible early and late human responses to radiation is shown in Box 32-1. In addition, many other radiation responses have been experimentally observed in animals. Most human responses have been observed to occur after exposure to rather large radiation doses. However, we are cautious and assume that even small doses are harmful.

Table 32-1 lists some of the human population groups in which many of these radiation responses have been observed.

BOX 32-1   Human Responses to Ionizing Radiation

EARLY EFFECTS OF RADIATION ON HUMANS
1. Acute radiation syndrome
   a. Hematologic syndrome
   b. Gastrointestinal syndrome
   c. Central nervous system syndrome
2. Local tissue damage
   a. Skin
   b. Gonads
   c. Extremities
3. Hematologic depression
4. Cytogenetic damage

LATE EFFECTS OF RADIATION ON HUMANS
1. Leukemia
2. Other malignant disease
   a. Bone cancer
   b. Lung cancer
   c. Thyroid cancer
   d. Breast cancer
3. Local tissue damage
   a. Skin
   b. Gonads
   c. Eyes
4. Shortening of life span
5. Genetic damage
   a. Cytogenetic damage
   b. Doubling of dose
   c. Genetically significant dose

EFFECTS OF FETAL IRRADIATION
1. Prenatal death
2. Neonatal death
3. Congenital malformation
4. Childhood malignancy
5. Diminished growth and development

 Radiobiology is the study of the effects of ionizing radiation on biologic tissue.

The ultimate goal of radiobiologic research is to accurately describe the effects of radiation on humans so that radiation can be used more safely in diagnosis and more effectively in therapy. Most radiobiologic research seeks to develop dose-response relationships so the effects of planned doses can be predicted and the response to accidental exposure managed.

COMPOSITION OF THE BODY

At its most basic level, the human body is composed of atoms; radiation interacts at the atomic level. The atomic composition of the body determines the character and degree of the radiation interaction that occurs. The molecular and tissue composition defines the nature of the radiation response. Box 32-2 summarizes the atomic composition of the body and shows that more than 85% of the body consists of hydrogen and oxygen.

CELL THEORY

Radiation interaction at the atomic level results in molecular change, which can produce a cell that is deficient in terms of normal growth and metabolism. Robert Hooke, the English schoolmaster, first named the **cell** as the biologic building block in 1665. Shortly

---

TABLE 32-1   Human Populations in Whom Radiation Effects Have Been Observed

Population	Effect
American radiologists	Leukemia, reduced life span
Atomic bomb survivors	Malignant disease
Radiation accident victims (e.g., Chernobyl)	Acute lethality
Marshall Islanders	Thyroid cancer
Uranium miners	Lung cancer
Radium watch-dial painters	Bone cancer
Patients treated with ^{131}I	Thyroid cancer
Children treated for enlarged thymus	Thyroid cancer
Children of Belarus (downwind from Chernobyl)	Thyroid cancer
Patients with ankylosing spondylitis	Leukemia
Patients who underwent Thorotrast studies	Liver cancer
Irradiation in utero	Childhood malignancy
Volunteer convicts	Fertility impairment
Cyclotron workers	Cataracts

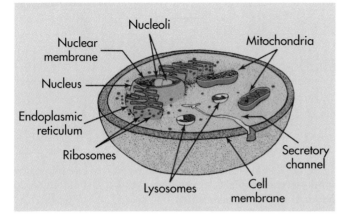

FIGURE 32-8 Schematic view of a human cell shows the principal structural components.

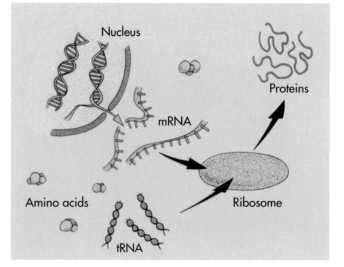

FIGURE 32-9 Protein synthesis is a complex process that involves many different molecules and cellular structures.

When a macromolecule is incorporated into the apparatus of a living cell, only a quantity of a few rads is necessary to produce a measurable biologic response. The lethal dose in some single-cell organisms, such as bacteria, is measured in kilorad, whereas human cells can be killed with a dose of less than 100 rad (1 Gy$_t$).

A number of experiments have shown that the nucleus is much more sensitive than the cytoplasm to the effects of radiation. Such experiments are conducted with the use of precise microbeams of electrons that can be focused and directed to a particular cell part, or through incorporation of the radioactive isotopes tritium (^{3}H) and carbon-14 (^{14}C) into cellular molecules that localize exclusively to the cytoplasm or the nucleus.

Cell Function

Every human cell has a specific function in supporting the total body. Some differences are obvious, as in nerve cells, blood cells, and muscle cells. Similarities are also somewhat obvious.

In addition to its specialized function, each cell to some extent absorbs all molecular nutrients through the cell membrane and uses these nutrients in energy production and molecular synthesis. If this molecular synthesis is damaged by radiation exposure, the cell may malfunction and die.

Protein synthesis is a good example of a critical cellular function necessary for survival (Figure 32-9). DNA, located in the nucleus, contains a molecular code that identifies which proteins the cell will make.

This code is determined by the sequence of base pairs (adenine–thymine and cytosine–guanine). A series of three base pairs, called a **codon,** identifies one of the 22 human amino acids available for protein synthesis.

This genetic message is transferred within the nucleus to a molecule of mRNA. mRNA leaves the nucleus by way of the endoplasmic reticulum and makes its way to a ribosome, where the genetic message is transferred to yet another RNA molecule (tRNA).

tRNA searches the cytoplasm for the amino acids for which it is coded. It attaches to the amino acid and carries it to the ribosome, where it is joined with other amino acids in sequence by peptide bonds to form the required protein molecule.

Interference with any phase of this procedure for protein synthesis could result in damage to the cell. Radiation interaction in which the molecule has primary control over protein synthesis (DNA) is more effective in producing a response than is radiation interaction with other molecules involved in protein synthesis.

Cell Proliferation

Although many thousands of rad (many gray) are necessary to produce physically measurable disruption of macromolecules in vitro, single ionizing events at a particularly sensitive site of a critical target molecule are thought to be capable of disrupting cell proliferation.

Cell proliferation is the act of a single cell or group of cells to reproduce and multiply in number.

The human body consists of two general types of cells: **somatic cells** and **genetic cells.** The genetic cells include the oogonium of the female and the spermatogonium of the male. All other cells of the body are somatic cells. When somatic cells proliferate or divide, they undergo **mitosis.** Genetic cells undergo **meiosis.**

Mitosis

The cell biologist and the geneticist view the cell cycle differently (Figure 32-10). Each cycle includes the various states of cell growth, development, and division. The geneticist considers only two phases of the cell cycle: **mitosis (M)** and **interphase.**

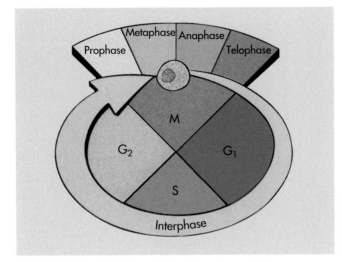

FIGURE 32-10 Progress of the cell through one cycle involves several phases.

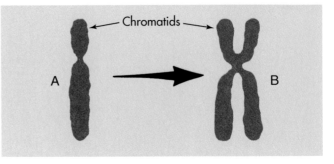

FIGURE 32-11 During the synthesis portion of interphase, the chromosomes replicate from a two-chromatid structure (**A**) to a four-chromatid structure (**B**).

Mitosis, the division phase, is characterized by four subphases: **prophase, metaphase, anaphase,** and **telophase.** The portion of the cell cycle between mitotic events is called *interphase.* Interphase is the period of growth of the cell between divisions.

The cell biologist usually identifies four phases of the cell cycle: M, G_1, S, and G_2. These phases of the cell cycle are characterized by the structure of the chromosomes, which contain the genetic material DNA. The **gap** in cell growth between M and S is G_1. G_1 is the pre-DNA synthesis phase.

The DNA synthesis phase is S. During this period, each DNA molecule is replicated into two identical daughter DNA molecules.

During S phase, the chromosome is transformed from a structure with two chromatids attached to a centromere to a structure with four chromatids attached to a centromere (Figure 32-11). The result is two pairs of homologous chromatids, that is, chromatids with precisely the same DNA content and structure.

The G_2 phase is the post-DNA synthesis gap of cell growth.

During interphase, the chromosomes are not visible; however, during mitosis, the DNA slowly takes the form of the chromosomes as seen microscopically. Figure 32-12 schematically depicts the process of mitosis.

During **prophase,** the nucleus swells and the DNA becomes more prominent and begins to take structural form. At **metaphase,** the chromosomes appear and are lined up along the equator of the nucleus. It is during metaphase that mitosis can be stopped and chromosomes can be studied carefully under the microscope.

 Radiation-induced chromosome damage is analyzed during metaphase.

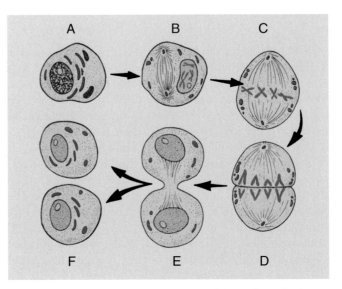

FIGURE 32-12 Mitosis is the phase of the cell cycle during which the chromosomes become visible, divide, and migrate to daughter cells. **A,** Interphase. **B,** Prophase. **C,** Metaphase. **D,** Anaphase. **E,** Telophase. **F,** Interphase.

Anaphase is characterized by splitting of each chromosome at the centromere, so that a centromere and two chromatids are connected by a fiber to the poles of the nucleus. These poles are called **spindles,** and the fibers are called **spindle fibers.** The number of chromatids per centromere has been reduced by half, and these newly formed chromosomes migrate slowly toward the spindle.

The final segment of mitosis, **telophase,** is characterized by the disappearance of structural chromosomes into a mass of DNA and the closing off of the nuclear membrane like a dumbbell into two nuclei. At the same time, the cytoplasm is divided into two equal parts, each of which accompanies one of the new nuclei.

Cell division is now complete. The two daughter cells look precisely the same as the parent and contain exactly the same genetic material.

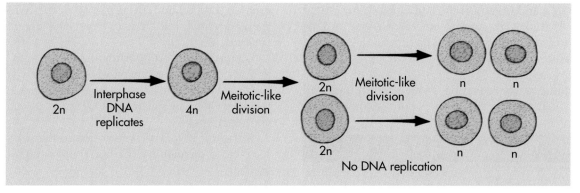

FIGURE 32-13 Meiosis is the process of reduction division, and it occurs only in reproductive cells. *n,* Number of similar chromosomes.

Meiosis

Genetic material can change during the division process of genetic cells, which is called **meiosis.** Genetic cells begin with the same number of chromosomes as somatic cells—23 pairs (46 chromosomes). However, for a genetic cell to be capable of marriage to another genetic cell, its complement of chromosomes must be reduced by half to 23, so that after conception and the union of two genetic cells, the daughter cells again will contain 46 chromosomes (Figure 32-13).

> Meiosis is the process whereby genetic cells undergo reduction division.

The genetic cell begins meiosis with 46 chromosomes that appear the same as in a somatic cell that has completed the G_2 phase. The cell then progresses through the phases of mitosis into two daughter cells, each containing 46 chromosomes of two chromatids each. The names of the subphases are the same for meiosis and mitosis.

Each of the daughter cells of this first division now progresses through a second division in which all cellular material, including chromosomes, is divided. However, the second division is not accompanied by an S phase. Therefore, no replication of DNA occurs; consequently, no chromosomes are duplicated. Each of the resulting granddaughter cells contains only 23 chromosomes.

Each parent has undergone two division processes, which have resulted in four daughter cells. During the second division, some chromosomal material is exchanged among chromatids through a process called **crossing over.** Crossing over results in changes in genetic constitution and changes in inheritable traits.

TISSUES AND ORGANS

During the development and maturation of a human from two united genetic cells, a number of different types of cells evolve. Collections of cells of similar structure and function form **tissues.** Box 32-4 is a breakdown of the composition of the body according to its tissue constituents.

These tissues in turn are precisely bound together to form **organs.** The tissues and the organs of the body serve as discrete units with specific functional responsibilities. Some tissues and organs combine into an overall integrated organization known as an **organ system.**

The principal organ systems of the body are the nervous system, the digestive system, the endocrine system, the respiratory system, and the reproductive system. Effects of radiation that appear at the whole-body level result from damage to these organ systems that occurs as the result of radiation injury to the cells of that system.

ORGAN SYSTEMS
- Nervous
- Reproductive
- Digestive
- Respiratory
- Endocrine

The cells of a tissue system are identified by their rate of proliferation and their stage of development. Immature cells are called **undifferentiated cells, precursor cells,** or **stem cells.** As a cell matures through growth and proliferation, it can pass through various stages of differentiation into a fully functional and mature cell.

> Stem cells are more sensitive to radiation than mature cells.

The sensitivity of the cell to radiation is determined somewhat by its state of maturity and its functional role. Table 32-2 lists a number of different types of cells in the body according to their degree of radiosensitivity.

The tissues and organs of the body include both stem cells and mature cells. Several types of tissue can be classified according to structural or functional features. These features influence the degree of radiosensitivity of the tissue.

Epithelium is the covering tissue, and it lines all exposed surfaces of the body, both exterior and interior. Epithelium covers the skin, the blood vessels, the abdominal and chest cavities, and the gastrointestinal tract.

Connective and **supporting tissues** are high in protein and are composed principally of fibers that are usually highly elastic. Connective tissue binds tissues and organs together. Bone ligaments and cartilage are examples of connective tissue.

Muscle is a special type of tissue that can contract. It is found throughout the body and is high in protein content.

Nervous tissue consists of specialized cells called **neurons** that have long, thin extensions from the cell to distant parts of the body. Nervous tissue is the avenue by which electrical impulses are transmitted throughout the body for control and response.

When these various types of tissue are combined to form an organ, they are identified according to two parts of the organ. The **parenchymal** part contains tissues that represent that particular organ, whereas the **stromal** part is composed of connective tissue and vasculature that provide structure to the organ.

The early effects of high-dose radiation may include observable organ damage. The various organs of the body exhibit a wide range of sensitivity to radiation. This radiosensitivity is determined by the function of the organ in the body, the rate at which cells mature within the organ, and the inherent radiosensitivity of the cell type.

Precise knowledge of these various organ radiosensitivities is unnecessary; however, knowledge of general levels of radiosensitivity is helpful toward understanding the effects of whole-body radiation exposure, particularly in the acute radiation syndrome (Table 32-3).

BOX 32-4   Tissue Composition of the Body

TISSUE	ABUNDANCE
• Muscle	• 43%
• Fat	• 14%
• Organs	• 12%
• Skeleton	• 10%
• Blood	• 8%
• Subcutaneous tissue	• 6%
• Bone marrow	• 4%
• Skin	• 3%

TABLE 32-2   Response to Radiation Is Related to Cell Type

Radiosensitivity	Cell Type
High	Lymphocytes
	Spermatogonia
	Erythroblasts
	Intestinal crypt cells
Intermediate	Endothelial cells
	Osteoblasts
	Spermatids
	Fibroblasts
Low	Muscle cells
	Nerve cells

TABLE 32-3   Relative Radiosensitivity of Tissues and Organs Based on Clinical Radiation Oncology

Level of Radiosensitivity*	Tissue or Organ	Effects
High: 200 to 1000 rad (2 to 10 Gy$_t$)	Lymphoid tissue	Atrophy
	Bone marrow	Hypoplasia
	Gonads	Atrophy
Intermediate: 1000 to 5000 rad (10 to 50 Gy$_t$)	Skin	Erythema
	Gastrointestinal tract	Ulcer
	Cornea	Cataract
	Growing bone	Growth arrest
	Kidney	Nephrosclerosis
	Liver	Ascites
	Thyroid	Atrophy
Low: >5000 rad (>50 Gy$_t$)	Muscle	Fibrosis
	Brain	Necrosis
	Spinal	Transection

*The minimum dose delivered at the rate of approximately 200 rad/day (2 Gy$_t$/day), which will produce a response.

SUMMARY

After radiation exposure, the human body responds in predictable ways. Radiobiology is the study of the effects of ionizing radiation on humans conducted to refine knowledge of the expected response.

If a response occurs within minutes or days of exposure, it is called an early effect of radiation. If an injury is not observable for months or years, it is called a late effect of radiation exposure.

The cell is the basic functional unit of all plants and animals. At the molecular level, the human body is composed primarily of water, protein, lipid, carbohydrate, and nucleic acid. The two important nucleic acids in human metabolism are DNA and RNA.

DNA contains all the hereditary information in the cell. If the cell is a genetic cell, the DNA contains the hereditary information of the whole individual. DNA is a macromolecule that is made up of two long chains of base sugar–phosphate combinations twisted into a double helix.

Major cellular function consists of protein synthesis and cell division. Mitosis is the growth, development, and division of cells. *Meiosis* is the term applied to the division of genetic cells.

Cells of similar structure bind together to form tissue. Tissues bind together to form organs. An overall integrated organization of tissue and organs is called an *organ system*.

The principal organ systems of the body are the nervous, digestive, endocrine, and reproductive systems. The radiosensitivity of various tissue and organ systems varies widely. Reproductive cells are highly radiosensitive, whereas nerve cells are less radiosensitive.

CHALLENGE QUESTIONS

1. Define or otherwise identify the following:
   a. ALARA
   b. Cell theory
   c. Anabolism
   d. Carbohydrate
   e. M, G_1, S, G_2
   f. Epithelium
   g. Cytoplasm
   h. Enzyme
   i. Organic molecule
   j. Late effect of radiation

2. At what structural level do x-rays interact with humans to produce a radiation response?
3. How does ionizing radiation affect an atom within a large molecule?
4. List five human groups in which radiation effects have been observed.
5. What are the effects of radiation on the populations mentioned in Question 4?
6. What is the most abundant atom and the most abundant molecule in the body?
7. What is a stem cell?
8. Why do we say that humans are basically a structured aqueous suspension?
9. What is the meaning of *epithelium?*
10. How do proteins function in the human body?
11. What do carbohydrates do for us?
12. DNA is the abbreviation for what molecule?
13. Which molecule is considered the genetic material of the cell?
14. What is the function of the endoplasmic reticulum?
15. What is the approximate dose of radiation required to produce a measurable physical change in a macromolecule?
16. List the stages of cell division of a somatic cell.
17. List the stages of cell reduction division of a genetic cell.
18. What cell type is the most radiosensitive?
19. What type of tissue is the least radiosensitive?
20. List three early radiation effects and three late radiation effects in humans.

The answers to the Challenge Questions can be found by logging on to our website at http://evolve.elsevier.com.

CHAPTER 33

Fundamental Principles of Radiobiology

OBJECTIVES

At the completion of this chapter, the student should be able to do the following:

1. State the law of Bergonie and Tribondeau
2. Describe the physical factors that affect radiation response
3. Describe the biologic factors that affect radiation response
4. Explain radiation dose-response relationships
5. Describe five types of radiation dose-response relationships

OUTLINE

Law of Bergonie and Tribondeau
Physical Factors That Affect Radiosensitivity
    Linear Energy Transfer
    Relative Biologic Effectiveness
    Protraction and Fractionation
Biologic Factors That Affect Radiosensitivity
    Oxygen Effect
    Age
    Recovery
    Chemical Agents
    Hormesis
Radiation Dose-Response Relationships
    Linear Dose-Response Relationships
    Nonlinear Dose-Response Relationships
    Constructing a Dose-Response Relationship

SOME TISSUES are more sensitive than others to radiation exposure. Such tissues usually respond more rapidly and to lower doses of radiation.

Reproductive cells are more sensitive than nerve cells. This and other radiobiologic concepts were detailed in 1906 by two French scientists.

Physical factors and biologic factors affect the radiobiologic response of tissue. Knowledge of these radiobiologic factors is essential for understanding the positive effects of radiation oncology and the potentially harmful effects of low-dose radiation exposure.

The principal aim of the study of radiobiology is to understand radiation dose–response relationships. A dose-response relationship is a mathematical and graphic function that relates radiation dose to observed response.

LAW OF BERGONIE AND TRIBONDEAU

In 1906, two French scientists, Bergonie and Tribondeau, theorized and observed that radiosensitivity was a function of the metabolic state of the tissue being irradiated. This has come to be known as the Law of Bergonie and Tribondeau and has been verified many times. Basically, the law states that the radiosensitivity of living tissue varies with maturation and metabolism (Box 33-1).

This law is principally interesting as a historical note in the development of radiobiology. It has found some application in radiation oncology. In diagnostic imaging, the law serves to remind us that the fetus is considerably more sensitive to radiation exposure than the child or the mature adult.

PHYSICAL FACTORS THAT AFFECT RADIOSENSITIVITY

When one irradiates tissue, the response of the tissue is determined principally by the amount of energy deposited per unit mass—the dose in rad (Gy_t). Even under controlled experimental conditions, however, when equal doses are delivered to equal specimens, the response may not be the same because of other modifying factors. A number of physical factors affect the degree of radiation response.

Linear Energy Transfer

Linear energy transfer (LET) is a measure of the rate at which energy is transferred from ionizing radiation to soft tissue. It is another method of expressing **radiation quality** and determining the value of the **radiation**

BOX 33-1 Law of Bergonie and Tribondeau

- Stem cells are radiosensitive; mature cells are radioresistant.
- Younger tissues and organs are radiosensitive.
- Tissues with high metabolic activity are radiosensitive.
- A high proliferation rate for cells and a high growth rate for tissues result in increased radiosensitivity.

weighting factor (W_R) used in radiation protection (see Chapter 37). LET is expressed in units of kiloelectron volt of energy transferred per micrometer of track length in soft tissue (keV/μm).

The LET of diagnostic x-rays is approximately 3 keV/μm.

The ability of ionizing radiation to produce a biologic response increases as the LET of radiation increases. When LET is high, ionizations occur frequently, increasing the probability of interaction with the target molecule.

Relative Biologic Effectiveness

As the LET of radiation increases, the ability to produce biologic damage also increases. This relative effect is quantitatively described by the relative biologic effectiveness (RBE).

RELATIVE BIOLOGIC EFFECTIVENESS

$$RBE = \frac{\text{Dose of standard radiation necessary to produce a given effect}}{\text{Dose of test radiation necessary to produce the same effect}}$$

The standard radiation, by convention, is orthovoltage x-radiation in the range of 200 to 250 kVp. This type of x-ray beam was used for many years in radiation oncology and in essentially all early radiobiologic research.

Diagnostic x-rays have an RBE of 1. Radiations with lower LET than diagnostic x-rays have an RBE less than 1, whereas radiations with higher LET have a higher RBE.

The RBE of diagnostic x-rays is 1.

Figure 33-1 shows the relationship between RBE and LET and identifies some of the more common types of radiation. Table 33-1 lists the approximate LET and RBE of various types of ionizing radiation.

TABLE 33-1	LET and RBE of Various Radiation Doses	
Type of Radiation	**LET (keV/μm)**	**RBE**
25 MV x-rays	0.2	0.8
^{60}Co gamma rays	0.3	0.9
1 MeV electrons	0.3	0.9
Diagnostic x-rays	3.0	1.0
10 MeV protons	4.0	5.0
Fast neutrons	50.0	10
5 MeV alpha particles	100.0	20
Heavy nuclei	1000.0	30

LET, Linear energy transfer; *RBE,* relative biologic effectiveness.

Question: When mice are irradiated with 250 kVp x-rays, death occurs at 650 rad (6.5 Gy$_t$). If similar mice are irradiated with fast neutrons, death occurs at only 210 rad (2.1 Gy$_t$). What is the RBE for the fast neutrons?

Answer:
$$RBE = \frac{650 \text{ rad}}{210 \text{ rad}} = 3.1$$

Protraction and Fractionation

If a dose of radiation is delivered over a long period of time rather than quickly, the effect of that dose is lessened. Stated differently, if the time of irradiation is lengthened, a higher dose is required to produce the same effect. This lengthening of time can be accomplished in two ways.

If the dose is delivered continuously but at a lower dose rate, it is said to be **protracted.** Six hundred rad (6 Gy$_t$) delivered in 3 min (200 rad/min [2 Gy$_t$/min]) is lethal for a mouse. However, when 600 rad is delivered at the rate of 1 rad/hr (10 mGy$_t$/hr) for a total time of 600 hr, the mouse will survive.

 Dose protraction and fractionation cause less effect because time is allowed for intracellular repair and tissue recovery.

If the 600 rad dose is delivered at the same dose rate, 200 rad/min, but in 12 equal fractions of 50 rad (500 mGy$_t$), all separated by 24 hr, the mouse will survive. In this situation, the dose is said to be **fractionated.**

Dose fractionation reduces effect because cells undergo repair and recovery between doses. Dose fractionation is used routinely in radiation oncology.

BIOLOGIC FACTORS THAT AFFECT RADIOSENSITIVITY

In addition to these physical factors, a number of biologic conditions alter the radiation response of tissue. Some of these factors, such as age and metabolic rate,

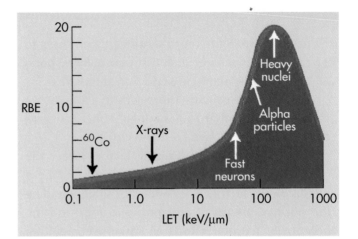

FIGURE 33-1 As linear energy transfer (LET) increases, relative biologic effectiveness (RBE) increases also, but a maximum value is reached followed by a lower RBE due to overkill.

have to do with the inherent state of tissue. Other factors are related to artificially introduced modifiers of the biologic system.

Oxygen Effect

Tissue is more sensitive to radiation when irradiated in the oxygenated, or aerobic, state than when irradiated under anoxic (without oxygen) or hypoxic (low-oxygen) conditions. This characteristic of tissue is called the *oxygen effect* and is described numerically by the **oxygen enhancement ratio (OER).**

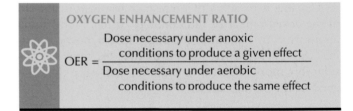

OXYGEN ENHANCEMENT RATIO
$$OER = \frac{\text{Dose necessary under anoxic conditions to produce a given effect}}{\text{Dose necessary under aerobic conditions to produce the same effect}}$$

Generally, tissue irradiation is conducted under conditions of full oxygenation. Hyperbaric (high-pressure) oxygen has been used in radiation oncology in an attempt to enhance the radiosensitivity of nodular, avascular tumors, which are less radiosensitive than tumors with an adequate blood supply.

 Diagnostic x-ray imaging is performed under conditions of full oxygenation.

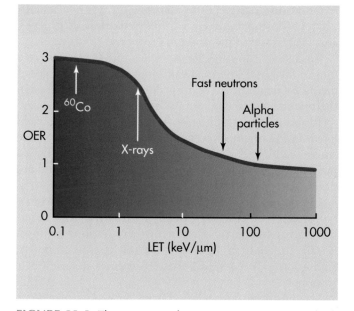

FIGURE 33-2 The oxygen enhancement ratio (OER) is high for low linear energy transfer (LET) radiation and decreases in value as the LET increases.

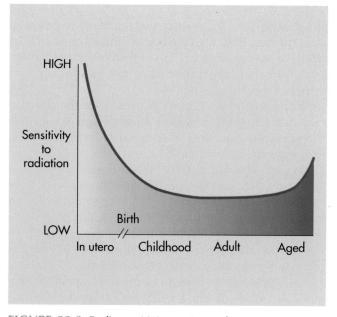

FIGURE 33-3 Radiosensitivity varies with age. Experiments with animals have shown that the very young and the very old are more sensitive to radiation.

Question: When experimental mouse mammary carcinomas are clamped and irradiated under hypoxic conditions, the tumor control dose is 10,600 rad (106 Gy_t). When these tumors are not clamped and are irradiated under aerobic conditions, the tumor control dose is 4050 rad (40.5 Gy_t). What is the OER for this system?

Answer:
$$OER = \frac{10,600}{4050} = 2.6$$

The OER is LET-dependent (Figure 33-2). The OER is highest for low-LET radiation, with a maximum value of approximately 3 that decreases to approximately 1 for high-LET radiation.

Age

The age of a biologic structure affects its radiosensitivity. The response of humans is characteristic of this age-related radiosensitivity (Figure 33-3). Humans are most sensitive before birth.

After birth, sensitivity decreases until maturity, at which time humans are most resistant to radiation effects. In old age, humans again become somewhat more radiosensitive.

Recovery

In vitro experiments show that human cells can recover from radiation damage. If the radiation dose is not sufficient to kill the cell before its next division (**interphase**

death), then given sufficient time, the cell will recover from the **sublethal radiation damage** it has sustained.

 Interphase death occurs when the cell dies before replicating.

This intracellular recovery is due to a **repair** mechanism inherent in the biochemistry of the cell. Some types of cells have greater capacity than others for repair of sublethal damage. At the whole-body level, this recovery from radiation damage is assisted through **repopulation** by surviving cells.

If a tissue or organ receives a sufficient radiation dose, it responds by shrinking. This is called **atrophy,** and it occurs because some cells die and disintegrate and are carried away as waste products.

If a sufficient number of cells sustain only sublethal damage and survive, they may proliferate and repopulate the irradiated tissue or organ.

The combined processes of intracellular repair and repopulation contribute to recovery from radiation damage.

RECOVERY
Recovery = Intracellular repair + Repopulation

Chemical Agents

Some chemicals can modify the radiation response of cells, tissues, and organs. For chemical agents to be effective, they must be present at the time of irradiation. Post-irradiation application does not usually alter the degree of radiation response.

Radiosensitizers. Agents that enhance the effect of radiation are called **sensitizing agents.** Examples include halogenated pyrimidines, methotrexate, actinomycin D, hydroxyurea, and vitamin K.

The halogenated pyrimidines become incorporated into the DNA of the cell and amplify the effects of radiation on that molecule. All radiosensitizers have an effectiveness ratio of approximately 2, that is, if 90% of a cell culture is killed by 200 rad (2 Gy_t), then in the presence of a sensitizing agent, only 100 rad (1 Gy_t) is required for the same percentage of lethality.

Radioprotectors. Radioprotective compounds include molecules that contain a sulfhydryl group (sulfur and hydrogen bound together), such as cysteine and cysteamine. Hundreds of others have been tested and found effective by a factor of approximately 2. For example, if 600 rad (6 Gy_t) is a lethal dose to a mouse, then in the presence of a radioprotective agent, 1200 rad (12 Gy_t) would be required to produce lethality.

Radioprotective agents have not found human application because, to be effective, they must be administered at toxic levels. The protective agent can be worse than the radiation!

Hormesis

A growing body of radiobiologic evidence suggests that a little bit of radiation is good for you. Studies have shown that animals given low radiation doses live longer than controls. The prevailing explanation is that a little radiation stimulates hormonal and immune responses to other toxic environmental agents.

Many nonradiation examples of hormesis can be found. In large quantities, fluoride is deadly. In small quantities, it is a known tooth preservative.

Regardless of radiation hormesis, we continue to practice ALARA ("as low as reasonably achievable") vigorously as a known safe approach to radiation management.

RADIATION DOSE-RESPONSE RELATIONSHIPS

Radiobiology is a relatively new science. Although some scientists were working with animals to observe the effects of radiation a few years after the discovery of x-rays, these studies were not experimentally sound, nor were their results applied. With the advent of the age of the atomic bomb in the 1940s, however, interest in radiobiology increased enormously.

The object of nearly all radiobiologic research is the establishment of radiation dose-response relationships.

A radiation dose-response relationship is a mathematical relationship between various radiation dose levels and magnitude of the observed response.

Radiation dose-response relationships have two important applications in radiology. First, these experimentally determined relationships are used to design therapeutic treatment routines for patients with cancer.

Radiobiologic studies also have been designed to yield information on the effects of low-dose irradiation. These studies and the dose-response relationships revealed provide the basis for radiation control activities and are particularly significant for diagnostic radiology.

Human responses to radiation exposure fall into two types: early or late, high dose or low dose, and deterministic or stochastic. **Deterministic** radiation responses usually follow high-dose exposure and an early response. Radiation-induced skin burns represent a deterministic response.

Stochastic responses are cancer, leukemia, or genetic effects. Such responses usually follow low radiation exposure and appear as a late radiation response.

Every radiation dose-response relationship has two characteristics. It is either linear or nonlinear, and it is either threshold or nonthreshold. These characteristics can be described mathematically or graphically. This discussion avoids the math.

Linear Dose-Response Relationships

Figure 33-4 shows examples of the linear dose-response relationship, which is so named because the response is directly proportionate to the dose. When the radiation

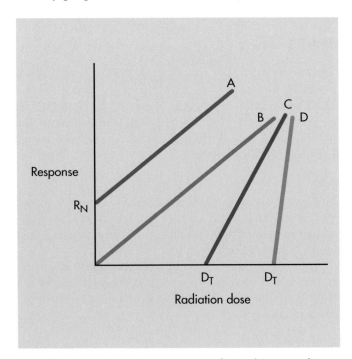

FIGURE 33-4 Linear dose-response relationships *A* and *B* are nonthreshold types; *C* and *D* are threshold types. R_N is the normal incidence or response with no radiation exposure.

dose is doubled, the response to radiation likewise is doubled.

Dose-response relationships *A* and *B* intersect the dose axis at zero or below (see Figure 33-4). These relationships are therefore the **linear, nonthreshold type.** In a nonthreshold dose-response relationship, any dose, regardless of its size, is expected to produce a response.

At zero dose, relationship A exhibits a measurable response, R_N. The level R_N, called the **natural** response level, indicates that even without radiation exposure, that type of response, such as cancer, occurs.

 Radiation-induced cancer, leukemia, and genetic effects follow a linear-nonthreshold dose-response relationship.

Dose-response relationships *C* and *D* are identified as **linear, threshold** because they intercept the dose axis at some value greater than zero. The threshold dose for *C* and *D* is D_T.

At radiation doses below D_T, no response is expected. Relationship *D* has a steeper slope than *C*; therefore, above the threshold dose, any increment of dose produces a larger response if that response follows relationship *D* rather than *C*.

Nonlinear Dose-Response Relationships

All other radiation dose-response relationships are nonlinear (Figure 33-5). Curves *A* and *B* are **nonlinear, nonthreshold.** Curve *A* shows that a large response results from a very small radiation dose. At high dose levels, radiation is not so efficient because an incremental dose at high levels results in less relative damage than the same incremental dose at low levels.

The dose-response relationship represented by curve *B* is just the opposite. Incremental doses in the low dose range produce very little response. At high doses, however, the same increment of dose produces a much larger response.

Curve *C* is a **nonlinear, threshold** relationship. At doses below D_T, no response is measured. As the dose is increased to above D_T, it becomes increasingly effective per increment of dose until the dose that corresponds to the inflection point of the curve is reached. This type of dose-response relationship is characteristic of a deterministic response.

The inflection point occurs when the curve stops bending up and begins bending down. Above this level, incremental doses become less effective. Relationship *C* is sometimes called an **S-type,** or **sigmoid-type,** radiation dose-response relationship.

 Skin effects resulting from high-dose fluoroscopy follow a sigmoid-type dose-response relationship.

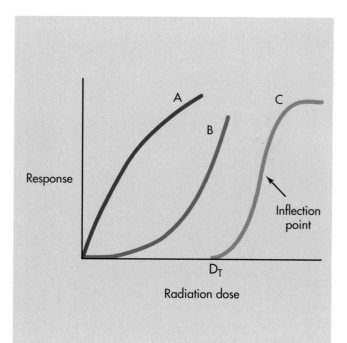

FIGURE 33-5 Nonlinear dose-response relationships can assume several shapes. Curve *A* is nonthreshold. Curves *B* and *C* are threshold. D_T, Threshold dose.

We shall refer to these general types of radiation dose-response relationships when discussing the type and degree of human radiation injury. Diagnostic radiology is concerned almost exclusively with the late effects of radiation exposure and therefore, with linear, nonthreshold dose-response relationships. For completeness, however, Chapter 35 briefly discusses early radiation damage.

Constructing a Dose-Response Relationship

Determining the radiation dose-response relationship for a whole-body response is tricky. It is very difficult to determine the degree of response, even that of early effects, because the number of experimental animals that can be used is usually small. It is nearly impossible to measure low-dose, late effects—the area of greatest interest in diagnostic imaging.

Therefore, we resort to irradiating a limited number of animals to very large doses of radiation in the hope of observing a statistically significant response. Figure 33-6 shows the results of such an experiment, in which four groups of animals were irradiated to a different dose. The observations on each group result in an ordered pair of data: a radiation dose and the associated biologic response.

The error bars in each ordered pair indicate the confidence associated with each data point. Error bars on the dose measurements are very narrow; thus, we can measure radiation dose very accurately. Error bars on the response, however, are very wide because of biologic variability and the limited number of observations at each dose.

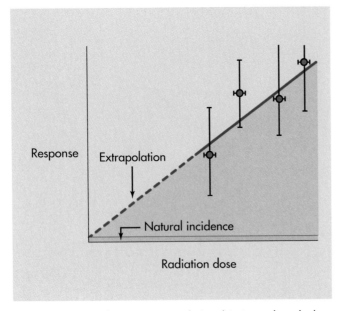

FIGURE 33-6 A dose-response relationship is produced when high-dose experimental data are extrapolated to low doses.

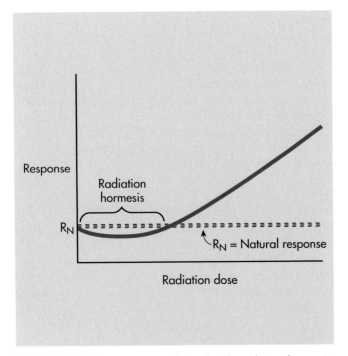

FIGURE 33-7 Dose-response relationship for radiation hormesis.

The principal interest in diagnostic imaging is to estimate response at very low radiation doses. Because this cannot be done directly, we **extrapolate** the dose-response relationship from the high-dose, known region into the low-dose, unknown region.

This extrapolation invariably results in a **linear, non-threshold** dose-response relationship. Such an extrapolation, however, may not be correct because of the many qualifying conditions on the experiment.

The radiation dose-response relationship that demonstrates radiation hormesis appears as in Figure 33-7. At very low doses, irradiated subjects experience less response than controls. The existence of radiation hormesis is a highly controversial topic in radiologic science. Regardless of its existence, no human radiation responses have been observed after doses less than 10 rad (100 mGy$_t$).

SUMMARY

In 1906, two French scientists first theorized that radiosensitivity was a function of the metabolic state of tissue being irradiated. Their theories, known as the Law of Bergonie and Tribondeau, state the following: (1) Stem cells are radiosensitive, mature cells are less so, (2) young tissue is more radiosensitive than older tissue, (3) high metabolic activity is radiosensitive, low metabolic rate is radioresistant, and (4) increases in proliferation and growth rates of cells make them more radiosensitive.

Physical and biologic factors affect tissue radiosensitivity. Physical factors include LET, RBE, fractionation (dose delivered over a long time), and protraction. Biologic factors that affect radiosensitivity include the oxygen effect, the age-related effect, and the recovery effect.

Some chemicals can modify cell response. These are called *radiosensitizers* and *radioprotectors*.

Radiobiologic research concentrates on radiation dose-response relationships. In linear dose-response relationships, the response is directly proportional to the dose. In nonlinear dose-response relationships, varied doses produce varied responses.

The threshold dose is the level below which there is no response. The nonthreshold dose-response relationship means that any dose is expected to produce a response. For establishing radiation protection guidelines for diagnostic imaging, the linear, nonthreshold dose-response model is used.

CHALLENGE QUESTIONS

1. Define or otherwise identify the following:
   a. Linear energy transfer
   b. Standard radiation
   c. Oxygen enhancement ratio
   d. Repopulation
   e. Extrapolation
   f. Threshold dose
   g. Interphase death
   h. Dose protraction
   i. Radiation weighting factor
   j. Tribondeau
2. Write the formula for relative biologic effectiveness.
3. Give an example of fractionated radiation.

4. Why is high-pressure (hyperbaric) oxygen used in radiation oncology?
5. Write the formula for the oxygen enhancement ratio.
6. How does age affect the radiosensitivity of tissue?
7. When a radiobiologic experiment is conducted in vitro, what does this mean?
8. Name three agents that enhance the effects of radiation.
9. Name three radioprotective agents.
10. Are radioprotective agents used for human application?
11. Explain the meaning of a radiation dose-response relationship.
12. What occurs in a nonlinear radiation dose-response relationship?
13. Explain why the linear, nonthreshold dose-response relationship is used as a model for diagnostic imaging radiation management.
14. State two of the corollaries to the law of Bergonie and Tribondeau.

15. Approximately 800 rad of 220 kVp x-rays is necessary to produce death in the armadillo. Cobalt-60 gamma rays have a lower LET than 220 kVp x-rays; therefore, 940 rad is required for armadillo lethality. What is the RBE of ^{60}CO compared with 220 kVp?
16. Under fully oxygenated conditions, 90% of human cells in culture will be killed by 150 rad x-rays. If cells are made anoxic, the dose required for 90% lethality is 400 rad. What is the OER?
17. What are the units of LET?
18. Describe how RBE and LET are related.
19. Is occupational radiation exposure fractionated, protracted, or continuous?
20. Describe how OER and LET are related.

The answers to the Challenge Questions can be found by logging on to our website at http://evolve.elsevier.com.

CHAPTER

34

Molecular and Cellular Radiobiology

OBJECTIVES

At the completion of this chapter, the student should be able to do the following:

1. Discuss three effects of in vitro irradiation of macromolecules
2. Explain the effects of radiation on DNA
3. Identify the chemical reactions involved in the radiolysis of water
4. Describe the effects of in vivo irradiation
5. Describe the principles of target theory
6. Discuss the kinetics of cell survival following irradiation

OUTLINE

Irradiation of Macromolecules
　　Main-Chain Scission
　　Cross-Linking
　　Point Lesions
　　Macromolecular Synthesis
　　Radiation Effects on DNA
Radiolysis of Water
Direct and Indirect Effects
Target Theory
Cell-Survival Kinetics
　　Single-Target, Single-Hit Model
　　Multitarget, Single-Hit Model
　　Recovery
Cell-Cycle Effects
LET, RBE, and OER

E VEN THOUGH the initial interaction between radiation and tissue occurs at the electron level, observable human radiation injury results from change at the molecular level. The occurrence of molecular lesions is categorized into effects on macromolecules and effects on water. This chapter discusses irradiation of macromolecules and radiolysis of water.

Because the human body is an aqueous solution that contains 80% water molecules, radiation interaction with water is the principal radiation interaction in the body. However, the ultimate damage occurs to the target molecule, DNA, which controls cellular metabolism and reproduction.

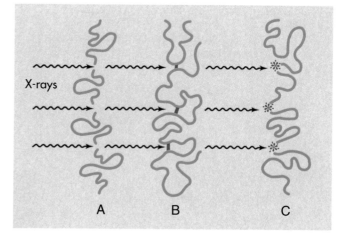

FIGURE 34-1 The results of irradiation of macromolecules. **A,** Main-chain scission. **B,** Cross-linking. **C,** Point lesions.

The effect of irradiation of macromolecules is quite different from that of irradiation of water. When macromolecules are irradiated **in vitro**, that is, outside the body or outside the cell, a considerable radiation dose is required to produce a measurable effect. Irradiation **in vivo**, that is, within the living cell, demonstrates that macromolecules are considerably more radiosensitive in their natural state.

 In vitro is irradiation outside of the cell or body. *In vivo* is irradiation within the body.

IRRADIATION OF MACROMOLECULES

A **solution** is a liquid that contains dissolved substances. A mixture of fluids such as water and alcohol is also a solution. When macromolecules are irradiated in solution in vitro, three major effects occur: main-chain scission, cross-linking, and point lesions (Figure 34-1).

Main-Chain Scission

Main-chain scission is the breakage of the backbone of the long-chain macromolecule. The result is the reduction of a long, single molecule into many smaller molecules, each of which may still be macromolecular.

Main-chain scission reduces not only the size of the macromolecule but also the **viscosity** of the solution. A viscous solution is one that is very thick and slow to flow, such as cold maple syrup. Tap water, on the other hand, has low viscosity. Measurements of viscosity determine the degree of main-chain scission.

Cross-Linking

Some macromolecules have small, spur-like side structures that extend off the main chain. Others produce these spurs as a consequence of irradiation.

These side structures can behave as though they had a sticky substance on the end, and they attach to a neighboring macromolecule or to another segment of the same molecule. This process is called **cross-linking.** Radiation-induced molecular cross-linking increases the viscosity of a macromolecular solution.

Point Lesions

Radiation interaction with macromolecules also can result in disruption of single chemical bonds, producing **point lesions.** Point lesions are not detectable, but they can cause a minor modification of the molecule, which in turn can cause it to malfunction within the cell.

 At low radiation doses, point lesions are considered to be the cellular radiation damage that results in the late radiation effects observed at the whole-body level.

Laboratory experiments have shown that all these types of radiation effects on macromolecules are reversible through intracellular repair and recovery.

Macromolecular Synthesis

Modern molecular biology has developed a generalized scheme for the function of a normal human cell. Molecular nutrients are brought to the cell and are diffused through the cell membrane, where they are broken down (**catabolism**) into smaller molecules with an accompanying release of energy.

This energy is used in several ways, but one of the more important ways is that they are used in the construction or **synthesis** of macromolecules from smaller molecules (**anabolism**). The synthesis of proteins and nucleic acids is critical to the survival of the cell and to its reproduction.

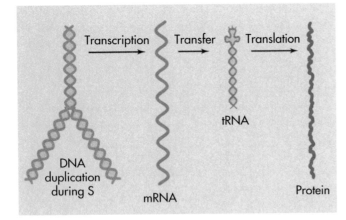

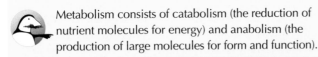

FIGURE 34-2 The genetic code of DNA is transcribed by messenger RNA (mRNA) and is transferred to transfer RNA (tRNA), which translates it into a protein.

> Metabolism consists of catabolism (the reduction of nutrient molecules for energy) and anabolism (the production of large molecules for form and function).

Chapter 32 describes the scheme of protein synthesis and its dependence on nucleic acids. Proteins are manufactured by **translation** of the genetic code from transfer RNA (tRNA), which had been **transferred** from messenger RNA (mRNA). The information carried by the mRNA was in turn **transcribed** from DNA. This chain of events is shown schematically in Figure 34-2.

Radiation damage to any of these macromolecules may result in cell death or late effects. Proteins are continuously synthesized throughout the cell cycle and occur in much more abundance than nucleic acids. Furthermore, multiple copies of specific protein molecules are always present in the cell. Consequently, proteins are less radiosensitive than nucleic acids.

Similarly, multiple copies of both types of RNA molecules are present in the cell, although they are less abundant than protein molecules. On the other hand, the DNA molecule, with its unique assembly of bases, is not so abundant.

>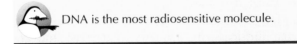
> DNA is the most radiosensitive molecule.

DNA is synthesized somewhat differently from proteins. During the G_1 portion of interphase, the deoxyribose, phosphate, and base molecules accumulate in the nucleus. These molecules combine to form a single large molecule that, during the S portion of interphase, is attached to an existing single chain of DNA (Figure 34-3). During G_1, molecular DNA is in the familiar double-helix form.

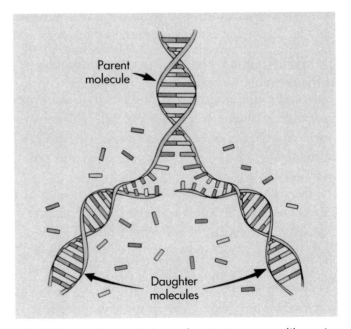

FIGURE 34-3 During S phase, the DNA separates like a zipper and two daughter DNA molecules are formed, each alike and each a replicate of the parent molecule.

>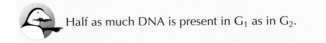
> Half as much DNA is present in G_1 as in G_2.

As the cell moves into S phase, the ladder begins to open up in the middle of each rung, much like a zipper. Now the DNA consists of only a single chain, and no pairing of bases occurs.

This state does not exist long, however, because the combined base sugar–phosphate molecule attaches to the single-strand DNA sequence, as determined by permitted base pairing. Consequently, where one double-helix DNA molecule was present, now two similar molecules exist, each a duplicate of the original. Parent DNA is said to be replicated into two duplicate DNA daughter molecules.

Radiation Effects on DNA

DNA is the most important molecule in the human body because it contains the genetic information for each cell. Each cell has a nucleus that contains DNA complexed with other molecules in the form of chromosomes. Chromosomes therefore control the growth and development of the cell; these in turn determine the characteristics of the individual (Figure 34-4).

If radiation damage to the DNA is severe enough, visible chromosome aberrations may be detected. Figure 34-5 is a representation of a normal chromosome and several distinct types of chromosome aberrations. Radiation-induced **chromosome aberrations** or **cytogenetic damage** is discussed more completely in Chapter 35.

The DNA molecule can be damaged without the production of a visible chromosome aberration. Although

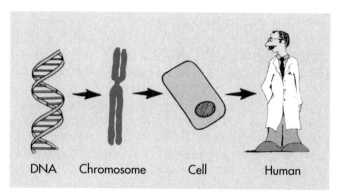

FIGURE 34-4 DNA is the target molecule for radiation damage. It forms chromosomes and controls cell and human growth and development.

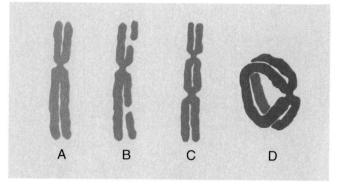

FIGURE 34-5 Normal and radiation-damaged human chromosomes. **A,** Normal. **B,** Terminal deletion. **C,** Dicentric formation. **D,** Ring formation.

such damage is reversible, it can lead to cell death. If enough cells of the same type respond similarly, then a particular tissue or organ can be destroyed.

Damage to the DNA also can result in abnormal metabolic activity. Uncontrolled rapid proliferation of cells is the principal characteristic of radiation-induced malignant disease. If damage to the DNA occurs within a germ cell, then it is possible that the response to radiation exposure will not be observed until the following generation, or even later.

The chromosome contains miles of DNA; therefore, when a visible aberration does appear, it signifies a considerable amount of radiation damage. Unobserved damage to the DNA also can produce responses at cellular and whole-body levels. The types of damage that can occur in the DNA molecule are as follows:

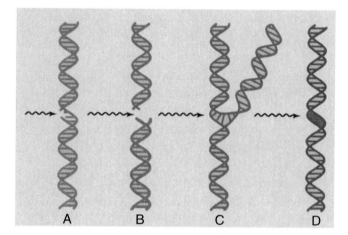

FIGURE 34-6 Types of damage that can occur in DNA. **A,** One side rail severed. **B,** Both side rails severed. **C,** Cross-linking. **D,** Rung breakage.

RADIATION RESPONSE OF DNA
- Main-chain scission with only one side rail severed
- Main-chain scission with both side rails severed
- Main-chain scission and subsequent cross-linking
- Rung breakage causing a separation of bases
- Change in or loss of a base

The gross structural radiation response of DNA is diagrammed schematically in Figure 34-6. Although each of these effects results in a structural change in the DNA molecule, they are all reversible. In some of these types of damage, the sequence of bases can be altered; therefore, the triplet code of codons may not remain intact. This represents a genetic mutation at the molecular level.

The fifth type of damage, the change or loss of a base, also destroys the triplet code and may not be reversible. This type of radiation damage is a molecular lesion of the DNA. These molecular lesions are called **point mutations,** and they can be of minor or major importance to the cell. One critical consequence of point mutations is the transfer

of the incorrect genetic code to one of the two daughter cells. This sequence of events is shown in Figure 34-7.

The three principal observable effects that may result from irradiation of DNA are cell death, malignant disease, and genetic damage. The latter two effects at the **molecular level** conform to the **linear, nonthreshold** dose-response relationship.

RADIOLYSIS OF WATER

Because the human body is an aqueous solution that contains approximately 80% water molecules, irradiation of water represents the principal radiation interaction in the body. When water is irradiated, it dissociates into other molecular products; this action is called **radiolysis of water** (Figure 34-8).

When an atom of water (H_2O) is irradiated, it is ionized and dissociates into two ions—an ion pair, as shown by the following:

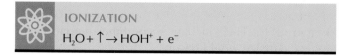

IONIZATION
$$H_2O + \uparrow \rightarrow HOH^+ + e^-$$

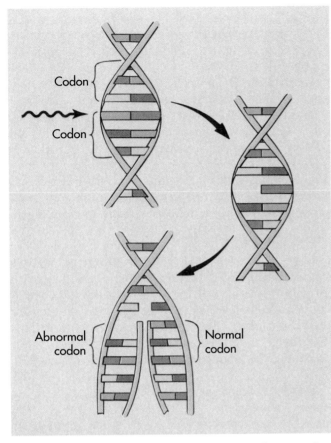

FIGURE 34-7 A point mutation results in the change or loss of a base, which creates an abnormal gene. This is therefore a genetic mutation that is passed to one of the daughter cells.

After this initial ionization, a number of reactions can happen. First, the ion pair may rejoin into a stable water molecule. In this case, no damage occurs. Second, if these ions do not rejoin, it is possible for the negative ion (the electron) to attach to another water molecule through the following reaction to produce yet a third type of ion.

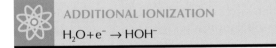

ADDITIONAL IONIZATION

$$H_2O + e^- \rightarrow HOH^-$$

The HOH and HOH⁻ ions are relatively unstable and can dissociate into still smaller molecules as follows:

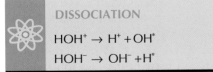

DISSOCIATION

$$HOH^+ \rightarrow H^+ + OH^*$$
$$HOH^- \rightarrow OH^- + H^*$$

The final result of the radiolysis of water is the formation of an ion pair, H⁺ and OH⁻, and two free radicals, H* and OH*. The ions can recombine; therefore, no biologic damage would occur.

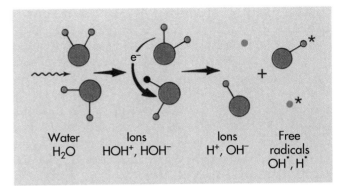

FIGURE 34-8 The radiolysis of water results in the formation of ions and free radicals.

These types of ions are not unusual. Many molecules in aqueous solution exist in a loosely ionized state because of their structure. Salt (NaCl), for instance, easily dissociates into Na⁺ and Cl⁻ ions. Even in the absence of radiation, water can dissociate into H⁺ and OH⁻ ions.

A free radical is an uncharged molecule that contains a single unpaired electron in the outer shell.

Free radicals are another story. They are highly reactive. Free radicals are unstable and therefore exist with a lifetime of less than 1 ms. During that time, however, they are capable of diffusion through the cell and interaction at a distant site. Free radicals contain excess energy that can be transferred to other molecules to disrupt bonds and produce point lesions at some distance from the initial ionizing event.

The H* and OH* molecules are not the only free radicals that are produced during the radiolysis of water. The OH* free radical can join with a similar molecule to form hydrogen peroxide.

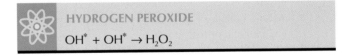

HYDROGEN PEROXIDE

$$OH^* + OH^* \rightarrow H_2O_2$$

Hydrogen peroxide is poisonous to the cell and therefore acts as a toxic agent.

The H* free radical can interact with molecular oxygen to form the hydroperoxyl radical as follows:

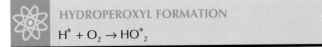

HYDROPEROXYL FORMATION

$$H^* + O_2 \rightarrow HO_2^*$$

The hydroperoxyl radical, along with hydrogen peroxide, is considered to be the principal damaging product after the radiolysis of water. Hydrogen peroxide also can be formed by the interaction of two hydroperoxyl radicals as follows:

HYDROGEN PEROXIDE FORMATION

$$HO_2^* + HO_2^* \rightarrow H_2O_2 + O_2$$

Some organic molecules, symbolized as RH, can become reactive free radicals as follows:

ORGANIC FREE RADICAL FORMATION

$$RH + \uparrow \rightarrow RH^* \rightarrow H^* + R^*$$

When oxygen is present, yet another species of free radical is possible as follows:

ORGANIC FREE RADICAL FORMATION

$$R^* + O_2 \rightarrow RO_2^*$$

Free radicals are energetic molecules because of their unique structure. This excess energy can be transferred to DNA, and this can result in bond breaks.

DIRECT AND INDIRECT EFFECTS

When biologic material is irradiated in vivo, the harmful effects of irradiation occur because of damage to a particularly sensitive molecule, such as DNA. Evidence for the direct effect of radiation comes from in vitro experiments wherein various molecules can be irradiated in solution. The effect is produced by ionization of the target molecule.

 If the initial ionizing event occurs on the target molecule, the effect of radiation is direct.

On the other hand, if the initial ionizing event occurs on a distant, noncritical molecule, which then transfers the energy of ionization to the target molecule, **indirect effect** has occurred. Free radicals, with their excess energy of reaction, are the intermediate molecules. They migrate to the target molecule and transfer their energy, which results in damage to that target molecule.

The principal effect of radiation on humans is indirect.

It is not possible to identify whether a given interaction with the target molecule resulted from direct or indirect effect. However, because the human body consists of approximately 80% water and less than 1% DNA, it is concluded that essentially all of the effects of irradiation in vivo result from indirect effect. When oxygen is present, as in living tissue, the indirect effects are amplified because of the additional types of free radicals that are formed.

TARGET THEORY

The cell contains many species of molecules, most of which exist in overabundance. Radiation damage to such molecules probably would not result in noticeable injury to the cell because similar molecules would be available to continue to support the cell.

On the other hand, some molecules in the cell are considered to be particularly necessary for normal cell function. These molecules are not abundant; in fact, there may be only one such molecule. Radiation damage to such a molecule could affect the cell severely because no similar molecules would be available as substitutes.

This concept of a sensitive key molecule serves as the basis for the **target theory**. According to the target theory, for a cell to die after radiation exposure, its target molecule must be inactivated (Figure 34-9).

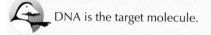 DNA is the target molecule.

The key molecular target is the DNA. Originally, the target theory was used to represent cell lethality. It can be used equally well, however, to describe nonlethal radiation-induced cell abnormalities.

In the target theory, the target is considered to be an area of the cell occupied by the target molecule or by a sensitive site on the target molecule. This area changes position with time because of intracellular molecular movement.

The interaction between radiation and cellular components is random; therefore, when an interaction does occur with a target, it occurs randomly. No favoritism is seen in radiation to the target molecule. Its sensitivity to radiation occurs simply because of its vital function in the cell.

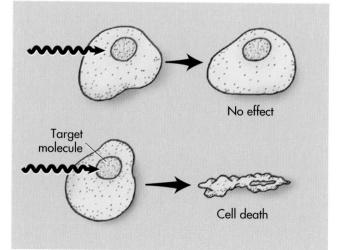

FIGURE 34-9 According to target theory, cell death will occur only if the target molecule is inactivated. DNA, the target molecule, is located within the cell nucleus.

When radiation does interact with the target, a **hit** is said to have occurred. Radiation interaction with molecules other than the target molecule also can result in a hit. It is not possible to distinguish between a direct and an indirect hit.

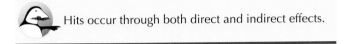

Hits occur through both direct and indirect effects.

When a hit occurs through indirect effect, the size of the target appears considerably larger because of the mobility of the free radicals. This increased target size contributes to the importance of the indirect effect of radiation.

Figure 34-10 illustrates some of the consequences of using target theory to explain the relationships among linear energy transfer (LET), the oxygen effect (oxygen enhancement ratio [OER]), and direct versus indirect effect. With low-LET radiation, in the absence of oxygen, the probability of a hit on the target molecule is low because of the relatively large distances between ionizing events.

If oxygen is present, free radicals are formed and the volume of effectiveness surrounding each ionization is enlarged. Consequently, the probability of a hit is increased.

When high-LET radiation is used, the distance between ionizations is so close that the probability of a hit by direct effect is high. When oxygen is added to the system and high-LET radiation is used, the added sphere of influence for each ionizing event, although

somewhat larger, does not result in additional hits. The maximum number of hits has already been produced by direct effect with high-LET radiation.

CELL-SURVIVAL KINETICS

Early radiation experiments at the cell level were conducted with simple cells, such as bacteria. It was not until the middle 1950s that laboratory techniques were developed to allow the growth and manipulation of human cells in vitro.

One technique for measuring the lethal effects of radiation on cells is shown in Figure 34-11. If normal cells are planted individually in a Petri dish and are incubated for 10 to 14 days, they divide many times and produce a visible **colony** that consists of many cells. This is cell **cloning.**

After irradiation of such single cells, some do not survive and, therefore, fewer colonies are formed. A higher radiation dose leads to the formation of fewer colonies.

The lethal effects of radiation are determined by observing cell survival, not cell death.

When a mathematical extension of target theory is used, two models of cell survival result. The **single-target, single-hit** model applies to biologic targets, such as enzymes, viruses, and simple cells like bacteria. The **multitarget, single-hit** model applies to more complicated biologic systems, such as human cells.

The following discussion concerns the equation of these models. The mathematics of these models is relatively unimportant but is given here for the interested student.

Single-Target, Single-Hit Model

Consider for a moment the situation illustrated in Figure 34-12. It is raining on a large concrete runway that contains 100 squares. A square is considered wet when one or more raindrops have fallen on it.

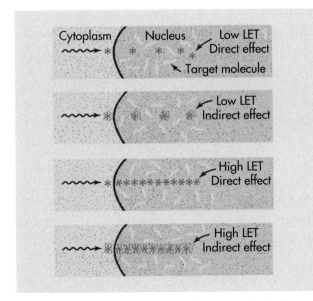

FIGURE 34-10 In the presence of oxygen, the indirect effect is amplified and the volume of action for low–linear energy transfer (LET) radiation is enlarged. The effective volume of action for high-LET radiation remains unchanged, in that maximum injury will have been inflicted by direct effect.

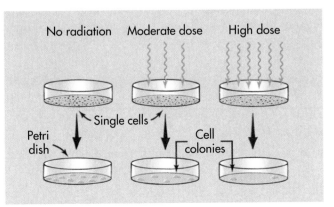

FIGURE 34-11 When single cells are planted in a Petri dish, they grow into visible colonies. Fewer colonies develop if the cells are irradiated.

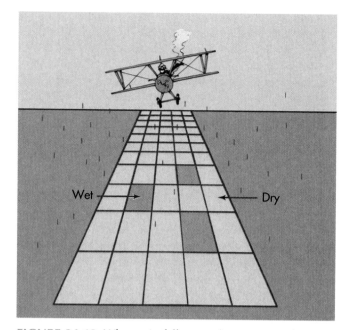

FIGURE 34-12 When rain falls on a dry pavement that consists of a large number of squares, the number of squares that remains dry decreases exponentially as the number of raindrops increases.

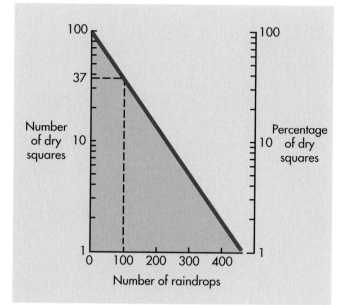

FIGURE 34-13 When the number of dry squares is plotted on semilogarithmic paper as a function of the number of raindrops, a straight line results, because when a few drops fall, some squares will be hit more than once.

When the first drop falls on the pavement, 1 of the 100 squares becomes wet. When the second drop falls, it will probably fall on a dry square and not on the one already wet. Consequently, 2 out of 100 squares will be wet.

When the third raindrop falls, there will probably be 3 wet and 97 dry squares. As the number of raindrops increases, however, it becomes more probable that a given square will be hit by 2 or more drops.

Because the raindrops are falling **randomly**, the probability that a square will become wet is governed by a statistical law called the **Poisson distribution**. According to this law, when the number of raindrops is equal to the number of squares (100 in this case), 63% of the squares will be wet and 37% of the squares will be dry. If the raindrops had fallen **uniformly**, all 100 squares would become wet with 100 raindrops.

 Radiation interacts randomly with matter.

Obviously, many of the 63 squares in this example have been hit twice or more. When the number of raindrops equals twice the number of squares, then 14 squares will be dry. After 300 raindrops, only 5 squares will remain dry.

Examine a graph of the number of dry squares as a function of the number of raindrops (Figure 34-13). If the number of squares exposed to the rain was large or unknown, the scale on the right, expressed in percent, would be used.

The wet squares analogy can be extended to the irradiation of a large number of biologic specimens—for example, 1000 bacteria. Bacteria presumably contain a single sensitive site, or **target,** that must be inactivated for the cell to die. As 1000 bacteria are irradiated with increasing increments of dose, a greater number are killed (Figure 34-14).

Just as with the wet squares, however, as the dose increases, some cells will suffer two or more hits. All hits per target in excess of one represent wasted radiation dose because the bacteria had been killed already by the first hit.

 A hit is not simply an ionizing event, but rather an ionization that inactivates the target molecule.

When the radiation dose reaches a level sufficient to kill 63% of the cells (37% survival), it is called D_{37}. Following a dose equal to $2 \times D_{37}$, 14% of the cells would survive, and so forth. D_{37} is a measure of the radiosensitivity of the cell. A low D_{37} indicates a highly radiosensitive cell, and a high D_{37} reveals radioresistance.

If there were no wasted hits (uniform interaction), D_{37} is the dose that would be sufficient to kill 100% of the cells.

The equation that describes the dose-response relationship represented by the graph in Figure 34-14 is

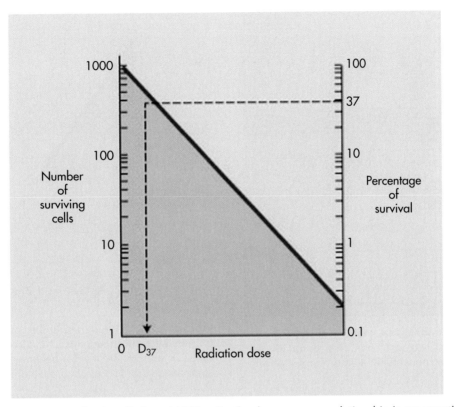

FIGURE 34-14 After irradiation of 1000 cells, the dose-response relationship is exponential. The D_{37} is that dose that results in 37% survival.

the **single-target, single-hit** model of radiation-induced lethality as follows:

> **SINGLE-TARGET, SINGLE-HIT MODEL**
>
> $S = N/N_0 = e^{-D/D_{37}}$
>
> where S is the surviving fraction, N is the number of cells surviving a dose D, N_0 is the initial number of cells, and D_{37} is a constant dose related to cell radiosensitivity.

Multitarget, Single-Hit Model

Returning to the wet squares analogy, suppose that each pavement square were divided into two equal parts, two targets (Figure 34-15). By definition, each half now must be hit with a raindrop for the square to be considered wet. The first few raindrops probably will hit only one half of any given square; therefore, after a very light rain, no squares may be wet.

Many raindrops must fall before any single square suffers a hit in both halves so that it can be considered wet. This represents a **threshold** because, according to our definition, a number of raindrops can fall and all squares will remain dry. As the number of raindrops increases, eventually some squares will have both halves hit and therefore will be considered wet.

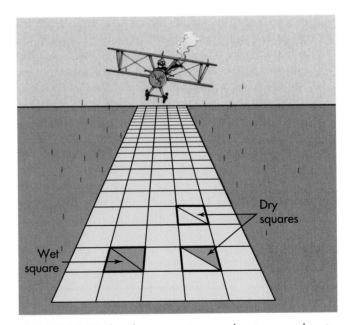

FIGURE 34-15 If each pavement square has two equal parts, each part must be hit for the square to be considered wet.

This portion of the curve is represented by region A in Figure 34-16.

When a large number of raindrops have fallen, region C will be reached, where every square will be at least half wet. When this occurs, each additional raindrop will produce a wet square. In region C, the

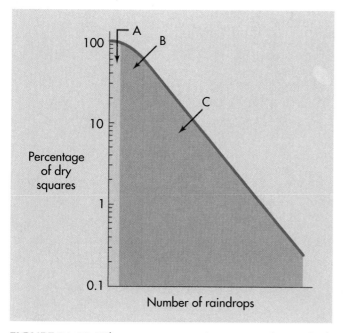

FIGURE 34-16 When a square contains two equal parts, both of which have to be hit to be considered wet, three regions of the dry square versus raindrops relationship can be identified.

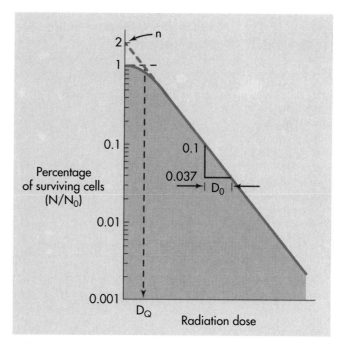

FIGURE 34-17 The multitarget, single-hit model of cell survival is characteristic of human cells that contain two targets.

relation between number of raindrops and wet squares is that described by the single-target, single-hit model. The intermediate region *B* is the region of accumulation of hits.

Complex biologic specimens such as human cells are thought to have more than a single critical target. Suppose that the human cell has two targets, each of which has to be inactivated for the cell to die. This would be analogous to the square having two halves, each of which had to be hit by rain for it to be considered wet. Figure 34-17 is a graph of single-cell survival for human cells that have two targets.

At very low radiation doses, cell survival is nearly 100%. As the radiation dose increases, fewer cells survive because more sustain a hit in both target molecules.

At a high radiation dose, all cells that survive have one target hit. Therefore, at still higher doses, the dose-response relationship would appear as the single-target, single-hit model.

The model of cell survival just described is the multitarget, single-hit model as follows:

MULTITARGET, SINGLE-HIT MODEL

$S = N/N_0 = 1 - (1 - e^{D/D_0})^n$

where *S* is the surviving fraction, *N* is the number of cells surviving a dose *D*, N_0 is the initial number of cells, D_0 is the dose necessary to reduce survival to 37% in the straight-line portion of the graph, and *n* is the *extrapolation number*.

The D_0 is called the **mean lethal dose** and is a constant related to the radiosensitivity of the cell. It is equal to D_{37} in the linear portion of the graph and therefore represents the dose that would result in one hit per target in the straight-line portion of the graph if no radiation were wasted.

 A large D_0 indicates radioresistant cells, and a small D_0 is characteristic of radiosensitive cells.

The **extrapolation number** is also called the **target number.** When this type of experiment was first conducted with human cells, the observed extrapolation number was 2. That result agreed with the hypothesis that similar regions on two homologous chromosomes (an identical pair) had to be inactivated to produce cell death. Because chromosomes come in pairs, the experimental results confirmed the hypothesis.

Subsequent experiments, however, have resulted in extrapolation numbers ranging from 2 to 12, and therefore the precise meaning of *n* is unknown.

The D_Q is called the **threshold dose.** It is a measure of the width of the shoulder of the multitarget, single-hit model and is related to the capacity of the cell to recover from sublethal damage. Table 34-1 lists reported values for D_0 and D_Q for various experimental cell lines.

A large D_Q indicates that the cell can recover readily from sublethal radiation damage.

TABLE 34-1	Doses for Various Experimental Mammalian Cell Lines	
Cell Type	**D_0 (rad)**	**D_Q (rad)**
Mouse oocytes	91	62
Mouse skin	135	350
Human bone marrow	137	100
Human fibroblasts	150	160
Mouse spermatogonia	180	270
Chinese hamster ovary	200	210
Human lymphocytes	400	100

D_0, Mean lethal dose; D_Q, threshold dose.

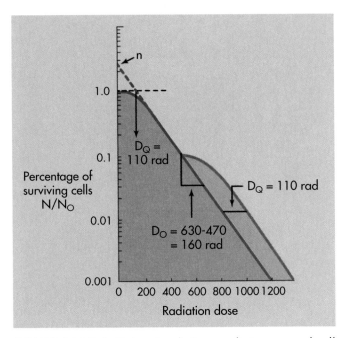

FIGURE 34-18 Split-dose irradiation results in a second cell survival curve with the same characteristics as the first and displaced along the dose axis by D_Q.

Recovery

The shoulder of the graph of the multitarget, single-hit model shows that for mammalian cells, some damage must be accumulated before the cell dies. This accumulated damage is called **sublethal damage.** The wider the shoulder, the more sublethal damage that can be sustained and the higher the value of D_Q.

Figure 34-18 demonstrates the results of a **split-dose irradiation** designed to describe the capacity of a cell to recover from sublethal damage. This illustration shows a rather typical human cell survival curve with $D_0 = 160$ rad (1.6 Gy_t), $D_Q = 110$ rad (1.1 Gy_t), and n = 2. If one takes those cells that survive any large dose (e.g., 470 rad [4.7 Gy_t]) and reincubates them in a growth medium, they will grow into another large population.

This new population of cells then can be used to perform a second cell survival experiment. When the cells that survived the first dose are subsequently subjected to additional incremental radiation doses, a second dose-response curve is generated that has precisely the same shape as the first.

After such a split occurs, the extrapolation number is the same and the mean lethal dose is the same, and the second dose-response curve is separated along the dose axis from the first dose-response curve by D_Q. For full recovery to occur, the time between such split doses must be at least as long as the cell generation time, usually 24 hours.

Such experiments show that cells that survive an initial radiation insult exhibit precisely the same characteristics as nonirradiated cells; therefore, the surviving cells have fully recovered from the sublethal damage produced by the initial irradiation.

 D_Q is a measure of the capacity to accumulate sublethal damage and the ability to recover from sublethal damage.

Question: From Figure 34-18, estimate the overall surviving fraction for a cell receiving a split dose of 400 rad followed by 400 rad (4 Gy_t).

Answer: At a dose of 400 rad, approximately 0.15 of the cells survive. Therefore, at a split dose of 400 rad and 400 rad, the surviving fraction should equal 0.15 × 0.15 = 0.023. The total dose is 800 rad (8 Gy_t), and the surviving fraction on the split-dose curve at 800 rad should equal 0.023, and it does. Had the 800 rad been delivered at one time, the surviving fraction would have been 0.012, as is shown by the single-dose curve of Figure 34-18.

CELL-CYCLE EFFECTS

When human cells replicate by mitosis, the average time from one mitosis to another is called the **cell-cycle time** or the **cell generation time.** Most human cells that are in a state of normal proliferation have generation times of approximately 24 hours.

Some specialized cells have generation times that extend to hundreds of hours, and other cells, such as neurons (nerve cells), do not normally replicate. Longer generation times primarily result from lengthening of the G_1 phase of the cell cycle.

G_1 is the most time variable of cell phases.

A randomly growing population of cells that are uniformly distributed in position throughout the cell cycle can be **synchronized** in various ways. A population of synchronized cells then can be subdivided into smaller populations and irradiated sequentially as they pass through the phases of the cell cycle.

Figure 34-19 represents results obtained from human fibroblasts. The fraction of cells that survive a given dose can vary by a factor of 10 from the most sensitive to the most resistant phase of the cell cycle.

This pattern of change in radiosensitivity as a function of phase in the cell cycle is the **age-response function,** and it varies among cells. Cells in mitosis are always most sensitive. The fraction of surviving cells is lowest in this phase. The next most sensitive phase of the cell cycle occurs at the G_1-S transition. The most resistant portion of the cell cycle is the late S phase.

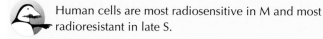

Human cells are most radiosensitive in M and most radioresistant in late S.

LET, RBE, AND OER

Mammalian cell survival experiments have been used extensively to measure the effects of various types of radiation and to determine the magnitude of various dose-modifying factors, such as oxygen. Because the mean lethal dose, D_0, is related to radiosensitivity, the ratio of D_0 for one condition of irradiation compared with another is a measure of the effectiveness of the dose modifier, whether it is physical or biologic.

If the same cell type is irradiated by two different radiations under identical conditions, results may appear as in Figure 34-20. At very high LET (as with alpha particles and neutrons), cell-survival kinetics follow the single-target, single-hit model. With low-LET radiation (x-rays), the multitarget, single-hit model applies.

The mean lethal dose after low-LET irradiation is always greater than that after high-LET irradiation. If the low-LET D_0 represents x-rays, then the ratio of one D_0 to another equals the relative biologic effectiveness (RBE) for the high-LET radiation as follows:

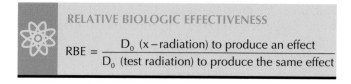

RELATIVE BIOLOGIC EFFECTIVENESS

$$RBE = \frac{D_0 \; (x-radiation) \; to \; produce \; an \; effect}{D_0 \; (test \; radiation) \; to \; produce \; the \; same \; effect}$$

Question: Figure 34-20 shows the radiation dose-response relationship of human fibroblasts exposed to x-rays and those exposed to 14 MeV neutrons. The D_0 after x-radiation is 170 rad (1.7 Gy_t); the D_0 for neutron irradiation is 100 rad (1 Gy_t). What is the RBE of 14 MeV neutrons relative to x-rays?

Answer: $$RBE = \frac{170 \; rad}{100 \; rad} = 1.7$$

Irradiation of mammalian cells with high-LET radiation follows the single-target, single-hit model.

The most completely studied dose modifier is oxygen. The presence of oxygen maximizes the effect of low-LET radiation. When anoxic cells are exposed, a considerably higher dose is required to produce a given effect.

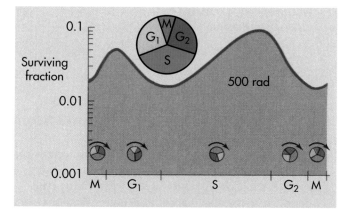

FIGURE 34-19 The age response of human fibroblasts after irradiation shows minimum survival during the M phase and maximum survival during the late S phase. Such cells are most radiosensitive during mitosis and most radioresistant during the late S phase.

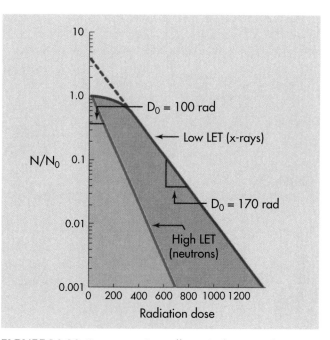

FIGURE 34-20 Representative cell-survival curves after exposure to 200 kVp x-rays and 14 MeV neutrons.

With high-LET radiation, little difference is noted between the response of oxygenated cells and that of anoxic cells. Figure 34-21 shows typical cell-survival curves for each of these combinations of LET and oxygen.

Such experiments are designed to measure the magnitude of the oxygen effect. The OER determined from single-cell survival experiments is defined as follows:

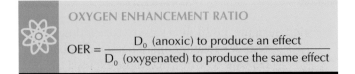

OXYGEN ENHANCEMENT RATIO

$$OER = \frac{D_0 \text{ (anoxic) to produce an effect}}{D_0 \text{ (oxygenated) to produce the same effect}}$$

Question: With reference to Figure 34-21, what is the estimated OER for human cells exposed to low-LET radiation and to high-LET radiation?

Answer: Low LET, no oxygen $D_0 = 340$ rad

Low LET, oxygen $D_0 = 140$ rad

$$OER = \frac{340 \text{ rad}}{140 \text{ rad}} = 2.4$$

High LET, no oxygen, $D_0 = 90$ rad

High LET, oxygen, $D_0 = 70$ rad

$$OER = \frac{90 \text{ rad}}{70 \text{ rad}} = 1.3$$

The interrelationships among LET, RBE, and OER are complex. However, it is LET that determines the magnitude of RBE and OER.

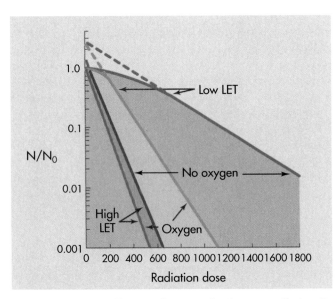

FIGURE 34-21 Cell-survival curves for human cells irradiated in the presence and the absence of oxygen with high- and low–linear energy transfer (LET) radiation.

SUMMARY

When macromolecules are irradiated in vitro, three major effects occur: (1) main-chain scission, (2) cross-linking, and (3) disruption of single chemical bonds in a macromolecule, causing point lesions. All three types of damage are reversible through intracellular repair and recovery.

DNA, with its unique assembly of bases, is not abundant in the cell. As a result, DNA is the most radiosensitive of all macromolecules. Chromosome aberrations or abnormal metabolic activity can result from DNA damage. DNA irradiation has three observable effects: cell death, malignant disease, and genetic damage.

Because the human body is 80% water, irradiation of water is the principal interaction that occurs in the body. Water dissociates into free radicals that are highly reactive and can diffuse through the cell to cause damage at some distance.

The initial ionizing event is said to be a direct effect if the interaction occurs with a DNA molecule. If the ionizing event occurs with water and transfers that energy to DNA, the event is said to be an indirect effect.

The concept of a sensitive key molecule within a cell serves as the basis for the target theory. For a cell to die after radiation exposure, the target molecule, DNA, must be inactivated.

Radiation exposure results in two models of cell survival. The single-target, single-hit model applies to simple cells such as bacteria. The multitarget, single-hit model implies a dose threshold. However, at higher doses, the relationship becomes a single-hit, single-target model. Experiments in cell recovery show that cells can recover from sublethal radiation damage.

CHALLENGE QUESTIONS

1. Define or otherwise identify the following:
   a. In vitro
   b. Cytogenetic damage
   c. Point mutation
   d. Free radical
   e. Target theory
   f. D_{37}
   g. Mean lethal dose
   h. Radiation hit
   i. Extrapolation number
   j. D_Q
2. List the effects of irradiation of macromolecules in solution in vitro.
3. How is solution viscosity used to determine the degree of radiation macromolecular damage?
4. What is the difference between catabolism and anabolism?
5. In what phase of the cell cycle does the DNA ladder open up in the middle of each rung and consist of only a single chain?

6. Name the three principal observable effects of DNA irradiation.
7. Differentiate between transcription, transfer, and translation when applied to molecular genetics.
8. Draw a diagram that illustrates the point mutations of DNA that transfer the incorrect genetic code to one of the two daughter cells.
9. Write the formula for radiolysis of water in which the atom of water is ionized and dissociates into two ions.
10. What happens to radiation-induced free radicals within the cell?
11. What is the target theory of radiobiology?
12. Does radiation interact with tissue uniformly or randomly?
13. Draw cell-survival curves to show the difference between irradiation with low LET and high-LET radiation.
14. What is the difference between in vitro and in vivo?

15. Complete the following chemical equations:
H_2O + Radiation → ?

HOH^+ (dissociation) → ?

HOH^- (dissociation) → ?

16. The D_{37} of a cellular species that follows the single-target, single-hit model is 150 rad. What percentage of cells will survive 450 rad?
17. What is the RBE of alpha radiation if the D_0 is 40 rad, compared with 180 rad for x-rays?
18. What is the difference between direct effect and indirect effect?
19. How does the radiosensitivity of human cells vary with stages of the cell cycle?
20. Draw cell-survival curves to show the difference between low-LET irradiation of aerobic cells and anoxic cells.

The answers to the Challenge Questions can be found by logging on to our website at http://evolve.elsevier.com.

CHAPTER 35

Early Effects of Radiation

OBJECTIVES

At the completion of this chapter, the student should be able to do the following:

1. Describe the three acute radiation syndromes
2. Identify the two stages that lead to acute radiation lethality
3. Define LD$_{50/60}$
4. Discuss local tissue damage after high-dose irradiation
5. Review the cytogenetic effects of radiation exposure

OUTLINE

Acute Radiation Lethality
   Prodromal Period
   Latent Period
   Manifest Illness
   LD$_{50/60}$
   Mean Survival Time
Local Tissue Damage
   Effects on Skin
   Effects on Gonads
Hematologic Effects
   Hemopoietic System
   Hemopoietic Cell Survival
Cytogenetic Effects
   Normal Karyotype
   Single-Hit Chromosome Aberrations
   Multi-Hit Chromosome Aberrations
   Kinetics of Chromosome Aberration

DURING THE 1920s and the 1930s, it would not have been unusual for a radiologic technologist to visit the hematology laboratory once a week for a routine blood examination. Before the introduction of personnel radiation monitors, periodic blood examination was the only way to monitor x-ray workers.

There was great concern over the danger of occupational radiation exposure. Today's occupational radiation exposures are quite low. Still, the radiologic technologist must understand the early effects of high radiation doses.

This chapter explores such early effects from the most severe (death) to the most worrisome today (skin effects). The chapter also reviews hematologic and cytogenetic effects.

To produce a radiation response in humans within a few days to months, the dose must be substantial. Such a response is called an *early effect of radiation exposure*. A dose of this magnitude is rare in diagnostic radiology.

These early effects have been studied extensively with laboratory animals, and some data have been obtained from observations of humans. This chapter considers only the more important effects as identified in Table 35-1, along with the minimum radiation dose necessary to produce each.

Early radiation responses are described as *deterministic*. Deterministic radiation responses are those that exhibit increasing severity with increasing radiation dose. Furthermore, there is usually a dose threshold.

ACUTE RADIATION LETHALITY

Death, of course, is the most devastating human response to radiation exposure. No cases of death after diagnostic x-ray exposure have ever been recorded, although some early x-ray pioneers died from the late effects of x-ray exposure. In each of these cases, however, the total radiation dose was extremely high by today's standards.

Acute radiation-induced human lethality is of only academic interest in diagnostic radiology. Diagnostic x-ray beams are neither intense enough nor large enough to cause death.

TABLE 35-1	Principal Early Effects of Radiation Exposure on Humans and the Approximate Threshold Dose		
Effect		**Anatomic Site**	**Threshold Dose**
Death		Whole body	200 rad/2 Gy$_t$
Hematologic depression		Whole body	25 rad/250 mGy$_t$
Skin erythema		Small field	200 rad/2 Gy$_t$
Epilation		Small field	300 rad/3 Gy$_t$
Chromosome aberration		Whole body	5 rad/50 mGy$_t$
Gonadal dysfunction		Local tissue	10 rad/100 mGy$_t$

Diagnostic x-ray beams always result in partial-body exposure, which is less harmful than whole-body exposure.

Some accidental exposures of persons in the nuclear weapons and nuclear energy fields have resulted in immediate death, but the number of such accidents has been small considering the length and activity of the atomic age. The unfortunate incident at Chernobyl in April 1986 is the one notable exception.

Thirty people at Chernobyl experienced the acute radiation syndrome and died. A number of minor late effects have been observed. No one died or was even seriously exposed in the March 1979 incident at the nuclear power reactor at Three Mile Island, Pennsylvania. Employment in the nuclear power industry is a safe occupation.

The sequence of events that follow high-level radiation exposure leading to death within days or weeks is called the **acute radiation syndrome**. There are, in fact, three separate syndromes that are dose related and that follow a rather distinct course of clinical responses.

These syndromes are **hematologic death, gastrointestinal (GI) death,** and **central nervous system (CNS) death.** The clinical signs and symptoms of each are outlined in Table 35-2. CNS death requires radiation doses in excess of 5000 rad (50 Gy$_t$) and results in death within hours. Hematologic death and GI death follow lower exposures and require a longer time for death to occur.

In addition to the three lethal syndromes, two periods are associated with acute radiation lethality. The **prodromal period** consists of acute clinical symptoms that occur within hours of exposure and continue for up to a day or two. After the prodromal period has ended, there may be a **latent period,** during which the subject is free of visible effects.

TABLE 35-2	Summary of Acute Radiation Lethality		
Period	Approximate Dose (rad)	Mean Survival Time (days)	Clinical Signs and Symptoms
Prodromal	>100	—	Nausea, vomiting, diarrhea
Latent	100 to 10,000	—	None
Hematologic	200 to 1000	10 to 60	Nausea, vomiting, diarrhea, anemia, leukopenia, hemorrhage, fever, infection
Gastrointestinal	1000 to 5000	4 to 10	Same as hematologic *plus* electrolyte imbalance, lethargy, fatigue, shock
Central nervous system	>5000	0 to 3	Same as gastrointestinal *plus* ataxia, edema, system vasculitis, meningitis

Prodromal Period

At radiation doses above approximately 100 rad (1Gy$_t$) delivered to the total body, signs and symptoms of radiation sickness may appear within minutes to hours. The symptoms of early radiation sickness most often take the form of nausea, vomiting, diarrhea, and a reduction in the white cells of the peripheral blood (leukopenia).

 This immediate response of radiation sickness is the prodromal period.

The prodromal period may last from a few hours to a couple of days. The severity of the symptoms is dose related; at doses in excess of 1000 rad (10 Gy$_t$), symptoms can be violent. At still higher doses, the duration of the prodromal syndrome becomes shorter, until it is difficult to separate the prodromal syndrome from the period of manifest illness.

Latent Period

After the period of initial radiation sickness, a period of apparent well-being occurs, which is called the *latent period*. The latent period extends from hours or less (at doses in excess of 5000 rad) to weeks (at doses from 100 to 500 rad).

 The latent period is the time after exposure during which there is no sign of radiation sickness.

The latent period is sometimes mistakenly thought to indicate an early recovery from a moderate radiation dose. It may be misleading, however, because it gives no indication of the extensive radiation response yet to follow.

Manifest Illness

The dose necessary to produce a given syndrome and the mean survival time are the principal quantitative measures of human radiation lethality (see Table 35-2). Although ranges of dose and resultant mean

survival times are given, there is rarely a precise difference in the dose and time-related sequence of events associated with each syndrome. At very high radiation doses, the latent period disappears altogether. At very low radiation doses, there may be no prodromal period at all.

Hematologic Syndrome. Radiation doses in the range of approximately 200 to 1000 rad (2 to 10 Gy$_t$) produce the hematologic syndrome. The patient initially experiences mild symptoms of the prodromal syndrome, which appear in a matter of a few hours and may persist for several days.

The latent period that follows can extend as long as 4 weeks and is characterized by a general feeling of wellness. There are no obvious signs of illness, although the number of cells in the peripheral blood declines during this time.

 The hematologic syndrome is characterized by a reduction in white cells, red cells, and platelets.

The period of **manifest illness** is characterized by possible vomiting, mild diarrhea, malaise, lethargy, and fever. Each of the types of blood cells follows a rather characteristic pattern of cell depletion. If the dose is not lethal, recovery begins in 2 to 4 weeks, but as long as 6 months may be required for full recovery.

If the radiation injury is severe enough, the reduction in blood cells continues unchecked until the body's defense against infection is nil. Just before death, hemorrhage and dehydration may be pronounced. Death occurs because of generalized infection, electrolyte imbalance, and dehydration.

Gastrointestinal (GI) Syndrome. Radiation doses of approximately 1000 to 5000 rad (10 to 50 Gy$_t$) result in the **GI syndrome**. The prodromal symptoms of vomiting and diarrhea occur within hours of exposure and persist for hours to as long as a day. A latent period of 3 to 5 days follows, during which no symptoms are present.

The manifest illness period begins with a second wave of nausea and vomiting, followed by diarrhea.

The victim experiences a loss of appetite (anorexia) and may become lethargic. The diarrhea persists and becomes more severe, leading to loose and then watery and bloody stools. Supportive therapy cannot prevent the rapid progression of symptoms that ultimately leads to death within 4 to 10 days of exposure.

 GI death occurs principally because of severe damage to the cells lining the intestines.

Intestinal cells are normally in a rapid state of proliferation and are continuously being replaced by new cells. The turnover time for this cell renewal system in a normal person is 3 to 5 days.

Radiation exposure kills the most sensitive cells—stem cells; this controls the length of time until death. When the intestinal lining is completely denuded of functional cells, fluids pass uncontrollably across the intestinal membrane, electrolyte balance is destroyed, and conditions promote infection.

At doses consistent with the GI syndrome, measurable and even severe hematologic changes occur. It takes a longer time for the cell renewal system of the blood to develop mature cells from the stem cell population; therefore, there is not enough time for maximum hematologic effects to occur.

Central Nervous System (CNS) Syndrome. After a radiation dose in excess of approximately 5000 rad (50 Gy_t) is received, a series of signs and symptoms occur that lead to death within a matter of hours to days. First, severe nausea and vomiting begins, usually within a few minutes of exposure.

During this initial onset, the patient may become extremely nervous and confused, may describe a burning sensation in the skin, may lose vision, and can even lose consciousness within the first hour. This may be followed by a latent period that lasts up to 12 hours, during which earlier symptoms subside or disappear.

The latent period is followed by the period of manifest illness, during which symptoms of the prodromal stage return but are more severe. The person becomes disoriented; loses muscle coordination; has difficulty breathing; may go into convulsive seizures; experiences loss of equilibrium, ataxia, and lethargy; lapses into a coma; and dies.

Regardless of the medical attention given the patient, the symptoms of manifest illness appear rather suddenly and always with extreme severity. At radiation doses high enough to produce CNS effects, the outcome is always death within a few days of exposure.

 The ultimate cause of death in CNS syndrome is elevated fluid content of the brain.

The CNS syndrome is characterized by increased intracranial pressure, inflammatory changes in the blood vessels of the brain (vasculitis), and inflammation of the meninges (meningitis). At doses sufficient to produce CNS damage, damage to all other organs of the body is equally severe. The classic radiation-induced changes in the GI tract and the hematologic system cannot occur because there is insufficient time between exposure and death for them to appear.

LD$_{50/60}$

If experimental animals are irradiated with varying doses of radiation, for example, 100 to 1000 rad (1 to 10 Gy_t), the plot of the percentage that die as a function of radiation dose would appear as in Figure 35-1. This figure illustrates the radiation dose-response relationship for acute human lethality.

 The LD$_{50/60}$ is the dose of radiation to the whole body that causes 50% of irradiated subjects to die within 60 days.

At the lower dose of approximately 100 rad (1 Gy_t), no one is expected to die. Above approximately 600 rad (6 Gy_t), all those irradiated die unless vigorous medical support is available. Above 1000 rad (10 Gy_t), even vigorous medical support does not prevent death.

 Acute radiation lethality follows a nonlinear, threshold dose-response relationship.

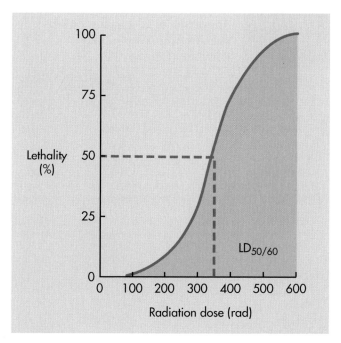

FIGURE 35-1 Radiation-induced death in humans follows a nonlinear, threshold dose-response relationship.

If death is to occur, it usually happens within 60 days of exposure. Acute radiation lethality is measured quantitatively by the $LD_{50/60}$, which is approximately 350 rad (3.5 Gy_t) for humans. With clinical support, humans can tolerate much higher doses; the maximum is reported to be 850 rad (8.5 Gy_t). Table 35-3 lists values of $LD_{50/60}$ for various species.

Question: From Figure 35-1, estimate the radiation dose that will produce 25% lethality in humans within 60 days.

Answer: First, draw a horizontal line from the 25% level on the y-axis until it intersects the S curve. Now, drop a vertical line from this point to the x-axis. This intersection with the x-axis occurs at the $LD_{25/60}$, which is approximately 250 rad (2.5 Gy_t).

Mean Survival Time

As the whole-body radiation dose increases, the average time between exposure and death decreases. This time is known as the **mean survival time.** A graph of radiation dose versus mean survival time is shown in Figure 35-2. This graph depicts three distinct regions associated with the three radiation syndromes.

As the radiation dose increases from 200 to 1000 rad (2 to 10 Gy_t), the mean survival time decreases from approximately 60 to 4 days; this region is consistent with death resulting from the hematologic syndrome. Mean survival time is dose dependent with the hematologic syndrome.

In the dose range associated with the GI syndrome, however, the mean survival time remains relatively constant, at 4 days. With larger doses, those associated with the CNS syndrome, the mean survival time is again dose dependent, varying from approximately 3 days to a matter of hours.

LOCAL TISSUE DAMAGE

When only part of the body is irradiated, in contrast with whole-body irradiation, a higher dose is required to produce a response. Every organ and tissue of the body can be affected by partial-body irradiation. The effect is cell death, which results in shrinkage of the organ or tissue. This effect can lead to total lack of function for that organ or tissue, or it can be followed by recovery.

> Atrophy is the shrinkage of an organ or tissue due to cell death.

There are many examples of local tissue damage immediately after radiation exposure. In fact, if the dose is high enough, any local tissue will respond. The manner in which local tissues respond depends on their intrinsic radiosensitivity and the kinetics of cell proliferation and maturation. Examples of local tissues that can be affected immediately are skin, gonads, and bone marrow.

All early radiation responses—local tissue damage is a good example—follow a threshold-type dose-response relationship. This is characteristic of a deterministic radiation response. A minimum dose is necessary to produce a deterministic response. Once that threshold

TABLE 35-3	Approximate $LD_{50/60}$ for Various Species After Whole-Body Radiation Exposure
Species	**$LD_{50/60}$ (rad)**
Pig	250
Dog	275
Human	350
Guinea pig	425
Monkey	475
Opossum	510
Mouse	620
Goldfish	700
Hamster	700
Rat	710
Rabbit	725
Gerbil	1050
Turtle	1500
Armadillo	2000
Newt	3000
Cockroach	10,000

$LD_{50/60}$, Dose of radiation to the whole body that causes 50% of irradiated subjects to die within 60 days.

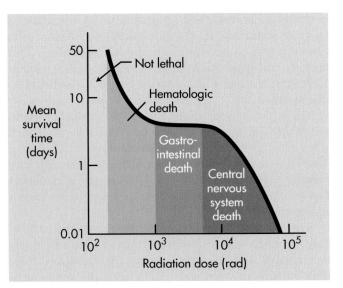

FIGURE 35-2 Mean survival time after radiation exposure shows three distinct regions. If death is due to hematologic or CNS effects, the mean survival time will vary with dose. If gastrointestinal (GI) effects cause death, it occurs in approximately 4 days.

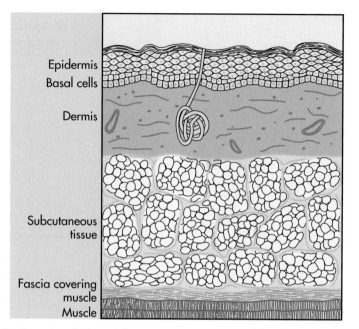

FIGURE 35-3 A sectional view of the anatomic structures of the skin. The basal cell layer is most radiosensitive.

dose has been exceeded, the severity of the response increases with increasing dose.

Effects on Skin

The tissue with which we have had the most experience is the skin. Normal skin consists of three layers: an outer layer (the epidermis), an intermediate layer of connective tissue (the dermis), and a subcutaneous layer of fat and connective tissue.

The skin has additional accessory structures, such as hair follicles, sweat glands, and sensory receptors (Figure 35-3). All cell layers and accessory structures participate in the response to radiation exposure.

The skin, similar to the lining of the intestine, represents a continuing cell renewal system, only with a much slower rate than that experienced by intestinal cells. Almost 50% of the cells lining the intestine are replaced every day, whereas skin cells are replaced at the rate of only approximately 2% per day.

The outer skin layer, the epidermis, consists of several layers of cells; the lowest layer consists of **basal cells.** Basal cells are the **stem cells** that mature as they migrate to the surface of the epidermis. Once these cells arrive at the surface as mature cells, they are slowly lost and have to be replaced by new cells from the basal layer.

> Damage to basal cells results in the earliest manifestation of radiation injury to the skin.

In earlier times, the tolerance of the patient's skin determined the limitations of radiation oncology with **orthovoltage x-rays** (200 to 300 kVp x-rays). The object

of x-ray therapy was to deposit energy in the tumor while sparing the surrounding normal tissue. Because the x-rays had to pass through the skin to reach the tumor, the skin was necessarily subjected to higher radiation doses than the tumor. The resultant skin damage was seen as **erythema** (a sunburn-like reddening of the skin), followed by **desquamation** (ulceration and denudation of the skin), which often required interruption of treatment.

After a single dose of 300 to 1000 rad (3 to 10 Gy_t), an initial mild erythema may occur within the first or second day. This first wave of erythema then subsides, only to be followed by a second wave that reaches maximum intensity in about 2 weeks.

At higher doses, this second wave of erythema is followed by a moist desquamation, which in turn may lead to a dry desquamation. Moist desquamation is known as **clinical tolerance** for radiation therapy.

During radiation therapy, the skin is exposed according to a fractionated scheme, usually approximately 200 rad/day (2 Gy_t/d), 5 days a week. To assist the radiation oncologist in planning patient treatment, isoeffect curves have been generated that accurately project the dose necessary to produce skin erythema or clinical tolerance after a prescribed treatment routine (Figure 35-4). Contemporary radiation oncology uses high-energy x-radiation from linear accelerators; this protects the skin from radiation damage.

Erythema was perhaps the first observed biologic response to radiation exposure. Many of the early x-ray pioneers, including Roentgen, suffered skin burns induced by x-rays.

One of the hazards to the patient during the early years of radiology was x-ray–induced erythema. During

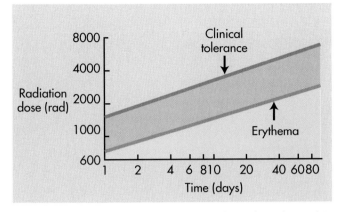

FIGURE 35-4 These isoeffect curves show the relationship between the number of daily fractions and the total radiation dose that will produce erythema or moist desquamation. As the fractionation of the dose increases, so does the total dose required.

TABLE 35-4	Potential Radiation Responses of Skin From High-Dose Fluoroscopy	
Potential Radiation Response	**Threshold Dose**	**Approximate Time of Onset**
Early transient erythema	200 rad/2 Gy_t	Hours
Main erythema	600 rad/6 Gy_t	10 days
Temporary epilation	300 rad/3 Gy_t	3 weeks
Permanent epilation	700 rad/7 Gy_t	3 weeks
Moist desquamation	1500 rad/15 Gy_t	4 weeks

those years, x-ray tube potentials were so low that it was usually necessary to position the tube very close to the patient's skin; exposures of 10 to 30 minutes were required. Often, the patient would return several days later with an x-ray burn.

These skin effects follow a nonlinear, threshold dose-response relationship similar to that described for radiation-induced lethality. Small doses of x-radiation do not cause erythema. Extremely high doses of x-radiation cause erythema in all persons so irradiated.

Whether intermediate radiation doses produce erythema depends on the individual's radiosensitivity, the dose rate, and the size of the irradiated skin field. Analysis of persons irradiated therapeutically with superficial x-rays has shown that the **skin erythema dose** required to affect 50% of those irradiated (**SED_{50}**), is about 500 rad (5 Gy_t).

Before the roentgen was defined and accurate radiation-measuring apparatus was developed, the skin was observed, and its response to radiation was used in formulating radiation protection practices. The unit used was the SED_{50}, and permissible radiation exposures were specified in fractions of SED_{50}.

Another response of the skin to radiation exposure is **epilation,** or loss of hair. For many years, soft x-rays (10 to 20 kVp), called **grenz rays,** were used as the treatment of choice for persons with skin diseases, such as tinea capitis (ringworm).

Tinea capitis of the scalp, not uncommon in children, was successfully treated by grenz radiation; unfortunately, the patient's hair would fall out for weeks or even months. Sometimes, an unnecessarily high dose of grenz rays resulted in permanent epilation.

High-dose fluoroscopy has focused more attention on the response of the skin to x-rays. The longer fluoroscopy times required for cardiovascular and interventional procedures, coupled with allowed exposure rates exceeding 20 R/min, are of great concern. Injuries to patients have been reported, and steps are being taken to establish better control over such exposures. Table 35-4 summarizes the potential effects of high-dose fluoroscopy.

Effects on Gonads

Human gonads are critically important target organs. As an example of local tissue effects, they are particularly sensitive to radiation. Responses to doses as low as 10 rad have been observed. Because these organs produce the germ cells that control fertility and heredity, their response to radiation has been studied extensively.

Much of what is known about the types of radiation response and about dose-response relationships has been derived from numerous animal experiments. Significant data are also available from human populations. Radiotherapy patients, radiation accident victims, and volunteer convicts all have provided data; this has resulted in a rather complete description of the gonadal response to radiation.

The cells of the testes (the male gonads) and the ovaries (the female gonads) respond differently to radiation because of differences in progression from the stem cell to the mature cell. Figure 35-5 illustrates this progression, indicating the most radiosensitive phase of cell maturation.

 Ovaries and testes produce oogonia and spermatogonia, which mature into ovum and sperm, respectively.

Germ cells are produced by both ovaries and testes, but they develop from the stem cell phase to the mature cell phase at different rates and at different times. This process of development is called **gametogenesis.**

The stem cells of the ovaries are the **oogonia,** and they multiply in number only before birth, during fetal life. The oogonia reach a maximum number of several

Male:

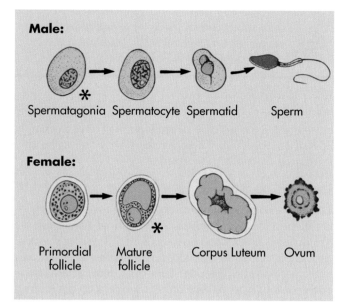

Spermatagonia   Spermatocyte   Spermatid   Sperm

Female:

Primordial   Mature   Corpus Luteum   Ovum
follicle   follicle

FIGURE 35-5 Progression of germ cells from the stem cell phase to the mature cell. Asterisk indicates the most radiosensitive cell.

TABLE 35-5	Response of Ovaries and Testes to Radiation
Approximate Dose	**Response**
10 rad/100 Gy$_t$	Minimal detectable response
200 rad/2 Gy$_t$	Temporary infertility
500 rad/5 Gy$_t$	Sterility

million and then begin to decline because of spontaneous degeneration.

During late fetal life, many **primordial follicles** grow to encapsulate the oogonia, which become **oocytes.** These follicle-containing oocytes remain in a suspended state of growth until puberty. By the time of prepuberty, the number of oocytes has been reduced to only several hundred thousand.

Commencing at puberty, the follicles rupture with regularity, ejecting a mature germ cell, the **ovum.** Only 400 to 500 such ova are available for fertilization (number of years of menstruation times 13 per year).

The germ cells of the testes are continually being produced from stem cells progressively through a number of stages to maturity, and similar to the ovaries, the testes provide a sustaining cell renewal system.

The male stem cell is the **spermatogonia,** which matures into the **spermatocyte.** The spermatocyte in turn multiplies and develops into a **spermatid,** which finally differentiates into the functionally mature germ cell, the **spermatozoa** or **sperm.** The maturation process from stem cell to spermatozoa requires 3 to 5 weeks.

Ovaries. Irradiation of the ovaries early in life reduces their size (atrophy) through germ cell death. After puberty, such irradiation also causes suppression and delay of menstruation.

The most radiosensitive cell during female germ cell development is the oocyte in the mature follicle.

Radiation effects on the ovaries depend somewhat on age. At fetal life and in early childhood, the ovaries are especially radiosensitive. They decline in radiosensitivity, reaching a minimum in the age range of 20 to 30 years, and then increase continually with age.

Doses as low as 10 rad (100 mGy$_t$) may delay or suppress menstruation in the mature female. A dose of approximately 200 rad (2 Gy$_t$) produces temporary infertility; approximately 500 rad (5 Gy$_t$) to the ovaries results in permanent sterility.

In addition to the destruction of fertility, irradiation of the ovaries of experimental animals has been shown to produce genetic mutations. Even moderate doses, such as 25 to 50 rad (250 to 500 mGy$_t$), have been associated with measurable increases in genetic mutations. Evidence also indicates that oocytes that survive such a modest dose can repair some genetic damage as they mature into ova.

Testes. The testes, similar to the ovaries, atrophy after high doses of radiation. A large volume of data on testicular damage has been gathered from observations of volunteer convicts and patients treated for carcinoma in one testis while the other was shielded. Many investigators have recorded normal births in such patients, whose remaining functioning testis received a radiation dose between 50 and 300 rad (0.5 and 3 Gy$_t$).

The spermatogonial stem cells signify the most sensitive phase in the gametogenesis of the spermatozoa. After irradiation of the testes, maturing cells, spermatocytes, and spermatids are relatively radioresistant and continue to mature. Consequently, no significant reduction in spermatozoa occurs until several weeks after exposure; therefore, fertility continues throughout this time, during which irradiated spermatogonia would have developed into mature spermatozoa had they survived.

Radiation doses as low as 10 rad (100 mGy$_t$) can reduce the number of spermatozoa (Table 35-5) in a manner reminiscent of the radiation response of the ovaries. With increasing dose, the depletion of spermatozoa increases and extends over a longer period.

Two hundred rad (2 Gy$_t$) produces temporary infertility, which commences approximately 2 months after irradiation and persists for up to 12 months. Five hundred rad (5 Gy$_t$) to the testes produces permanent sterility. Even after doses sufficient to produce

permanent sterility, the male normally retains his ability to engage in sexual intercourse.

Male gametogenesis is a self-renewing system; some evidence suggests that the most hazardous mutations are the genetic ones induced in surviving postspermatogonial cells. Consequently, after testicular irradiation of doses exceeding approximately 10 rad (100 mGy$_t$), the male should refrain from procreation for 2 to 4 months until all cells that were in the spermatogonial and postspermatogonial stages at the time of irradiation have matured and disappeared.

This reduces but probably does not eliminate any increase in genetic mutations caused by the persistence of the stem cell. Evidence from animal experiments suggests that genetic mutations undergo some repair even when the stem cell is irradiated.

HEMATOLOGIC EFFECTS

If you were a radiologic technologist in practice during the 1920s and the 1930s, you might have visited the hematology laboratory once a week for a routine blood examination. Before the introduction of personnel radiation monitors, periodic blood examination was the only monitoring performed on x-ray and radium workers. This examination included total cell counts and a white cell (leukocyte) differential count.

Most institutions had a radiation safety regulation such that, if the leukocytes were depressed by greater than 25% of normal level, the employee was given time off or was assigned to nonradiation activities until the count returned to normal.

 Under no circumstances is a periodic blood examination recommended as a feature of any current radiation protection program.

What was not entirely understood at that time was that the minimum whole-body dose necessary to produce a measurable hematologic depression was approximately 25 rad (250 mGy$_t$). These workers were being heavily irradiated by today's standards.

Hemopoietic System

The hemopoietic system consists of bone marrow, circulating blood, and lymphoid tissue. Lymphoid tissues are the lymph nodes, spleen, and thymus. With this system, the principal effect of radiation is a depressed number of blood cells in the peripheral circulation. Time- and dose-related effects on the various types of circulating blood cells are determined by the normal growth and maturation of these cells.

All cells of the hemopoietic system apparently develop from a single type of stem cell (Figure 35-6). This stem cell is called a **pluripotential stem cell** because it can develop into several different types of mature cells.

Although the spleen and the thymus manufacture one type of leukocyte (the lymphocyte), most circulating blood cells, including lymphocytes, are manufactured in the bone marrow. In a child, the bone marrow is rather uniformly distributed throughout the skeleton. In an adult, the active bone marrow responsible for producing circulating cells is restricted to flat bones, such as the ribs, sternum, and skull, and the ends of long bones.

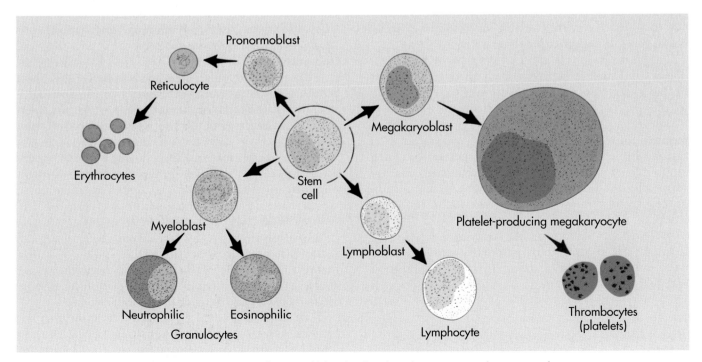

FIGURE 35-6 Four principal types of blood cells—lymphocytes, granulocytes, erythrocytes, and thrombocytes—develop and mature from a single pluripotential stem cell.

From the single pluripotential stem cell, a number of cell types are produced. Principally, these are **lymphocytes** (those involved in the immune response), **granulocytes** (scavenger type of cells used to fight bacteria), **thrombocytes** (also called *platelets* and involved in the clotting of blood to prevent hemorrhage), and **erythrocytes** (red blood cells that are the transportation agents for oxygen). These cell lines develop at different rates in the bone marrow and are released to the peripheral blood as mature cells.

While in the bone marrow, the cells proliferate in number, differentiate in function, and mature. Developing granulocytes and erythrocytes spend about 8 to 10 days in the bone marrow. Thrombocytes have a lifetime of approximately 5 days in the bone marrow.

Lymphocytes are produced over varying times and have varying lifetimes in the peripheral blood. Some are thought to have lives measured in terms of hours and others in terms of years. In the peripheral blood, granulocytes have a lifetime of only a couple of days. Thrombocytes have a lifetime of approximately 1 week, and erythrocytes a lifetime of nearly 4 months.

The hemopoietic system, therefore, is another example of a cell renewal system. Normal cell growth and development determine the effects of radiation on this system.

Hemopoietic Cell Survival

The principal response of the hemopoietic system to radiation exposure is a decrease in the numbers of all types of blood cells in the circulating peripheral blood. Lethal injury to the stem cells causes depletion of these mature circulating cells.

Figure 35-7 shows the radiation response of three circulating cell types. Examples are given for low, moderate, and high radiation doses, showing that the degree of cell depletion increases with increasing dose. These figures are the results of observations on experimental animals, radiotherapy patients, and the few radiation accident victims.

After exposure, the first cells to become affected are the lymphocytes. These cells are reduced in number (**lymphopenia**) within minutes or hours after exposure, and they are very slow to recover. Because the response is so immediate, the radiation effect is apparently a direct one on the lymphocytes themselves rather than on the stem cells.

> The lymphocytes and the spermatogonia are the most radiosensitive cells in the body.

Granulocytes experience a rapid rise in number (granulocytosis), followed first by a rapid decrease and then a slower decrease in number (granulocytopenia). If the radiation dose is moderate, then an abortive rise in granulocyte count may occur 15 to 20 days after irradiation. Minimum granulocyte levels are reached approximately 30 days after irradiation. Recovery, if it is to occur, takes approximately 2 months.

The depletion of platelets (thrombocytopenia) after irradiation develops more slowly, again because of the longer time required for the more sensitive precursor cells to reach maturity. Thrombocytes reach a minimum

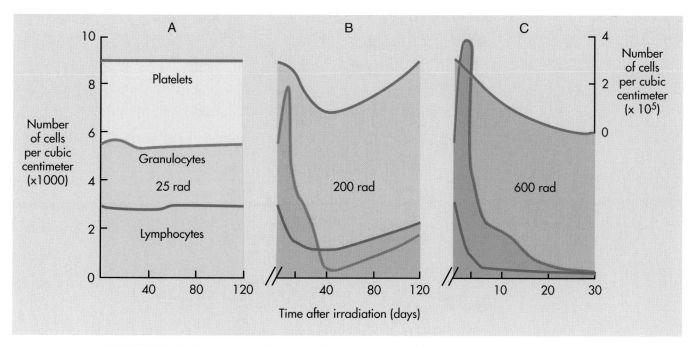

FIGURE 35-7 These graphs show the radiation response of the major circulating blood cells. **A,** 25 rad. **B,** 200 rad. **C,** 600 rad.

in about 30 days and recover in approximately 2 months, similar to the response kinetics of granulocytes.

Erythrocytes are less sensitive than the other blood cells, apparently because of their very long lifetime in the peripheral blood. Injury to these cells is not apparent for a matter of weeks. Total recovery may take 6 months to a year.

CYTOGENETIC EFFECTS

A technique developed in the early 1950s contributed enormously to human genetic analysis and radiation genetics. The technique calls for a culture of human cells to be prepared and treated so that the chromosomes of each cell can be easily observed and studied. This has resulted in many observations on radiation-induced chromosome damage.

 Cytogenetics is the study of the genetics of cells, particularly cell chromosomes.

The photomicrograph shown in Figure 35-8 shows the chromosomes of a human cancer cell following radiation therapy. The many chromosome aberrations represent a high degree of damage.

Radiation cytogenetic studies have shown that nearly every type of chromosome aberration can be radiation induced, and that some aberrations may be specific to radiation. The rate of induction of chromosome aberrations is related in a complex way to the radiation dose and differs among the various types of aberrations.

Radiation-induced chromosome aberrations follow a nonthreshold dose-response relationship.

Attempts to measure chromosome aberrations in patients after diagnostic x-ray examination have been largely unsuccessful. However, some studies involving high-dose fluoroscopy have shown radiation-induced chromosome aberrations soon after the examination was performed.

Without question, high doses of radiation cause chromosome aberrations. Low doses no doubt also do so, but it is technically difficult to observe aberrations at doses that are less than approximately 10 rad (100 mGy$_t$). An even more difficult task is to identify the link between radiation-induced chromosome aberrations and latent illness or disease.

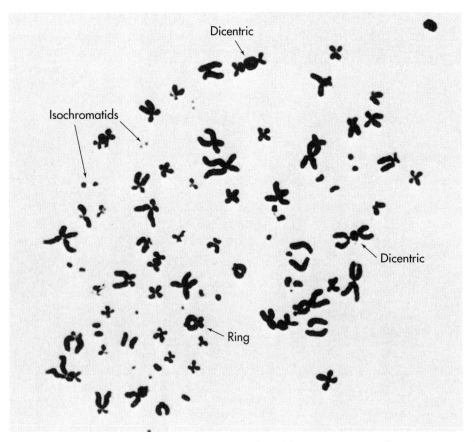

FIGURE 35-8 Chromosome damage in an irradiated human cancer cell. (Courtesy Neil Wald, University of Pittsburgh.)

When the body is irradiated, all cells can suffer cytogenetic damage. Such damage is classified here as an early response to radiation because, if the cell survives, the damage manifests during the next mitosis after the radiation exposure.

Human peripheral lymphocytes are most often used for cytogenetic analysis, and these lymphocytes do not move into mitosis until stimulated in vitro by an appropriate laboratory technique.

Cytogenetic damage to the stem cells is sustained immediately but may not be manifested for the considerable time required for that stem cell to reach maturity as a circulating lymphocyte.

Although chromosome damage occurs at the time of irradiation, it can be months and even years before the damage is measured. For this reason, chromosome abnormalities in circulating lymphocytes persist in some workers who were irradiated in industrial accidents 20 years ago.

Normal Karyotype

The human chromosome consists of many long strings of DNA mixed with a protein and folded back on itself many times. Refer back to Figure 32-11, which shows a normal chromosome as it would appear in the G_1 phase of the cell cycle, when only two chromatids are present, and in the G_2 phase of the cell cycle after DNA replication. The chromosome structure of four chromatids represented for the G_2 phase is that which is visualized in the metaphase portion of mitosis.

For certain types of cytogenetic analysis of chromosomes, photographs are taken and enlarged so that each chromosome can be cut out like a paper doll and paired with its sister into a chromosome map, which is called a **karyotype** (Figure 35-9).

> Each cell consists of 22 pairs of autosomes and a pair of sex chromosomes—the X chromosome from the female and the Y chromosome from the male.

Structural radiation damage to individual chromosomes can be visualized without constructing a karyotype. These are the single- and double-hit chromosome aberrations. Reciprocal translocations require a karyotype for detection. Point genetic mutations are undetectable even with karyotype construction.

Single-Hit Chromosome Aberrations

When radiation interacts with chromosomes, the interaction can occur through direct or indirect effect. In either mode, these interactions result in a **hit**. The hit, however, is somewhat different from the hit described previously in radiation interaction with DNA.

The DNA hit results in an invisible disruption of the molecular structure of the DNA. A chromosome hit, on the other hand, produces a visible derangement of the chromosome. Because the chromosomes contain DNA, this indicates that such a hit has disrupted many molecular bonds and has severed many chains of DNA.

> A chromosome hit represents severe damage to the DNA.

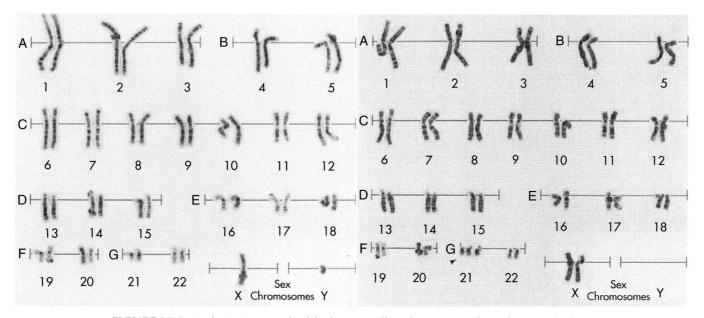

FIGURE 35-9 A photomicrograph of the human cell nucleus at metaphase shows each chromosome distinctly. The karyotype is made by cutting and pasting each chromosome similar to paper dolls and aligning them largest to smallest. The left karyotype is male, the right female. (Courtesy Carolyn Caskey Goodner, Identigene, Inc.)

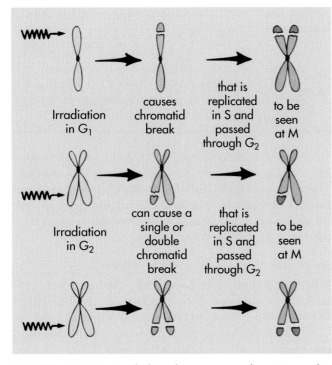

FIGURE 35-10 Single-hit chromosome aberrations after irradiation in G_1 and G_2. The aberrations are visualized and recorded during the M phase.

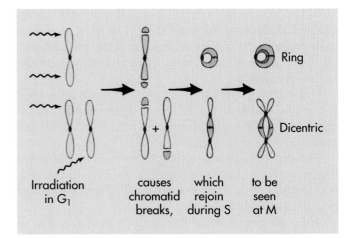

FIGURE 35-11 Multi-hit chromosome aberrations after irradiation in G_1 result in ring and dicentric chromosomes, in addition to chromatid fragments. Similar aberrations can be produced by irradiation during G_2, but they are rarer.

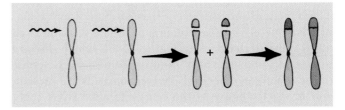

FIGURE 35-12 Radiation-induced reciprocal translocations are multi-hit chromosome aberrations that require karyotypic analysis for detection.

Single-hit effects produced by radiation during the G_1 phase of the cell cycle are shown in Figure 35-10. The breakage of a chromatid is called **chromatid deletion.** During S phase, both the remaining chromosome and the deletion are replicated.

The chromosome aberration visualized at metaphase consists of a chromosome with material missing from the ends of two sister chromatids and two acentric (without a centromere) fragments. These fragments are called **isochromatids.**

Chromosome aberrations also can be produced by single-hit events during the G_2 phase of the cell cycle (see Figure 35-10). The probability that ionizing radiation will pass through sister chromatids to produce isochromatids is low. Usually, radiation produces a chromatid deletion in only one arm of the chromosome. The result is a chromosome with an arm that is obviously missing genetic material and a chromatid fragment.

Multi-Hit Chromosome Aberrations

A single chromosome can sustain more than one hit. Multi-hit aberrations are not uncommon (Figure 35-11).

In the G_1 phase of the cell cycle, ring chromosomes are produced if the two hits occur on the same chromosome. Dicentrics are produced when adjacent chromosomes each suffer one hit and recombine. The mechanism for the joining of chromatids depends on a condition called **stickiness** that is radiation-induced and appears at the site of the severed chromosome.

Similar aberrations can be produced in the G_2 phase of the cell cycle; however, such aberrations again require that (1) either the same chromosome be hit two or more times, or (2) adjacent chromosomes be hit and joined together. However, these events are rare.

Reciprocal Translocations. The multi-hit chromosome aberrations previously described represent rather severe damage to the cell. At mitosis, the acentric fragments are lost or are attracted to only one of the daughter cells because they are unattached to a spindle fiber. Consequently, one or both of the daughter cells can be missing considerable genetic material.

Reciprocal translocations are multi-hit chromosome aberrations that require karyotypic analysis for detection (Figure 35-12). Radiation-induced reciprocal translocations result in no loss of genetic material, simply a rearrangement of the genes. Consequently, all or nearly all genetic codes are available; they simply may be organized in an incorrect sequence.

Kinetics of Chromosome Aberration

At very low doses of radiation, only single-hit aberrations occur. When the radiation dose exceeds approximately 100 rad (1 Gy_t), the frequency of multi-hit aberrations increases more rapidly.

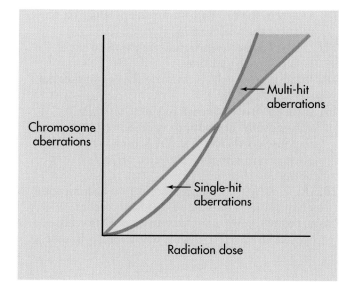

FIGURE 35-13   Dose-response relationships for single-hit aberrations are linear, nonthreshold, whereas those for multi-hit aberrations are nonlinear, nonthreshold.

The general dose-response relationship for production of single- and multi-hit aberrations is shown in Figure 35-13. Single-hit aberrations are produced with a **linear, nonthreshold** dose-response relationship. Multi-hit aberrations are produced following a **nonlinear, nonthreshold** relationship. A number of investigators have experimentally characterized these relationships.

RADIATION DOSE-RESPONSE RELATIONSHIPS FOR CYTOGENETIC DAMAGE
Single-hit: $Y = a + bD$
Multi-hit: $Y = a + bD + cD^2$

where Y is the number of single- or multi-hit chromosome aberrations, a is the naturally occurring frequency of chromosome aberrations, and b and c are radiation dose (D) coefficients of damage for single- and multi-hit aberrations, respectively.

Some laboratories use cytogenetic analysis as a biologic radiation dosimeter. Multi-hit aberrations are considered to be the most significant in terms of latent human damage. If the radiation dose is unknown yet is not life threatening, the approximate chromosome aberration frequency is two single-hit aberrations per rad per 1000 cells and one multi-hit aberration per 10 rad per 1000 cells.

SUMMARY

After exposure to a high radiation dose, humans can experience a response within a few days to a few weeks. This immediate response is called an *early effect of radiation exposure*. Such early effects are usually deterministic, that is, the severity of response is dose related and there is a dose threshold.

The sequence of events that follows high-dose radiation exposure leading to death within days or weeks is called the *acute radiation syndrome*, which includes the hematologic syndrome, the GI syndrome, and the CNS syndrome. These syndromes are dose related.

$LD_{50/60}$ is the dose of radiation to the whole body in which 50% of subjects will die within 60 days. For humans, this dose is estimated at 350 rad (3.5 Gy_t). As radiation dose increases, the time between exposure and death decreases.

When only part of the body is irradiated, higher doses are tolerated. Examples of local tissue damage include effects on the skin, gonads, and bone marrow. The first manifestation of radiation injury to the skin is damage to the basal cells. Resultant skin damage occurs as erythema, desquamation, or epilation.

Radiation of the male testes can result in a reduction of spermatozoa. A dose of 200 rad (2 Gy_t) produces temporary infertility. A dose of 500 rad (5 Gy_t) to the testes produces permanent sterility. In the male as in the female, the stem cell is the most radiosensitive phase.

The hemopoietic system consists of bone marrow, circulating blood, and lymphoid tissue. The principal effect of radiation on this system is fewer blood cells in the peripheral circulation. Radiation exposure decreases the numbers of all precursor cells; this reduces the number of mature cells in the circulating blood. Lymphocytes and spermatogonia are considered the most radiosensitive cells in the body.

The study of chromosome damage from radiation exposure is called *cytogenetics*. Chromosome damage takes on the following different forms: (1) chromatid deletion, (2) dicentric chromosome aberration, and (3) reciprocal translocations.

CHALLENGE QUESTIONS

1. Define or otherwise identify the following:
   a. GI death
   b. Latent period
   c. $LD_{50/60}$
   d. Erythema
   e. Clinical tolerance
   f. Primordial follicle
   g. Erythrocyte
   h. Karyotype
   i. Epilation
   j. Multi-hit aberration
2. What is the minimum dose that results in reddening of the skin?
3. Explain the prodromal syndrome.
4. Clinical signs and symptoms of the manifest illness stage of acute radiation lethality are classified into what three groups?

5. During which stage of the acute radiation syndrome is recovery stimulated?
6. What dose of radiation results in the gastrointestinal syndrome?
7. Why does death occur with the GI syndrome?
8. Identify the cause of death from the CNS syndrome.
9. Describe the stages of gametogenesis in the female. Identify the most radiosensitive phases.
10. What cells of the hemopoietic system arise from pluripotential stem cells?
11. Discuss the maturation of basal cells in the epidermis.
12. What two cells are the most radiosensitive cells in the human body?
13. Describe the changes in mean survival time associated with increasing dose.
14. What are the approximate values of $LD_{50/60}$ and SED_{50} in humans?
15. What are the four principal blood cell lines and what is the function of each?

16. Diagram the mechanism for the production of a reciprocal translocation.
17. List the clinical signs and symptoms of the hematologic syndrome.
18. What mature cells form from the omnipotential stem cell?
19. If the normal incidence of single hit–type chromosome aberrations is 0.15 per 100 cells and the dose coefficient is 0.0094, how many such aberrations would be expected after a dose of 38 rad?
20. If the normal incidence of multi-hit chromosome aberrations is 0.082 and the dose coefficient is 0.0047, how many dicentrics per 100 cells would be expected after a whole-body dose of 16 rad?

The answers to the Challenge Questions can be found by logging on to our website at http://evolve.elsevier.com.

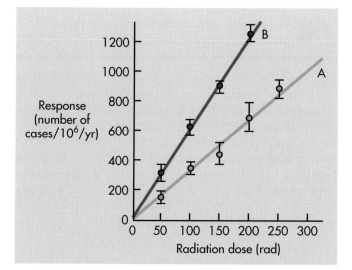

FIGURE 36-4 Slope of the linear, nonthreshold dose-response relationship is equal to the absolute risk. *A* and *B* show absolute risks of 3.4 and 6.2 cases per 10^6 persons/rad/year, respectively.

Answer:
$$5 \times 10^{-4}\,\text{rem}^{-1} = \frac{5}{10,000 \times rem}$$
$$= \frac{5}{100,000 \times 100\ mrem}$$
$$= 5\ fatal\ cancers$$

Question: There are approximately 300,000 American radiologic technologists, and they receive an annual effective dose of 50 mrem (0.5 mSv). What is the expected number of annual deaths because of this occupational exposure?

Answer:
$$5 \times 10^{-4}\,\text{rem}^{-1} = \frac{5}{10,000 \times rem}$$
$$= \frac{25}{1,000,000 \times 50\ mrem}$$

Therefore in 300,000 RTs

$$= 7.5\ deaths\ from\ malignant\ disease$$

The reader should realize that death from malignant disease occurs in approximately 20% of the population.

RADIATION-INDUCED MALIGNANCY

All the late effects, including radiation-induced malignancy, have been observed in experimental animals, and on the basis of these animal experiments, dose-response relationships have been developed. At the human level, these late effects have been observed, but often, data are insufficient to allow precise identification of the dose-response relationship. Consequently, some of the conclusions drawn regarding human responses are based in part on animal data.

TABLE 36-4	Summary of the Incidence of Leukemia in Atomic Bomb Survivors		
	Hiroshima	Nagasaki	Total
Total number of survivors in study	74,356	25,037	99,393
Observed cases	102	42	144 of leukemia
Expected cases	39	13	52 of leukemia

Most of these late effects are stochastic effects. A stochastic effect is one that has no dose threshold. Even the smallest radiation dose can produce an effect. With increasing dose, the incidence, not the severity, of the response increases. All radiation-induced malignancies are stochastic.

Leukemia

When one considers radiation-induced leukemia in laboratory animals, there is no question that this response is real and that the incidence increases with increasing radiation dose. The form of the dose-response relationship is linear and nonthreshold. A number of human population groups have exhibited an elevated incidence of leukemia after radiation exposure—atomic bomb survivors, American radiologists, radiotherapy patients, and children irradiated in utero, to name a few.

Atomic Bomb Survivors. Probably the greatest wealth of information that we have accumulated regarding radiation-induced leukemia in humans has been drawn from observations of survivors of the atomic bombings of Hiroshima and Nagasaki. At the time of the bombings, approximately 300,000 people lived in those two cities. Nearly 100,000 were killed from the blast and from early effects of radiation. Another 100,000 people received significant doses of radiation and survived. The remainder were unaffected because their radiation dose was less than 10 rad (100 mGy$_t$).

After World War II, scientists of the Atomic Bomb Casualty Commission (**ABCC**), now known as the Radiation Effects Research Foundation (**RERF**), attempted to determine the radiation dose received by each of the atomic bomb survivors in both cities. They estimated the dose to each survivor by considering not only distance from the explosion but also terrain, type of bomb, type of building construction if the survivor was inside, and other factors that might influence dose.

A summary of the data obtained through these investigations is given in Table 36-4, and the data analysis is shown graphically in Figure 36-5. After high doses were delivered by these bombs, the leukemia incidence was as much as 100 times that in the nonirradiated population. Even though large error bars are seen at each dose increment, the response appears linear, nonthreshold.

If, however, one expands the data in the low-dose region (e.g., below 200 rad), one could conclude that a threshold exists in the neighborhood of 50 rad (500m Gy_t). Nevertheless, neither this information nor other available information is interpreted to support a threshold response.

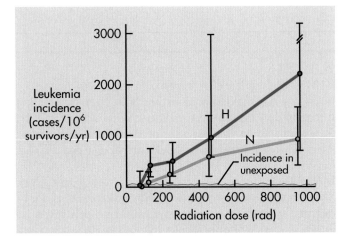

FIGURE 36-5 Data from the atomic bomb survivors of Hiroshima (H) and Nagasaki (N) suggest a linear, nonthreshold dose-response relationship.

 Radiation-induced leukemia follows a linear, nonthreshold dose-response relationship.

Figure 36-6 demonstrates the temporal distribution of the onset of leukemia among atomic bomb survivors for the 40 years after the bombings. The data are presented as cases per 100,000 and include for comparison the leukemia rate in the population at large and in the nonexposed populations of the bombed cities. A rather rapid rise in leukemia incidence reached a plateau after approximately 5 years. The incidence declined slowly for approximately 20 years, when it reached the natural level experienced by the nonexposed.

Radiation-induced leukemia is considered to have a latent period of 4 to 7 years and an at-risk period of approximately 20 years.

The at-risk period is that time after irradiation during which one might expect the radiation effect to occur. The at-risk period for radiation-induced cancer is lifetime.

Data from atomic bomb survivors show without a doubt that radiation exposure to those survivors caused the later development of leukemia. It is interesting,

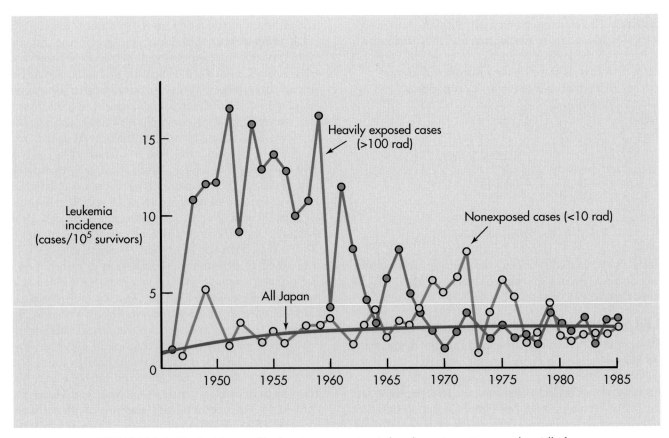

FIGURE 36-6 The incidence of leukemia among atomic bomb survivors increased rapidly for the first few years, then declined to natural incidence by approximately 1975.

however, to reflect on some additional aspects of these events.

Of the 300,000 total residents, 335 persons are estimated to have survived doses in excess of 600 rad (6 Gy). The leukemia risk estimates are based on only 144 cases in the total exposed population. Acute leukemia and chronic myelocytic leukemia were observed most often among atomic bomb survivors.

 Chronic lymphocytic leukemia is rare and therefore is not considered to be a form of radiation-induced leukemia.

Taken to the final analysis, data from the atomic bomb survivors pointed to an absolute risk of 5×10^{-4} rem^{-1} (5×10^{-2} Sv^{-1}). The overall relative risk based on the total number of observed leukemia deaths (144) versus the number of expected leukemia deaths (52) is approximately 3:1.

Radiologists. By the second decade of radiology, reports of pernicious anemia and leukemia in radiologists began to appear. In the early 1940s, several investigators reviewed the incidence of leukemia in American radiologists and found it alarmingly high. These early radiologists functioned without the benefit of modern radiation protection devices and procedures, and many served as both radiation oncologists and diagnostic radiologists.

It has been estimated that some of these early radiologists received doses exceeding 100 rad/yr (1 Gy$_t$/yr). Currently, American radiologists do not exhibit an elevated incidence of leukemia compared with other physician specialists.

A rather exhaustive study of mortality among radiologists in Great Britain during the period from the turn of the century to 1960 did not show an elevated risk of leukemia. The reasons for such a different experience between American and British radiologists are unknown.

Studies of radiation-induced leukemia among American radiologic technologists consistently show no evidence of any radiation effect.

Patients With Ankylosing Spondylitis. In the 1940s and 1950s, particularly in Great Britain, it was common practice to treat patients with ankylosing spondylitis with radiation. Ankylosing spondylitis is an arthritis-like condition of the vertebral column.

Patients cannot walk upright or move except with great difficulty. For relief, they would be given fairly high doses of radiation to the spinal column, and the treatment was quite successful. Patients who previously had been hunched over were able to stand erect.

Radiation therapy was a permanent cure and remained the treatment of choice for approximately 20 years, until it was discovered that some who had been cured by radiation were dying from leukemia. Graphic

results on the observations of these patients are shown in Figure 36-7.

During the period from 1935 to 1955, 14,554 male patients were treated at 81 different radiation therapy centers in Great Britain. Review of treatment records showed that the dose to the bone marrow of the spinal column ranged from 100 to 4000 rad (1 to 40 Gy).

Fifty-two cases of leukemia occurred in this population. When this incidence of leukemia is compared with that of the general population, the relative risk is 10:1.

Absolute risk can be obtained from these data by determining the slope of the best-fit line through the data points (Figure 36-7). Such an analysis yields a result of approximately 8×10^{-4} rem^{-1} (8×10^{-2} Sv^{-1}). If 95% confidence limits are placed on the data, one cannot rule out the possibility of a threshold dose at approximately 300 rad (3 Gy$_t$).

Leukemia in Other Populations. Several studies have been designed to link leukemia incidence with environmental radiation. Natural background radiation levels increase in general with altitude and with latitude, but the range of levels observed is not sufficient to demonstrate a causal relationship with leukemia.

Other population groups that have provided evidence, both positive and negative, regarding the leukemia-inducing action of radiation include radium watch-dial painters, children receiving superficial x-ray treatment, and some additional adult radiation therapy groups.

Cancer

What has been discussed regarding radiation-induced leukemia also can be reported for radiation-induced cancer. We do not have similar quantities of human data regarding cancer as we do for leukemia. Nevertheless, it can be said without question that radiation can cause cancer.

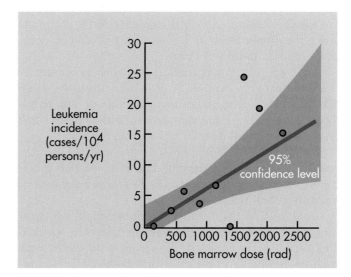

FIGURE 36-7 Results of observations of leukemia in patients with ankylosing spondylitis treated with x-ray therapy suggest a linear, nonthreshold dose-response relationship.

The relative risks and absolute risks have been shown to be similar to those reported for leukemia. Many types of cancer have been implicated as radiation induced, and a discussion of the more important ones is in order.

It is not possible to link any case of cancer to a previous radiation exposure, regardless of its magnitude, because cancer is so common. Approximately 20% of all deaths are caused by cancer; therefore, any radiation-induced cancers are obscured. Leukemia, on the other hand, is a relatively rare disease; this makes analysis of radiation-induced leukemia easier.

Thyroid Cancer. Thyroid cancer has been shown to develop in three groups of patients whose thyroid glands were irradiated in childhood. The first two groups, called the Ann Arbor series and the Rochester series, consisted of individuals who, in the 1940s and early 1950s, were treated shortly after birth for thymic enlargement. The thymus is a gland lying just below the thyroid gland that can enlarge shortly after birth in response to infection.

At these facilities, radiation was often the treatment of choice. After a dose of up to 500 rad (5 Gy$_t$), the thymus gland would shrink so that all enlargement disappeared. No additional problems were evident until up to 20 years later, when thyroid nodules and thyroid cancer began to develop in some of these patients.

Another group included 21 children who were natives of the Rongelap Atoll in 1954; they were subjected to high levels of fallout during a hydrogen bomb test. The winds shifted during the test, carrying the fallout over an adjacent inhabited island rather than one that had been evacuated. These children received radiation doses to the thyroid gland from both external exposure and internal ingestion of approximately 1200 rad (12 Gy$_t$).

If one computes the incidence of thyroid nodularity, considered **preneoplastic**, in these three groups and plots this incidence as a function of estimated dose, the result is that shown in Figure 36-8. Admittedly, the error bars on the dose data and on the incidence levels are large. Still, the implication of a linear, nonthreshold dose-response relationship is clear.

Data are just now becoming available on the nearly 100,000 persons exposed to radiation from the 1989 Chernobyl incident. No excess leukemia or cancer has been observed in this population, although a small increase in thyroid nodularity has been noted.

Bone Cancer. Two population groups have contributed an enormous quantity of data showing that radiation can cause bone cancer. The first group consists of radium watch-dial painters.

In the 1920s and 1930s, various small laboratories hired employees, most often female, who worked at benches painting watch dials with paint laden with radium sulfate. To prepare a fine point on the paintbrushes, the employees would touch the tip of the brush to the tongue. In this manner, substantial quantities of radium were ingested.

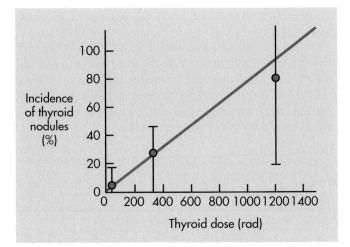

FIGURE 36-8 Radiation-induced preneoplastic thyroid nodularity in three groups of persons whose thyroid glands were irradiated in childhood follows a linear, nonthreshold dose-response relationship.

Radium salts were used because the emitted radiation, principally alpha and beta particles, would continuously excite the luminous compounds so the watch dial would glow in the dark. Current technology uses harmlessly low levels of tritium (^{3}H) and promethium (^{147}Pm) for this purpose.

When ingested, the radium would behave metabolically similar to calcium and deposit in bone. Because of radium's long half-life (1620 years) and alpha emission, these employees received radiation doses to bone of up to 50,000 rad (500 Gy$_t$).

Seventy-two bone cancers in approximately 800 persons have been observed during a follow-up period in excess of 50 years. Analysis of these data has disclosed an overall relative risk of 122:1. The absolute risk is equal to 1×10^{-4} rem^{-1} (1×10^{-2} Sv^{-1}).

Another population in whom excess bone cancer developed consisted of patients treated with radium salts for a variety of diseases, from arthritis to tuberculosis. Such treatments were common practice in many parts of the world until about 1950.

Skin Cancer. Skin cancer usually begins with the development of a radiodermatitis. Significant data have been developed from several reports of skin cancer induced in radiation therapy recipients treated with orthovoltage (200 to 300 kVp) or superficial x-rays (50 to 150 kVp).

Radiation-induced skin cancer follows a threshold dose-response relationship.

From these data, we conclude that the latent period is approximately 5 to 10 years, but we do not have enough data to assign absolute risk values. When the dose delivered to the skin was in the range of

500 to 2000 rad (5 to 20 Gy_t), the relative risk of developing skin cancer was 4:1. If the dose was 4000 to 6000 rad (40 to 60 Gy_t) or 6000 to 10,000 rad (60 to 100 Gy_t), the relative risks were 14:1 and 27:1, respectively.

Breast Cancer. In Chapter 19, some of the radiographic techniques used in mammography were discussed. The radiation dose to mammography patients is considered in a later chapter. Here, we discuss the risk of radiation-induced breast cancer.

Controversy is ongoing regarding the risk of radiation-induced breast cancer, with implications for breast cancer detection by x-ray mammography. Concern over such risk first surfaced in the mid-1960s, after reports were published of breast cancer developing in patients with tuberculosis.

Tuberculosis was for many years treated by isolation in a sanitarium. During the patient's stay, one mode of therapy was to induce a pneumothorax in the affected lung; this was done under non–image-intensified fluoroscopy. Many patients received multiple treatments and up to several hundred fluoroscopic examinations.

Precise dose determinations are not possible, but levels of several hundred rad would have been common. In some of these patient populations, the relative risk for radiation-induced breast cancer was shown to be as high as 10:1.

One such population exhibited no excess risk. This finding, however, was explained as a consequence of the fluoroscopic technique. In the positive studies, the patient faced away from the radiologist, toward the fluoroscopic x-ray tube, during exposure. In the study that reported negative findings, patients were imaged while facing the radiologist so that the radiation beam entered posteriorly. The breast tissue was exposed only to the low-intensity beam that exited the patient.

Additional studies have produced results suggesting that radiation-induced breast cancer developed in patients treated with x-rays for acute postpartum mastitis. The dose to these patients ranged from 75 to 1000 rad (0.75 to 10 Gy_t). The relative risk factor in this population was approximately 3:1.

Radiation-induced breast cancer has also been observed among atomic bomb survivors. Through 1980, observations on nearly 12,000 women who received radiation doses to the breasts of 10 rad or more showed a relative risk of 4:1.

In some of these studies, only one breast was irradiated. In nearly every such case, breast cancer developed only in the irradiated breast. These patients have now been followed for up to 35 years. On the basis of all available data regarding radiation-induced breast cancer, the best estimate for absolute risk is 6 cases/10^6 persons/rad/yr.

Lung Cancer. Early in the 20th century, it was observed that approximately 50% of workers in the Bohemian pitchblende mines of Germany died of lung cancer. Lung cancer incidence in the general population was negligible by comparison. The dusty mine environment was considered to be the cause of this lung cancer. Now it is known that radiation exposure from radon in the mines contributed to the incidence of lung cancer in these miners.

Observations of American uranium miners active in the Colorado plateau in the 1950s and 1960s have also shown elevated levels of lung cancer. The peak of this activity occurred in the early 1960s, when approximately 5000 miners were active in nearly 500 underground mines and 150 open-pit mines. Most of the mines were worked by fewer than 10 men; therefore, for such a small operation, one could expect a lack of proper ventilation.

The radiation exposure in these mines occurred because of the high concentration of uranium ore. Uranium, which is radioactive with a very long half-life of 10^9 years, decays through a series of radioactive nuclides by successive alpha and beta emissions, each accompanied by gamma radiation.

One of the decay products of uranium is **radon** (^{222}Rn). This radionuclide is a gas that emanates through the rock to produce a high concentration in air. When breathed, radon can be deposited in the lung, where it undergoes an additional successive series of decay to a stable isotope of lead. During these subsequent decay actions, several alpha particles are released, resulting in a rather high local dose. Also, alpha particles emit high-LET radiation and therefore have a high RBE.

To date, more than 4000 uranium miners have been observed, and they have received estimated doses to lung tissue as high as 3000 rad (30 Gy_t); on this basis, the relative risk was approximately 8:1. It is interesting to note that smoking uranium miners have a relative risk of approximately 20:1.

Liver Cancer. Thorium dioxide (ThO_2) in a colloidal suspension known as **Thorotrast** was widely used in diagnostic radiology between 1925 and 1945 as a contrast agent for angiography. Thorotrast was approximately 25% ThO_2 by weight, and it contained several radioactive isotopes of thorium and its decay products. Radiation that was emitted produced a dose in the ratio of approximately 100:10:1 of alpha, beta, and gamma radiation, respectively.

The use of Thorotrast has been shown to be responsible for several types of carcinoma after a latent period of approximately 15 to 20 years. After extravascular injection, it is carcinogenic at the site of the injection. After intravascular injection, ThO_2 particles are deposited in phagocytic cells of the reticuloendothelial system and are concentrated in the liver and spleen. Its half-life and high alpha radiation dose have resulted in many cases of cancer in these organs.

TOTAL RISK OF MALIGNANCY

On the basis of many of these observations on human population groups after exposure to low-level radiation, and considering all the risk estimates taken collectively for leukemia and cancer, a number of simplified conclusions can be made. The overall absolute risk for induction of malignancy is approximately 8 cases/10,000/rad (8×10^{-2} Sv^{-1}), with the at-risk period extending for 20 to 25 years after exposure.

Lethality from radiation-induced malignant disease is projected at approximately 50%. Five deaths from radiation-induced malignancy can be expected after an exposure of 1 rad to 10,000 persons. The risk of death from radiation-induced malignant disease is 5/10,000/rad (5×10^{-2} Sv^{-1}).

Three Mile Island

To make these values somewhat more meaningful, we can consider the celebrated Three Mile Island incident in 1979. Approximately 2,000,000 people resided within an 80-km (50-mile) radius of Three Mile Island, on the Susquehanna River, in Pennsylvania.

On the basis of population statistics, one would expect to observe approximately 330,000 cancer deaths in these persons. During the total period of the radiation incident, the average dose to persons living within a 160-km (100-mile) radius was 1.5 mrad (15 µGy$_t$); to those within the 80-km (50-mile) radius, it was 8 mrad (80 µGy$_t$).

By applying 1.5 mrad as the population dose, one can predict that the Three Mile Island incident will result in no more than two additional malignant deaths as a result of this population radiation exposure. Clearly, this response is not detectable in the face of approximately 400,000 natural cancer deaths in this population.

> **PREDICTED RADIATION-INDUCED DEATHS AT THREE MILE ISLAND**
>
> 2×10^6 people × 5 deaths/10^4 people/rad
> × 0.0015 rad = 1.5 deaths

BEIR Committee

The Committee on the Biologic Effects of Ionizing Radiation (BEIR), an arm of the National Academy of Sciences, has reviewed the data on late effects of low-dose, low-LET radiation. This report showed the results summarized in Table 36-5, which are considered authoritative.

BEIR committee members examined three situations. First, they estimated the excess mortality from malignant disease after a one-time accidental exposure to 10 rad; such a situation is highly unlikely in radiology. Second, they considered the response to a dose of 1 rad/yr for life; this situation is possible in diagnostic radiology but rare. Finally, they considered excess radiation-induced cancer mortality after a continuous dose of 100 mrad/yr.

TABLE 36-5	BEIR Committee Estimated Excess Mortality From Malignant Disease in 100,000 People	
	Male	**Female**
Normal expectation Excess cases	20,560	16,680
Single exposure to 10 rad (100 mGy$_t$)	770	810
Continuous exposure to 1 rad/yr (10 mGy$_t$/yr)	2880	3070
Continuous exposure to 100 mrad/yr (1 mGy$_t$/yr)	520	600

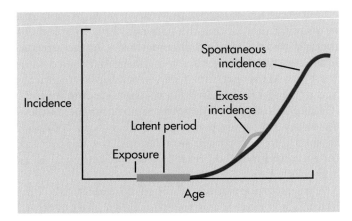

FIGURE 36-9 Exposure at an early age can result in an excess bulge of cancer after a latent period.

This is still considerably higher than the experience of most radiologic technologists but can serve as a good upper limit of occupational radiation risk.

When a linear, nonthreshold dose-response relationship was assumed, these analyses showed an additional 800 cases of malignant disease death in a population of 100,000 after 10 rad and an additional 550 deaths after 100 mrad/yr. These cases represent an addition to the normal incidence of cancer death, which is approximately 20,000 per 100,000 persons.

> The BEIR Committee has further stated that because of the uncertainty in its analysis, less than 1 rad/yr may not be harmful.

The BEIR Committee also has analyzed available human data with regard to age at exposure, a limited time of expression of effects, and whether the response was **absolute** or **relative**. This requires additional definitions of these terms.

If one is irradiated at an early age and the response is limited in time, radiation-induced excess malignant disease appears as a bulge on the age-response relationship (Figure 36-9). Childhood leukemia is a good example.

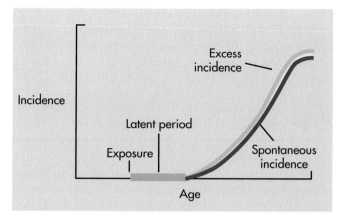

FIGURE 36-10 The absolute risk model predicts that the excess radiation-induced cancer risk is constant for life.

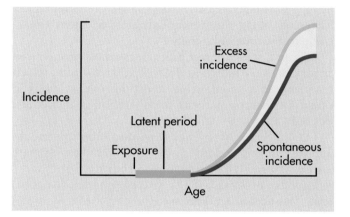

FIGURE 36-11 The relative risk model predicts that the excess radiation-induced cancer risk is proportional to the natural incidence.

An absolute age-response relationship is shown in Figure 36-10. Here, the increased incidence of cancer is seen as a constant number of cases after a minimal latent period. Most subscribe to a relative age-response relationship, in which the increased incidence of cancer is proportional to the natural incidence (Figure 36-11).

Perhaps the best way to present these radiation risk data is to compare them with other known causes of death. As one might imagine, volumes of tables are available that analyze risk. This information is presented in simplified form in Table 36-6.

Note that in these common situations, risk from radiation exposure is near the bottom of the list. Our actual occupational risk is even less because we use protective apparel during fluoroscopy and the radiation risk estimate assumes whole-body exposure.

RADIATION AND PREGNANCY

Since the first medical applications of x-rays, concern and apprehension have arisen regarding the effects of radiation before, during, and after pregnancy. Before

TABLE 36-6	Average Annual Risk of Death From Various Causes
Cause	**Your Chance of Dying This Year**
All causes (all ages)	1 in 100
20 cigarettes per day	1 in 280
Heart disease	1 in 300
Cancer	1 in 520
All causes (25-year-old)	1 in 700
Stroke	1 in 1200
Motor vehicle accident	1 in 4000
Drowning	1 in 30,000
Alcohol (light drinker)	1 in 50,000
Air travel	1 in 100,000
Radiation, 100 mrad	1 in 100,000
Texas Gulf Coast hurricane	1 in 4,500,000
Being a rodeo cowboy	1 in 6,200,000

pregnancy, the concern is interrupted fertility. During pregnancy, concern is directed to possible congenital effects in newborns. Postpregnancy concerns are related to suspected genetic effects. All these effects have been demonstrated in animals, and some have been observed in humans.

Effects on Fertility

The early effect of high-level radiation on the interruption of fertility in both men and women is discussed in Chapter 35. Ample evidence shows that such an effect does occur and is dose related. The effects of low-dose, long-term irradiation on fertility, however, are less well defined.

Animal data in this area are lacking. Those that are available indicate that, even when radiation is delivered at the rate of 100 rad per year, no noticeable depression in fertility is noted.

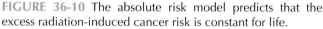 Low-dose, chronic irradiation does not impair fertility.

The health effects analysis of 150,000 American radiologic technologists mentioned earlier has revealed no effect on fertility. The number of births that occurred during a 12-year sampling period equaled the number expected.

Irradiation In Utero

Irradiation in utero concerns the following two types of exposures: that of the radiation worker and that of the patient. Recommended techniques and radiation control procedures associated with these exposed persons are considered fully in Chapter 40. Here, we consider the biologic effects of such irradiation.

Substantial animal data are available to describe fairly completely the effects of relatively high doses of radiation delivered during various periods of gestation. Because the embryo is a rapidly developing cell system, it is particularly sensitive to radiation. With age, the embryo (and then the fetus) becomes less sensitive to the effects of radiation, and this pattern continues into adulthood.

After maturity has been reached, radiosensitivity increases with age. Figure 36-12 summarizes the observed $LD_{50/60}$ in mice exposed at various times, showing this aggregated radiosensitivity. Such findings are of particular concern because diagnostic x-ray exposure often occurs when pregnancy is unknown.

All observations point to the first trimester during pregnancy as the most radiosensitive period.

The effects of radiation in utero are time related and dose related. They include prenatal death, neonatal death, congenital abnormalities, malignancy induction, general impairment of growth, genetic effects, and mental retardation. Figure 36-13 has been redrawn from studies designed to observe the effects of a 200-rad (2-Gy_t) dose delivered at various stages in utero in mice. The scale along the x-axis indicates the approximate comparable time in humans.

Within 2 weeks of fertilization, the most pronounced effect of a high radiation dose is prenatal death, which manifests as a spontaneous abortion. Observations in radiation therapy patients have confirmed this effect, but only after very high doses.

On the basis of animal experimentation, it would appear that this response is very rare. Our best estimate is that a 10-rad (100-mGy_t) dose during the first 2 weeks will induce perhaps a 0.1% rate of spontaneous abortion. This occurs in addition to the 25% to 50% normal incidence of spontaneous abortions.

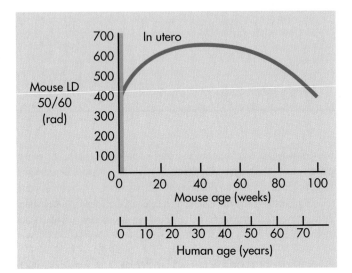

FIGURE 36-12 $LD_{50/60}$ of mice in relation to age at time of irradiation.

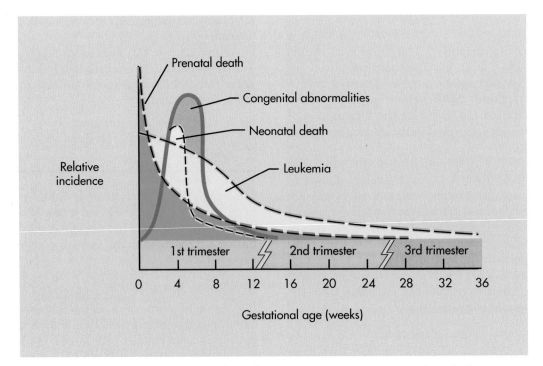

FIGURE 36-13 After 200 rad are delivered at various times in utero, a number of effects can be observed.

Fortunately, this response is of the all-or-none variety: Either a radiation-induced abortion occurs, or the pregnancy is carried to term with no ill effect.

> The first 2 weeks of pregnancy may be of least concern because the response is all-or-nothing.

During the period of **major organogenesis,** from the 2nd through the 10th week, two effects may occur. Early in this period, skeletal and organ abnormalities can be induced. As major organogenesis continues, congenital abnormalities of the central nervous system may be observed if the pregnancy is carried to term.

If radiation-induced congenital abnormalities are severe enough, the result will be neonatal death. After a dose of 200 rad (2 Gy$_t$) to the mouse, nearly 100% of fetuses suffered significant abnormalities. In 80%, this was sufficient to cause neonatal death.

Such effects are rare after diagnostic levels of exposure and are essentially undetectable after radiation doses of less than 10 rad (100 mGy$_t$). A dose of 10 rad (100 mGy$_t$) during organogenesis is expected to increase the incidence of congenital abnormalities by 1% above the natural incidence. To complicate matters, an approximate 5% incidence of naturally occurring congenital abnormalities occurs in the unexposed population.

Irradiation in utero at the human level has been associated with childhood malignancy by a number of investigators. Perhaps the most complete study of this effect was conducted by Alice Stewart and coworkers in a project known as the Oxford Survey, a study of childhood malignancy in England, Scotland, and Wales.

Nearly every such case of childhood malignancy in these countries since 1946 has been investigated. Each case was first identified and then investigated by interview with the mother, review of the hospital charts, and review of the physician records.

Each "case" of childhood malignancy was matched with a "control" for age, sex, place of birth, socioeconomic status, and other demographic factors. The control subject was a child who matched with the "case" in all respects, except that the control did not have cancer or leukemia. The Oxford Survey is being continued at this time and has now considered more than 10,000 cases and a like number of matched control subjects.

Although the Oxford Survey has reviewed all malignancies, it is the findings of radiation-induced leukemia that have been of particular importance. Table 36-7 shows the results of this survey in terms of relative risk.

> The relative risk of childhood leukemia after irradiation in utero is 1.5.

A relative risk of 1.5 for the development of childhood leukemia after irradiation in utero is significant. This indicates an increase of 50% over the nonirradiated rate. The number of cases involved, however, is small.

The incidence of childhood leukemia in the population at large is approximately 9 cases per 100,000 live births. According to the Oxford Survey, if all 100,000 had been irradiated in utero, perhaps 14 cases of leukemia would have resulted. Although these findings have been substantiated in several American populations, no consensus has been reached among radiobiologists that this effect after such low doses is indeed real.

Other effects after irradiation in utero have been studied rather fully in animals and have been observed in some human populations. An unexpected finding in the offspring of atomic bomb survivors is mental retardation. Children of exposed mothers performed poorly on IQ tests and demonstrated poor scholastic performance compared with unexposed Japanese children.

These differences are marginal, yet significant. When assessment is based on test scores, measurable mental retardation is apparent in approximately 6% of all children. A 10-rad dose in utero is expected to increase this incidence by an additional 0.5%.

Radiation exposure in utero does retard the growth and development of the newborn. Irradiation in utero, principally during the period of major organogenesis, has been associated with microcephaly (small head) and, as discussed, mental retardation.

Human data bearing on these effects have been obtained from patients irradiated medically, atomic bomb survivors, and residents of the Marshall Islands who were exposed to radioactive fallout in 1954 during weapons testing. For instance, heavily irradiated children at Hiroshima are, on average, 2.25 cm (0.9 in) shorter, 3 kg (6.6 lb) lighter, and 1.1 cm (0.4 in) smaller in head circumference than members of nonirradiated control groups.

These effects, as well as mental retardation, have been observed principally in those receiving doses in excess of 100 rad (1 Gy$_t$) in utero. The lack of appropriate and sensitive tests of mental function makes it impossible to draw similar conclusions at doses below 100 rad (1 Gy$_t$).

TABLE 36-7	Relative Risk of Childhood Leukemia After Irradiation In Utero by Trimester	
Time of X-Ray Examination		**Relative Risk**
First trimester		8.3
Second trimester		1.5
Third trimester		1.4
Total		**1.5**

population's radiation dose is not known. Relative risk is computed by comparing the number of persons in the exposed population with late effects versus the number in an unexposed population in whom the same condition developed. Excess risk determines the magnitude of the late effect as the difference between cases and control subjects.

The effects of low-dose, long-term irradiation in utero can include the following: prenatal death, neonatal death, congenital abnormalities, malignancy, impaired growth, genetic effects, and mental retardation. However, these abnormalities are based on doses greater than 100 rad, with minimum reported doses in animal experiments at approximately 10 rad. No evidence at the human or animal level indicates that the levels of radiation exposure currently experienced occupationally or medically are responsible for any such effects on fetal growth or development.

CHALLENGE QUESTIONS

1. Define or otherwise identify the following:
   a. Epidemiology
   b. In utero
   c. ABCC-RERF
   d. Thorotrast
   e. Major organogenesis
   f. The Oxford Survey
   g. H.J. Muller
   h. Doubling dose
   i. Radon (^{222}Rn)
   j. Radium watch-dial painters
2. What population experienced radiation-induced cataracts?
3. What is the risk of life span shortening for radiation workers?
4. What is the significance of the change in death statistics of American radiologists from the 1935 to 1944 time period to the 1955 to 1958 time period?
5. Approximately 300,000 radiologic technologists are working in the United States, and their annual exposure is 50 mrem (0.5 mSv). If a 40-year working period is assumed, how many are likely to die from occupational radiation exposure?
6. What is the absolute risk when three cases of radiation-induced leukemia develop per year in 100,000 persons after an average dose of 2 rad?
7. When should excess risk be used as the preferable risk index?
8. Twenty million people in Scandinavia were exposed to an average 0.7 mrad as a result of Chernobyl. If an absolute risk of 10 cases/10^6/rad/yr over a 30-year period is assumed, how many malignancies will be induced?

9. What is the suspected reason why American radiologists have an elevated risk for leukemia?
10. Discuss the experience of radiation-induced leukemia in patients with ankylosing spondylitis.
11. Why was the thymus gland irradiated in the Ann Arbor and Rochester series? What were the late effects of the thymus irradiation?
12. Discuss the way that bone cancer developed in watch-dial painters in the 1920s and 1930s.
13. Explain the risk of radon gas to uranium miners.
14. During the period of the Three Mile Island incident, what was the average dose to persons living within a 100-mile radius of the nuclear plant?
15. What are the effects on fertility caused by low-dose, long-term irradiation?
16. Is it true that most radiation-induced mutations are recessive?
17. In a population of 30,367 irradiated persons, 13 cases of leukemia developed; in a control population of 86,672 persons, 31 cases of leukemia developed. What was the relative risk?
18. What is the absolute risk if 32 cases of leukemia develop per year in 100,000 persons after an average dose of 2 rad?
19. How many cases of radiation-induced leukemia are suspected to have occurred among atomic bomb survivors?
20. What is the difference between relative risk and excess risk?

The answers to the Challenge Questions can be found by logging on to our website at http://evolve.elsevier.com.

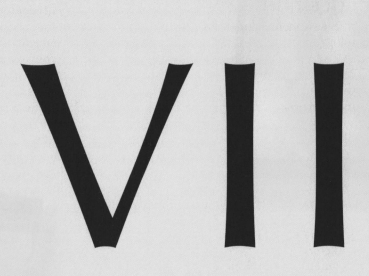

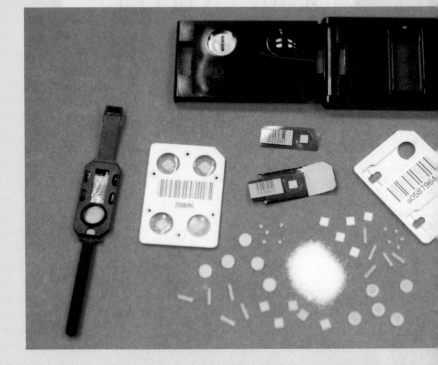

RADIATION PROTECTION

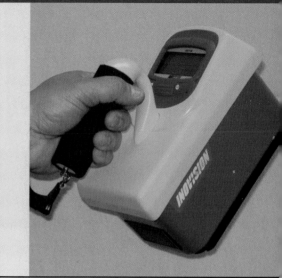

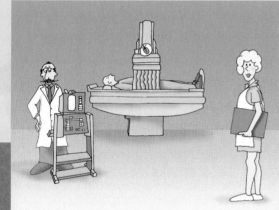

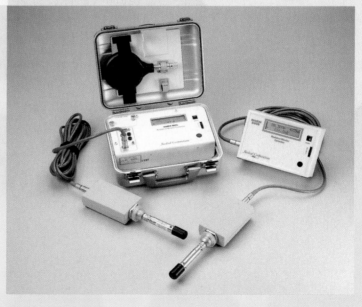

Health Physics

OBJECTIVES

At the completion of this chapter, the student should be able
to do the following:

1. Define health physics
2. List the cardinal principles of radiation protection and discuss
   the ALARA concept
3. Explain the meaning of NCRP and the concept of dose limits
4. Name the recommended dose limits for radiation workers and
   the public
5. Discuss the radiosensitivity of the stages of pregnancy
6. Describe the recommended management procedures for pregnant
   radiation workers and for the pregnant patient

OUTLINE

Radiation and Health
Cardinal Principles of Radiation Protection
    Minimize Time
    Maximize Distance
    Use Shielding
Effective Dose
    Patient Effective Dose
    Radiologic Technologist Effective Dose
Radiologic Terrorism
    Radiologic Device
    Radiation Protection Guidance
    Radiation Detection and Measurement Equipment

level of exposure at any other distance, behind any shielding, for any length of time can be calculated. The order in which these calculations are made makes no difference.

Question: The kVp of a radiographic imaging system rarely exceeds 100 kVp. The output intensity is 4.6 mR/mAs at 100-cm SID. The distance to a desk on the other side of the wall to which the x-ray beam is directed is 200 cm. The wall contains 0.96 mm Pb, and 300 mAs is anticipated daily. If the exposure is to be restricted to 2 mR/wk, how long each day may the desk be occupied?

Answer: Daily x-ray output at 100 cm =

$$(4.6 \text{ mR/mAs})(300 \text{ mAs}) = 1380 \text{ mR}$$

Daily output at 200 cm =

$$(1380)(100/200)^2 = 345 \text{ mR}$$

Daily output behind 0.96 mm Pb or 4

$$\text{HVLs} = 22 \text{ mR}$$
$$= 110 \text{ mR/wk}$$

$$\text{Time allowed} = \frac{2\text{mR}}{110 \text{ mR/wk}} = 0.018 \text{ week}$$
$$= 43 \text{ minutes}$$

However, this analysis does not take into account the x-ray beam attenuation by the patient, which is approximately 2 TVLs or 0.01. Therefore,

Daily output behind 0.96 mm Pb and the

$$\text{patient} = (110 \text{ mR})(0.01) = 1.1 \text{ mR}$$

$$\text{Time allowed} = \frac{2 \text{ mR}}{1.1 \text{ mR/wk}} =$$
$$1.8 \text{ wk (unlimited)}$$

Question: Suppose an analysis shows that if an administrator remains at her desk for longer than 24 minutes each week, the occupational dose limit will be exceeded. How much additional protective lead would be required?

Answer:

Full occupancy is 40 hr × 60 min/hr = 2400 min

$$\frac{2400 \text{ min}}{24 \text{ min}} = 100$$

That is, 2 TVLs or an additional 1.6 mm Pb.

Figure 37-3 illustrates the use of these cardinal principles of radiation protection during a typical clinical situation.

EFFECTIVE DOSE

It is relatively easy to measure patient radiation exposure and dose during medical x-ray imaging. However, x-ray imaging involves partial-body exposure. Radiographic images are collimated to the tissue of importance; therefore, the total body is not exposed.

Radiation risk coefficients are based on total body radiation exposure, as for the atomic bomb survivors of Hiroshima and Nagasaki. When only part of the body is exposed, as in medical x-ray imaging, the risk of a stochastic radiation response is not proportional to the tissue dose but rather to the effective dose (E).

> Effective dose is the equivalent whole-body dose.

The equivalent whole-body dose is the weighted average of the radiation dose to various organs and tissues. The National Committee on Radiation Protection (NCRP) has identified various tissues and organs and the relative radiosensitivity of each (Table 37-2).

Effective dose is the weighted average dose to each of the tissues in Table 37-1.

$$E = \Sigma \, D_i \, W_t$$

Patient Effective Dose

Consider, for example, the relationship between patient dose and effective dose in computed tomography (CT) (Figure 37-4). CT examination of the pelvis results in a rather uniform dose of 2000 mrad (20 mGy) to the tissues of the pelvis. Other tissues are not irradiated.

The exercise shown in Box 37-2 illustrates the manner in which one arrives at patient effective dose. This exercise shows that the effective dose for pelvic CT is 740 mrad.

Another example, as shown in Figure 37-5, posterior-anterior chest radiography, should help explain this concept. Entrance skin dose for this examination is approximately 10 mrad. If one assumes an average tissue dose of half the entrance skin dose, 5 mrad, the effective dose is 1.35 mrem, as computed in Box 37-3.

Radiologic Technologist Effective Dose

We receive essentially all of our occupational radiation exposure during fluoroscopy. During radiography and mammography, the radiographer is positioned behind a protective barrier, resulting in zero occupational radiation exposure.

During fluoroscopy, we position our occupational radiation monitor at the collar, as shown in Figure 37-6, to

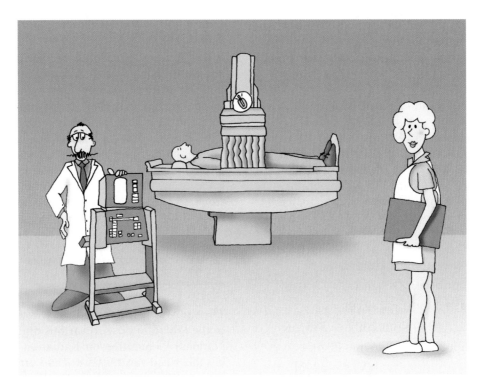

FIGURE 37-3 Application of the cardinal principles of radiation protection in radiology.

TABLE 37-2	Weighting Factors for Various Tissues
Tissue	**Tissue Weighting Factor (W_t)**
Gonad	0.20
Active bone marrow	0.12
Colon	0.12
Lung	0.12
Stomach	0.12
Bladder	0.05
Breast	0.05
Esophagus	0.05
Liver	0.05
Thyroid	0.05
Bone surface	0.01
Skin	0.01

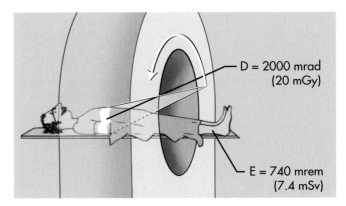

FIGURE 37-4 The relationship between tissue dose and effective dose during computed tomography.

estimate dose to the tissues of the head and neck. The tissues of the trunk of the body receive essentially zero dose; the protective apron does what it is designed to do.

So the estimation of effective occupational dose is shown in Box 37-4 for an occupation monitor response of 100 mrem (1 mSv). The result of this exercise is an occupational effective dose of 5 mrem.

> We assume the occupational effective dose to be 10% of the monitor dose.

Assuming an effective dose of 10% of the occupational monitor dose is conservative. In actual fact, it is something less than 10%.

We will return to the concept of effective dose in Chapters 39 and 40. Be reminded that it is effective dose that should be used for radiation risk estimation.

RADIOLOGIC TERRORISM

Emergency response to a radiologic incident conducted by terrorists, an exceptionally rare event, must be dealt with quickly and competently in order to save life and limit property and environmental damage. **Emergency responders** are those individuals who must make the first decisions and take the first steps in the early stages of such an event.

The first emergency responders are likely to be police, fire, or emergency medical personnel. In the setting of a health care facility, radiologic technologists may likely be the first emergency responders.

BOX 37-2 Effective Dose During Computed Tomography

Computed tomography of the abdomen and pelvis results in a tissue dose of 2000 mrad (20 m Gy_t). What is the effective dose?

$$E = \Sigma\, D_i\, W_i$$
$$= (2000)(0.2)\ \text{gonads}$$
$$+ (2000)(0.12)\ \text{colon}$$
$$+ (2000)(0.05)\ \text{liver}$$

All other organs listed in Table 37-2 receive essentially zero dose.
$$= 400\ \text{gonads}$$
$$+ 240\ \text{colon}$$
$$+ 100\ \text{liver}$$
$$= 740\ \text{mrad}$$

BOX 37-3 Effective Dose During PA Chest Radiography

A PA chest radiograph results in an entrance skin dose of 10 mrad, an exit dose of 0.1 mrad, and an average tissue dose of 5 mrad. What is the effective dose?

$$E = \Sigma\, D_i\, W_i$$
$$= (5)(0.12)\ \text{lung}$$
$$+ (5)(0.05)\ \text{breast}$$
$$+ (5)(0.05)\ \text{esophagus}$$
$$+ (5)(0.05)\ \text{thyroid}$$

All other tissues receive essentially zero dose.
$$= 0.6\ \text{lung}$$
$$+ 0.25\ \text{breast}$$
$$+ 0.25\ \text{esophagus}$$
$$+ 0.25\ \text{thyroid}$$
$$= 1.35\ \text{mrad}$$

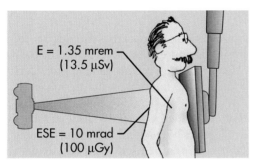

FIGURE 37-5 Effective dose during posterior-anterior chest radiography.

 Rescue and medical emergencies should be attended to before radiologic concerns are addressed.

The first task of emergency responders is to prevent injury and death and to attend to the medical needs of victims. Such immediate responses include limiting acute, high-intensity radiation exposure and limiting low-intensity radiation exposure that could result in late stochastic effects. This is an ALARA exercise and will involve the application of the cardinal principles of radiation protection: Reduce time of exposure, increase distance from the source, and impose shielding between the source and the victim.

Radiologic Device

The malevolent use of radiologic material by terrorists can be described as one of three devices: a radiation exposure device (RED), a radiologic dispersal device (RDD), and an improvised nuclear device (IND). Dealing with the effect of such devices requires specific response techniques for each.

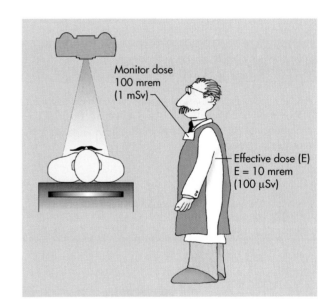

FIGURE 37-6 Effective dose for occupational radiation exposure is based on the occupational radiation monitor.

 Radiologic terrorism can be addressed safely with an emergency responder's equipment kit.

An RED is a sealed source of radioactive material that directly exposes people. An RED will not disperse radioactive material; therefore, decontamination of an RED is not required.

An RDD is a bomb that when exploded disperses radioactive contamination over a wide area. Although the contamination can be particularly troublesome, it is not usually life threatening. The RDD may not be explosive, but rather, radioactive material. It may be dispersed by hand in the form of powder, mist, or gas into a water supply or ventilation system.

An IND contains nuclear material that can produce a nuclear explosion. An IND is indeed a nuclear weapon; therefore, it is unlikely to be the form of attack used by a terrorist. However, should an IND be employed, the death and devastation would be extreme.

Radiation Protection Guidance

Protection against exposure to external radiation, exposure from photon and particle radiation, and internal radioactive contamination transferred from surface radioactive contamination must be considered. This is accomplished by establishing boundaries for known levels of radiation exposure and radioactive contamination.

With the use of radiation monitoring instruments, an inner boundary is established at an exposure rate of 10 R/hr (100 Gy$_a$/hr). Inside of this boundary, one should assume that levels of radioactive contamination are high, until it is proved otherwise.

BOX 37-4 Occupational/Radiation Effective Dose

An occupational radiation monitor records a dose of 100 mrem (1 mSv). What is the effective dose if the occupational dose is received during fluoroscopy when a protective apron is worn?

$E = \Sigma\, D_i\, W_i$

$\quad = (100)(0.05)$ thyroid

All other tissues receive essentially zero dose.

$\quad = 5$ mrem

 Being exposed to radiation does not make an individual radioactive.

An outer boundary should be established when exposure exceeds 10 mR/hr (100 μ Gy$_a$/hr) or when radioactive contamination is detectable.

Radiation Detection and Measurement Equipment

Radiation detection equipment with specific capacity should be readily available to the first responder. It is recommended that such equipment be stored in the nuclear medicine laboratory and identified to all technologists and radiologists who might be pressed into emergency response.

Radioactive contamination is rarely life threatening.

Radiation detection apparatus should be capable of measuring radiation exposure levels to 50 R/hr (500 m Gy$_a$/hr). Further, it is recommended that such instruments should emit unambiguous alarms at 10 mR/hr (100 μ Gy$_a$/hr), 10 R/hr (100 m Gy$_a$/hr), and 50 R/hr (500 m Gy$_a$/hr). (Such a specially designed instrument is shown in Figure 37-7.) An additional instrument should be available that can be used to clearly detect the presence of alpha and beta radioactive contamination.

Emergency responders should have available standard protective coveralls and shoe covers to protect against radioactive contamination of the responder. Protective respiratory devices may be needed in the case of aerosol radioactive contamination. Decontamination of victims

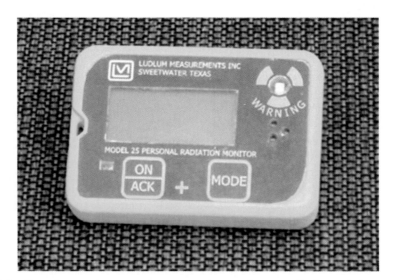

FIGURE 37-7 Radiation detection instrument designed especially for radiologic terrorism. (Courtesy Ian Hamilton, Ludlum Instruments.)

may be necessary, and an area should be cordoned off for such activity, so that a contaminated-to-clean step-off pad is provided.

The Radiation Safety Officer of a hospital should assign an individual to be responsible for establishing the emergency response equipment store and for seeing that adequate continuing education is provided for those who might be called upon to perform as emergency responders.

SUMMARY

Health physics is concerned with the research, teaching, and operational aspects of radiation control. The three cardinal principles developed for radiation workers are as follows: Minimize time of radiation exposure, maximize distance from the radiation source, and use shielding to reduce radiation exposure. ALARA (as low as reasonably achievable) defines the principal concept of radiation protection.

Effective dose is that which should be used to estimate radiation risk to the patient or the radiologic technologist. Assuming that effective dose is 10% of a collar-positioned monitor is conservative and results in overestimation of stochastic response.

Radiologic terrorism is possible with three principal devices: a radiation exposure device, a radiologic dispersal device, and an improvised nuclear device.

CHALLENGE QUESTIONS

1. Define or otherwise identify the following:
   a. Health physics
   b. TVL
   c. NCRP
   d. Effective dose
   e. ALARA
   f. Tissue weighting factor (W_r)
   g. First responder
   h. Clarence Dally
   i. Manhattan Project
   j. LNT

2. Write the equation for the radiation dose as a function of time of exposure.
3. What is the function of the 5-minute reset timer on a fluoroscopy imaging system?
4. A fluoroscope emits 3.5 R/mA-minute at the tabletop for every mA of operation. What is the approximate patient entrance skin exposure (ESE) after a 3.2-minute fluoroscopic examination of 1.5 mA?
5. What are the three cardinal principles of radiation protection?
6. The output intensity of a radiographic unit is 4.2 mR/mAs. What is the total output after a 200-ms exposure at 300 mA?
7. At the exposure rate in #6, what is the approximate patient skin dose after a 3.2-minute fluoroscopic examination of 1.5 mA?
8. How can the three cardinal principles of radiation protection be best applied in diagnostic radiology?
9. What exposure will a radiologic technologist receive when exposed for 10 minutes at 4 m from a source with intensity of 100 mR/hr at 1 m while wearing a protective apron equivalent to 2 HVLs?
10. What wartime effort coined the term *health physicist*?
11. The collar-positioned monitor of a fluoroscopist records 90 mrem (0.9 mSv) over the course of a month. This represents approximately what effective dose (E)?
12. Describe the change in longevity that occurred during the 20th century and the impact of radiation on that change.
13. How many half-value layers are included in a tenth-value layer?
14. What should first responders do in the event of a radiologic emergency?
15. Discuss the concept of effective dose.

The answers to the Challenge Questions can be found by logging on to our website at http://evolve.elsevier.com.

CHAPTER 38

Designing for Radiation Protection

OBJECTIVES

At the completion of this chapter, the student should be able
to do the following:

1. Name the leakage radiation limit for x-ray tubes
2. List nine radiation protection features of a radiographic imaging system
3. List nine radiation protection features of a fluoroscopic imaging system
4. Discuss the design of primary and secondary radiation barriers
5. Describe the three types of radiation dosimeters used in diagnostic imaging

OUTLINE

Radiographic Protection Features
Protective X-Ray Tube
  Housing
Control Panel
Source-to-Image Receptor
  Distance Indicator
Collimation
Positive-Beam Limitation
Beam Alignment
Filtration
Reproducibility
Linearity
Operator Shield
Mobile X-ray Imaging System
Fluoroscopic Protection Features
Source-to-Skin Distance
Primary Protective Barrier
Filtration
Collimation
Exposure Control
Bucky Slot Cover
Protective Curtain
Cumulative Timer
Dose Area Product

Design of Protective Barriers
Type of Radiation
Factors That Affect Barrier
  Thickness
**Radiation Detection and
Measurement**
Gas-Filled Detectors
Scintillation Detectors
Thermoluminescence Dosimetry
Optically Stimulated
  Luminescence Dosimetry

A NUMBER of features of modern x-ray imaging systems designed to improve radiographic quality have been discussed in previous chapters. Many of these features are also designed to reduce patient radiation dose during x-ray examinations. For instance, proper beam collimation contributes to improved image contrast and is effective in reducing patient dose.

More than 100 individual radiation protection devices and accessories are associated with modern x-ray imaging systems. Some are characteristic of either radiographic or fluoroscopic imaging systems, and some are mandated by federal regulation for all diagnostic x-ray imaging systems. A description of the devices required for all diagnostic x-ray imaging systems follows.

RADIOGRAPHIC PROTECTION FEATURES

Many radiation protection devices and accessories are associated with modern x-ray imaging systems. Two that are appropriate for all diagnostic x-ray imaging systems relate to the protective housing of the x-ray tube and to the control panel.

Protective X-ray Tube Housing

Every x-ray tube must be contained within protective housing that reduces leakage radiation during use.

> Leakage radiation must be less than 100 mR/hr (1 mGy$_a$/hr) at a distance of 1 m from the protective housing.

Control Panel

The control panel must indicate the conditions of exposure and must positively indicate when the x-ray tube is energized. These requirements are usually satisfied with the use of kVp and mA indicators. Sometimes, visible or audible signals indicate when the x-ray beam is energized.

> X-ray beam on must be positively and clearly indicated to the radiologic technologist.

Source-to-Image Receptor Distance Indicator

A source-to-image receptor distance (SID) indicator must be provided. This can be as simple as a tape measure attached to the tube housing, or as advanced as lasers.

> The SID indicator must be accurate to within 2% of the indicated SID.

Collimation

Light-localized, variable-aperture rectangular collimators should be provided. Cones and diaphragms may replace the collimator for special examinations. Attenuation of the useful beam by collimator shutters must be equivalent to attenuation by the protective housing.

> The x-ray beam and the light beam must coincide to within 2% of the SID.

Question: Most radiographs are taken at an SID of 100 cm. How much difference is allowed between the projection of the light field and the x-ray beam at the image receptor?

Answer: 2% of 100 cm = 2 cm

Positive-Beam Limitation

Automatic, light-localized, variable-aperture collimators were required on all but special x-ray imaging systems manufactured in the United States between 1974 and 1994. These positive-beam–limiting (PBL) devices are no longer required but continue to be a part of most new radiographic imaging systems. They must be adjusted so that with any image receptor size in use and at all standard SIDs, the collimator shutters automatically provide an x-ray beam equal to the image receptor.

> The PBL must be accurate to within 2% of the SID.

Beam Alignment

In addition to proper collimation, each radiographic tube should be provided with a mechanism to ensure proper alignment of the x-ray beam and the image receptor. It does no good to align the light field and the x-ray beam if the image receptor is not also aligned.

Filtration

All general purpose diagnostic x-ray beams must have a total filtration (inherent plus added) of at least 2.5 mm Al when operated above 70 kVp. Radiographic tubes operated between 50 and 70 kVp must have at least 1.5 mm Al. Below 50 kVp, a minimum of 0.5 mm Al total filtration is required. X-ray tubes designed for mammography usually have 30 μm Mo or 60 μm Rh filtration.

As was discussed in Chapter 9, it is not normally possible physically to examine and measure the thickness of each component of total filtration. An accurate measurement of half-value layer (HVL) is sufficient. If the HVL is equal to or greater than the values given in Table 9-3 at various kVp levels, total filtration is adequate.

Question: The following data are obtained on a three-phase radiographic imaging system operating at 70 kVp, 100 mA, 100 ms. Is the filtration adequate?

Added filtration (mm Al)	0	0.5	1.0	1.5	2.0	3.0	4.0	5.0
Exposure (mR)	87	74	65	56	49	39	31	25

Answer: A plot of these data (Figure 38-1) indicates an HVL of 2.0 mm Al. Table 9-3 shows that at 70 kVp, an HVL of 2.0 mm Al or greater is sufficient. The filtration is adequate.

Reproducibility

For any given radiographic technique, the output radiation intensity should be constant from one exposure to another. This is checked by making repeated radiation exposures through the same technique and observing the average variation in radiation intensity.

 The variation in x-ray intensity should not exceed 5%.

Linearity

When adjacent mA stations are used, for example, 100 mA and 200 mA, and exposure time is adjusted for constant mAs, the output radiation intensity should remain constant. When the exposure time remains constant, causing

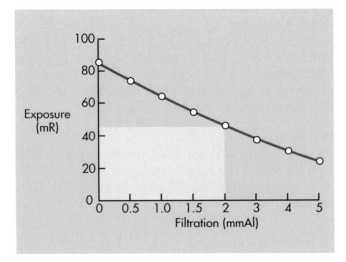

FIGURE 38-1 Measurement of x-ray beam intensity as a function of added filtration results in a half-value layer (HVL) of 2.0 mmAl.

the mAs to increase in proportion to the increase in mA, radiation intensity should be proportional to mAs.

 The maximum acceptable variation in linearity is 10% from one mA station to an adjacent mA station.

This takes any inaccuracy in the exposure timer out of the analysis. Radiation intensity is expressed in units of mR/mAs (mGy$_a$/mAs).

Operator Shield

It must not be possible to expose an image receptor while the radiologic technologist stands unprotected outside a fixed protective barrier, usually the console booth. The exposure control should be fixed to the operating console and not to a long cord. The radiologic technologist may be in the examination room during exposure, but only if protective apparel is worn.

Mobile X-ray Imaging System

A protective lead apron should be assigned to each mobile x-ray imaging system. The exposure switch of such an imaging system must allow the operator to remain at least 2 m from the x-ray tube during exposure. Of course, the useful beam must be directed away from the radiologic technologist while positioned at this minimum distance.

FLUOROSCOPIC PROTECTION FEATURES

The features of fluoroscopic imaging systems that follow are intended primarily to reduce patient radiation dose. Usually, when patient radiation dose is reduced, personnel exposure is reduced similarly.

Source-to-Skin Distance

One would think that increasing the distance between any x-ray tube and the patient would result in reduced patient dose because of the increased distance. This is true, but to maintain exposure to the image intensifier, the mA must be increased to compensate for the increased distance. Because of the divergence of the x-ray beam, the entrance skin exposure (ESE) is lessened for the required exit exposure as the source-to-skin distance (SSD) is increased.

 The SSD must be not less than 38 cm on stationary fluoroscopes and not less than 30 cm on mobile fluoroscopes.

Review Figure 38-2, where a 20-cm abdomen is 5 HVLs thick. If the fluoroscopic x-ray tube is moved from 40 cm SSD to 20 cm SSD, the ESE is greatly increased. The exposure required at the image intensifier is 1 mR.

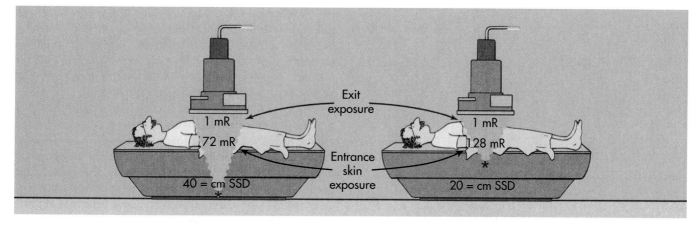

FIGURE 38-2 Patient entrance skin exposure (ESE) is considerably higher when the fluoroscopic x-ray tube is too close to the tabletop.

BOX 38-1 Effect of SSD on ESE

On the basis of x-ray beam divergence alone at 40 cm SSD:

$$\frac{I_1}{I_2} = \frac{d_2^2}{d_1^2}$$

$$\frac{I_1}{1} = \frac{60^2}{40^2}$$

$$I_1 = 2.25\,mR$$

at 20 cm SSD:

$$\frac{I_1}{1} = \frac{40^2}{20^2}$$

$$I_1 = 4.0\,mR$$

Additive HVL due to the 20-cm patient:
at 40 cm SID:

$$2.25 \times 2^5 = 2.25 \times 32$$
$$= 72\,mR\ at\ 20\,cm\,SSD$$
$$4.0 \times 2^5 = 128\,mR$$

ESE, Entrance skin exposure; *HVL,* half-value layer; *SID,* source-to-image receptor distance; *SSD,* source-to-skin distance.

The ESEs will be 2.25 mR and 4.0 mR, respectively, solely because of the divergence of the x-ray beam—the inverse square law. Add the x-ray attenuation of 5 HVLs for each geometry, and the respective ESEs become 72 mR and 128 mR (Box 38-1).

Primary Protective Barrier

The fluoroscopic image receptor assembly serves as a primary protective barrier and must be 2 mm Pb equivalent. It must be coupled with the x-ray tube and interlocked so that the fluoroscopic x-ray tube cannot be energized when the image receptor is in the parked position.

Filtration

The total filtration of the fluoroscopic x-ray beam must be at least 2.5 mm Al equivalent. The tabletop, patient cradle, or other material positioned between the x-ray tube and the tabletop are included as part of the total filtration. When the filtration is unknown, the HVL should be measured. The minimum HVL reported in Table 18-3 must be met so that adequate filtration can be assumed.

Collimation

Fluoroscopic x-ray beam collimators must be adjusted so that an unexposed border is visible on the image monitor when the input phosphor of the image intensifier is positioned 35 cm above the tabletop and the collimators are fully open. For automatic collimating devices, such an unexposed border should be visible at all heights above the tabletop. The collimator shutters should track with height above the tabletop.

Exposure Control

The fluoroscopic exposure control should be of the dead man type; that is, if the operator should drop dead or just release the pressure, the exposure would be terminated—unless, of course, he or she falls on the switch! The conventional foot pedal or pressure switch on the fluoroscopic image receptor satisfies this condition.

Bucky Slot Cover

During fluoroscopy, the Bucky tray is moved to the end of the examination table, leaving an opening in the side of the table approximately 5 cm wide at gonadal level. This opening should be covered automatically with at least 0.25 mm Pb equivalent.

Protective Curtain

A protective curtain or panel of at least 0.25 mm Pb equivalent should be positioned between the fluoroscopist and the patient. Figure 38-3 shows the typical isoexposure distribution for a fluoroscope. Without

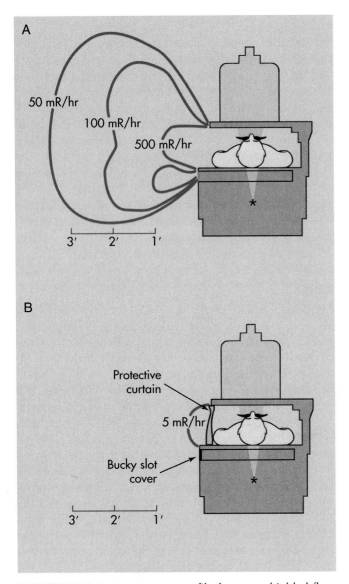

FIGURE 38-3 **A,** Isoexposure profile for an unshielded fluoroscope demonstrates the need for protective curtains and Bucky slot covers. **B,** Isoexposure profile with these protective devices.

the curtain and the Bucky slot cover, the exposure of radiology personnel is many times higher.

Cumulative Timer

A cumulative timer that produces an audible signal when the fluoroscopic time has exceeded 5 minutes must be provided. This device is designed to ensure that the radiologist is aware of the relative beam-on time during each procedure. The assisting radiologic technologist should record total fluoroscopy beam-on time for each examination.

Dose Area Product

The intensity of the x-ray beam at the tabletop of a fluoroscope should not exceed 2.1 R/min (21 mGy$_a$/min) for each mA of operation at 80 kVp. If there is no optional

high-level control, the intensity must not exceed 10 R/min (100 mGy$_a$/min) during fluoroscopy. If an optional *high-level control* is provided, the maximum tabletop intensity allowed is *20 R/min (200 mGy$_a$/min)*. There is no limit on x-ray intensity when the image is recorded, as in cineradiography or videography.

The overall carcinogenic risk (stochastic effect) to a patient depends on effective radiation dose (E), which is related to tissue radiation dose and to the volume of tissue exposed. Tissue radiation dose, which refers to the energy deposited locally, is the quantity that best reflects the potential for injury to that tissue (deterministic effect).

Dose area product (DAP) is a quantity that reflects not only the dose but also the volume of tissue irradiated; therefore, it may be a better indicator of risk than dose. DAP is expressed in R-cm^2 (cGy-cm^2).

DAP increases with increasing field size even if the dose remains unchanged. Smaller field size results in lower DAP, and thus less risk, because a smaller amount of tissue is exposed.

DAP may be used to monitor radiation output from radiographic and fluoroscopic imaging systems. DAP meters are becoming more common on x-ray imaging systems. Typically, the radiolucent device is placed near the x-ray source below the collimator, before the beam enters the patient.

The risk for injury to the skin where the beam enters the patient can be derived by dividing the DAP measurement by the area of the beam at the skin. Using DAP to monitor radiation intensity is a good way to implement radiation management procedures and keep patient exposures low.

DESIGN OF PROTECTIVE BARRIERS

In designing a radiology department or an individual x-ray examination room, it is not sufficient to consider only general architectural characteristics. Great attention must be given to the location of the x-ray imaging system in the examination room.

The use of adjoining rooms is also of great importance when the design is geared toward radiation safety. It is often necessary to include protective barriers, usually sheets of lead, in the walls of x-ray examination rooms. If the radiology facility is located on an upper floor, then it may be necessary to shield the floor as well.

A great number of factors are considered when a protective barrier is designed. This discussion touches only on the fundamentals and some basic definitions. Whenever new x-ray facilities are being designed or old ones renovated, a medical physicist must be consulted for assistance in the design of proper radiation shielding.

Type of Radiation

For the purpose of protective barrier design, three types of radiation are considered (Figure 38-4). Primary radiation is the most intense and therefore the most hazardous and the most difficult to shield.

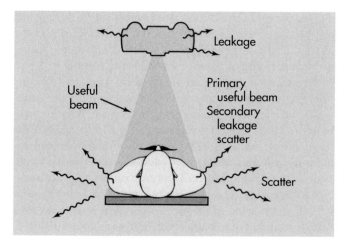

FIGURE 38-4 Three types of radiation—the useful beam, leakage radiation, and scatter radiation—must be considered when the protective barriers of an x-ray room are designed.

When a chest board is positioned on a given wall, it is sometimes necessary to provide shielding directly behind the chest board, in addition to that specified for the rest of the wall. Any wall to which the useful beam can be directed is designated a **primary protective barrier.**

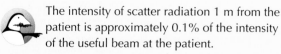

Primary radiation is the useful beam.

Lead bonded to sheet rock or wood paneling is used most often as a primary protective barrier. Such lead shielding is available in various thicknesses and is specified for architects and contractors in units of pounds per square foot (lb/ft²).

Concrete, concrete block, or brick may be used instead of lead. As a rule of thumb, 4 inches of masonry is equivalent to 1/16 inch of lead. Table 38-1 shows available lead thicknesses and equivalent thicknesses of concrete.

There are two types of secondary radiation: **scatter radiation** and **leakage radiation.** Scatter radiation results when the useful beam intercepts any object, causing some x-rays to be scattered. For the purpose of protective shielding calculations, the scattering

object can be regarded as a new source of radiation. During radiography and fluoroscopy, the patient is the single most important scattering object.

> The intensity of scatter radiation 1 m from the patient is approximately 0.1% of the intensity of the useful beam at the patient.

Question: The patient ESE is 410 mR (4.1 mGy$_a$) for a kidney, ureter, and bladder (KUB) examination. What will be the approximate radiation exposure at 1 m from the patient? At 3 m from the patient?

Answer: At 1 m: 410 mR × 0.1% = 410 mR × 0.001
= 0.41 mR = 410 μR

At 3 m: 0.41 mR × (1/3)² = 0.41 mR (1/9)
= 0.046 mR = 46 μR

Leakage radiation is that radiation emitted from the x-ray tube housing in all directions other than that of the useful beam. If the x-ray tube housing is designed properly, the leakage radiation will never exceed the regulatory limit of 100 mR/hr (1 mGy$_a$/hr) at 1 m. Although in practice, leakage radiation levels are much lower than this limit, 100 mR/hr at 1 m is used for protective barrier calculations.

Protective barriers designed to shield areas from secondary radiation are called **secondary protective barriers.** Secondary protective barriers are always less thick than primary protective barriers.

Often, lead is not required for secondary protective barriers because the computation usually results in less than 0.4 mm Pb. In such cases, conventional gypsum board, glass, or lead acrylic is adequate.

Many walls that are secondary protective barriers can be protected adequately with four thicknesses of 5/8-inch gypsum board. Operating console barriers are secondary protective barriers—the useful beam is never directed at the operating console booth. Four thicknesses of gypsum board and 1/2-inch plate glass may be all that is necessary. Sometimes glass walls 1/2 to 1 inch thick can be used as control booth barriers. Table 38-2 gives equivalent thicknesses for secondary protective barrier materials.

TABLE 38-1	Lead and Concrete Equivalents for Primary Protective Barrier				
LEAD				**CONCRETE**	
mm	in	lb/ft²		cm	in
0.4	1/64	1		2.4	1 3/8
0.8	1/32	2		4.8	1 7/8
1.2	3/64	3		7.2	2 7/8
1.6	1/16	4		9.6	3 3/4

Question: What percentage of the recommended 100-mrem/wk (1-mSv/wk) public dose limit will be incident on a control booth barrier located 3 m from the x-ray tube and the patient? Assume that the x-ray output is 3 mR/mAs and that the weekly beam-on time is 5 minutes at an average 100 mA—a generous assumption.

Answer: From scatter radiation, the barrier will receive:

Total primary beam = 3 mR/mAs × 10 mA × 5 min × 60 s/min
= 90,000 mR

Scatter radiation = 90,000 mR × 1/1000 × $(1/3)^2$
= 10 mR

From leakage radiation, the barrier will receive:

Leakage radiation at 1 m = 100 mR/hr × 5/60 hr = 8.3 mR

Leakage radiation = 8.3 mR $(1/3)^2$
= 0.9 mR

Total secondary radiation = 10 mR + 0.9 mR
= 10.9 mR or 11% of the recommended dose limit

This analysis is representative of the clinical environment. The estimated exposure occurs to the control booth barrier—not to the radiologic technologist. The composition of the barrier and the additional distance reduce technologist exposure even further. This is the reason why personnel radiation exposure during radiography is very low.

Radiologic technologists receive most of their occupational radiation exposure during fluoroscopy.

Factors That Affect Barrier Thickness

Many factors must be taken into consideration when the required protective barrier thickness is calculated. A thorough discussion of these factors is beyond the scope of this book; however, a definition of each is useful for an understanding of the problems involved.

Distance. The thickness of a barrier naturally depends on the distance between the source of radiation and the barrier. The distance is that to the adjacent occupied area, not to the inside of the wall of the x-ray room.

A wall along which an x-ray imaging system is positioned probably requires more shielding than the other walls of the room. In such a case, the leakage radiation may be more hazardous than the scatter radiation or even the useful beam. It may be desirable to position the x-ray imaging system in the middle of the room because then no single wall is subjected to especially intense radiation exposure.

Occupancy. The use of the area that is being protected is of principal importance. If the area were a rarely occupied closet or storeroom, the required shielding would be less than if it were an office or laboratory that was occupied 40 hours per week.

This concept reflects the **time of occupancy factor (T).** Table 38-3 reports the occupancy levels of various areas as suggested by the National Council on Radiation Protection and Measurements (NCRP).

Control. An area that is occupied primarily by radiology personnel and patients is called a **controlled area.** The design limits for a controlled area are based on the recommended occupational dose limit; therefore, the barrier is required to reduce the exposure to a worker in the area to less than 100 mrem per week (1 mSv/wk).

Design limits for a controlled area are based on the annual recommended occupational dose limit of 5000 mrem/yr (50 mSv/yr).

An **uncontrolled area** can be occupied by anyone; therefore, the maximum exposure rate allowed is based on the recommended dose limit for the public of 100 mrem/yr (1 mSv/yr). This is equivalent to 2 mrem/wk (20 μSv/wk), which is the design limit for an uncontrolled area. Furthermore, the protective barrier should ensure that no individual will receive more than 2.5 mrem (25 μSv) in any single hour.

Workload. The shielding required for an x-ray examination room depends on the level of radiation activity in that room. The greater the number of examinations performed each week, the thicker the shielding that is required.

TABLE 38-2	Equivalent Material Thicknesses for Secondary Barriers			
	SUBSTITUTES			
Computed Lead Required	**Steel (mm)**	**Glass (mm)**	**Gypsum (mm)**	**Wood (mm)**
0.1	0.5	1.2	2.8	19
0.2	1.2	2.5	5.9	33
0.3	1.8	3.7	8.8	44
0.4	2.5	4.8	12	53

TABLE 38-3	Levels of Occupancy of Areas That May Be Adjacent to X-ray Rooms, as Suggested by the NCRP
Occupancy	**Area**
Full	Work areas (e.g., offices, laboratories, shops, wards, and nurses' stations), living quarters, children's play areas, and occupied space in nearby buildings
Frequent	Corridors, restrooms, patient rooms
Occasional	Waiting rooms, stairways, unattended elevators, janitors' closets, outside area

This characteristic is called **workload (W)** and is expressed in units of milliampere-minutes per week (mAmin/wk). A busy, general purpose x-ray room may have a workload of 500 mAmin/wk. Rooms in private offices have workloads of less than 100 mAmin/wk.

Question: The plans for a community hospital call for two x-ray examination rooms. The estimated patient load for each room is 15 patients per day, and each patient will average 3 films taken at 80 kVp, 70 mAs. What is the projected workload of each room?

Answer:

15 patients/day × 5 days/wk

$$= 75 \text{ patients/wk}$$

75 patients/wk × 3 films/pt

$$= 225 \text{ films/wk}$$

225 films/wk × 70 mAs/film

$$= 15,750 \text{ mAs/wk}$$

$$15,750 \text{ mAs/wk} \times \frac{1 \text{ min}}{60 \text{ sec}}$$

$$= 262.5 \text{ mAmin/wk}$$

For combination radiographic/fluoroscopic imaging systems, usually only the radiographic workload need be considered for barrier calculations. When the fluoroscopic x-ray tube is energized, a primary protective barrier in the form of the fluoroscopic screen always intercepts the useful x-ray beam. Consequently, the primary barrier requirements are always much less for fluoroscopic x-ray beams than for radiographic x-ray beams.

Use Factor. The percentage of time during which the x-ray beam is on and directed toward a particular protective barrier is called the **use factor** (**U**) for that barrier. The NCRP recommends that walls be assigned a use factor of 1/4 and the floor a use factor of 1.

Studies have shown these recommendations to be high and therefore very conservative. Many medical physicists suggest that primary barriers in fact do not exist. All barriers are secondary because the useful beam always is intercepted by the patient and the image receptor.

If an x-ray room has a special design, other use factors may be assigned. A room designed strictly for chest radiography has one wall with a use factor of 1. All others have a use factor of zero for primary radiation and thus would be considered secondary radiation barriers.

The ceiling nearly always is considered a secondary protective barrier. For a secondary barrier, leakage and scatter radiation are present 100% of the time that the x-ray tube is energized.

> The use factor for secondary barriers is always 1.

kVp. The final consideration in the design of an x-ray protective barrier is the penetrability of the x-ray beam. For protective barrier calculations, kVp is used as the measure of penetrability. Most modern x-ray imaging systems are designed to operate at up to 150 kVp. Most examinations, however, are conducted at an average of 75 kVp.

Usually, constant operation is assumed at a kVp greater than that actually used: 100 kVp for general radiography, 30 kVp for mammography. Therefore, it is more likely that the protective barrier will be too thick than too thin.

Alternatively, a workload distribution such as those shown in Figure 38-5 may be used. Workload distribution results in a more precise determination of required barrier thickness, but it is a considerably more difficult computation to perform.

Measurements of radiation exposure outside the x-ray examination room always result in radiation levels far less than those anticipated by calculation. The total beam-on time is always less than that assumed. The average kVp is usually closer to 75 kVp than to 100 kVp.

Calculations do not account for the fact that the patient and the image receptor always intercept the useful beam. Therefore, although the calculations are intended to result in a dose limit of 100 mrem/wk (1 mSv/wk) or 2 mrem/wk (20 μSv/wk) outside the x-ray room, rarely will the actual exposure exceed 1/10 of those dose limits. To confirm this for yourself, keep records for 1 week of kVp, mAs, and beam direction.

RADIATION DETECTION AND MEASUREMENT

Instruments are designed to detect radiation or to measure radiation, or to do both. Those designed for detection usually operate in the **pulse** or **rate** mode and are used to indicate the presence of radiation. In the pulse mode, the presence of radiation is indicated by a ticking, chirping, or beeping sound. In the rate

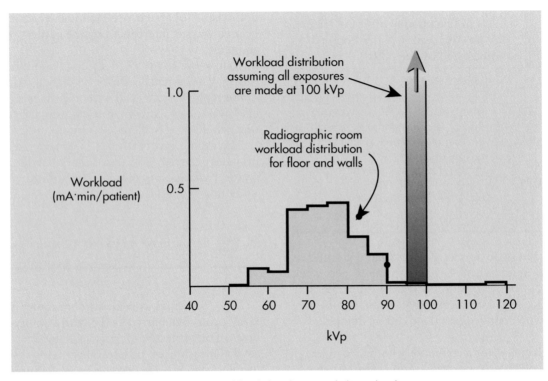

FIGURE 38-5 Workload distribution of clinical voltage.

mode, the instrument response is expressed in mR/hr (mGy$_a$/hr) or R/hr (Gy$_a$/hr).

Instruments designed to measure the intensity of radiation usually operate in the **integrate** mode. They accumulate the signal and respond with a total exposure (mR or R). Such application is called **dosimetry,** and the radiation measuring devices are called **dosimeters.**

The earliest radiation detection device was the photographic emulsion; it is still a primary means of radiation detection and measurement. However, other devices have been developed that have more favorable characteristics than the photographic emulsion for some applications. Table 38-4 lists most of the currently available radiation detection and measurement devices, along with some of their principal characteristics and uses.

It is apparent that film has two principal applications in diagnostic radiology: the making of a radiograph and the radiation monitoring of personnel (film badge). The photographic process was discussed in Chapters 11 and 12. Use of film as a radiation monitor is covered in Chapter 40.

Four other types of radiation detection devices are of particular importance in diagnostic radiology. The gas-filled radiation detector is used widely as a device to measure radiation intensity and to detect radioactive contamination. Thermoluminescence dosimetry (TLD) and optically stimulated luminescence (OSL) dosimetry are used for both patient and personnel radiation monitoring. Scintillation detection is the basis for the gamma camera, an imaging device used in nuclear medicine; it

TABLE 38-4	Radiation Detection and Measuring Device Characteristics and Uses
Device	**Characteristics—Uses**
Photographic	Limited range, sensitive, energy dependent— personnel monitoring, emulsion imaging
Ionization chamber	Wide range, accurate, portable—survey for radiation levels 1 mR/hr
Proportional counter	Laboratory instrument, accurate, sensitive—assay of small quantities of radionuclides
Geiger-Muller counter	Limited to 100 mR/hr, portable—survey for low radiation levels and radioactive contamination
Thermoluminescence dosimetry	Wide range, accurate, sensitive—personnel monitoring, stationary, area monitoring
Optically stimulated luminescence dosimetry	Wide range, accurate, sensitive—newest personnel monitoring device
Scintillation detection	Limited range, very sensitive, stationary or portable instruments—photon spectroscopy, imaging

is also used in computed tomography (CT) and digital radiography imaging systems.

Gas-Filled Detectors

Three types of gas-filled radiation detectors are used: ionization chambers, proportional counters, and Geiger-Muller detectors. Although these are different in terms of response characteristics, each is based on the same principle of operation. As radiation passes through gas, it ionizes atoms of the gas. The electrons released in ionization are detected as an electrical signal that is proportional to the radiation intensity.

> The ionization of gas is the basis for gas-filled radiation detectors.

Consider an ideal gas-filled detector as shown schematically in Figure 38-6. It consists of a cylinder filled with air or any of a number of other gases.

Along the central axis of the cylinder a rigid wire called the **central electrode** is positioned. If a voltage is impressed between the central electrode and the wall such that the wire is positive and the wall negative, then any electrons liberated in the chamber by ionization will be attracted to the central electrode.

These electrons form an electrical signal, either as a pulse of electrons or as a continuous current. This electric signal then is amplified and measured. Its intensity is proportional to the radiation intensity that caused it.

In general, the larger the chamber, the more gas molecules are available for ionization, and therefore, the more sensitive is the instrument. Similarly, if the chamber is pressurized, then a greater number of molecules are available for ionization, and even higher sensitivity results.

> High sensitivity means that an instrument can detect very low radiation intensities.

Sensitivity is not the same as **accuracy**. A high level of accuracy means that an instrument can detect and **precisely measure** the intensity of a radiation field. Instrument accuracy is controlled by the overall electronic design of the device.

Region of Recombination. If the voltage across the chamber of the ideal gas-filled detector is increased slowly from zero to a high level, the resulting electrical signal in the presence of fixed radiation intensity will increase in stages (Figure 38-7). During the first stage, when the voltage is very low, no electrons are attracted to the central electrode. The ion pairs produced in the chamber recombine. This is known as the **region of recombination,** shown as stage *R* in Figure 38-7.

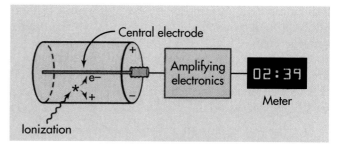

FIGURE 38-6 The ideal gas-filled detector consists of a cylinder of gas and a central collecting electrode. When a voltage is maintained between the central electrode and the wall of the chamber, electrons produced in ionization can be collected and measured.

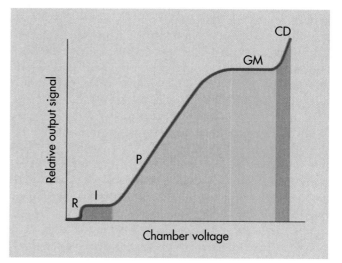

FIGURE 38-7 The amplitude of the signal from a gas-filled detector increases in stages as the voltage across the chamber is increased.

Ion Chamber Region. As the chamber voltage is increased, a condition is reached whereby every electron released by ionization is attracted to the central electrode and collected. The voltage at which this occurs varies according to the design of the chamber, but for most conventional instruments, it occurs in the range of 100 to 300 V.

This portion of the gas-filled detector performance curve is known as the **ionization region,** indicated by *I* in the Figure 38-7. Ion chambers are operated in this region.

Several different types of ion chambers are used in radiology; the most familiar of these is the portable survey instrument (Figure 38-8). This instrument is used principally for area radiation surveys. It can measure a wide range of radiation intensities, from 1 mR/hr (10 μGy_a/hr) to several thousand R/hr (Gy_a/hr).

The ion chamber is the instrument of choice for measuring radiation intensity in areas around a fluoroscope, around radionuclide generators and syringes, in the vicinity of patients with therapeutic quantities of radioactive materials, and outside of protective barriers. Other, more accurate ion chambers are used for precise calibration of the output intensity of diagnostic x-ray imaging systems (Figure 38-9).

Another application of a precision ion chamber is the dose calibrator (Figure 38-10). These devices find daily use in nuclear medicine laboratories for the assay of radioactive material.

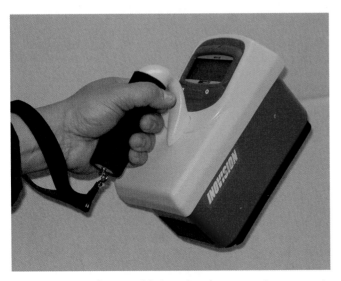

FIGURE 38-8 This portable ion chamber survey instrument is useful for radiation surveys when exposure levels are in excess of 1 mR/hr. (Courtesy Cardinal Health, Inc.)

Proportional Region. As the chamber voltage of the ideal gas-filled detector is increased still farther above the ionization region, electrons of the filling gas released by primary ionization are accelerated more rapidly to the central electrode. The faster these electrons travel, the greater is the probability that they will produce additional ionization on their way to the central electrode. These additional ionizations result in additional electrons called **secondary electrons.**

Secondary electrons also are attracted to the central electrode and collected. The total number of electrons collected in this fashion increases with increasing chamber voltage. The result is a rather large electron pulse for each primary ionization. This stage of the voltage response curve is known as the **proportional region.**

Proportional counters are sensitive instruments that are used primarily as stationary laboratory instruments for the assay of small quantities of radioactivity. One characteristic of proportional counters that makes them particularly useful is their ability to distinguish between alpha and beta radiation. Nevertheless, proportional counters find few applications in clinical radiology.

Geiger-Muller Region. The fourth region of the voltage response curve for the ideal gas-filled chamber is the **Geiger-Muller (G-M) region.** This is the region in which Geiger counters operate.

In the G-M region, the voltage across the ionization chamber is sufficiently high that, when a single ionizing

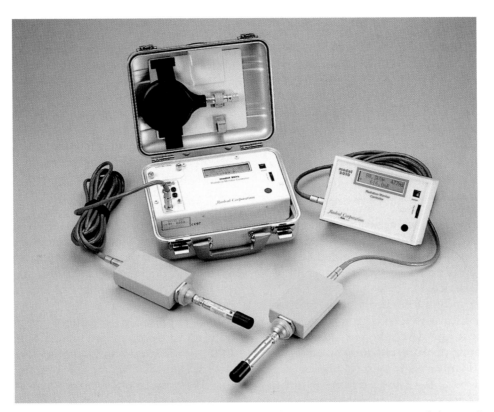

FIGURE 38-9 This ion chamber dosimeter is used for accurate measurement of diagnostic x-ray beams. (Courtesy Radcal Corp.)

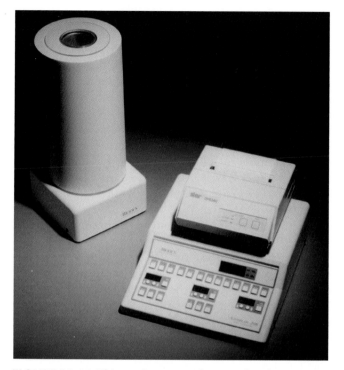

FIGURE 38-10 This configuration of an ion chamber is called a *dose calibrator*. It is used in nuclear medicine to measure accurately quantities of radioactive material. (Courtesy Biodex Medical Systems, Inc.)

event occurs, a cascade of secondary electrons is produced in a fashion similar to a very brief, yet violent, chain reaction. The effect is that nearly all molecules of the gas are ionized, liberating a large number of electrons. This results in a large electron pulse.

When sequential ionizing events occur soon after one another, the detector may not be capable of responding to a second event if the filling gas has not been restored to its initial condition. Therefore, a **quenching agent** is added to the filling gas of the Geiger counter to enable the chamber to return to its original condition; subsequent ionizing events then can be detected. The minimum time between ionizations that can be detected is known as the **resolving time.**

Geiger counters are used for contamination control in nuclear medicine laboratories. As portable survey instruments, they are used to detect the presence of radioactive contamination on work surfaces and laboratory apparatus.

They are not particularly useful as dosimeters because they are difficult to calibrate for varying conditions of radiation. Geiger counters are sensitive instruments that are capable of detecting and indicating single ionizing events. If they are equipped with an audio amplifier and a speaker, one can even hear the crackle of individual ionizations.

The Geiger counter does not have a very wide range. Most instruments are limited to less than 100 mR/hr (1 mGy$_a$/hr).

Region of Continuous Charge. If the voltage across the gas-filled chamber is increased still further, a condition is reached whereby a single ionizing event completely discharges the chamber, as in operation in the G-M region. Because of the high voltage, however, electrons continue to be stripped from atoms of the filling gas, producing a continuous current or signal from the chamber.

In this condition of continuous discharge, the instrument is useless for the detection of radiation, and continued operation in this region results in damage. The region of continuous discharge is indicated as *CD* in Figure 38-7.

Scintillation Detectors

Scintillation detectors are used in several areas of radiologic science. The scintillation detector is the basis for the gamma camera in nuclear medicine and is used in the detector arrays of CT imaging systems; it is the image receptor for several types of digital imaging systems.

The Scintillation Process. Some types of material scintillate when irradiated, that is, they emit a flash of light immediately in response to absorption of an x-ray. The amount of light emitted is proportional to the amount of energy absorbed by the material.

Consider, for example, the two x-ray interactions diagrammed in Figure 38-11. If a 50-keV x-ray interacts photoelectrically in the crystal, all the energy (50 keV) will reappear as light. If, however, that same x-ray interacts through a Compton scattering event in which only 20 keV of energy is absorbed, then a proportionately lower quantity of light will be emitted in the scintillation.

Only those materials with a particular crystalline structure scintillate. At the atomic level, the process involves the rearrangement of valence electrons into traps. The return of the electron from the trap to its normal position is immediate in scintillation and delayed in luminescence. This property was considered under an earlier discussion of luminescence (see Chapter 13).

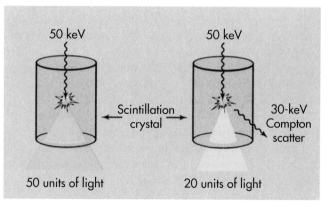

FIGURE 38-11 During scintillation, the intensity of light emitted is proportional to the amount of energy absorbed in the crystal.

Types of Scintillation Phosphors. Many different types of liquids, gases, and solids can respond to ionizing radiation by scintillation. Scintillation detectors are used most often to indicate individual ionizing events and are incorporated into fixed or portable radiation detection devices. They can be used to measure radiation in the rate mode or the integrate mode.

Nearly all the noble gases can be made to respond to radiation by scintillation. Such applications are rare, however, because the detection efficiency is very low and the probability of interaction therefore is small.

Liquid scintillation detectors are used frequently in the research laboratory to detect low-energy beta emissions from carbon-14 (^{14}C) and tritium (^3H). Because they present a relatively harmless radiation hazard and are incorporated easily into biologic molecules, ^{14}C and ^3H are useful research radionuclides.

These radionuclides emit low-energy beta particles with no associated gamma rays. This makes them difficult to detect. With liquid scintillation counting, however, biologic molecules can be mixed with a liquid scintillation phosphor so that the beta emission interacts directly with the phosphor, causing a flash of light to be emitted. Liquid scintillation counters have nearly 100% detection efficiency for beta radiation.

By far, the most widely used scintillation phosphors are the inorganic crystals—thallium-activated sodium iodide (NaI:Tl) and thallium-activated cesium iodide (CsI:Tl). The **activator atoms** of thallium are impurities grown into the crystal to control the spectrum of the light emitted and to enhance its intensity.

NaI:Tl crystals are incorporated into gamma cameras; CsI:Tl is the phosphor that is incorporated into image-intensifier tubes as the input phosphor and into flat panel digital radiography image receptors. Both types of crystals have been incorporated into CT imaging system detector arrays. However, many of today's CT imaging systems use cadmium tungstate ($CdWO_4$) or a ceramic as the scintillation detector.

The Scintillation Detector Assembly. Light produced during scintillation is emitted isotopically, that is, with equal intensity in all directions. Consequently, when used as radiation detectors, scintillation crystals are enclosed in aluminum with a polished inner surface in contact with the crystal. This allows the light flash to be reflected internally to the one face of a crystal that is not enclosed, which is called the **window.**

Aluminum containment is also necessary to seal the crystal hermetically. A **hermetic seal** is one that prevents the crystal from coming into contact with air or moisture. This is necessary because many scintillation crystals are **hygroscopic,** that is, they absorb moisture. When moisture is absorbed, the crystals swell and crack. Cracked crystals are not useful because the crack produces an interface that reflects and attenuates the scintillation.

Figure 38-12 shows the basic components of a single crystal–photomultiplier (PM) tube assembly representative of the type used in the portable survey instrument. The detector portion of the assembly is the NaI:Tl crystal contained in the aluminum hermetic seal. Coupled to the window of the crystal is a PM tube that converts light flashes from the scintillator into an electrical signal of pulses.

The PM tube is an electron vacuum tube that contains a number of elements. The tube consists of a **glass envelope,** which provides structural support for the internal elements and maintains the vacuum inside the tube.

The portion of the glass envelope that is coupled to the scintillation crystal is called the **window of the tube.** The crystal window and the PM tube window are sandwiched together with a silicone grease, which provides **optical coupling,** so that the light emitted by the scintillator is transmitted to the interior of the PM tube with minimum loss.

As light passes from the crystal into the PM tube, it is incident on a thin metal coating called a **photocathode,** which consists of a compound of cesium, antimony, and bismuth. Electrons are emitted from the photocathode by a process called **photoemission,** which is similar to thermionic emission in the filament of an x-ray tube, except that the stimulus is light rather than heat.

> A photocathode is a device that emits electrons when illuminated.

The flash of light from the scintillation crystal therefore is incident on the photocathode, and electrons are released by photoemission. The number of electrons emitted is directly proportional to the intensity of the light.

These photoelectrons are accelerated to the first of a series of plate-like elements called **dynodes.** Each dynode serves to amplify the electron pulse through **secondary electron emission.** For each electron incident on the dynode, several secondary electrons are emitted and directed

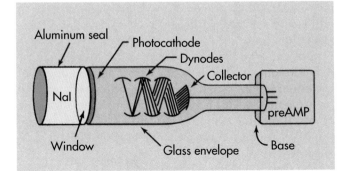

FIGURE 38-12 Scintillation detector assembly characteristics of the type used in a portable survey instrument.

to the next stage. Consequently, an electron gain occurs for each dynode in the PM tube.

 The dynode gain is the ratio of secondary electrons to incident electrons.

The number of dynodes and the gain of each dynode determine the overall electron gain of the PM tube. Photomultiplier tube gain is the dynode gain raised to the power of the number of dynodes.

PHOTOMULTIPLIER TUBE GAIN

PM tube gain = g^n
where dynode gain is g, and n is equal to the number of dynodes.

Question: An eight-stage PM tube (eight dynodes) has a dynode gain of three (three electrons emitted for each incident electron). What is the PM tube gain?

Answer: PM tube gain = 3^8 = 6561

The last plate-like element of the PM tube is the collecting electrode or **collector**. The collector absorbs the electron pulse from the last dynode and conducts it to the **preamplifier**. The preamplifier provides an initial state of pulse amplification. It is attached to the **base** of the PM tube, a structure that provides support for the glass envelope and internal structures.

The overall result of scintillation detection is that a single photon interaction produces a burst of light; this, in turn, produces photoelectron emission, which then is amplified to produce a relatively large electron pulse.

 The size of the electron pulse is proportional to the energy absorbed by the crystal from the incident photon.

It is this property of scintillation detection that promotes its use as an energy-sensitive device for **gamma spectrometry** that uses **pulse height analysis**. Through such an application, unknown gamma emitters can be identified and more sensitive radioisotope imaging can be accomplished by counting only those pulses with energy that represents total gamma ray absorption.

Scintillation detectors are sensitive devices for x-rays and gamma rays. They are capable of measuring radiation intensities as low as single-photon interactions. This property of scintillation detectors results in their use as portable radiation devices in much the same manner as Geiger counters are used.

A portable scintillation detector is more sensitive than a Geiger counter because it has much higher detection efficiency. For this application, the scintillation detector would be used to monitor the presence of contamination and perhaps low levels of radiation.

Thermoluminescence Dosimetry

Some materials glow when heated, thus exhibiting thermally stimulated emission of visible light, called *thermoluminescence*. In the early 1960s, Cameron and coworkers at the University of Wisconsin experimented with some thermoluminescent materials and were able to show that exposure to ionizing radiation caused some materials to glow particularly brightly when subsequently heated.

 TLD is the emission of light by a thermally stimulated crystal following irradiation.

Radiation-induced thermoluminescence has been developed into a sensitive and accurate method of radiation dosimetry for personnel radiation monitoring and for measurement of patient dose during diagnostic and therapeutic radiation procedures. Personnel and patient radiation monitoring is discussed later; however, at this time, it is important to discuss some of the basic principles of TLD (Figure 38-13).

After irradiation, the TLD phosphor is placed on a special dish or planchet for analysis in an instrument called a *TLD analyzer*. The temperature of the planchet can be controlled carefully. Directly viewing the planchet is a PM tube. The PM tube is the same type of light-sensitive and light-measuring vacuum tube that was described previously as a major component of scintillation detectors.

The PM tube–planchet assembly is placed in a chamber with a light-tight seal. The output signal from the PM tube is amplified and displayed.

The Glow Curve. As the temperature of the planchet is increased, the amount of light emitted by the TLD

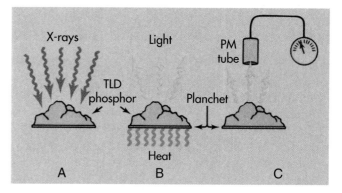

FIGURE 38-13 Thermoluminescence dosimetry is a multistep process. **A,** Exposure to ionizing radiation. **B,** Subsequent heating. **C,** Measurement of the intensity of emitted light.

increases in an irregular manner. Figure 38-14 shows the light output from lithium fluoride (LiF) as temperature increases. Several prominent peaks can be seen on the graph; each occurs because of a specific electron transition within the thermoluminescent crystals.

Such a graph is known as a **glow curve;** each type of thermoluminescent material has a characteristic glow curve. The height of the highest temperature peak and the total area under the curve are directly proportional to the energy deposited in the TLD by ionizing radiation. TLD analyzers are electronic instruments that are designed to measure the height of the glow curve or the area under the curve and relate this to exposure or dose through a conversion factor.

Types of Thermoluminescence Dosimetry Material. Many materials, including some body tissues, exhibit the property of radiation-induced thermoluminescence. Materials that are used for TLD, however, are somewhat limited in number and are principally types of inorganic crystals. Lithium fluoride (LiF) is the most widely used TLD material. It has an atomic number of 8.2 and therefore exhibits x-ray absorption properties similar to those of soft tissue.

LiF is relatively sensitive. It can measure doses as low as 5 mrad (50 μGy_t) with modest accuracy, and at doses exceeding 10 rad (100 mGy_t), its accuracy is better than 5%.

> Lithium fluoride is a nearly tissue-equivalent radiation dosimeter.

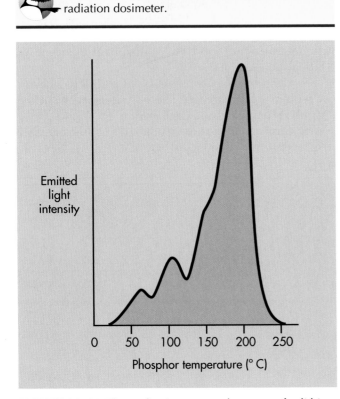

FIGURE 38-14 Thermoluminescence glow curve for lithium fluoride (LiF).

Calcium fluoride (CaF) activated with manganese (CaF_2:Mn) has a higher effective atomic number (Z = 16.3) than LiF; this makes it considerably more sensitive to ionizing radiation. CaF_2:Mn can measure radiation doses of less than 1 mrad (10 μGy_t) with moderate accuracy. Other types of TLDs are available; Table 38-5 lists some thermoluminescent phosphors and their principal characteristics and applications.

Properties of Thermoluminescence Dosimetry. A particular advantage of TLD is size. The TLD can be obtained in several solid crystal shapes and sizes. Rectangular rods measuring 1 x 1 x 6 mm and flat chips measuring 3 x 1 mm are the most popular sizes. The TLD also can be obtained in powder form; this allows irradiation in nearly any configuration. TLDs are also available with the phosphor matrixed with Teflon or plated onto a wire and sealed in glass.

The TLD is reusable. With irradiation, the energy absorbed by the TLD remains stored until released as visible light by heat during analysis. Heating restores the crystal to its original condition and makes it ready for another exposure.

The TLD responds proportionately to dose. If the dose is doubled, the TLD response also is doubled.

The TLD is rugged, and its small size makes it useful for monitoring dose in small areas, such as body cavities. The TLD does not respond to individual ionizing events; therefore, it cannot be used in a rate meter type of instrument. The TLD is suitable only for integral dose measurements, but it does not give immediate results. It must be analyzed after irradiation for dosimetry results.

Optically Stimulated Luminescence Dosimetry

An additional radiation dosimeter especially adapted for personnel monitoring was developed by Landauer in the late 1990s (Figure 38-15). The process is called *optically stimulated luminescence* (OSL) and uses aluminum oxide (Al_2O_3) as the radiation detector.

Irradiation of Al_2O_3 stimulates some electrons into an excited state. During processing, laser light stimulates these electrons, causing them to return to their ground state with the emission of visible light. The intensity of the visible light emission is proportional to the radiation dose received by the Al_2O_3.

The OSL process is not unlike TLD. Both are based on stimulated luminescence. However, OSL has several advantages over TLD, especially as applied to occupational radiation monitoring.

With a minimum reportable dose of 1 mrad, OSL is more sensitive than TLD. OSL has a precision of 1 mrad, which beats TLD. Other features of OSL include reanalysis for confirmation of dose, qualitative information about exposure conditions, wide dynamic range, and excellent long-term stability.

TABLE 38-5	Some Thermoluminescent Phosphors and Their Characteristics and Uses			
	Lithium Fluoride	**Lithium Borate**	**Calcium Fluoride**	**Calcium Sulfate**
Composition	LiF	$Li_2B_4O_7$:Mn	CaF_2:Mn	$CaSO_4$:Dy
Density 10^3 (kg/m³)	2.64	2.5	3.18	2.61
Effective atomic number	8.2	7.4	16.3	15.3
Temperature of main peak (° C)	195	200	260	220
Principal use	Patient and personnel dose	Research	Environmental monitoring	Environmental monitoring

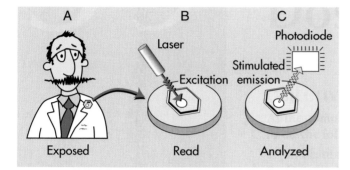

FIGURE 38-15 Optically stimulated luminescence dosimetry is a multistep process. **A,** Exposure to ionizing radiation. **B,** Laser illumination. **C,** Measurement of the intensity of stimulated light emission.

SUMMARY

Many radiation protection devices, accessories, and protocols are associated with modern x-ray imaging systems. This chapter discusses the radiation protection devices that are common to all radiographic and fluoroscopic imaging systems. Many of these devices are federally mandated; others exhibit features added by manufacturers.

Leakage radiation emitted by the x-ray tube during exposure must be contained by a protective x-ray tube housing. The limit of leakage must be no more than 100 mR per hour at a distance of 1 m from the housing. The control panel must indicate exposure by kVp and mA meters or visible and audible signals.

Great attention is given to the design of radiographic rooms, to the placement of x-ray imaging systems, and to the use of adjoining rooms. Two types of protective barriers are used: primary barriers and secondary barriers. Primary barriers intercept the useful x-ray beam and require the greatest amount of lead or concrete. Secondary barriers protect personnel from scatter and leakage radiation.

Dosimeters are instruments designed to detect and measure radiation. Other than photographic emulsion, four types of highly accurate devices are used to measure radiation. Gas-filled detectors include the ionization chamber, the proportional counter, and the Geiger-Muller counter. The scintillation detector is a very sensitive device that is used in nuclear medicine. Two other radiation detection devices used especially for occupational radiation monitoring are thermoluminescence dosimetry and optically stimulated luminescence dosimetry.

CHALLENGE QUESTIONS

1. Define or otherwise identify the following:
   a. TLD
   b. Use factor
   c. Diagnostic protective x-ray tube housing
   d. Glow curve
   e. Primary protective barrier
   f. X-ray linearity
   g. Secondary radiation
   h. Occupancy factor
   i. Geiger-Muller region
   j. Resolving time
2. What do audible and visible signals indicate on the radiographic control console?
3. List as many devices used for radiation protection on radiographic equipment as you can.
4. What is the result if the x-ray beam and the film are not properly aligned?
5. What filtration is used for mammography equipment operated below 30 kVp?
6. How are reproducibility and linearity different when the intensity of the x-ray beam is measured?
7. What characteristics of fluoroscopic equipment are designed for radiation protection?
8. How can filtration be measured if the amount of inherent and added filtration is unknown?
9. Name the three types of radiation exposure that are of concern when protective barriers are designed.
10. List four factors that are taken into consideration when a barrier for a radiographic room is designed.

ALL MEDICAL health physics activity is directed in some way toward minimizing the radiation exposure of radiologic personnel and the radiation dose to patients during x-ray examination. Radiation exposure of radiologists and radiologic technologists is measured with the use of occupational radiation monitors. Patient dose usually is estimated by conducting simulated x-ray examinations with human phantoms and test objects.

If radiation control procedures are adopted, occupational radiation exposure and patient dose can be kept acceptably low. Health physicists subscribe to ALARA—keep radiation exposure *as low as reasonably achievable*. Radiologic technologists should follow this guide as well.

PATIENT DOSE DESCRIPTIONS

Exposure of patients to medical x-rays is commanding increasing attention in our society for two reasons.

First, the frequency of x-ray examination is increasing among all age groups, at a rate of approximately 18% per year in the United States. This indicates that physicians are relying more and more on x-ray diagnosis to assist them in patient care, even taking into account the newer imaging modalities.

This is to be expected. X-ray diagnosis is considered much more accurate today than in the past. More rigorous training programs required of radiologists and radiologic technologists and improvements in diagnostic x-ray imaging systems allow for more difficult, but more substantive, x-ray examinations. Efficacy and diagnostic accuracy are much improved.

Second, concern among public health officials and radiation scientists is increasing regarding the risk that is associated with medical x-ray exposure. Acute effects on superficial tissues after angiointerventional procedures are reported with increasing frequency.

The possible late effects of diagnostic x-ray exposure are of concern; therefore, attention must be given to good radiation control practices. When a diagnosis can be obtained with a low radiation dose, it should be used because of reduced risk. This is in keeping with **ALARA.**

Estimation of Patient Dose

Patient dose from diagnostic x-rays usually is reported in one of three ways. Exposure to the entrance surface, or **entrance skin exposure (ESE)**, is reported most often because it is easy to measure.

The **gonadal dose** is important because of possible genetic responses to medical x-ray exposure. The dose to the gonads is not difficult to measure or estimate.

The dose to the **bone marrow** is important because bone marrow is the target organ believed responsible for radiation-induced leukemia. Bone marrow dose cannot be measured directly; it is estimated from ESE.

> Patient radiation dose is expressed as entrance skin exposure, gonadal dose, and bone marrow dose.

Table 39-1 presents some representative values of ESE and gonadal dose for various x-ray examinations. The mean marrow dose for each procedure also is presented. Note that these are only approximate values and should not be used to estimate patient dose at any facility.

In any given x-ray facility, actual doses delivered may be considerably different. Efficiency of x-ray production and image receptor speed are the most important variables. These values provide for relative dose comparisons among various radiologic examinations. Doses during fluoroscopy are too dependent on technique, equipment, and beam-on time to be estimated easily. Usually, such doses must be measured.

TABLE 39-1	Representative Radiation Quantities From Various Diagnostic X-ray Procedures			
Examination	Technique (kVp/mAs)	Entrance Skin Exposure (mR)	Mean Marrow Dose (mrad)	Gonad Dose (mrad)
Skull	76/50	200	10	<1
Chest	110/3	10	2	<1
Cervical spine	70/40	150	10	<1
Lumbar spine	72/60	300	60	225
Abdomen	74/60	400	30	125
Pelvis	70/50	150	20	150
Extremity	60/5	50	2	<1
CT (head)	125/300	4000	20	50
CT (pelvis)	125/400	2000	50	2000

CT, Computed tomography.

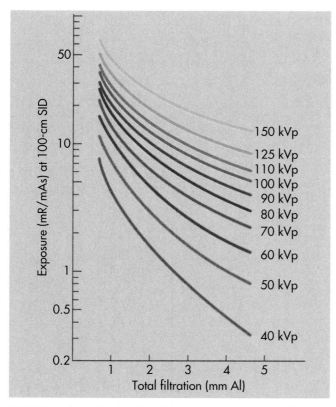

FIGURE 39-1 This family of curves is a nomogram for estimating output x-ray intensity from a single-phase radiographic unit. (Courtesy John R. Cameron,[†] University of Wisconsin.)

Entrance Skin Exposure. ESE most often is referred to as the *patient dose.* It is used widely because it is easy to measure, and reasonably accurate estimates can be made in the absence of measurements.

Thermoluminescence dosimeters (TLDs) are used most often. The size, sensitivity, and accuracy of TLDs make them very satisfactory patient radiation monitors.

A small grouping or pack of 3 to 10 TLDs can be taped easily to the patient's skin in the center of the x-ray field. Because the response of the TLD is proportional to exposure and dose, the TLD can be used to measure all levels experienced in diagnostic radiology. With proper laboratory technique, the results of such measurements are accurate to within 5%.

Two rather straightforward methods for estimating ESE are available in the absence of patient measurements. The first requires the use of a nomogram such as that shown in Figure 39-1. This figure contains a family of curves from which one can estimate the output intensity of a radiographic unit if the technique is known or assumed. The output intensity of different x-ray imaging systems varies widely, so the use of this nomogram method is good only to perhaps 50%.

Use of this nomogram first requires knowledge of the total filtration in the x-ray beam. This is usually available from the medical physics report, but if not,

3 mm Al is a good estimate. Next, the kVp and mAs of the intended examination should be identified.

A vertical line rising from the value of total filtration should be drawn until it intersects with the kVp of the examination. From this intersection, a horizontal line is drawn to the left until it intersects the mR/mAs axis. The resultant mR/mAs value is the approximate output intensity of the radiographic unit. This value should be multiplied with the examination mAs value to obtain the approximate patient exposure.

Question: With reference to Figure 39-1, estimate the ESE from a lateral cervical spine image made at 66 kVp, 150 mAs, with a radiographic unit having 2.5 mm Al total filtration.

Answer: Estimate the intersection between a vertical line rising from 2.5 mm Al and a horizontal line through 66 kVp. Extend the horizontal line to the y-axis and read 3.8 mR/mAs.
3.8 mR/mAs × 150 = 570 mR

A better approach requires that a medical physicist construct a nomogram such as that shown in Figure 39-2 for each radiographic unit. A straight edge between any kVp and mAs value will cross the ESE scale at the correct mR value.

Question: Using the nomogram in Figure 39-2, identify the ESE when a radiographic exposure is made at 66 kVp, 150 mAs.

Answer: The line is drawn as shown and crosses the ESE scale at 1000 mR.

A third method for estimating ESE requires that one know the output intensity for at least one operating condition. During the annual or special radiation control survey and calibration of an x-ray imaging system, the medical physicist measures this output intensity, usually in units of mR/mAs at 80 cm—the approximate source-to-skin distance (SSD)—or at 100 cm—the source-to-image receptor distance (SID). At 70 kVp, radiographic output intensity varies from approximately 2 to 10 mR/mAs at 80 cm SSD.

With this calibration value available, one first would make adjustment for a different SSD by applying the inverse square law.

Question: The output intensity of a radiographic unit is reported as 3.7 mR/mAs (37 μGy$_a$/mAs) at 100 cm SID. What is the intensity at 75 cm SSD?

Answer: At 75 cm SSD, the intensity will be greater by $(100/75)^2 = (1.32)^2 = 1.78$
3.7 mR/mAs × 1.78 = 6.6 mR/mAs

With the ESE, one scales this according to the kVp and mAs of the examination. Output intensity varies according to the square of the ratio in terms of the change in kVp. Refer to Chapter 9 to review this relationship.

Question: The output intensity at 70 kVp and 75 cm SSD is 6.6 mR/mAs (66 μGy$_a$/mAs). What is the output intensity at 76 kVp?

Answer: At higher kVp, the output intensity is greater by the square of the ratio of the kVp.

$$(76/70)^2 = (1.09)^2$$
$$= 1.18$$
$$6.6 \text{ mR/mAs} \times 1.18 = 7.8 \text{ mR/mAs}$$

The final step in estimating ESE is to multiply the output intensity in mR/mAs by the examination mAs value because these values are proportional.

Question: If the radiographic technique for an intravenous pyelogram calls for 80 mAs, what is the ESE when the output intensity is 7.8 mR/mAs (78 μGy$_a$/mAs)?

Answer: 7.8 mR/mAs × 80 mAs = 624 mR

These steps can be combined into a single calculation, as illustrated in the following example.

Question: The output intensity for a radiographic unit is 4.5 mR/mAs (4.5 μGy$_a$/mAs) at 70 kVp and 80 cm. If a lateral skull film is taken at 66 kVp, 150 mAs, what will be the ESE at an 80-cm SSD? What would be the skin dose at a 90-cm SSD?

Answer: At 80 cm SSD

$$\text{Dose} = (4.5 \text{ mR/mAs})\left(\frac{66 \text{ kVp}}{70 \text{ kVp}}\right)^2 (150 \text{ mAs})$$

$$= 600 \text{ mR}$$

At 90 cm SSD

$$\text{Dose} = (600 \text{ mR})\left(\frac{80}{90}\right)^2 = 474 \text{ mR}$$

ESE in fluoroscopy is much more difficult to estimate because the x-ray field moves and sometimes varies in size. If the field were of one size and stationary, ESE would be directly related to exposure time.

For the average fluoroscopic examination, one can assume an ESE of 4 R/min.

Question: A fluoroscopic procedure requires 2.5 min at 90 kVp, 2 mA. What is the approximate ESE?

Answer: ESE = (4 R/min) (2.5 min) = 10 R

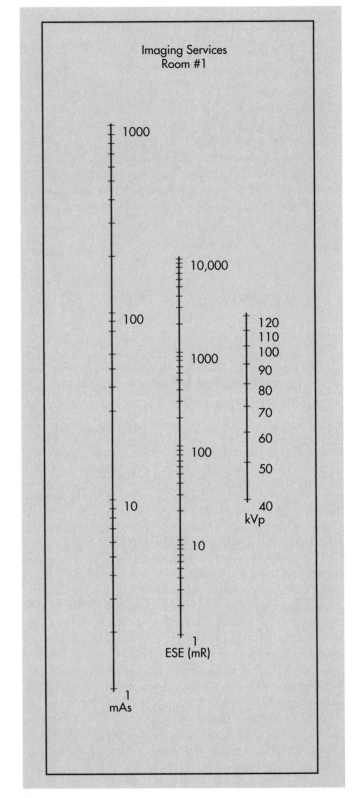

FIGURE 39-2 This type of nomogram is very accurate but must be fashioned individually for each radiographic unit. (Courtesy Michael D. Harpen, University of South Alabama.)

TABLE 39-2	Distribution of Active Bone Marrow in Adults	
Anatomic Site	**Percentage of Bone Marrow**	
Head	10	
Upper limb girdle	8	
Sternum	3	
Ribs	11	
Cervical vertebrae	4	
Thoracic vertebrae	13	
Lumbar vertebrae	11	
Sacrum	11	
Lower limb girdle	29	
Total	**100**	

TABLE 39-3	Genetically Significant Dose Estimated From Diagnostic X-ray Examination	
Population	**Genetically Significant Dose (mrad)**	
Denmark	22	
Great Britain	12	
Japan	27	
New Zealand	12	
Sweden	72	
United States	20	

Mean Marrow Dose. The hematologic effects of radiation are rarely experienced in diagnostic radiology. It is appropriate, however, that we understand the mean marrow dose, which is one measure of patient dose during diagnostic procedures.

The mean marrow dose is the average radiation dose to the entire active bone marrow. For instance, if during a particular examination, 50% of the active bone marrow were in the primary beam and received an average dose of 25 mrad (250 µGy$_t$), the mean marrow dose would be 12.5 mrad (125 µGy$_t$).

Table 39-1 includes the approximate mean marrow dose in adults for various radiographic examinations. In children, these levels generally would be lower because the radiographic techniques used are considerably less. Table 39-2 shows the distribution of active bone marrow in the adult, and this gives some clue as to which diagnostic x-ray procedures involve exposure to large amounts of bone marrow.

In the United States, the mean marrow dose from diagnostic x-ray examinations averaged over the entire population is approximately 100 mrad/yr (1 mGy$_t$/yr). Such a dose never results in the hematologic responses described in Chapter 35. It is a dose concept, however, that is used to estimate, on a population basis, the risk of one late effect of radiation—leukemia.

Genetically Significant Dose. Measurements and estimates of gonad dose are important because of the suspected genetic effects of radiation. Although the gonad dose from diagnostic x-rays is low for each individual, this may have some significance in terms of population effects.

The population gonad dose of importance is the **GSD,** the radiation dose to the population gene pool. Thus, it is a weighted-average gonad dose. It takes into account those persons who are irradiated and those who are not, with averaging of the results. The GSD can be estimated only through large-scale epidemiologic studies.

GENETICALLY SIGNIFICANT DOSE

$$GSD = \frac{\Sigma DN_X P}{\Sigma N_T P}$$

where Σ is the mathematical symbol meaning to sum or add values, D is the average gonad dose per examination, N_X signifies the number of persons receiving x-ray examinations, N_T is the total number of persons in the population, and P (progeny) is the expected future number of children per person.

For computational purposes, therefore, the GSD considers the age, sex, and expected number of children for each person examined with x-rays. It also acknowledges the various types of examinations and the gonadal dose per examination type.

Estimates of GSD have been conducted in many different countries (Table 39-3). The estimate reported by the U.S. Public Health Service is 20 mrad/yr (0.2 mGy$_t$/yr). Thus, this is a genetic radiation burden over and above the existing natural background radiation level of approximately 100 mrad/yr (1 mGy$_t$/yr). The genetic effects of this total GSD—120 mrad/yr (1.2 mGy$_t$/yr)—are not detectable.

Patient Dose in Special Examinations

Dose in Mammography. Because of the considerable application of x-rays for examination of the female breast and concern for the induction of breast cancer by radiation, it is imperative that we have some understanding of the radiation doses involved in such examinations.

The genetically significant dose (GSD) is the gonad dose that, if received by every member of the population, would produce the total genetic effect on the population as the sum of the individual doses actually received.

Screen-film and digital mammography currently are the only acceptable techniques.

An ESE of approximately 800 mR/view (8 mGy$_a$/view) is normal. Increasing the x-ray tube potential much beyond 26 kVp degrades the image unacceptably; therefore, further dose reduction by technique manipulation is unlikely.

Radiographic grids are used in most screen-film mammography examinations. Grid ratios of 4:1 and 5:1 are most popular. The contrast enhancement produced by the use of such grids is significant, but so is the increase in patient dose. Patient dose is increased by approximately two times with the use of such grids compared with the nongrid technique.

The values stated for patient dose in mammography can be misleading. Because of the low x-ray energies used in mammography, the dose falls off very rapidly as the x-ray beam penetrates the breast. If the ESE for a craniocaudad view is 800 mR (8 mGy$_a$), the dose to the midline of the breast may be only 100 mrad (1.0 mGy$_t$).

Fortunately, it is known that the risk of an adverse biologic response from mammography is small. Certainly, it is nothing about which a patient should be concerned. Any possible response, however, is related to the average radiation dose to glandular tissue, and not to skin exposure. **Glandular dose** (D_g) varies in a complicated way, with variations noted in x-ray beam quality and quantity.

Glandular dose is approximately 15% of the ESE.

Specification of an ESE can be misleading when one considers a two-view examination, such as that used for screening (Figure 39-3). Consider an examination that consists of craniocaudad and mediolateral oblique views, each of which produces an ESE of 800 mR (8 mGy$_a$).

It would be incorrect to describe this total examination procedure as resulting in an ESE of 1.6 R (16 mGy$_a$). Skin exposures from different projections cannot be added. We must specify the skin exposure for each view or attempt to estimate the total D_g.

Total D_g can be estimated by approximating that the contribution from each view will be 15% of the ESE. Consequently, the total D_g would be the sum of (0.15 × 800 = 120 mrad [1.2 mGy$_t$]) as the contribution from each of the craniocaudad and mediolateral oblique views. The total D_g would, therefore, be 240 mrad (2.4 mGy$_t$).

Glandular dose should not exceed 100 mrad/view with contact mammography and 300 mrad/view with a grid.

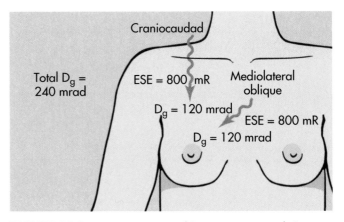

FIGURE 39-3 Two mammographic exposures result in a total glandular dose that is the sum of the individual glandular doses.

From this discussion, it would seem that patient dose in mammography can be considerably reduced if the number of views is restricted. The axillary view should not be done routinely. For screening programs, no more than two views per breast are advisable. Digital mammography should result in lower D_g than that attained with screen-film mammography.

Dose in Computed Tomography Imaging. An important consideration in computed tomography (CT) imaging, as with any x-ray procedure, is not only the skin dose but also the distribution of dose to internal organs and tissues during imaging. On the basis of skin dose, CT results in a higher dose than other diagnostic x-ray procedures. The skin dose delivered by a series of contiguous CT slices is much higher than that delivered by a single radiographic view. A typical radiographic head or body examination, however, often involves several views.

Because of increasing use of multislice spiral CT, CT must be considered a high-dose procedure. U.S. Public Health Service data suggest that 10% of all x-ray examinations are now CT, yet CT accounts for 70% of total patient effective dose. The CT tissue dose is approximately equal to the average fluoroscopic dose.

As was pointed out in Chapter 23, CT differs in many important ways from other x-ray examinations. A radiograph can be likened to a photograph taken with a flash in that the patient is "floodlighted" with x-rays to directly expose the image receptor.

On the other hand, CT images the patient with a fine, collimated beam of x-rays. This difference in radiation delivery also means that the **dose distribution** from CT is different from that in radiographic procedures.

The CT dose is nearly uniform throughout the imaging volume for a head examination. The CT dose is approximately 50% of the ESE for body CT. Radiographic and fluoroscopic doses are high at the entrance surface and very low at the exit surface.

Part of the dose efficiency of CT is attributable to the precise collimation of the x-ray beam. Scatter radiation

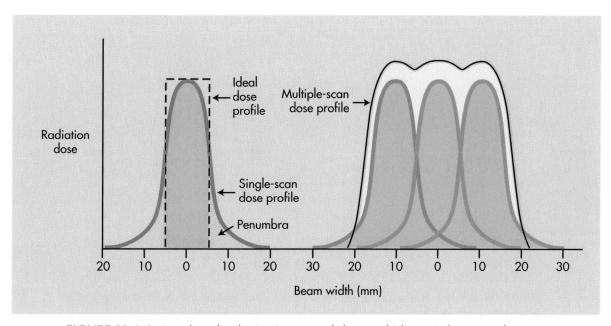

FIGURE 39-4 Patient dose distribution in step-and-shoot multislice spiral computed tomography is complicated because the profile of the x-ray beam cannot be made sharp.

increases patient dose and reduces radiographic contrast. Because CT uses narrow, well-collimated x-ray beams, scatter radiation is reduced significantly, and contrast resolution is improved significantly. Thus, a larger percentage of the x-ray beam contributes usefully to the image.

The precise collimation used in CT means that only a well-defined volume of tissue is irradiated for each image. The ideal x-ray beam for CT would have sharp boundaries. No overlap between adjacent images would be seen. Thus, the dose delivered to a patient from a series of ideal contiguous CT images should be the same as that from a single slice.

Figure 39-4 illustrates, however, why this ideal situation cannot be attained in practice. The size of the focal spot of the x-ray tube blurs the sharp boundaries of the section. Also, the x-ray beam is not precisely parallel, and some spreading occurs as the beam crosses the image field.

If a series of adjacent images is performed with an automatically indexed patient couch, the couch movement must be precise. If the couch moves too much between images, some tissue will be missed. If it moves too little, some tissue in each image will be doubled-exposed.

> It is essential that CT collimators be monitored periodically for proper adjustment.

Multislice spiral CT results in lower patient dose than conventional step-and-shoot CT because fewer tails are seen on the dose profile for a given volume of tissue. The dose profile tail is called a *penumbra*.

Typical CT doses range from 3000 to 5000 mrad (30 to 50 mGy$_t$) during head imaging and from 2000 to 4000 mrad (20 to 40 mGy$_t$) during body imaging. These values are only approximate and vary widely depending on the type of CT imaging system and the examination technique used. The effective dose for each examination is approximately 1000 mrem (10 mSv).

A 64-slice CT imaging system will result in a lower patient dose than fewer slices because a lower contribution is made from the penumbra for the same volume of tissue (Figure 39-5). Additional patient dose saving occurs when the same beam width is imaged with combined pixel rows (Figure 39-6) because the mA can be reduced without compromising image noise and therefore contrast resolution.

> The higher the multislice value, the lower the patient dose will be.

Because the CT x-ray beam is well collimated, the area of irradiation can be precisely controlled. Thus, radiosensitive organs such as the eyes can be avoided selectively. Shields as protection from the primary x-ray beam in CT are of little use. Not only does the metal from shields produce artifacts in the image, but the rotational scheme of the x-ray source greatly reduces their effectiveness.

Patient dose during spiral CT is somewhat more difficult to assess than the dose during conventional step-and-shoot CT. At a pitch of 1.0:1, the patient dose is approximately the same. At a higher pitch, the dose is reduced compared with conventional CT. At a lower pitch, patient dose is increased.

As with any radiographic procedure, many factors influence patient dose. For CT imaging, a generalization is possible.

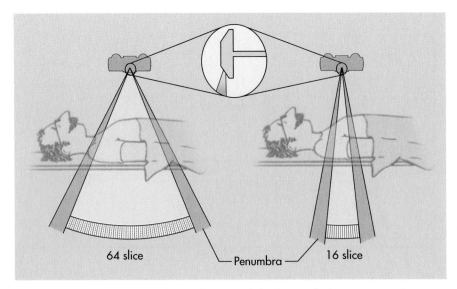

FIGURE 39-5 Patient radiation dose is lower with higher multislice computed tomography because the beam penumbra is less for a given imaged anatomy.

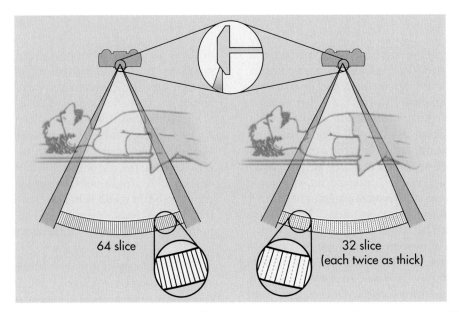

FIGURE 39-6 When two detector rows are combined for the same beam width, patient dose will be lower.

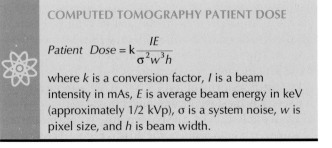

COMPUTED TOMOGRAPHY PATIENT DOSE

$$Patient\ Dose = k\frac{IE}{\sigma^2 w^3 h}$$

where k is a conversion factor, I is a beam intensity in mAs, E is average beam energy in keV (approximately 1/2 kVp), σ is a system noise, w is pixel size, and h is beam width.

Note that, as with radiography, patient dose is proportional to x-ray beam intensity. It is also directly proportional to the average beam energy. Other factors are variables that are unique to CT imaging.

Sigma (σ) is noise. This is equivalent to quantum mottle in screen-film radiography and represents random statistical variations in CT numbers. The w stands for the pixel size, one of the determinants of spatial resolution. The last factor, h, is the beam width.

> A reduction in the noise or beam width, while other factors remain constant, increases patient dose.

All other factors being equal, a low-noise, high-resolution CT image results in higher patient dose. The challenge with CT, as indeed with all x-ray imaging, is not so much to deliver fantastically good resolution and low noise (because this could be achieved at the cost of very high patient dose) but to use the x-ray beam efficiently, producing the best possible image at a reasonable dose to the patient.

REDUCTION OF UNNECESSARY PATIENT DOSE

The radiologic technologist has considerable control over many sources of unnecessary patient dose. Unnecessary patient dose is defined as any radiation dose that is not required for the patient's well-being or for proper management and care.

Unnecessary Examinations

The radiologic technologist has practically no control over what some consider the largest source of unnecessary patient dose, that is, the unnecessary x-ray examination. This is almost exclusively the radiologist's or the clinician's responsibility. Radiologic technologists can help by asking whether the patient has had a previous x-ray examination. If so, perhaps those images should be obtained for review before any other steps are taken.

Unfortunately, this source of unnecessary patient dose presents a serious dilemma for the radiologist and the clinician. Many x-ray examinations are requested when it is known that the yield of helpful information may be extremely low or nonexistent. When such an examination is performed, the benefit to the patient in no way compensates for the radiation dose.

If the examination is not performed, however, the clinician and the radiologist may be criticized severely if management of the patient's condition results in failure. Even though the examination in question would have contributed little, if anything, to effective patient management, the radiologist may even be sued. In such situations, the radiologist is caught between the proverbial "rock and a hard place."

Routine x-ray examinations should not be performed when there is no precise medical indication. Substantial evidence shows that such examinations are of little benefit because they are not cost-effective and the disease detection rate is very low. Examples of such cases are discussed in the following sections.

Mass Screening for Tuberculosis. General screening by chest x-ray examination has not been found to be effective. Better methods of tuberculosis testing are now available. Some x-ray screening in high-risk groups (e.g., medical and paramedical personnel), in service personnel posing a potential community hazard (e.g., food handlers, teachers), and in special occupational groups (e.g., miners, workers having contact with beryllium, asbestos, glass, or silica) may be appropriate.

Hospital Admission. Chest x-ray examinations should not be performed for routine hospital admission when no clinical indication of chest disease is found.

Among patients who might be candidates for such examination are those admitted to the pulmonary service.

Preemployment Physicals. Chest and lower back x-ray examinations are not justified because the knowledge gained about previous injury or disease through this approach is nil.

Periodic Health Examinations. Many physicians and health care organizations promote annual or biannual physical examinations. Certainly, when such an examination is conducted on an asymptomatic patient, it should not include x-ray examination, especially fluoroscopic examination.

Emergency Room CT. CT has passed radiography as the first line of diagnostic imaging. This overutilization must be controlled because of the rapidly rising population effective dose.

Whole-Body Multislice Spiral CT Screening. Some facilities now offer this procedure to the public for self-referral. Until evidence reveals a significant disease detection rate, this should not be done. The radiation dose is too high.

Repeat Examinations

One area of unnecessary radiation exposure that the radiologic technologist can influence is that of repeat examinations. The frequency of repeat examinations has been estimated variously to range as high as 10% of all examinations. In the typical busy hospital facility, the rate of repeat examinations should not normally exceed 5%. Examinations with the highest repeat rates include lumbar spine, thoracic spine, and abdomen.

> It should never be necessary to repeat a digital radiographic examination.

Some repeat examinations are performed because of equipment malfunction. However, most are caused by radiologic technologist error. Studies of causes of repeat examinations have shown that improper positioning and poor radiographic technique resulting in an image that is too light or too dark are primarily responsible for repeats.

Motion and improper collimation are responsible for some repeats. Infrequent errors that contribute to repeat examinations include dirty screens, use of improperly loaded cassettes, light leaks, chemical fog, artifacts caused by a dirty processor, wrong projection, improper patient preparation, grid errors, and multiple exposures.

Radiographic Technique

In general, the use of high-kVp technique results in reduced patient dose. Increasing the kVp is always associated with a reduction in mAs to obtain an acceptable radiographic optical density; this, in turn, results in reduced patient dose.

This dose reduction occurs because the patient dose is linearly related to the mAs but is related to approximately the square of the kVp. An area of radiography for which high-kVp technique is widely accepted is examination of the chest.

Question: A lateral skull radiograph is obtained at 64 kVp, 80 mAs, and results in an ESE of 400 mR (4 mGy$_a$). If the tube potential is increased to 74 kVp (15% increase) and the mAs is reduced by half, to 40 mAs, the optical density will remain the same. What will be the new ESE?

Answer:
$$Dose = (400 \text{ mR})\left(\frac{40 \text{ mAs}}{80 \text{ mAs}}\right)\left(\frac{74 \text{ kVp}}{64 \text{ kVp}}\right)^2$$

$$= (400 \text{ mR})(0.5)(1.34)$$

$$= 268 \text{ mR}$$

Of course, the radiologist must be the final judge of radiographic quality. Increasing kVp even slightly may result in images with contrast that is too low for proper interpretation by the radiologist.

 Digital radiography can be conducted at higher kVp, resulting in lower patient dose.

Proper collimation is essential to good radiographic technique. Positive beam limitation does not prevent the radiologic technologist from reducing field size still further through collimation. With the use of collimation, not only is patient effective dose reduced, but image quality is improved with enhanced contrast resolution because scatter radiation also is reduced.

Image Receptor

The image receptor should be selected first for the type of examination that is being performed, and second for the radiation dose necessary to produce a good-quality image. It should be kept in mind that it is screen speed rather than film speed that principally controls patient dose.

 The fastest-speed screen-film combination consistent with the nature of the examination should be used.

Rare Earth and other fast screens should be used when possible. The routine application of such screens in orthopedic, chest, and magnification radiography is appropriate. In some applications, the use of such fast systems may result in bothersome quantum mottle, but this again must be decided by the radiologist. Usually, 400-speed systems are used now for general radiography.

Digital radiographic (DR) image receptors are inherently faster than screen-film. Patient dose should be lower with the use of DR because of increased speed and increased kVp accompanied by reduced mAs.

Patient Positioning

When the upper extremities or the breast is examined, especially with the patient in a seated position, care should be taken that the useful beam does not intercept the gonads. Position the patient lateral to the useful beam and provide a protective apron as a shield.

Specific Area Shielding

X-ray examinations result in partial-body exposure, although most radiation protection guides and radiation response information are based on whole-body exposure. The partial-body nature of the x-ray examination is controlled by proper beam collimation and the use of specific area shielding.

Use of specific area shielding is indicated when a particularly sensitive tissue or organ is in or near the useful beam. The lens of the eye, the breasts, and the gonads frequently are shielded from the primary radiation beam. Two types of specific area shielding devices are used: the **contact shield** and the **shadow shield.**

Lens shields are always of the contact type. The contact shielding device is positioned directly on the patient. Gonad shields, on the other hand, can be of the contact or shadow type.

Breast shields are contact shields that are recommended for use during scoliosis examinations. Such examinations often consist of an anterior-posterior (AP) projection, which subjects juvenile breasts to primary beam x-irradiation. The posterior-anterior (PA) projection, however, is equally satisfactory because magnification is of little importance. The PA projection results in a breast dose of only approximately 1% of the AP projection.

Figure 39-7 shows some examples of contact gonad shields. When such contact shields are not purchased commercially, a properly cut piece of protective material is perfectly adequate. Shapes such as hearts, diamonds, triangles, and squares have been used effectively, especially for children.

An example of the shadow shield is shown in Figure 39-8. This type of shield is just as effective as the contact shield and is more acceptable for use with adult patients. The use of such devices, however, requires careful attention on the part of the radiologic technologist.

The shield must shadow the gonads without interfering with the desired anatomy. Improper positioning of the shadow shield can result in a repeat examination and increased patient dose. Shadow shields are particularly useful during surgery for which sterile procedure is required. Box 39-1 lists the main points of gonadal shielding.

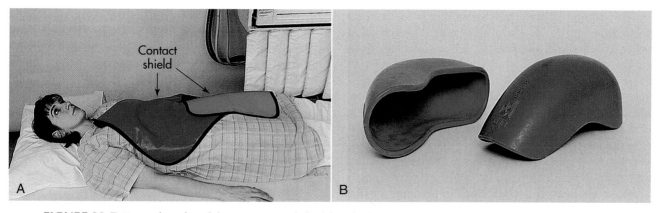

FIGURE 39-7 Examples of useful contact gonad shields, which can be a piece of vinyl lead (**A**) or shaped (**B**).

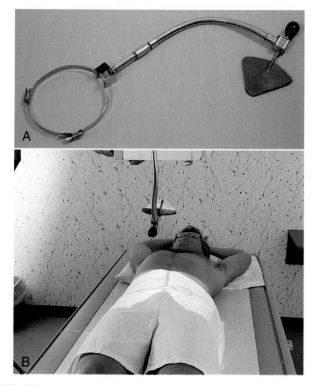

FIGURE 39-8 **A,** Shadow shield. **B,** Shadow shield suspended above the beam-defining system casts a shadow over the gonads. (Courtesy Fluke Biomedical.)

BOX 39-1   Gonad Shielding

- Gonad shielding should be considered for all patients, especially children and those who are potentially reproductive. As an administrative procedure, this would include all patients younger than 40 years of age and perhaps even older men.
- Gonad shielding should be used when the gonads lie in or near the useful beam.
- Proper patient positioning and beam collimation should not be relaxed when gonad shields are in use.
- Gonad shielding should be used only when it does not interfere with obtaining the required diagnostic information.

THE PREGNANT PATIENT

Two situations in diagnostic radiology require particular care and action. Both are associated with pregnancy. Their importance is obvious from both a physical and an emotional standpoint.

Radiobiologic Considerations

The severity of the potential response to radiation exposure in utero is both time related and dose related, as was discussed in Chapter 36. Unquestionably, the period most sensitive to radiation exposure occurs before birth. Furthermore, the fetus is more sensitive early in pregnancy than late in pregnancy. As a general rule, the higher the radiation dose, the more severe will be the radiation response.

Time Dependence. A grave misunderstanding is that the most critical time for irradiation is during the first 2 weeks, when it is most unlikely that the expectant mother knows of her condition. In fact, this is the time during pregnancy when such irradiation is least hazardous. Pregnancies fail during this period for reasons other than exposure to radiation.

The most likely biologic response to irradiation during the first 2 weeks of pregnancy is resorption of the embryo, and therefore no pregnancy. No other response is likely.

No concern has been expressed over the possibility of induction of congenital abnormalities during the first 2 weeks of pregnancy. Such a response has not been demonstrated in experimental animals or in humans after any level of radiation dose.

The time from approximately the second week to the tenth week of pregnancy is called the period of **major organogenesis**. During this time, the major organ systems of the fetus are developing. If the radiation dose is sufficiently high, congenital abnormalities may result.

Early in organogenesis, the most likely congenital abnormalities are associated with skeletal deformities. Later in this period, neurologic deficiencies are more likely to occur.

During the second and third trimesters of pregnancy, the responses previously noted are unlikely. The results of numerous investigations strongly suggest that if a response occurs after diagnostic irradiation during the latter two trimesters, the principal response would be the appearance of malignant disease during childhood.

These responses to irradiation during pregnancy require a very high radiation dose before the risk of occurrence is significant. No such responses would occur at less than 25 rad (250 mGy).

Such dose levels are highly unlikely, yet they are possible with patients who receive multiple x-ray examinations of the abdomen or pelvis. They are essentially impossible with radiologic technologists because their occupational exposures are so low. No other significant responses have been reported after irradiation in utero.

Dose Dependence. As one might imagine, virtually no information is available at the human level to construct dose-response relationships for irradiation in utero. However, a large body of data on animal irradiation, particularly that in rats and mice, serves as the basis from which such relationships can be estimated. The statements that follow, although attributed to human exposure, represent estimates based on extrapolation from animal studies.

After an in utero radiation dose of 200 rad (2 Gy), it is nearly certain that each of the effects noted previously will occur. The likelihood is small, however, that an exposure of this magnitude would be experienced in diagnostic radiology.

Spontaneous abortion after irradiation during the first 2 weeks of pregnancy is unlikely at radiation doses less than 25 rad (250 mGy). The precise nature of the dose-response relationship is unknown, but a reasonable estimate of risk suggests that 0.1% of all conceptions would be resorbed after a dose of 10 rad (100 mGy).

The response at lower doses would be proportionately lower. Keep in mind, however, that the incidence of spontaneous abortion in the absence of radiation exposure is estimated to be in the 25% to 50% range.

In the absence of radiation exposure, approximately 5% of all live births exhibit a manifest congenital abnormality. A 1% increase in congenital abnormalities is estimated to follow a 10-rad (100-mGy) fetal dose, with a proportionately lower increase at lower doses.

The induction of a childhood malignancy after irradiation in utero is difficult to assess. Risk estimates are even lower than those reported for spontaneous abortion and congenital abnormalities. The best approach to assessing risk of childhood malignancy is to use a relative risk estimate.

During the first trimester, the relative risk of radiation-induced childhood malignancy is in the range of 5 to 10; it drops to approximately 1.4 during the third trimester. The overall relative risk is accepted to be 1.5—a 50% increase over the naturally occurring incidence.

Patient Information

Safeguards against accidental irradiation early in pregnancy present complex administrative problems. This situation is particularly critical during the first 2 months of pregnancy, when such a condition may not be suspected, and when the fetus is particularly sensitive to radiation exposure. After 2 months, the risk of irradiating an unknown pregnancy becomes small because the patient is usually aware of her condition.

If the state of pregnancy is known, then under some circumstances, the radiologic examination should not be conducted. One should never knowingly examine a pregnant patient with x-rays unless a documented decision to do so has been made. When such an examination does proceed, it should be conducted with all of the previously discussed techniques for minimizing patient dose.

When a pregnant patient must be examined, the examination should be done with precisely collimated beams and carefully positioned protective shields. The use of high-kVp technique is most appropriate in such situations. The administrative protocols that can be used to ensure that we do not irradiate pregnant patients vary from complex (elective booking) to simple (posting).

Elective Booking. The most direct way to ensure against the irradiation of an unsuspected pregnancy is to institute **elective booking.** This requires that the clinician, radiologist, or radiologic technologist determine the time of the patient's previous menstrual cycle. X-ray examinations in which the fetus is not in or near the primary beam may be allowed, but they should be accompanied by pelvic shielding.

Ideally, the referring physician should be responsible for determining the menstrual cycle and for withholding the examination request if there is any question about its necessity. This may require a radiologist-sponsored educational program that can be conducted easily at regularly scheduled medical staff meetings.

Patient Questionnaire. An alternative procedure is to have the patient herself indicate her menstrual cycle. In many diagnostic imaging departments, the patient must complete an information form before undergoing examination.

X-Ray Consent for Women of Childbearing Age

X-ray examinations of abdomen and pelvis exposing the uterus to radiation are:

Abdomen (KUB)	Colon (barium enema)	Pyelograms (IVP and retrograde)
Stomach (UGI)	Gallbladder	Cystograms
Small Intestine (SI)	Hips, sacrum, coccyx	Lumbar spine and pelvis
All nuclear medicine studies		

The 10 days after onset of menstural period are generally considered safe for x-ray examinations.

Onset of last menstural period   Date _____   Date today _____

I am pregnant   Yes _____   No _____   Don't know _____
I have had a hysterectomy   Yes _____   No _____   Don't know _____
I use an IUD   Yes _____   No _____   Don't know _____

I recognize that if I am pregnant and have radiation to the abdomen, there is a possibility of injury to the fetus. However, I understand that the likelihood of such injury is slight and that my physician feels that the information to be gained from this examination is important to my health. I therefore wish to have this x-ray examination performed now.

_____
Name of examination

_____
Signature of patient

_____
Witness

FIGURE 39-9 X-ray consent for women of childbearing age.

These forms often include questions such as, "Are you or could you be pregnant?" and "What was the date of your last menstrual period?" Figure 39-9 is an example of such a simple, yet effective questionnaire for protecting against irradiation of a pregnant patient.

Posting. If neither elective booking nor the request form seems appropriate to a diagnostic imaging service, an equally successful method is to post signs of caution in the waiting room. Such signs could read, "Are you pregnant or could you be? If so, inform the radiologic technologist," or "Warning—special precautions are necessary if you are pregnant," or "Caution—if there is any possibility that you are pregnant, it is very important that you inform the radiologic technologist before you have an x-ray examination."

We meet our responsibility to the pregnant patient by posting signs in the waiting room.

Figure 39-10 is a helpful poster that is available from the National Center for Devices and Radiological Health.

Such posting satisfies our responsibility to the patient and to the health care facility.

It has been estimated that less than 1% of all women referred for x-ray examination are potentially pregnant. If a pregnant patient escapes detection and is irradiated, however, what is the subsequent responsibility of the radiology service to the patient, and what should be done?

The first step is to estimate the fetal dose. The medical physicist should be consulted immediately and requested to estimate the fetal dose. If a preliminary review of the examination techniques used (i.e., type of examination, kVp, and mAs) determines that the dose may have exceeded 1 rad (10 mGy$_t$), a more complete dosimetric evaluation should be conducted.

Table 39-4 presents representative fetal dose levels for many examinations. With knowledge of the types of examinations performed and the techniques and apparatus used, the medical physicist can accurately determine the fetal dose. Test objects and dosimetry materials are available to ensure that this determination can be made with confidence.

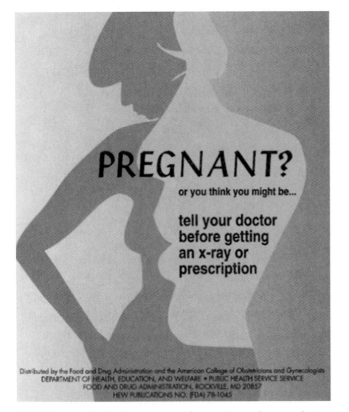

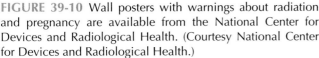

FIGURE 39-10 Wall posters with warnings about radiation and pregnancy are available from the National Center for Devices and Radiological Health. (Courtesy National Center for Devices and Radiological Health.)

TABLE 39-4	Representative Entrance Exposures and Fetal Doses for Radiographic Examinations Frequently Performed With a 400-Speed Image Receptor	
Examination	**Entrance Skin Exposure (mR)**	**Fetal Dose (mrad)**
Skull (lateral)	70	0
Cervical spine (AP)	110	0
Shoulder	90	0
Chest (PA)	10	0
Thoracic spine (AP)	180	1
Cholecystogram (PA)	150	1
Lumbosacral spine (AP)*	250	80
Abdomen or KUB (AP)*	220	70
Intravenous pyelogram (IVP)*	210	60
Hip*	220	50
Wrist or foot	5	0

AP, Anteroposterior; *IVP,* intravenous pyelogram; *KUB,* kidneys, ureters, bladder; *PA,* posterior-anterior.

*Gonadal shields should be used if possible.

Once the fetal dose is known, the referring physician and the radiologist should determine the stage of gestation at which x-ray exposure occurred. With this information, only two alternatives are possible: Allow the patient to continue to term, or terminate the pregnancy.

Recommendation for abortion after diagnostic x-ray exposure is rarely indicated. Because the natural incidence of congenital anomalies is approximately 5%, no such effects can reasonably be considered a consequence of diagnostic x-ray doses. Manifest damage to the newborn is unlikely at fetal doses below 25 rad (250 mGy$_t$), although some suggest that lower doses may cause mental developmental abnormalities.

In view of the available evidence, a reasonable approach is to apply a 10- to 25-rad rule. Below 10 rad (100 mGy$_t$), a therapeutic abortion is not indicated unless additional risk factors are involved. Above 25 rad (250 mGy$_t$), the risk of latent injury may justify a therapeutic abortion.

Between 10 and 25 rad, the precise time of irradiation, the emotional state of the patient, the effect an additional child would have on the family, and other social and economic factors must be considered carefully.

Fortunately, experience with such situations has shown that fetal doses have been consistently low. The fetal dose rarely exceeds 5 rad (50 mGy$_t$) after a series of x-ray examinations.

PATIENT DOSE TRENDS

The National Council on Radiation Protection and Measurements (NCRP) issues scientific reports on various aspects of radiation control, including patient radiation dose. The data shown in the pie chart in Figure 1-23 were published in 1990. They show a total annual radiation dose of 3.6 mSv, of which 0.53 mSv results from patient diagnostic radiation exposure.

Figure 39-11 is from data in a soon-to-be published NCRP report showing the current estimated human radiation exposure profile. Natural sources of radiation exposure remain at 3 mSv, but look what's happening to medical imaging, 3.2 mSv! The contribution from computed tomography is soaring and represents the overutilization of this imaging modality.

This increase in patient radiation dose requires that radiologic technologists and radiologists exercise more control over medical imaging, especially computed tomography, in keeping with ALARA. We must be more aware of appropriateness criteria for diagnostic imaging and gain more control over unnecessary x-ray imaging.

With the introduction of digital imaging we are in a better position to automatically estimate the patient effective dose for each x-ray examination and record that to a continuing patient dose file. We monitor our occupational radiation exposure for life; we will be instituting protocols to do the same for our medical radiation exposure.

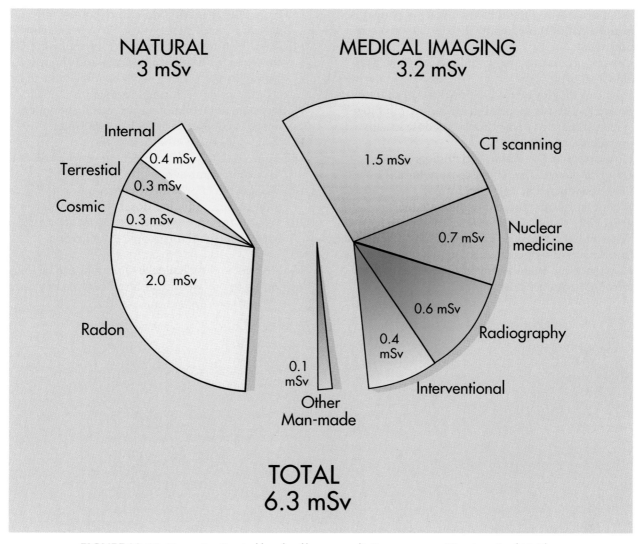

FIGURE 39-11 Current estimated levels of human radiation exposure. (Courtesy Fred Mettler, University of New Mexico.)

SUMMARY

Patient dose from diagnostic x-rays usually is recorded in one of the following three ways: (1) ESE, (2) mean marrow dose, or (3) gonadal dose. TLDs are the monitor of choice for patient radiation dose. By knowing the output intensity of at least one x-ray technique and the SSD, the medical physicist can estimate the ESE for any patient examination. For fluoroscopic examination, a good general assumption for the ESE is 4 R/min.

Patient radiation dose can be reduced easily by eliminating unnecessary examinations and repeat examinations, and by ensuring proper radiographic technique and patient positioning. The radiobiology of pregnancy requires particular attention to the pregnant patient. By posting the waiting room and the examination room with educational signs, we meet our responsibility to the pregnant patient.

CHALLENGE QUESTIONS

1. Define or otherwise identify the following:
   a. ALARA
   b. Fetal DL
   c. Major organogenesis
   d. Elective booking
   e. GSD
   f. penumbra
   g. shadow shield
   h. ESE
   i. CT beam width
   j. MMD
2. What is the embryo's response to irradiation above 25 rad during the first 2 weeks after conception?
3. During the fetal period of major organogenesis, what radiation responses are possible?

4. What procedure should be followed if a patient is examined and subsequently discovers that she is pregnant?

5. List five procedures that could result in a measurable fetal dose.

6. How can the three cardinal principles of radiation protection best be applied in diagnostic radiology?

7. What estimate of patient radiation dose usually is measured and reported?

8. How does one use a radiation nomogram?

9. Estimate the entrance skin exposure for a PA chest image conducted at 110 kVp/2 mAs.

10. What factors are required to estimate the genetically significant dose?

11. What radiation dose description is most important for x-ray mammography?

12. How do x-ray beam width and beam penumbra affect patient dose during CT?

13. How does the term "dose distribution" affect specification of patient dose in x-ray imaging?

14. Describe how patient dose during multislice CT compares with that during step-and-shoot CT.

15. Name three screening x-ray examinations that should not be performed regularly.

16. Estimate the fetal dose after an AP abdominal image is conducted at 76 kVp/40 mAs.

17. What does the symbol Σ mean?

18. Approximately what percentage of the ESE is D_g for mammography?

19. What is the approximate contribution of CT to total patient radiation dose?

20. What is the approximate fetal dose after a 3.5-min barium enema fluoroscopic examination?

The answers to the Challenge Questions can be found by logging on to our website at http://evolve.elsevier.com.

CHAPTER 40

Occupational Radiation Dose Management

OBJECTIVES

At the completion of this chapter, the student should be able to do the following:

1. Discuss the units and concepts of occupational radiation exposure
2. Discuss ways to reduce occupational radiation exposure
3. Explain occupational radiation monitors and where they should be positioned
4. Discuss personnel radiation monitoring reports
5. List the available thicknesses of protective apparel

OUTLINE

Occupational Radiation Exposure
   Fluoroscopy
   Interventional Radiology
   Mammography
   Computed Tomography
   Surgery
   Mobile Radiology
Radiation Dose Limits
   Whole-Body Dose Limits
   Dose Limits for Tissues and Organs
   Public Exposure
   Educational Considerations
Reduction of Occupational Radiation Exposure
   Occupational Radiation Monitoring
   Occupational Radiation Monitoring Report
   Protective Apparel
   Position
   Patient Holding
   Pregnant Technologist/Radiologist
   Management Principles

RADIATION DOSE is measured in units of rads (Gy_t). Radiation exposure is measured in roentgens (Gy_a). When the exposure is to radiologic technologists and radiologists, the proper unit is the rem (Sv).

The rem is the unit of effective dose; it is used for radiation protection purposes. Although exposure, dose, and effective dose have precise and different meanings, they often are used interchangeably in radiology because they have approximately the same numeric value following whole-body exposure.

When properly used, exposure (R, Gy_a) refers to radiation intensity in air. Dose (rad, Gy_t) measures the radiation energy absorbed as a result of radiation exposure; it is used to identify irradiation of patients. Effective dose (rem, Sv) identifies the biologic effectiveness of the radiation energy absorbed. This unit is applied to occupationally exposed persons and to population exposure, and the SI unit the sievert (Sv) is preferred because all regulations are expressed in sievert.

TABLE 40-1	Occupational Radiation Exposure of Radiologic Personnel
Exposure Category	**Value**
Average whole-body dose	0.7 mSv/yr
Those receiving less than the minimum detectable dose	53%
Those receiving <1 mSv/yr	88%
Those receiving >50 mSv/yr	0.05%

to allow the technologist to leave the immediate examination area. The radiologic technologist should wear a protective apron for each such mobile examination.

During fluoroscopy, both radiologist and radiologic technologist are exposed to relatively high levels of radiation. Personnel exposure, however, is related directly to the x-ray beam-on time. With care, personnel exposures can be kept as low as reasonably achievable (ALARA).

Question: A barium enema examination requires 2.5 minutes of fluoroscopic x-ray beam time. If the radiographer is exposed to 250 mR/hr, what will be his or her occupational radiation exposure?

Answer: Exposure = Exposure rate × Time
= 250 mR/hr × 2.5 minutes
= 250 mR/hr × 0.0417 hour
= 10.4 mR

Remote fluoroscopy results in low personnel exposures because personnel are not in the x-ray examination room with the patient. With some fluoroscopes, the x-ray tube is over the table and the image receptor under the table. This geometry offers some advantage in terms of image quality, but personnel exposures are higher because secondary radiation (scatter and leakage) levels are higher.

This condition should be kept in mind during mobile and C-arm fluoroscopy. It is best to position the x-ray tube under the patient during mobile and C-arm fluoroscopy (Figure 40-1).

Interventional Radiology

Personnel engaged in interventional radiology procedures often receive higher exposures than do those in general radiologic practice because of longer fluoroscopic x-ray beam-on time. The frequent absence of a protective curtain on the image-intensifier tower and the use of cineradiography also contribute to higher personnel exposure.

Extremity exposure during interventional radiology procedures may be significant. Even with protective gloves, exposure of the forearm can approach the recommended dose limit of 500 mSv/yr (50 rem/yr) if care

OCCUPATIONAL RADIATION EXPOSURE

Although the recommended dose limit for radiologic personnel is 50 mSv/yr (5000 mrem/yr), experience has shown that considerably lower exposures than this are routine. The occupational radiation exposure of radiologic personnel engaged in general x-ray activity normally should not exceed 1 mSv/yr (100 mrem/yr).

Radiologists usually receive slightly higher exposures than radiologic technologists. This is because the radiologist receives most of his or her exposure during fluoroscopy and is usually closer to the radiation source—the patient—during such procedures. Table 40-1 reports the results of an analysis of the annual occupational radiation exposure of radiologic personnel. Clearly, the radiation exposures are low.

Fluoroscopy

Unquestionably, the highest occupational exposure of diagnostic x-ray personnel occurs during fluoroscopy and mobile radiography. During radiographic exposure, the radiologist is rarely present and the radiologic technologist is behind the console protective barrier.

When fixed protective barriers are not available, such as during mobile examination, the mobile x-ray imaging system is equipped with an exposure cord long enough

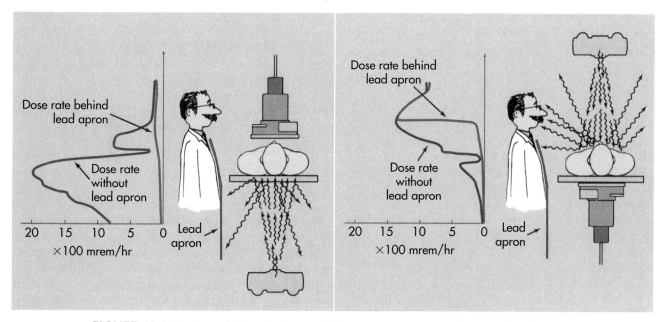

FIGURE 40-1 Scatter radiation during portable fluoroscopy is more intense with the x-ray tube over the patient. (Courtesy Stephen Balter, Columbia University Medical Center.)

is not taken. Without protective gloves, excessive hand exposures are possible.

> Extremity monitoring must be provided for interventional radiologists.

Mammography

Personnel exposures associated with mammography are low because the low kVp of operation results in less scatter radiation. Usually, a long exposure cord and a conventional wall or window wall are sufficient to provide adequate protection.

Rarely does a room that is used strictly for mammography require protective lead shielding. Dedicated mammography x-ray units have personnel protective barriers made of lead glass, lead acrylic, and even plate glass as an integral component. Usually, such barriers are totally adequate.

Computed Tomography

Personnel exposures in computed tomography (CT) facilities are low. Because the CT x-ray beam is finely collimated and only secondary radiation is present in the examination room, radiation levels are low compared with those experienced in fluoroscopy. Figure 40-2 shows the isoexposure profiles for the horizontal and vertical planes of a multislice spiral CT imaging system. These data are given as mR/360 degrees rotation, and they show that personnel can be permitted to remain in the room during imaging. However, protective apparel should always be worn in such situations.

Question: It is necessary for a radiologic technologist to remain in the CT room at midtable position during a 20-rotation examination. What would be the occupational exposure if no protective apron were worn?

Answer: From Figure 40-2, we may assume an exposure of 0.1 mR/scan.

Occupational exposure = 0.1 mR/scan × 2 = 2 mR
Of course, with a protective apron the trunk of the body would receive essentially zero exposure.

Surgery

Nursing personnel and others working in the operating room and in intensive care units are sometimes exposed to radiation from mobile x-ray imaging systems and C-arm fluoroscopes. Although these personnel are often anxious about such exposures, many studies have shown that their occupational exposure is near zero and certainly is no cause for concern. It usually is not necessary to provide occupational radiation monitors for such personnel.

Mobile Radiology

Occupational radiation monitors are not necessary during mobile radiography, except as used with the radiologic technologist and anyone who is required to immobilize or hold patients. Personnel who regularly operate or are in the immediate vicinity of a C-arm fluoroscope should wear an occupational radiation monitor, in addition to protective apparel. During C-arm fluoroscopy, the x-ray beam may be on for a relatively long time, and the beam can be pointed in virtually any direction.

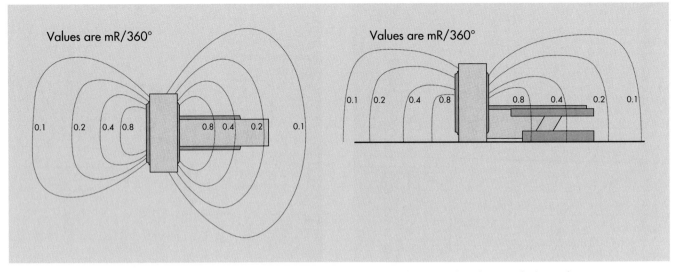

FIGURE 40-2 Isoexposure profiles (in mR/360 degrees) in horizontal and vertical planes for multislice spiral computed tomography.

It should **never** be necessary for radiologic personnel to exceed 50 mSv/yr (5000 mrem/yr). In smaller hospitals, emergency centers, and private clinics, occupational exposures rarely exceed 5 mSv/yr (500 mrem/yr). As Table 40-1 reported, average exposures in most facilities are less than 1 mSv/yr (100 mrem/yr).

RADIATION DOSE LIMITS

A continuing effort of health physicists has been the description and identification of occupational dose limits. For many years, a **maximum permissible dose (MPD)** was specified. The MPD was the dose of radiation that would be expected to produce no significant radiation effects.

At radiation doses below the MPD, no responses should occur. At the level of the MPD, the risk is not zero, but it is small—lower than the risk associated with other occupations and reasonable in light of the benefits derived. The concept of MPD is now obsolete and has been replaced by dose limits (DLs).

Whole-Body Dose Limits

To establish DLs, the National Council on Radiation Protection (NCRP) assessed risk on the basis of data from reports of the National Academy of Sciences (Biologic Effects of Ionizing Radiation [BEIR] Committee) and the National Safety Council (Table 40-2). State and federal government agencies routinely adopt these recommended dose limits as law. Current DLs are prescribed for various organs as well as for the whole body, and for various working conditions. If one received the DL each year, the lifetime risk would not exceed 10^{-4} yr^{-1}.

DLs imply that if received annually, the risk of death would be less than 1 in 10,000.

TABLE 40-2	Fatal Accident Rates in Various Industries
Industry	**Rate (10^{-4} yr^{-1})**
Trade	0.4
Manufacture	0.4
Service	0.4
Government	0.9
Radiation workers	0.9
All groups	0.9
Transport	2.2
Public utilities	2.2
Construction	3.1
Mining	4.3
Agriculture	4.4

The value 10^{-4} yr^{-1} represents the approximate risk of death for those working in safe industries. The DLs recommended by the NCRP ensure that radiation workers have the same risk as those in safe industries.

Question: Suppose all 300,000 American radiologic technologists receive the DL (50 mSv) this year. How many would be expected to die prematurely?

Answer: $(300,000)(10^{-4}) = 30$
But of course, they actually receive approximately 0.5 mSv/yr; therefore, the expected mortality is as follows:
$$30\left(\frac{0.5}{50}\right) = 0.3;\ \text{less than 1!}$$

Particular care is taken to ensure that no **radiation worker** receives a radiation dose in excess of the DL. The DL is specified only for occupational exposure. It should not be confused with medical x-ray exposure

TABLE 40-3	Historical Review of Dose Limits for Occupational Exposure		
Year	Recommendation	Approximate Daily Dose Limit (mrem)	Source
1902	Dose limited by fogging of a photographic plate after 7-minute contact exposure	10,000	Rollins
1915	Lead shielding of tube needed (no numeric British Roentgen Society exposure levels given)		
1921	General methods to reduce exposure		British X-ray and Radium Protection Committee
1925	"It is entirely safe if an operator does not receive every thirty days a dose exceeding 1/100 of an erythema dose."	200	Mutscheller
1925	10% of SED per year	200	Sievert
1926	One SED per 90,000 working hours	40	Dutch Board of Health
1928	0.000028 of SED per day	175	Barclay and Cox
1928	0.001 of SED per month 5 R per day permissible for the hands	150	Kaye
1931	Limit exposure to 0.2 R per day	200	Advisory Committee on X-ray and Radium Protection of the United States
1932	0.001 of SED per month	30	Failla
1934	5 R per day permissible for the hands	5000	Advisory Committee on X-ray and Radium Protection of the United States
1936	0.1 R per day	100	Advisory Committee on X-ray and Radium Protection of the United States
1941	0.02 R per day	20	Taylor
1943	200 mR per day is acceptable	200	Patterson
1959	5 rem per year, 5 (N-18) rem accumulated	20	National Council on Radiation Protection and Measurements
1987	50 mSv per year, 10 × N mSv cumulative	20	National Council on Radiation Protection and Measurements
1991	20 mSv per year	8	International Commission on Radiation Protection

SED, Skin erythema dose.

received as a patient. Although patient dose should be kept low, there is no patient DL.

The first DL— 500 mSv/wk (50,000 mrem/wk)—was recommended in 1902. The current DL is 1 mSv/wk (100 mrem/wk). Through the years, a downward revision of the DL has occurred. The history of these continuing recommendations is given in Table 40-3 and is shown graphically in Figure 40-3.

In the early years of radiology, the DL consisted of a single value that was considered the safe working level for whole-body exposure. It was based primarily on the known acute response to radiation exposure and presumed that a threshold dose existed.

Today, the DL is specified not only for whole-body exposure but also for partial-body exposure, organ exposure, and exposure of the general population, again excluding medical exposure as a patient and exposure from natural sources (Table 40-4). The DLs included in Table 40-4 were published first by the NCRP in 1987

and were refined in 1993. They replaced the previous MPDs, which had been in effect since 1959. These DLs have been adopted by state and federal regulatory agencies and are now the law of the United States. Note that International System (SI) units are preferred.

The basic annual DL is 50 mSv/yr (5000 mrem/yr). The DL for the lens of the eye is 150 mSv/yr (15 rem/yr), and that for other organs is 500 mSv/yr (50 rem/yr).

The cumulative whole-body DL is 10 mSv (1000 mrem) times age in years. The DL during pregnancy is 5 mSv (500 mrem), but once pregnancy has been declared, monthly exposure shall not exceed 0.5 mSv (50 mrem).

Current DLs are based on a *linear, nonthreshold dose-response relationship;* they are considered to represent an acceptable level of occupational radiation exposure.

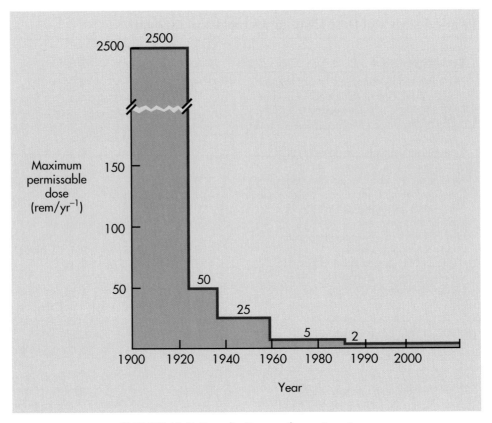

FIGURE 40-3 Dose limits over the past century.

In practice, at least in diagnostic radiology, it is seldom necessary to exceed even ¹/₁₀ the appropriate DL. However, because the basis for the DL assumes a linear, non-threshold dose-response relationship, **all unnecessary** radiation exposure should be avoided.

Occupational exposure is described as *dose equivalent* in units of millisievert (millirem). DLs are specified as *effective dose (E)*. This scheme has been adopted to afford enhanced precision in radiation protection practices.

The effective dose (E) concept accounts for different types of radiation because of their varying relative biologic effectiveness. Effective dose also considers the relative radiosensitivity of various tissues and organs.

These are particularly important considerations when a protective apron is worn. Wearing a protective apron reduces radiation dose to many tissues and organs to near zero. Therefore, effective dose is much less than that recorded by a collar-positioned radiation monitor.

EFFECTIVE DOSE

Effective dose (E) = Radiation weighting factor
(W_r) × Tissue weighting factor (W_t) × Absorbed dose

Adoption of this scheme is progressing. For our purposes, effective dose (E) is the quantity of importance. It is expressed in mSv (mrem) and forms the basis for our DLs.

As can be seen in Table 40-5, the radiation weighting factor (W_r) is equal to 1 for the types of radiation used in medicine. The value of W_r for other types of radiation depends on the linear energy transfer (LET) of that radiation.

The tissue weighting factor (W_t) accounts for the relative radiosensitivity of various tissues and organs. Tissues with a higher value of W_t are more radiosensitive. These are shown in Table 40-6.

Practical implementation of these DLs and weighting factors does not change our previous approach. The DL is sufficiently high that it rarely, if ever, is exceeded in diagnostic radiology.

With a collar-positioned radiation monitor, a change in procedure is necessary to estimate effective dose (E). Because essentially all of our radiation exposure occurs during fluoroscopy and the trunk is shielded by a lead apron, the response of the monitor overestimates the effective dose (E).

A conversion factor of 0.3 should be applied to the collar monitor–reported value to estimate effective dose (E). If a protective apron is not worn (e.g., by a radiographer who does no fluoroscopy), then the monitor response may be considered the effective dose.

Dose Limits for Tissues and Organs

The whole-body DL of 50 mSv/yr (5000 mrem/yr) is an effective dose, which takes into account the weighted average to various tissues and organs. In addition, the

TABLE 40-4	Dose Limits Recommended by the National Council on Radiation Protection and Measurements

A. Occupational exposures
   1. Effective dose
      a. Annual: 50 mSv (5000 mrem)
      b. Cumulative: 10 mSv × age (1000 mrem × age)
   2. Equivalent annual dose for tissues and organs
      a. Lens of the eye: 150 mSv (15 rem)
      b. Thyroid, skin, hands, and feet: 500 mSv (50 rem)
B. Public exposures (annual)
   1. Effective dose, frequent exposure: 1 mSv
      (100 mrem)
   2. Equivalent dose for tissues and organs
      a. Lens of eye: 15 mSv (1500 mrem)
      b. Skin, hands, and feet: 50 mSv (5000 mrem)
C. Education and training exposures (annual)
   1. Effective dose: 1 mSv (100 mrem)
   2. Equivalent dose for tissues and organs
      a. Lens of eye: 15 mSv (1500 mrem)
      b. Skin, hands, and feet: 50 mSv (5000 mrem)
D. Embryo–fetus exposures
   1. Total equivalent dose: 5 mSv (500 mrem)
   2. Equivalent dose in 1 month: 0.5 mSv (50 mrem)
E. Negligible individual dose (annual): 0.01 mSv (10 mrem)

TABLE 40-5	Weighting Factors for Various Types of Radiation

Type of Energy Range	Radiation Weighting Factor (W_r)
X- and gamma rays, electrons	1
Neutrons, energy < 10 keV	5
10 keV to 100 keV	10
>100 keV to 2 MeV	20
> 2 MeV to 20 MeV	10
>20 MeV	5
Protons	2
Alpha particles	20

TABLE 40-6	Weighting Factors for Various Tissues

Tissue	Tissue Weighting Factor (W_t)
Gonad	0.20
Active bone marrow	0.12
Colon	0.12
Lung	0.12
Stomach	0.12
Bladder	0.05
Breast	0.05
Esophagus	0.05
Liver	0.05
Thyroid	0.05
Bone surface	0.01
Skin	0.01

NCRP has identified several specific tissues and organs with specific recommended dose limits.

Skin. Some organs of the body have a higher DL than the whole-body DL. The DL for the skin is 500 mSv/yr (50 rem/yr).

This limit is not normally of concern in diagnostic radiology because it applies to nonpenetrating radiation such as alpha and beta radiation and very soft x-rays. Radiologic technologists exclusively engaged in mammography or nuclear medicine are highly unlikely to sustain radiation exposure to the skin in excess of 10 mSv/yr (1000 mrem/yr).

Extremities. Radiologists often have their hands near the primary fluoroscopic radiation beam; therefore, extremity exposure may be of concern. The DL for the extremities is the same as that for the skin—500 mSv/yr (50 rem/yr).

These radiation levels are quite high and under normal circumstances should not even be approached. For certain occupational groups, such as interventional radiologists and nuclear medicine technologists, extremity personnel monitors should be provided. Such devices are worn on the wrist or the finger.

Lens. Because radiation is known to produce cataracts, a DL is specified for the lens of the eye. This DL is 150 mSv/yr (15 rem/yr) and it should never be approached, much less exceeded, in x-ray imaging. The response of a collar-positioned can be used as the lens dose.

Public Exposure

Individuals in the general population are limited to 1 mSv/yr (100 mrem/yr). For hospital workers who are not radiology employees but who may regularly visit x-ray rooms, the DL is 1 mSv/yr (100 mrem/yr).

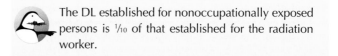 The DL established for nonoccupationally exposed persons is ¹/₁₀ of that established for the radiation worker.

This value of 1 mSv/yr is the DL that medical physicists use when computing the thickness of protective barriers. If a barrier separates an x-ray examining room from an area occupied by the general public, the shielding is designed so that the annual exposure of an individual in the adjacent area cannot exceed 1 mSv/yr (100 mrem/yr).

If the adjacent area is occupied by radiation workers, the shielding must be sufficient to maintain an annual exposure level less than 10 mSv/yr (1000 mrem/yr). This approach to shielding derives from the 10 mSv × N cumulative DL.

Radiation exposure of the general public or of individuals in this population is measured rarely because this process is not necessary. Most radiology personnel do not receive even this level of exposure.

Educational Considerations

Several special situations are associated with whole-body occupational DL. Students younger than 18 years of age may not receive more than 1 mSv/yr (100 mrem/yr) during the course of their educational activities. This is included in and is not added to the 1 mSv (100 mrem) permitted each year as a nonoccupational exposure.

Consequently, student radiologic technologists younger than 18 years of age may be engaged in x-ray imaging, but their exposure must be monitored and must remain below 1 mSv/yr (100 mrem/yr). Because of this, it is general practice not to accept underage persons into schools of radiologic technology unless their 18th birthday is within sight.

In keeping with **ALARA**, even more changes in DL are on the way. The International Commission on Radiological Protection (ICRP) has issued several recommendations, including an annual whole-body DL of 20 mSv (2000 mrem). Such a reduction is currently under consideration in the United States.

REDUCTION OF OCCUPATIONAL RADIATION EXPOSURE

The radiologic technologist can do much to minimize occupational radiation exposure. Most exposure control procedures do not require sophisticated equipment or especially rigorous training, but simply a conscientious attitude regarding the performance of assigned duties. Most equipment characteristics, technique changes, and administrative procedures designed to minimize patient dose also reduce occupational exposure.

In diagnostic radiology, at least 95% of the radiologic technologist's occupational radiation exposure comes from fluoroscopy and mobile radiography. Attention to the cardinal principles of radiation protection (time, distance, and shielding) and ALARA are the most important aspects of occupational radiation control.

During fluoroscopy, the radiologist should minimize x-ray beam-on time. This can be done through careful technique, which includes intermittent activation of fluoroscopic views rather than one long period of x-ray beam-on time. It is a common radiation protection practice to maintain a log of fluoroscopy time by recording x-ray beam-on time with the 5-minute reset timer.

During fluoroscopy, the radiologic technologist should step back from the table when his or her immediate presence and assistance are not required. The radiologic technologist also should take maximum advantage of all protective shielding, including apron, curtain, and Bucky slot cover, as well as the **radiologist.**

 Each mobile x-ray unit should have a protective apron assigned to it.

The radiologic technologist should wear a protective apron during all mobile examinations and should maintain maximum distance from the source. The primary beam should never be pointed at the radiologic technologist or other nearby personnel.

The exposure cord on a portable x-ray unit must be at least 2 m long.

During radiography, the radiologic technologist is positioned behind a control booth barrier. Such barriers usually are considered secondary barriers because they intercept only leakage and scatter radiation. Consequently, leaded glass and leaded gypsum board are often unnecessary for such barriers.

The useful beam should never be directed toward the operating console.

Other work assignments in diagnostic imaging, such as scheduling, darkroom duties, and filing, result in essentially no occupational radiation exposure.

Occupational Radiation Monitoring

The level of occupational exposure to radiologists and radiologic technologists depends on the type and frequency of activity in which they are engaged. Determining the quantity of radiation they receive requires a program of occupational radiation monitoring. Occupational radiation monitoring refers to procedures instituted to estimate the amount of radiation received by individuals who work in a radiation environment.

Occupational radiation monitoring is required when there is any likelihood that an individual will receive more than 1/10 of the recommended dose limit.

Most clinical diagnostic imaging personnel must be monitored; however, it usually is not necessary to monitor diagnostic radiology secretaries and file clerks. Furthermore, it usually is not necessary to monitor operating room personnel, except perhaps those routinely involved in cystoscopy and C-arm fluoroscopy.

The occupational radiation monitor offers no protection against radiation exposure!

The occupational radiation monitor simply measures the quantity of radiation to which the monitor was exposed; therefore, it is simply an indicator of exposure to the wearer. Basically, three types of personnel monitors are used in diagnostic radiology: film badges, thermoluminescence dosimeters (TLDs), and optically stimulated luminescence dosimeters (OSLs).

Regardless of the type of monitor used, it is essential that it be obtained from a certified laboratory. In-house processing of radiation monitors should not be attempted.

Film Badges. Film badges came into general use during the 1940s and have been used widely in diagnostic radiology ever since. Film badges are specially designed devices in which a film similar to dental radiographic film is sandwiched between metal filters inside a plastic holder. Figure 40-4 presents a view of two typical occupational radiation monitors.

The film incorporated into a film badge is special radiation dosimetry film that is particularly sensitive to x-rays. The optical density on the exposed and processed film is related to the exposure received by the film badge.

Carefully controlled calibration, processing, and analyzing conditions are necessary for the film badge to measure accurately occupational radiation exposure. Usually, exposures less than 10 mR (100 μGy_a) are not measured by film badge monitors, and the film badge vendor will report only that a minimum exposure (M) was received. When higher exposures are received, they can be reported accurately.

The metal filters, along with the window in the plastic film holder, allow estimation of the x-ray energy. The usual filters are made of aluminum and copper.

When the radiation exposure is a result of penetrating x-rays, the image of the filters on the processed film is faint, and there may be no image at all of the window in the plastic holder. If the badge is exposed to soft x-rays, the filters are well imaged and the optical densities under the filters allow estimation of x-ray energy.

Often, the filters to the front of the film badge differ in shape from the filters to the back of the film badge. Radiation that had entered through the back of the film badge normally would indicate that the person wearing the badge received considerably higher exposure than indicated, because the x-rays would have penetrated through the body before interacting with the film badge.

 Film badges must be worn with the appropriate side to the front.

Several advantages of film badge occupational radiation monitors continue to make them popular. They are inexpensive, easy to handle, easy to process, and reasonably accurate, and they have been in use for several decades.

Film badge monitors also have disadvantages. They cannot be reused, and because they incorporate film as

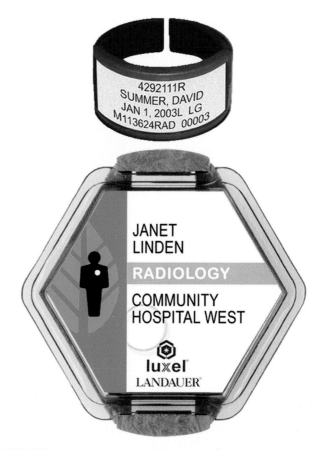

FIGURE 40-4 Some representative radiation monitors. In many, metal filters are incorporated to help identify the type of radiation and its energy. (Courtesy Landauer, Inc.)

the sensing device, they cannot be worn for longer than 1 month because of possible fogging caused by temperature and humidity.

Film badge monitors should never be left in an enclosed car or other area where excessive temperatures may occur. The fogging produced by elevated temperature and humidity results in a falsely high evaluation of radiation exposure.

Thermoluminescence Dosimeters. The sensitive material of the TLD monitor (Figure 40-5) is lithium fluoride (LiF) in crystalline form, either as a powder or more often as a small chip approximately 3 mm square and 1 mm thick. When exposed to x-rays, the TLD absorbs energy and stores it in the form of excited electrons in the crystalline lattice.

When heated, these excited electrons fall back to their normal state with the emission of visible light. The intensity of visible light is measured with a photomultiplier tube or photodiode and is proportional to the radiation dose received by the crystal. This sequence was described in Chapter 38.

The TLD occupational radiation monitor offers several advantages over film. It is more sensitive and more accurate than a film badge monitor. Properly calibrated TLD monitors can measure exposure as low as 5 mR (50 μGy_a).

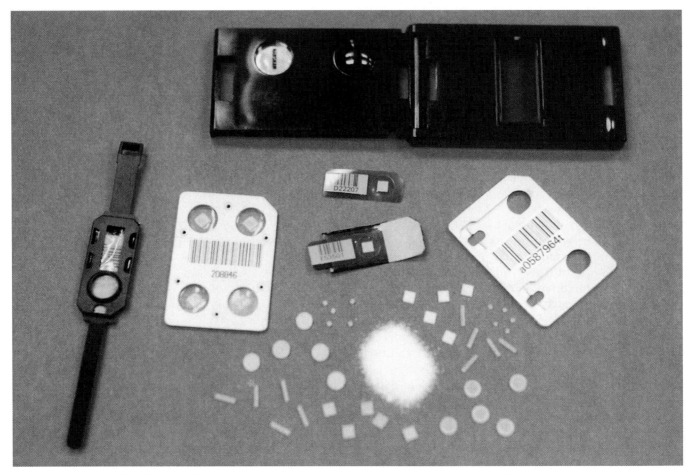

FIGURE 40-5 Thermoluminescence dosimeters are available as chips, discs, rods, and powder. These are used for area and environmental radiation monitoring, and especially for occupational radiation monitoring. (Courtesy Bicron.)

The TLD monitor does not suffer from loss of information after it is exposed to excessive heat or humidity.

 TLDs can be worn for intervals up to 1 year.

The primary disadvantage of TLD personnel monitoring is cost. The price of a typical TLD monitoring service is perhaps twice that of film badge monitoring. If the frequency of monitoring is quarterly, however, the cost is about the same.

Optically Stimulated Luminescence. OSL dosimeters (Figure 40-6) are worn and handled just as film badges and TLDs are, and they are approximately the same size. OSL dosimeters have one advantage over TLDs. They are more sensitive, measuring as low as 1 mR (10 μGy_a).

Where to Wear the Occupational Radiation Monitor. Much discussion and research in health physics have gone into providing precise recommendations about where a radiologic technologist should wear the occupational radiation monitor. Official publications of

the NCRP offer suggestions that have been adopted as regulations in most states.

Many radiologic technologists wear their personnel monitors in front at waist or chest level because it is convenient to clip the badge over a belt or a shirt pocket. If the technologist is not involved in fluoroscopic procedures, these locations are acceptable.

 If the radiologic technologist participates in fluoroscopy, the occupational radiation monitor should be positioned on the collar above the protective apron.

The recommended dose limit of 50 mSv/yr (5000 mrem/yr) refers to the effective dose (E). It has been shown that during fluoroscopy, when a protective apron is worn, exposure to the collar region is approximately 20 times greater than that to the trunk of the body beneath the protective apron. So, if the occupational radiation monitor is worn beneath the protective apron, it will record a falsely low exposure and will not indicate what could be excessive exposure to unprotected body parts.

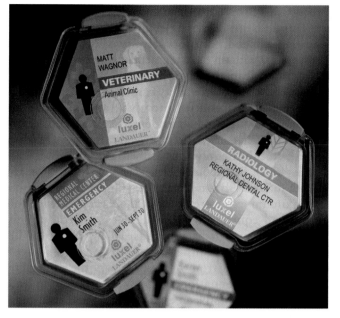

FIGURE 40-6 Optically stimulated luminescence dosimeters. (Courtesy Landauer, Inc.)

In some clinical situations, for example, during pregnancy and with extremity monitoring, it may be advisable to wear more than one radiation monitor. The abdomen should be monitored during pregnancy. The extremities should be monitored during interventional procedures when the radiologist's hands are in close proximity to the useful beam. Nuclear medicine technologists should wear extremity monitors when handling millicurie quantities of radioactive material.

Occupational Radiation Monitoring Report

State and federal regulations require that results of the occupational radiation monitoring program be recorded in a precise fashion and maintained for review. Annual, quarterly, monthly, or weekly monitoring periods are acceptable.

The occupational radiation monitoring report must contain a number of specific items of information (Figure 40-7). These various items are identified in the headers of the columns.

Exposure data that must be included on the form include current exposure and cumulative annual exposure. Separate radiation monitors, such as extremity monitors or fetal monitors, are identified separately from the whole-body monitor.

LANDAUER®

SAMPLE ORGANIZATION
RADIATION SAFETY OFFICER
2 SCIENCE ROAD
GLENWOOD, IL 60425

Landauer, Inc. 2 Science Road Glenwood, Illinois 60425-1586
Telephone: (708) 755-7000 Facsimile: (708) 755-7016
www.landauerinc.com

luxel®

RADIATION DOSIMETRY REPORT

ACCOUNT NO.	SERIES CODE	ANALYTICAL WORK ORDER	REPORT DATE	DOSIMETER RECEIVED	REPORT TIME IN WORK DAYS	PAGE NO.
103702	RAD	992150087	07/16/00	07/12/00	4	1

PARTICIPANT NUMBER	NAME			DOSIMETER	USE	RADIATION QUALITY	DOSE EQUIVALENT (MREM) FOR PERIODS SHOWN BELOW			YEAR TO DATE DOSE EQUIVALENT (MREM)			LIFETIME DOSE EQUIVALENT (MREM)			RECORDS FOR YEAR	INCEPTION DATE (MM/YY)
	ID NUMBER	BIRTH DATE	SEX				DEEP DDE	EYE LDE	SHALLOW SDE	DEEP DDE	EYE LDE	SHALLOW SDE	DEEP DDE	EYE LDE	SHALLOW SDE		
FOR MONITORING PERIOD:							05/01/00 - 06/30/00			2000							
0000H	CONTROL			J	CNTRL		M	M	M							5	07/97
	CONTROL			P	CNTRL		M	M	M								07/97
	CONTROL			U	CNTRL			M	M								07/97
00191	ADAMS, JANE		F	P	WHBODY		M	M	M	9	10	12	9	10	12	5	07/98
00191	ADDISON, JOHN		M	J	WHBODY	PN	90	90	90	100	100	100	200	200	200	5	07/97
						P	60	60	60	70	70	70	170	170	170		
						NF	30	30	30	30	30	30	30	30	30		
00197	EDWARDS, CHRIS		M	P	WHBODY		M	M	M	M	M	M	M	M	M	5	01/98
00202	HARRIS, KATHY		F	P	WHBODY		M	M	M	M	M	M	M	M	M	4	02/99
				U	RFINGR				M			30			30		02/99
00192	JORGENSON, MIKE		M	P	WHBODY		M	M	M	M	M	M	M	M	M	5	07/97
				U	RFINGR				M			70			100		07/97
00200	MEYER, STEVE		M	P	COLLAR	PL	105	105	105	316	327	334	1206	1247	1284	5	08/98
				P	WAIST		M	M	M	M	M	M	M	M	M		08/98
					ASSIGN		4		105	11	327	334	51	1247	1284		
					NOTE		ASSIGNED DOSE BASED ON EDE 1 CALCULATION										
				U	RFINGR				140			690			2180		08/98
00193	THOMAS, LEE		M	P	WHBODY		ABSENT			M	M	M	M	M	M	5	07/97
				U	RFINGR		ABSENT					M			M		07/97
00196	WALKER, JANE		F	P	WHBODY		3	3	3	12	11	11	22	21	21	5	11/97
00198	ZERR, ROBERT		M	P	WHBODY		40	40	40	200	200	200	240	240	240	5	07/98
					NOTE		CALCULATED										

M: MINIMAL REPORTING SERVICE OF 1 MREM
ELECTRONIC MEDIA TO FOLLOW THIS REPORT

QUALITY CONTROL RELEASE: LMR

1 - PR 6774 - RPT131 - N1

- 21587

Accredited by the National Institute of Standards and Technology through NVLAP®*

FIGURE 40-7 Occupational radiation monitoring report must include the items of information shown here. (Courtesy Landauer, Inc.)

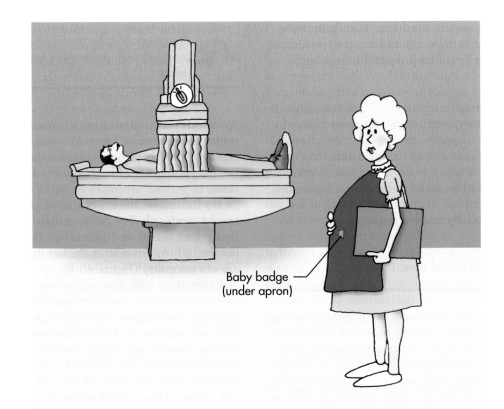

Baby badge
(under apron)

FIGURE 40-8 When the fluoroscopist is pregnant, a second "baby monitor" should be positioned under the protective apron.

New Employee Notification

This is to certify that _____ , a new employee of this radiologic facility, has received instructions regarding mutual responsibilities should she become pregnant during this employment.

In addition to personal counseling by _____ , she has been given to read several documents dealing with pregnancy in diagnostic radiology. Furthermore, the additional reading material that follows is available in the departmental office:

1. *Review of NCRP radiation dose limit for embryo and fetus in occupationally-exposed women*, NCRP Report No 53, Washington, DC, 1977, National Council on Radiation Protection and Measures.
2. *Medical radiation exposure of pregnant and potentially pregnant women*, NCRP Report No 54, Washington, DC, 1977, National Council on Radiation Protection and Measures.
3. Wagner, LK et al: *Exposure of the pregnant patient to diagnostic radiation*, Philadelphia, 1985, JB Lippincott.
4. *The effects on populations of exposure to low levels of ionizing radiation*, Washington, DC, 1990, National Academy of Sciences.

I understand that should I become pregnant and I decide to declare my pregnancy, it is my responsibility to inform my supervisor of my condition so that additional protective measures can be taken.

_____   _____
Supervisor   Employee

_____
Date

FIGURE 40-9 Form for new employee notification.

Bucky factor (B)   Ratio of incident radiation to transmitted radiation through a grid; ratio of patient dose with and without a grid.

Bucky slot cover   Protective cover that automatically shields the Bucky slot opening during fluoroscopic examinations when the Bucky tray is at the foot of the table.

Buffer   Acetate added to the fixer to maintain a constant pH.

Buffering agent   Alkali compound in the developer that enhances the action of the developing agent by controlling the concentration of hydrogen ions.

Byte   Group of eight bits; represents one character or digit.

Calipers   Instrument with two bent or curved legs used for measuring the thickness of a solid.

Calorie (c)   Energy necessary to raise the temperature of 1 g of water by 1°C.

C-arm fluoroscope   Portable device for fluoroscopy. The opposite ends of the C-shaped support arm hold the image intensifier and the x-ray tube.

Cassette   Rigid holder that contains the film and screens.

Cassette-loaded spot film   Conventional method of capturing images with image-intensified fluoroscopes.

Catabolism   Process that creates energy for a cell by breaking down molecular nutrients that are brought to and diffused through the cell membrane.

Cathode   Negative side of the x-ray tube; contains the filament and the focusing cup.

Cathode rays   Stream of electrons.

Cathode ray tube (CRT)   Electron beam tube designed for a two-dimensional display of signals.

Cell   Basic unit of all living matter.

Cell cloning   Process by which normal cells produce a visible colony in a short time.

Cell cycle time   Average time from one mitosis to another.

Cell theory   Principle that all plants and animals contain cells as their basic functional units.

Center for Diseases and Radiological Health (CDRH)   Agency responsible for a national electronic radiation control program. Known as the Bureau of Radiological Health (BRH) before 1982.

Central axis x-ray beam   X-ray beam composed of x-rays that travel along the center of the useful x-ray beam.

Central nervous system (CNS) syndrome   Form of acute radiation syndrome caused by radiation doses of 50 Gy (5000 rad) or more of ionizing radiation that results in failure of the central nervous system, followed by death within a few hours to several days.

Central processing unit (CPU)   Processing hardware in large computers.

Central ray   Center of the x-ray beam that interacts with the image receptor.

Centrifugal force   Force that causes an electron to travel straight and leave the atom.

Centripetal force   Force that keeps an electron in orbit.

Characteristic curve   Graph of optical density versus log relative response; H & D curve.

Characteristic x-ray   X-ray released as a result of the photoelectric effect; its discrete energies are determined by the respective electron binding energy.

Charge-coupled device (CCD)   Solid-state device that converts visible light photons to electrons.

Chelate   Sequestering agent.

Chemical energy   Energy released by a chemical reaction.

Chemical fog   Artifact produced by chemical contamination of the developer.

Chemical symbol   Alphabetic abbreviation for an element.

Chip   Tiny piece of semiconductor material.

Chromatid deletion   Breakage of a chromatid.

Cine film   Film used in cinefluorography.

Cinefluorography   Recording of fluoroscopic images on movie film.

Classical scattering   Scattering of x-rays with no loss of energy. Also called *coherent*, *Rayleigh*, or *Thompson scattering*.

Clearing agent   A chemical, usually ammonium thiosulfate, that is added to the fixer to remove undeveloped silver bromine from the emulsion.

Clinical tolerance   Moist desquamation in radiation therapy.

Closed-core transformer   Square core of ferromagnetic material built up of laminated layers of iron; it helps to reduce energy losses caused by eddy currents.

Coast time   Time it takes the rotor to rest after use.

Codon   Series of three base pairs in the DNA.

Collimation   Restriction of the useful x-ray beam to reduce patient dose and improve image contrast.

Collimator   Device used to restrict x-ray beam size and shape.

Commutator   Device that acts like a switch, converting an alternating-current generator to a direct-current generator.

Compensating filter   Material inserted between an x-ray source and a patient to shape the intensity of the x-ray beam. An x-ray beam filter is designed to make the remnant beam more uniform in intensity.

Compression   The act of flattening soft tissue to improve optical density.

Compression device   Device that maintains close screen-film contact when the cassette is closed and latched.

Compton effect   Scattering of x-rays that results in ionization and loss of energy.

Compton scattering   Interaction between an x-ray and a loosely bound outer-shell electron that results in ionization and x-ray scattering.

Computed radiography (CR) Radiographic technique that uses a photostimulable phosphor as the image receptor and an area beam.

Computed tomography (CT) Creation of a cross-sectional tomographic section of the body with a rotating fan beam, a detector array, and computed reconstruction.

Computed tomography dose index (CTDI) Radiation dose in a single slice over a 10-cm length so that dose delivered beyond the selected slice thickness is included.

Conduction Transfer of heat by molecular agitation.

Conductor Material that allows heat or electric current to flow.

Cone Circular metal tube that attaches to x-ray tube housing to limit the beam size and shape.

Cone cutting Misalignment of cones that causes one side of the radiograph to not be exposed because the edge of the cone may interfere with the x-ray beam.

Cones and cylinders Modifications of the aperture diaphragm.

Connective tissue Tissue that binds tissue and organs together.

Contact shields Shields that are flat and are placed directly on the patient's gonads.

Continuous quality improvement (CQI) Program that includes administrative protocols for the continual improvement of mammographic quality.

Contrast Degree of difference between the light and dark areas of a radiograph.

Contrast agent Compound used as an aid for imaging internal organs with x-rays.

Contrast improvement factor Ratio of radiographic contrast with a grid to that without a grid.

Contrast index Difference between the step with an average optical density closest to 2.2 and the step with an average optical density closest to, but not less than, 0.5.

Contrast medium Agent that enhances differences between anatomic structures.

Contrast resolution Ability to distinguish between and to image similar tissues.

Controlled area Area where personnel occupancy and activity are subject to control and supervision for the purpose of radiation protection.

Convection Transfer of heat by the movement of hot matter to a colder place.

Conversion efficiency (CE) Rate at which x-ray energy is transformed into light in an intensifying screen.

Conversion factor Ratio of illumination intensity at the output phosphor to radiation intensity incident on the input phosphor.

Coolidge tube Type of vacuum tube in use today that allows x-ray intensity and energy to be selected separately and accurately.

Cosmic rays Particulate and electromagnetic radiation emitted by the sun and the stars.

Coulomb (C) SI unit of electric charge.

Coulomb per kilogram (C/kg) SI unit of radiation exposure: 2.58×10^{-4} C/kg = 1 R.

Coupling Joining of magnetic fields produced by the primary and secondary coils.

Covalent bond Chemical union between atoms formed by sharing one or more pairs of electrons.

Covering power The more efficient use of silver in an emulsion to produce the same optical density per unit exposure.

Crookes tube Forerunner of modern fluorescent, neon, and x-ray tubes.

Crossed grid Grid on which lead strips run parallel to the long and short axes.

Cross-linking Process of side spurs created by irradiation and attached to a neighboring macromolecule or to another segment of the same molecule.

Crossover Process that occurs during meiosis wherein chromatids exchange chromosomal material.

Crossover rack Device in an automatic processor that transports film from one tank to the next.

Cryogen Extremely cold liquid.

Crystal lattice Three-dimensional, cross-linked structure of silver, bromine, and iodine atoms.

Curie (Ci) Former unit of radioactivity. Expressed as 1 Ci = 3.7×10^{10} disintegrations per second 3.7×10^{10} Bq.

Cutie pie Nickname for an ionization chamber–type survey meter.

Cytoplasm Protoplasm that exists outside the cell's nucleus.

Cytosine Nitrogenous organic base that attaches to a deoxyribose molecule.

Data acquisition system (DAS) Computer-controlled electronic amplifier and switching device to which the signal from each radiation detector of a multislice spiral computed tomographic scanning system is connected.

Decimal system System of numbers based on multiples of 10.

Densitometer Instrument that measures the optical density of exposed film.

Density difference (DD) The difference between the step with an average optical density closest to 2.2 and the step with an average optical density closest to, but not less than, 0.5.

Deoxyribonucleic acid (DNA) Molecule that carries the genetic information necessary for cell replication; the target molecule of radiobiology.

Derived quantities Any secondary quantity derived from a combination of one or more of three base quantities, such as mass, length, and time.

Desquamation Ulceration and denudation of the skin.

Detail Degree of sharpness of structural lines on a radiograph.

Detective quantum efficiency (DQE) Percentage of x-rays absorbed by the screen by the image receptor.

Detector array Group of detectors and the interspace material used to separate them; the image receptor in computed tomography.

Deterministic effect Biologic response whose severity varies with radiation dose. A dose threshold usually exists.

Developing Stage of processing during which the latent image is converted to a manifest image.

Developing agent A chemical, usually phenidone, hydroquinone, or Metol, that reduces exposed silver ions to atomic silver.

Development fog Artifact that results from reduction of crystals that had not been exposed to metallic silver caused by the lack of a restrainer.

Diagnostic mammography Examination performed on patients with symptoms or elevated risk factors for breast cancer.

Diagnostic-type protective tube housing Lead-lined housing enclosing an x-ray tube that shields leakage radiation to less than 100 mR/hr at 1 m.

Diaphragm Device that restricts an x-ray beam to a fixed size.

Dichroic stain Two-colored stain that appears as a curtain effect on the radiograph.

DICOM Digital Imaging and Communications in Medicine Standard that enables imaging systems from different manufacturers to communicate.

Differential absorption Different degrees of absorption in different tissues that result in image contrast and formation of the x-ray image.

Digital fluoroscopy (DF) Digital x-ray imaging system that produces a series of dynamic images with the use of an area x-ray beam and an image intensifier.

Digital radiography (DR) Static images produced with a fan x-ray beam intercepted by a linear array of radiation detectors or an area x-ray beam intercepted by a photostimulable phosphor plate or a direct-capture solid-state device.

Dimagnetic Nonmagnetic materials that are unaffected when brought into a magnetic field.

Dimensional stability Property that allows the base of radiographic film to maintain its size and shape during use and processing, so it does not contribute to image distortion.

Diode Vacuum tube with two electrodes—a cathode and an anode.

Dipolar Referring to a molecule with areas of opposing electric charge.

Direct current (DC) Flow of electricity in only one direction within a conductor.

Direct-current motor Electric motor in which many turns of wire are used for the current loop and many bar magnets are used to create the external magnetic field.

Direct effect Effect of radiation that occurs when ionizing radiation interacts directly with a particularly radiosensitive molecule.

Direct-exposure film Film used without intensifying screens.

Disaccharide A sugar.

Dissociation Process of separating a whole into parts.

Distortion Unequal magnification of different portions of the same object.

Dose Amount of radiant energy absorbed by an irradiated object.

Dose equivalent (H) Radiation quantity that is used for radiation protection and that expresses dose on a common scale for all radiation. Expressed in rem or sievert (Sv).

Dose length product (DLP) Product of computed tomography dose index (CTDI) and slice thickness. Depends only on selected computed tomography (CT) parameters and does not reflect patient dose.

Dose limit (DL) Maximum permissible occupational radiation dose.

Dosimeter Instrument that detects and measures exposure to ionizing radiation.

Dosimetry The practice of measuring the intensity of radiation.

Double-contrast examination Examination of the colon that uses air and barium for contrast.

Double-emulsion film Radiographic film that has an emulsion coating on both sides of the base and a layer of supercoat over each emulsion.

Double-helix Configuration of DNA that is shaped like a ladder twisted about an imaginary axis like a spring.

Doubling dose That dose of radiation that is expected to double the number of genetic mutations in a generation.

Duplicating film Single-emulsion film that is exposed to ultraviolet light or blue light through the existing radiograph to produce a copy.

Dynamic range Range of values that can be displayed by an imaging system; shades of gray.

Early effect Radiation response that occurs within minutes or days after radiation exposure.

Eddy current Current that opposes the magnetic field that induced it, creating a loss of transformer efficiency.

Edge enhancement Accentuation of the interface between different tissues.

Edge response function (ERF) Mathematical expression of the ability of the computed tomographic scanner to reproduce a high-contrast edge with accuracy.

Effective atomic number Weighted average atomic number for the different elements of a material.

Effective dose (E) Sum of specified tissues of the products of equivalent dose in a tissue (H_T) and the weighting factor for the tissue (W_T). Effective dose is a method of converting a nonuniform radiation dose, as when a protective apron is worn, to a dose, with respect to risk, as if the whole body were exposed.

Effective dose equivalent (H_E) Sum of the products of the dose equivalent to a tissue (H_T) and the weighting factors (W_T) applicable to each of the tissues irradiated. The values (W_T) are different for effective dose and effective dose equivalent.

Effective focal-spot size Area projected onto the patient and the image receptor.

Elective booking Safeguard against the irradiation of an unsuspected pregnancy.

Electric circuit Path of electron flow from the generating source through the various components and back again.

Electric current Flow of electrons.

Electric field Lines of force exerted on charged ions in the tissues by the electrodes that cause charged particles to move from one pole to another.

Electrical energy Work that can be done when an electron or an electronic charge moves through an electric potential.

Electricity Form of energy created by the activity of electrons and other subatomic particles in motion.

Electrification Process of adding or removing electrons from a substance.

Electrified object Object that has too few or too many electrons.

Electrode Electrical terminal or connector.

Electromagnet Coil or wire wrapped around an iron core that intensifies the magnetic field.

Electromagnetic energy Type of energy in x-rays, radio waves, microwaves, and visible light.

Electromagnetic radiation Oscillating electric and magnetic fields that travel in a vacuum with the velocity of light. Includes x-rays, gamma rays, and some nonionizing radiation (such as ultraviolet, visible, infrared, and radio waves).

Electromagnetic spectrum Continuum of electromagnetic energy.

Electromotive force Electric potential; measured in volts (V).

Electron Elementary particle with one negative charge. Electrons surround the positively charged nucleus and determine the chemical properties of the atom.

Electron binding energy Strength of attachment of an electron to the nucleus.

Electron optics Engineering aspects of maintaining proper electron travel.

Electron spin Momentum of a particle of an atom in a fixed pattern.

Electron volt (eV) Unit of energy equal to that which an electron acquires from a potential difference of 1 V.

Electrostatics Study of fixed or stationary electric charge.

Element Atom that has the same atomic number and the same chemical properties. Substance that cannot be broken down further without changing its chemical properties.

Elemental mass Characteristic mass of an element, determined by the relative abundance of isotopes and their respective atomic masses.

Elongation Image that is made to appear longer than it really is because the inclined object is not located on the central x-ray beam.

Embryologic effect Damage that occurs as the result of exposure of an organism to ionizing radiation during its embryonic stage of development.

Emulsion Material with which x-rays or light photons from screens interact and transfer information.

Endoplasmic reticulum Channel or series of channels that allows the nucleus to communicate with the cytoplasm.

Energy Ability to do work; measured in joules (J).

Energy levels Orbits around the nucleus that contain a designated number of electrons.

Energy subtraction Technique that uses the two x-ray beams alternately to provide a subtraction image that results from differences in photoelectric interaction.

Entrance roller Roller that grips the film to begin its trip through the processor.

Entrance skin exposure (ESE) X-ray exposure to the skin; expressed in milliroentgen (mR).

Enzyme Molecule that is needed in small quantities to allow a biochemical reaction to continue, even though it does not directly enter into the reaction.

Epidemiology Study of the occurrence, distribution, and causes of disease in humans.

Epilation Loss of hair.

Epithelium Covering tissue that lines all exposed surfaces of the body, both exterior and interior.

Erg (Joule) Unit of energy and work.

Erythema Sunburn-like reddening of the skin.

Erythrocyte Red blood cell.

EUR/OPE *E*lectrons *u*sed in *r*eduction/*o*xidation *p*roduces *e*lectrons.

Excess risk Difference between observed and expected numbers of cases.

Excitation Addition of energy to a system achieved by raising the energy of electrons with the use of x-rays.

Exit radiation X-rays that remain after the beam exits through the patient.

Exponent Superscript or power to which 10 is raised in scientific notation.

Exponential form Power-of-10 notation.

Exposed matter Matter that intercepts radiation and absorbs part or all of it; irradiated matter.

Exposure Measure of the ionization produced in air by x-rays or gamma rays. Quantity of radiation intensity expressed in roentgen (R), Coulombs per kilogram (C/kg), or air kerma (Gy).

Exposure factors Factors that influence and determine the quantity and quality of x-radiation to which the patient is exposed.

Exposure linearity   Ability of a radiographic unit to produce a constant radiation output for various combinations of mA and exposure time.

Extinction time   Time required to end an exposure.

Extrafocal radiation, off-focus radiation   Electrons that bounce off the focal spot and land on other areas of the target.

Extrapolation   Estimation of a value beyond the range of known values.

Falling-load generator   Design in which exposure factors are adjusted automatically to the highest mA at the shortest exposure time allowed by the high-voltage generator.

Fan beam   X-ray beam pattern used in computed tomography and digital radiography; projected as a slit.

Feed tray   The start of the transport system, where the film to be processed is inserted into the automatic processor in the darkroom.

Ferromagnetic material   Material that is strongly attracted by a magnet and that usually can be permanently magnetized by exposure to a magnetic field.

Field   Interactions among different energies, forces, or masses that cannot be seen but can be described mathematically.

Field of view (FOV)   Image matrix size provided by digital x-ray imaging systems.

Fifteen percent rule   Principle that states that if the optical density on a radiograph is to be increased with the use of kVp, an increase in kVp by 15% is equivalent to doubling of the mAs.

Filament   Part of the cathode that emits electrons, resulting in a tube current.

File   Collection of data or information that is treated as a unit by the computer.

Film badge   Pack of photographic film used for approximate measurement of radiation exposure to radiation workers. It is the most widely used and most economical type of personnel radiation monitor.

Film graininess   Distribution of silver halide grains in an emulsion.

Filtered back projection   Process by which an image acquired during computed tomography and stored in computer memory is reconstructed.

Filtration   Removal of low-energy x-rays from the useful beam with aluminum or another metal. It results in increased beam quality and reduced patient dose.

First-generation computed tomographic scanner   Finely collimated x-ray beam, single-detector assembly that translates across the patient and rotates between successive translations.

Five-percent rule   Principle that states that an increase of 5% in the kVp may be accompanied by a 30% reduction in the mAs to produce the same optical density at a slightly reduced contrast scale.

Fixing   Stage of processing during which the silver halide not exposed to radiation is dissolved and removed from the emulsion.

Fluorescence   Emission of visible light only during stimulation.

Fluorescent screen   Cycle in a television picture tube whereby the electron beam creates the television optical signal and then immediately fades.

Fluoroscope   Device used to image moving anatomic structures with x-rays.

Fluoroscopy   Imaging modality that provides a continuous image of the motion of internal structures while the x-ray tube is energized. Real-time imaging.

Flux gain   Ratio of the number of light photons at the output phosphor to the number of x-rays at the input phosphor.

Focal spot   Region of the anode target in which electrons interact to produce x-rays.

Focal-spot blur   Blurred region on the radiograph over which the technologist has little control.

Focused grid   Radiographic grid constructed so that the grid strips converge on an imaginary line.

Focusing cup   Metal shroud that surrounds the filament.

Fog   Unintended optical density on a radiograph that reduces contrast through light or chemical contamination.

Fog density   Development of silver grain that contains no useful information.

Force   That which changes the motion of an object; a push or a pull. Expressed in newtons (N).

Foreshortening   Reduction in image size; related to the angle of inclination of the object.

4% voltage ripple   Three-phase, 12-pulse power whose voltage supplied to the x-ray tube never falls below 96% of peak value.

14% ripple   Three-phase, six-pulse power whose voltage supplied to the x-ray tube never falls below 86% of peak value.

Fourth-generation computed tomographic scanner   Unit in which the x-ray source rotates but the detector assembly does not.

Fraction   Numeric value expressed by dividing one number by another.

Fractionated   Radiation dose delivered at the same dose in equal portions at regular intervals.

Free radical   Uncharged molecule that contains a single unpaired electron in the valence shell.

Frequency   Number of cycles or wavelengths of a simple harmonic motion per unit time. Expressed in Hertz (Hz). 1 Hz = 1 cycle/s.

Fulcrum   Imaginary pivot point about which the x-ray tube and the image receptor move.

Full-wave rectification   Circuit in which the negative half-cycle corresponding to the inverse voltage is reversed, so a positive voltage is always directed across the x-ray tube.

Full width at half maximum (FWHM)   Width of the profile at half its maximum value.

Fundamental laws of motion   The three principles of inertia, force, and action/reaction established by Isaac Newton.

Fundamental particles   The three primary constituents of an atom: electrons, photons, and neutrons.

Gantry   Portion of the computed tomographic or magnetic resonance imaging system that accommodates the patient and source or the detector assemblies.

Gastrointestinal (GI) syndrome   Form of acute radiation syndrome that appears in humans at a threshold dose of about 10 Gy (1000 rad). It is characterized by nausea, diarrhea, and damage to the cells lining the intestines.

Geiger-Muller (G-M) counter   Radiation detection and radiation measuring instrument that detects individual ionizations. It is the primary radiation survey instrument for nuclear medicine facilities.

Gelatin   Part of the emulsion that provides mechanical support for the silver halide crystals by holding them uniformly dispersed in place.

Generation time   *See* Cell cycle time.

Genetically significant dose (GSD)   Average gonadal dose given to members of the population who are of childbearing age.

Genetic cell   Oogonium or spermatogonium.

Genetic effect   Effect of radiation that is seen in an individual and in subsequent unexposed generations.

Germ cell   Reproductive cell.

Glandular dose   Average radiation dose to glandular tissue.

Glow curve   Graph that shows the relationship of light output to temperature change.

Glycogen   Human polysaccharide.

Gonadal dose   Exposure to the reproductive organs.

Gradient   Slope of the tangent at any point on the characteristic curve.

Granulocyte   Scavenger cell used to fight bacteria.

Gray (Gy)   Special name for the SI unit of absorbed dose and air kerma. 1 Gy = 1 J/kg = 100 rad.

Gray scale   Image display in which intensity is recorded as variations in brightness.

Grid   Device used to reduce the intensity of scatter radiation in the remnant x-ray beam.

Grid cleanup   Ability of a grid to absorb scatter radiation.

Grid-controlled tube   X-ray tube designed to be turned on and off very rapidly for situations that require multiple exposures at precise exposure times.

Grid cutoff   Absence of optical density on a radiograph caused by unintended x-ray absorption in a grid.

Grid frequency   Number of grid lines per inch or centimeter.

Grid lines   Series of sections of radiopaque material.

Grid ratio   Ratio of grid height to grid strip separation.

Guanine   Nitrogenous organic base that attaches to a deoxyribose molecule.

Guide shoe   Device in an automatic processor that is used to steer film around bends.

Guidewire   Device that allows the safe introduction of the catheter into the vessel.

Halation   Reflection of screen light transmitted through the emulsion and base.

Half-life   Time required for a quantity of radioactivity to be reduced to half its original value.

Half-value layer (HVL)   Thickness of absorber necessary to reduce an x-ray beam to half its original intensity.

Half-wave rectification   Condition in which the voltage is not allowed to swing negatively during the negative half of its cycle.

Hard copy   Permanent image on film or paper, as opposed to an image on a cathode ray tube, a disc, or magnetic tape.

Hardener   A chemical, usually potassium glutaraldehyde alum in the fixer, that is used to stiffen and shrink the emulsion.

Hard x-ray   X-ray that has high penetrability and therefore is of high quality.

Hardware   Visible parts of the computer.

Health physics   The science that is concerned with the recognition, evaluation, and control of radiation hazards.

Heel effect   Absorption of x-rays in the heel of the target, resulting in reduced x-ray intensity to the anode side of the central axis.

Hematologic syndrome   Form of acute radiation syndrome that develops after whole-body exposure to doses ranging from approximately 1 to 10 Gy (100 to 1000 rad). It is characterized by reduction in white cells, red cells, and platelets in circulating blood.

Hertz (Hz)   Unit of frequency; the number of cycles or oscillations that occur each second during simple harmonic motion.

Hexadecimal number system   Number system used by low-level applications to represent a set of four bits.

High-contrast resolution   Ability to image small objects with high subject contrast; spatial resolution.

High-voltage generator   One of three principal parts of an x-ray imaging system; it is always close to the x-ray tube.

Hit   Radiation interaction with the target.

Homeostasis   a. State of equilibrium among tissue and organs. b. Ability of the body to return to normal function despite infection and environmental changes.

Hormone   Protein manufactured by various endocrine glands and carried by the blood to regulate body functions such as growth and development.

Horsepower (hp)   British unit of power.

Hounsfield unit (HU)   Scale of computed tomographic numbers used to assess the nature of tissue.

Hybrid subtraction   Technique that combines temporal and energy subtraction.

Hydroquinone   Principal compound used in the chemical composition of film developers.

Hypersthenic   Referring to a body habitus of a patient who is large in frame and overweight.

Hypo   Sodium thiosulfate, a fixing agent that removes unexposed and undeveloped silver halide crystals from the emulsion.

Hypo retention   Undesirable retention of the fixer in emulsion.

Hyposthenic   Referring to a body habitus of a patient who is thin but healthy looking.

Hysteresis   Additional resistance created by the alternate reversal of the magnetic field caused by the alternating current.

Image detail   Sharpness of small structures on the radiograph.

Image-forming x-ray   X-ray that exits from the patient and enters the image receptor.

Image intensifier   Electronic vacuum tube that amplifies a fluoroscopic image to reduce patient dose.

Image matrix   Layout of cells in rows and columns.

Image noise   Deterioration of the radiographic image.

Image receptor (IR)   Medium that transforms the x-ray beam into a visible image; radiographic film or a phosphorescent screen.

Image receptor contrast   Contrast that is inherent in the film and is influenced by processing of the film. *See also* Subject contrast.

Improper fraction   Fraction in which the quotient is greater than 1.

Indirect effect   Effect of radiation that results from the production of free radicals produced by the interaction of radiation with water.

Induction   Process of making ferromagnetic material magnetic.

Induction motor   Electric motor in which the rotor is a series of wire loops but the external magnetic field is supplied by several fixed electromagnets called *stators*.

Inertia   Property of matter that resists change in motion or at rest.

Infrared light   Light that consists of photons with wavelengths longer than those of visible light but shorter than those of microwaves.

Infrared radiation   Electromagnetic radiation just lower in energy than visible light, with a wavelength in the range of 0.7 to 1000 µm.

Inherent filtration   Filtration of useful x-ray beams provided by the permanently installed components of an x-ray tube housing assembly and the glass window of an x-ray tube.

Initiation time   Time required to start an exposure.

Input   Process of transferring information into primary memory.

Insulator   Material that inhibits the flow of electrons within a conductor or during heat transfer.

Integrate mode   Function of an instrument designed to measure the total accumulated intensity of radiation over time.

Intensification factor (IF)   Ratio of exposure without screens to that with screens to produce the same optical density.

Intensifying screen   Sensitive phosphor that converts x-rays to light to shorten exposure time and reduce patient dose.

Intensity profile   Projection formed by the intensity of radiation detected according to the attenuation pattern.

Internally deposited radionuclide   Naturally occurring radionuclide in the human body.

International System of Units (SI)   Standard system of units based on the meter, the kilogram, and the second; it has been adopted by all countries and is used in all branches of science.

Interface   Hardware and software that enable imaging systems to interconnect and to connect with printers.

Interphase   Period of growth of the cell between divisions.

Interpolation   Estimation of a value between two known values.

Interrogation time   Time during which the signal from an image detector is sampled.

Interspace material   Sections of radiolucent material in a grid.

Interstitial   Referring to the area between cells.

Inverse square law   Law that states that the intensity of radiation at a location is inversely proportional to the square of its distance from the source of radiation.

Inverse voltage   Current that flows from the anode to the cathode.

Inverter   High-speed switches that convert direct current into a series of square pulses.

In vivo   In the living cell.

Ion   Atom with too many or too few electrons; an electrically charged particle.

Ion chamber   Instrument that detects and measures the radiation intensity in areas outside of protective barriers.

Ion pair   Two oppositely charged particles.

Ionic bond   Bonding that occurs because of an electrostatic force between ions.

Ionization   Removal of an orbital electron from an atom.

Ionization potential   Amount of energy (34 eV) necessary to ionize tissue atoms.

Ionized   Referring to an atom that has an extra electron or has had an electron removed.

Ionizing radiation   Radiation capable of ionization.

Irradiated   Referring to matter that intercepts radiation and absorbs part or all of it; exposed.

Isobars   Atoms that have the same number of nucleons but different numbers of protons and neutrons.

Isochromatid   Fragment in a chromosome aberration.

Isomers   Atoms that have the same numbers of protons and neutrons but a different nuclear energy state.

Isotones   Atoms that have the same number of neutrons.

Isotopes   Atoms that have the same number of protons but a different number of neutrons.

Isotropic   Equal intensity in all directions; having the same properties in all directions.

Joule (J) Unit of energy; the work done when a force of 1 N acts on an object along a distance of 1 m.

Karotype Chromosome map.

Kerma (k) Energy absorbed per unit mass from the initial kinetic energy released in matter of all the electrons liberated by x-rays or gamma rays. Expressed in gray (Gy). 1 Gy = 1 J/kg.

Kilo- Prefix meaning "one thousand."

Kiloelectron volt (keV) The kinetic energy of an electron equivalent to 1000 eV. 1 keV = 1000 eV.

Kilogram (kg) Scientific unit of mass that is unrelated to gravitational effects; 1000 g.

Kilovolt (kV) Electric potential equal to 1000 V.

Kinetic energy Energy of motion.

Kilovolt peak (kVp) Measure of the maximum electrical potential across an x-ray tube; expressed in kilovolts.

Lag Phosphorescence.

Laser disc Removable disc that uses laser technology to write and read data.

Late effect Radiation response that is not observed for 6 months or longer after exposure.

Latent image Unobservable image stored in the silver halide emulsion; it is made manifest by processing.

Latent image center Sensitivity center that has many silver ions attracted to it.

Latent period Period after the prodromal stage of the acute radiation syndrome during which no sign of radiation sickness is apparent.

Lateral decentering Improper positioning of the grid that results in cutoff.

Latitude Range of x-ray exposure over which a radiograph is acceptable.

Law of Bergonié and Tribondeau Principle that states that the radiosensitivity of cells is directly proportional to their reproductive activity and inversely proportional to their degree of differentiation.

Law of conservation of energy Principle that states that energy may be transformed from one form to another but cannot be created or destroyed; the total amount of energy is constant.

Law of conservation of matter Principle that states that matter can be neither created nor destroyed.

Law of inertia Principle that states that a body will remain at rest or will continue to move with a constant velocity in a straight line unless acted on by an external force.

LD$_{50/60}$ Dose of radiation expected to cause death within 60 days to 50% of those exposed.

Leakage radiation Secondary radiation emitted through the tube housing.

Limiting resolution Spatial frequency at a modulation transfer function equal to 0.1.

Line focus Projection of an inclined line onto a surface, resulting in a smaller size.

Line focus principle Design incorporated into x-ray tube targets to allow a large area for heating while a small focal spot is maintained.

Line pair One bar and its interspace of equal width.

Linear energy transfer (LET) Measure of the rate at which energy is transferred from ionizing radiation to soft tissue. Expressed in kiloelectron volts per micrometer of soft tissue.

Linear, nonthreshold Referring to the dose-response relationship that intersects the dose axis at or below zero.

Linear, threshold Referring to the dose-response relationship that intercepts the dose axis at a value greater than zero.

Linear tomography Imaging modality in which the x-ray tube is mechanically attached to the image receptor and moves in one direction as the image receptor moves in the opposite direction.

Lodestone A leading stone.

Log relative exposure (LRE) Change in optical density over each exposure interval.

Logic function Computer-recognized command that evaluates an intermediate result and performs subsequent computations in accordance with that result.

Long gray scale Low-contrast radiograph that has many shades of gray.

Look-up table (LUT) Matrix of data that manipulates the values of gray levels, converting an image input value to a different output value.

Low-contrast resolution Ability to image objects with similar subject contrast.

Luminescence Emission of visible light.

Lymphocyte White blood cell that plays an active role in providing immunity for the body by producing antibodies; it is the most radiosensitive blood cell.

Lysosome Cell that contains enzymes capable of digesting cellular fragments.

Magnetic dipole Current that flows in an infinitesimally small loop.

Magnetic dipole moment Vector with a magnitude equal to the product of the current that flows in a loop and the area of the current loop.

Magnetic domain An accumulation of many atomic magnets with their dipoles aligned.

Magnetic permeability Property of a material that causes it to attract the imaginary lines of the magnetic field.

Magnetic susceptibility The ease with which a substance can be magnetized.

Magnetite The magnetic oxide of iron.

Magnetism The polarization of a material.

Magnetization Relative magnetic flux density in a material compared with that in a vacuum.

Magnification Condition in which the images on the radiograph are larger than the object they represent.

Magnitude Number that represents a quantity.

Main-chain scission Breakage of the long-chain macromolecule that divides the long, single molecule into smaller ones.

Mainframe computer A fast, medium to large, large-capacity system that has multiple microprocessors.

Mammographer A radiologic technologist who specializes in breast x-ray studies.

Mammography Radiographic examination of the breast using low kilovoltage.

Manifest illness Stage of acute radiation syndrome during which signs and symptoms are apparent.

Manifest image The observable image that is formed when the latent image undergoes proper chemical processing.

Man-made radiation X-rays and artificially produced radionuclides used for nuclear medicine.

Mask image Image obtained from mask mode.

Mask mode Method of temporal subtraction that results in successive subtraction images of contrast-filled vessels.

Masking The act of ensuring that no extraneous light from the viewbox enters the viewer's eyes.

Mass A quantity of matter; expressed in kilograms.

Mass density Quantity of matter per unit volume.

Mass-energy equivalence Energy equals mass multiplied by the square of the speed of light.

Matrix Rows and columns of pixels displayed on a digital image.

Matter Anything that occupies space and has form or shape.

Maximum-intensity projection (MIP) Reconstruction of an image through selection of the highest-value pixels along any arbitrary line in the data set; only those pixels are exhibited.

Maximum permissible dose (MPD) Dose of occupational radiation that would be expected to produce no significant radiation effects. An old expression. Replaced by Dose Limit.

Mean lethal dose Constant related to the radiosensitivity of a cell.

Mean marrow dose (MMD) Average radiation dose to the entire active bone marrow.

Mean survival time Average time between exposure and death.

Mechanical energy Ability of an object to do work. *See also* Kinetic energy and Potential energy.

Medical physicist Physicist who examines and monitors the performance of imaging equipment.

Meiosis Process of germ cell division that reduces the chromosomes in each daughter cell to half the number of chromosomes in the parent cell.

Metabolism Anabolism and catabolism.

Metaphase Phase of cell division during which the chromosomes are divisible.

Metol Secondary constituent used in the chemical composition of developing agents.

Microcalcifications Calcific deposits that appear as small grains of varying sizes on the x-ray film.

Microcomputer Personal computer or electronic organizer.

Microcontroller Tiny computer installed in an appliance.

Microfocus tube Tube that has a very small focal spot and that is specifically designed for imaging very small microcalcifications at relatively short source-to-image distances.

Microwave Short-wavelength radiofrequency.

Mid-density (MD) step Step that has an average optical density closest to, but not less than, 1.2.

Milliampere (mA) Measure of x-ray tube current.

Milliampere-second (mAs) Product of exposure time and x-ray tube current; measure of the total number of electrons.

Minification gain Ratio of the square of the diameter of the input phosphor to the square of the diameter of the output phosphor.

Misregistration Misalignment of two or more images because of patient motion between image acquisitions.

Mitochondrion Structure that digests macromolecules to produce energy for the cell.

Mitosis (M) Process of somatic cell division wherein a parent cell divides to form two daughter cells identical to the parent cell.

Modem Device that converts digital information into analog information.

Modulation Changing of the magnitude of a video signal; the magnitude is directly proportional to the light intensity received by the television camera tube.

Modulation transfer function (MTF) Mathematical procedure for measuring resolution.

Molecule Group of atoms of various elements held together by chemical forces; the smallest unit of a compound that can exist by itself and retain all its chemical properties.

Molybdenum Target material for x-ray tubes that is used in mammography.

Momentum Product of the mass of an object and its velocity.

Monoenergetic Beam that contains x-rays or gamma rays that all have the same energy.

Monosaccharide A sugar.

Motherboard Main circuit board in a system unit.

Motion blur Blurring of the image that results from movement of the patient or the x-ray tube during exposure.

Moving grid Grid that moves while the x-ray exposure is being made.

Multiplanar reformation (MPR) Process by which transverse images are stacked to form a three-dimensional data set.

Multislice computed tomography Imaging modality that uses two detector arrays to produce two spiral slices at the same time.

Multitarget or single-hit model Model of radiation dose-response relationship for more complicated biologic systems, such as human cells.

Muscle Tissue that is capable of contracting.

Mutual induction   Process of producing electricity in a secondary coil by passing an alternating current through a nearby primary coil.

National Council on Radiation Protection and Measurement (NCRP)   Organization that continuously reviews recommended dose limits.

Natural environmental radiation   Naturally occurring ionizing radiation, including cosmic rays, terrestrial radiation, and internally deposited radionuclides.

Natural magnet   Magnet that gets its magnetism from the Earth.

Nervous tissue   Tissue that consists of neurons and serves as the avenue through which electrical impulses are transmitted throughout the body for control and response.

Neuron   Cell of the nervous system that has long, thin extensions from the cell to distant parts of the body.

Neutron   Uncharged elementary particle, with a mass slightly greater than that of the proton, that is found in the nucleus of every atom heavier than hydrogen.

Newton (N)   Unit of force in the SI system; $1 N = 0.22$ lb.

Node   One of many stations or terminals of a computer network.

Noise   **a.** Grainy or uneven appearance of an image caused by an insufficient number of primary x-rays. **b.** Uniform signal produced by scattered x-rays.

Nonionizing radiation   Radiation for which the mechanism of action in tissue does not directly ionize atomic or molecular systems through a single interaction.

Nonlinear, nonthreshold   Referring to varied responses that are produced from varied doses, with any dose expected to produce a response.

Nonlinear, threshold   Referring to varied responses that are produced from varied doses, with a particular level below which there is no response.

Nonscheduled maintenance   Maintenance that becomes necessary because of a failure in the system that necessitates processor repair.

Nonstochastic effects   Biologic effects of ionizing radiation that demonstrate the existence of a threshold. Severity of biologic damage increases with increased dose. (See Determination Effects.)

North pole   Magnetic pole that has a positive electrostatic charge.

Nuclear energy   Energy contained within the nucleus of an atom.

Nucleolus   Rounded structure that often is attached to the nuclear membrane and controls the passage of molecules, especially RNA, from the nucleus to the cytoplasm.

Nucleon   A proton or a neutron.

Nucleotide   Unit formed from a nitrogenous base, a five-carbon sugar molecule, and a phosphate molecule.

Nucleus   **a.** Center of a living cell; spherical mass of protoplasm that contains the genetic material (DNA) that is stored in its molecular structure. **b.** Center of an atom that contains neutrons and protons.

Nuclide   General term that refers to all known isotopes, both stable and unstable, of chemical elements.

Object plane   Plane in which the anatomic structures that are to be imaged lie.

Object-to-image receptor distance (OID)   Distance from the image receptor to the object that is to be imaged.

Occupational dose   Dose received by an individual in a restricted area during the course of employment in which the individual's assigned duties involve exposure to radiation.

Occupational exposure   Radiation exposure received by radiation workers.

Off-focus radiation   X-rays produced in the anode but not at the focal spot.

Off-level grid   Artifact produced by an improperly positioned radiographic tube—not by an improperly positioned grid.

1% voltage ripple   High-frequency generators that have higher x-ray quantity and quality.

100% voltage ripple   Single-phase power in which the voltage varies from zero to its maximum value.

Oocytes   Primordial follicles that grow to encapsulate oogonia.

Opaque   Surface that does not allow the passage of light.

Open filament   Condition that results when the filament becomes thinner and breaks.

Operating console   Console that allows the radiologic technologist to control the x-ray tube current and voltage so that the useful x-ray beam is of proper quantity and quality.

Operating system   Series of instructions that organizes the course of data through the computer to solve a particular problem.

Optical density   Degree of blackening of a radiograph.

Optical disc   Removable disc that uses laser technology to write and read data.

Ordered pairs   Notation for coordinates in which the first number of the pair represents a distance along the x-axis and the second number indicates a distance up the y-axis.

Origin   Point at which two axes meet on a graph.

Organs   Collection of tissues of similar structure and function.

Organ system   Combination of tissues and organs that forms an overall integrated organization.

Organic molecule   Molecule that is life supporting and contains carbon.

Orthochromatic   Referring to blue- or green-sensitive film; usually exposed with rare Earth screen.

Outcome analysis   Image interpretation that involves reconciling the patient's ultimate disease condition with the radiologist's diagnosis.

Output   Process of transferring the results of a computation from primary memory to storage or to the user.

Overcoat   Protective covering of gelatin that encloses the emulsion.

Overexposed   Referring to a radiograph that is too dark because too much x-radiation reached the image receptor.

Ovum   Mature germ cell in a female.

Oxidation   Reaction that produces an electron.

Oxygen enhancement ratio (OER)   Ratio of the dose necessary to produce a given effect under anoxic conditions to the dose necessary to produce the same effect under aerobic conditions.

Pair production   Interaction between the x-ray and the nuclear electric field that causes the x-ray to disappear and that causes two electrons—one positive and one negative—to take its place.

Panchromatic   Referring to film that is sensitive to the entire visible light spectrum.

Parallel circuit   Circuit that contains elements that bridge conductors rather than lie in a line along a conductor.

Parallel grid   Simple grid in which all lead grid strips are parallel.

Paramagnetic   Referring to materials slightly attracted to a magnet and loosely influenced by an external magnetic field.

Parenchymal   Referring to part of the organ that contains tissues representative of that particular organ.

Partial volume effect   Distortion of signal intensity from a tissue because it extends partially into an adjacent slice thickness.

Particle accelerator   An atom "smasher." Cyclotron. Linear Accelerator.

Particulate radiation   Radiation distinct from x-rays and gamma rays; examples include alpha particles, electrons, neutrons, and protons.

Penetrability   Ability of an x-ray to penetrate tissue; range in tissue; x-ray quality.

Penetrometer   Aluminum step wedge.

Penumbra   Image blur that results from the size of the focal spot; geometric unsharpness.

Permanent magnet   Magnet whose magnetism is induced artificially.

Phantom   Device that simulates some parameters of the human body for evaluation of imaging system performance.

Phenidone   Secondary constituent in the chemical composition of developing agents.

Phosphor   Active layer of the radiographic intensifying screen closest to the radiographic film.

Phosphorescence   Emission of visible light during and after stimulation.

Photoconductor   Material that conducts electrons when illuminated.

Photodiode   Solid-state device that converts light into an electric current.

Photodisintegration   Process by which very high-energy x-rays can escape interaction with electrons and the nuclear electric field and can be absorbed directly by the nucleus.

Photoelectron   Electron that has been removed during the process of photoelectric absorption.

Photoelectric effect   Absorption of an x-ray by ionization.

Photoemission   Electron emission after light stimulation.

Photographic effect   Formation of the latent image.

Photometer   Instrument that measures light intensity.

Photomultiplier tube   Electron tube that converts visible light into an electrical signal.

Photon   Electromagnetic radiation that has neither mass nor electric charge but interacts with matter as though it is a particle; x-rays and gamma rays.

Photospot camera   Camera that exposes only one frame when active, receiving its image from the output phosphor of the image-intensifier tube.

Photostimulation   Emission of visible light after excitation by laser light.

Photothermographic   Printing process by which film is exposed to light, thereby forming a latent image that is made visible by heat.

Phototimer   Device that allows automatic exposure control.

Pitch   *See* Spiral pitch ratio.

Pixel   Picture element; the cell of a digital image matrix.

Planck's constant (h)   Fundamental physical constant that relates the energy of radiation to its frequency.

Planetary rollers   Rollers positioned outside the master roller and guide shoes.

Pluripotential stem cell   Stem cell that has the ability to develop into several different types of mature cells.

Pocket ionization chamber (pocket dosimeter)   Personnel radiation monitoring device.

Point lesion   Any change that results in impairment or loss of function at the point of a single chemical bond.

Point mutation   Molecular lesion caused by the change or loss of a base that destroys the triplet code and may not be reversible.

Polarity   Existence of opposing negative and positive charges.

Pole   Magnetically charged end of a material.

Polyenergetic   Referring to radiation, such as x-rays, with a spectrum of energies.

Polysaccharide   Large carbohydrate that includes starches and glycogen.

Positive beam limiting (PBL)   Feature of radiographic collimators that automatically adjusts the radiation field to the size of the image receptor.

Potassium bromide   Compound used as a restrainer in the developer.

Potassium iodide   Compound used as a restrainer in the developer.

Potential energy   Ability to do work by virtue of position.

Power   Time rate at which work (W) is done. 1 W = 1 J/s.

Power-of-10 notation   Exponential form.

Precursor cell   An immature cell.

Predetector collimator   Collimator that restricts the x-ray beam viewed by the detector array.

Prepatient collimator Collimator that consists of several sections so that a nearly parallel x-ray beam results.

Prereading voltmeter A kVp meter that registers even though an exposure is not being made and no current is flowing within the circuit; this allows the voltage to be monitored before an exposure.

Preservative Chemical additive, usually sodium sulfide, that maintains the chemical balance of the developer and fixer.

Preventive maintenance Planned program of parts replacement at regular intervals.

Primary coil The first coil through which the varying current in an electromagnet is passed.

Primary protective barrier Any wall to which the useful beam can be directed.

Processing Chemical treatment of the emulsion of a radiographic film to change a latent image to a manifest image.

Processor Electronic circuitry that does the actual computations and the memory that supports it.

Prodromal period First stage of the acute radiation syndrome; occurs within hours after radiation exposure.

Proper fraction Fraction in which the quotient is less than 1.

Prophase Phase of cell division during which the nucleus and the chromosomes enlarge and the DNA begins to take structural form.

Proportion The relation of one part to another.

Proportional counter Sensitive instrument that is used primarily as stationary laboratory instrument for the assay of small quantities of radioactivity.

Protective coating Layer of the radiographic intensifying screen closest to the radiographic film.

Protective housing Lead-lined metal container into which the x-ray tube is fitted.

Protein synthesis Metabolic production of proteins.

Proton Elementary particle with a positive electric charge equal to that of an electron and a mass approximately equal to that of a neutron. It is located within the nucleus of an atom.

Protracted dose Dose of radiation that is delivered continuously but at a lower dose rate.

Pulse mode/rate mode Instruments designed to detect the presence of radiation.

Quality assurance (QA) All planned and systematic actions necessary to provide adequate confidence that a facility, system, or administrative component will perform safely and satisfactorily in service to a patient. It includes scheduling, preparation, and promptness in examination or treatment, reporting of results, and quality control.

Quality control (QC) All actions necessary to control and verify the performance of equipment; part of quality assurance.

Quantum An x-ray photon.

Quantum mottle Radiographic noise produced by the random interaction of x-rays with an intensifying screen. This effect is more noticeable when very high rare Earth systems are used at a high kVp.

Quantum theory Theory in the physics of matter smaller than an atom and of electromagnetic radiation.

Rad (radiation absorbed dose) Special unit for absorbed dose and air kerma. 1 rad = 100 erg/g = 0.01 Gy.

Radiation Energy emitted and transferred through matter.

Radiation biology Branch of biology that is concerned with the effects of ionizing radiation on living systems.

Radiation exposure X-ray quantity or intensity; measured in roentgens.

Radiation fog Artifact caused by unintentional exposure to radiation.

Radiation hormesis Theory that suggests that very low radiation doses may be beneficial.

Radiation quality Relative penetrability of an x-ray beam determined by its average energy; usually measured by half-value layer or kilovolt peak.

Radiation quantity Intensity of radiation; usually measured in milliroentgen (mR).

Radiation standards Recommendations, rules, and regulations regarding permissible concentrations, as well as safe handling techniques, transportation, and industrial control of radioactive material.

Radiation (thermal) Transfer of heat by the emission of infrared electromagnetic radiation.

Radiation weighting factor (W_R) Factor used for radiation protection that accounts for differences in biologic effectiveness between different radiations. Formerly called **quality factor.**

Radioactive decay Naturally occurring process whereby an unstable atomic nucleus relieves its instability through the emission of one or more energetic particles.

Radioactive disintegration Process by which the nucleus spontaneously emits particles and energy and transforms itself into another atom to reach stability.

Radioactive half-life Time required for a radioisotope to decay to half its original activity.

Radioactivity Rate of decay or disintegration of radioactive material. Expressed in curie (Ci) or becquerel (Bq). 1 Ci = 3.7 × 10^{10} Bq.

Radiofrequency (RF) Electromagnetic radiation with frequencies from 0.3 kHz to 300 GHz; magnetic resonance imaging uses RF in the range of approximately 1 to 100 mHz.

Radiographer Radiologic technologist who deals specifically with x-ray imaging.

Radiographic contrast Combined result of image receptor contrast and subject contrast.

Radiographic intensifying screen Device that converts the energy of the x-ray beam into visible light to increase the brightness of an x-ray image.

Radiographic noise Undesirable fluctuation in the optical density of the image.

Radiographic technique Combination of settings selected on the control panel of the x-ray imaging system to produce a quality image on the radiograph.

Radiographic technique chart Guide that describes standard methods for consistently producing high-quality images.

Radiography Imaging modality that uses x-ray film and usually an x-ray tube mounted from the ceiling on a track that allows the tube to be moved in any direction; provides fixed images.

Radioisotopes Radioactive atoms that have the same number of protons. They are changed into a different atomic species by disintegration of the nucleus accompanied by the emission of ionizing radiation.

Radiological Society of North America (RSNA) Scientific society of radiologists and medical physicists.

Radiologist Physician who specializes in medical imaging with the use of x-rays, ultrasound, and magnetic resonance imaging.

Radiolucent Referring to a tissue or material that transmits x-rays and appears dark on a radiograph.

Radiolysis of water Dissociation of water into other molecular products as a result of irradiation.

Radionuclides Any nucleus that emits radiation.

Radiopaque Referring to a tissue or material that absorbs x-rays and appears bright on a radiograph.

Radiosensitivity Relative susceptibility of cells, tissues, and organs to the harmful action of ionizing radiation.

Radon Colorless, odorless, naturally occurring radioactive gas (^{222}Ra) that decays via alpha emission and has a half-life of 3.8 days.

RAID (redundant array of inexpensive discs) system System that consists of at least disc drives within a single cabinet that collectively act as a single storage system.

Random access memory (RAM) Data that can be stored or accessed at random from anywhere in main memory in approximately equal amounts of time, regardless of where they are located.

Rare Earth element Element that is a transitional metal found in low abundance in nature.

Rare Earth screen Radiographic intensifying screen made from rare Earth elements, which make it more useful for radiographic imaging.

Raster pattern Pattern produced on the screen of a television picture tube by the movement of an electron beam or on film by a laser scan.

Ratio Mathematical relationship between similar quantities.

Read-only memory (ROM) Data storage device that contains information supplied by the manufacturer that cannot be written on or erased.

Real time Display for which the image is continuously renewed, often to view anatomic motion, in fluoroscopy and ultrasound.

Reciprocity law Principle that states that optical density on a radiograph is proportional only to the total energy imparted to the radiographic film.

Reconstruction Creation of an image from data.

Reconstruction time Time needed for the computer to present a digital image after an examination has been completed.

Recorded detail Degree of sharpness of structural lines on a radiograph.

Recovery Repair and repopulation.

Rectification Process of converting alternating current to direct current.

Rectifier Electronic device that allows current flow in only one direction.

Red filter Filter that transmits light only above 600 nm; it is used with both green- and blue-sensitive film.

Redox Simultaneous reduction and oxidation reactions.

Reducing agent Chemical responsible for reduction.

Reduction Process by which an electron is given up by a chemical to neutralize a positive ion.

Reflection Return or reentry of an x-ray.

Reflective layer Layer of the intensifying screen that intercepts light headed in other directions and redirects it to the film.

Refraction Deviation of course that occurs when photons of visible light traveling in straight lines pass from one transparent medium to another.

Region of interest (ROI) Area of an anatomic structure on a reconstructed digital image as defined by the operator using a cursor.

Relative age-response relationship Increased incidence of a disease proportional to its natural incidence.

Relative biologic effectiveness (RBE) Ratio of the dose of standard radiation necessary to produce a given effect to the dose of test radiation needed for the same effect.

Relative risk Estimation of late radiation effects in large populations without precise knowledge of their radiation dose.

Relay Electrical device based on electromagnetic induction that serves as a switch.

Rem (radiation equivalent man) Special unit for dose equivalent and effective dose. It has been replaced by the sievert (Sv) in the SI system. 1 rem = 0.01 Sv.

Remnant radiation X-rays that pass through the patient and interact with the image receptor.

Replenishment Replacement of developer and of fixer in the automatic processing of film.

Repopulation Replication by surviving cells.

Resistance Opposition to a force.

Resolution Measure of the ability of a system to image two separate objects and visually distinguish one from the other.

Restrainer Compound that restricts the action of the developing agent to only irradiated silver halide crystals.

Ribonucleic acid (RNA) Molecules that are involved in the growth and development of a cell through a number of small, spherical cytoplasmic organelles that attach to the endoplasmic reticulum.

Ribosomes The site of protein synthesis.

Right-hand rule Rule by which the direction of magnetic field lines can be determined.

Roller subassembly One of three principal film-transport subsystems in an imaging system.

Rotating anode Anode used in general purpose x-ray tubes because the tubes must be capable of producing high-intensity x-ray beams in a short time.

Rotor Rotating part of an electromagnetic induction motor that is located inside the glass envelope.

Saccharide A carbohydrate.

Safe industry Industry that has an associated annual fatality accident rate of no more than 1 per 10,000 workers.

Safelight Incandescent lamp with a color filter that provides sufficient illumination in the darkroom while ensuring that the film remains unexposed.

Sagittal plane Any anterior-posterior plane parallel to the long axis of the body.

Saturation current Filament current that has risen to its maximum value because all available electrons have been used.

Scalar Referring to a quantity or a measurement that has only magnitude.

Scanned projection radiography (SPR) Generalized method of making a digital radiograph; used in computed tomography for precise localization.

Scatter radiation X-rays scattered back in the direction of the incident x-ray beam.

Scheduled maintenance Procedures performed on a routine basis.

Scientific notation Exponential form.

Scintillation detector Instrument used in the detector arrays of many computed tomographic scanners.

Screen lag The phosphorescence in an intensifying screen.

Screen speed Relative number used to identify the efficiency of conversion of x-rays into usable light.

Screen-film The most commonly used film; used with intensifying screens.

Screening mammography Imaging examination that is performed on the breasts of asymptomatic women with a two-view protocol, to detect unsuspected cancer.

Second (s) Standard unit of time.

Secondary coil Coil in which induced current in an electromagnet flows.

Secondary electron Electron ejected from the outer shell of an atom.

Secondary memory Data stored on tape drives, diskettes, and hard disc drives.

Secondary protective barrier Barrier designed to shield an area from secondary radiation.

Secondary radiation Leakage and scatter reaction.

Second-generation computed tomographic scanner Unit that incorporates the natural extension of the single detector to a multiple-detector assembly that intercepts a fan-shaped rather than a pencil-shaped x-ray beam.

Section thickness The thickness of tissue that will not be blurred by tomography.

Selectivity Ratio of primary radiation to scattered radiation transmitted through the grid.

Self-induction Magnetic field produced in a coil of wire that opposes the alternating current being conducted.

Self-rectified system Imaging system in which the x-ray tube serves as the vacuum-tube rectifier.

Semiconductor Material that can serve both as a conductor and as an insulator of electricity.

Sensitivity Ability of an image receptor to respond to x-rays.

Sensitivity center Physical imperfections in the lattice of the emulsion layer that occur during the film manufacturing process.

Sensitivity profile Slice thickness.

Sensitizing agent Agent that enhances the effect of radiation.

Sensitometer Optical step wedge that is used to construct a characteristic curve.

Sensitometry Study of the response of an image receptor to x-rays.

Sequestering agent Agent introduced into the developer to form stable complexes with metallic ions and salts.

Shaded surface display (SSD) Computer-aided technique that identifies a narrow range of values as belonging to the object to be imaged and displays that range.

Shadow dose equivalent (HS) Dose of radiation to which the external skin or an extremity is exposed.

Shadow shield Shield that is suspended over the region of interest; it casts a shadow over the patient's reproductive organs.

Shape distortion Type of distortion caused by elongation or foreshortening.

Shells Orbital energy levels that surround the nucleus of an atom.

Shell-type transformer Transformer that confines more of the magnet field lines of the primary winding because there are essentially two closed cores.

Short gray scale High-contrast radiograph that exhibits black to white in just a few apparent steps.

Sievert (Sv) Special name for the SI unit of dose equivalent and effective dose. 1 Sv = 1 Jkg = 100 rem.

Sigmoid-type (S-type) dose-response relationship Nonlinear, threshold radiation dose-response relationship.

Silver bromide Material that makes up 98% of the silver halide crystals in a typical emulsion.

Silver halide crystals Active ingredient of the radiographic emulsion. It is instrumental in creating a latent image on the radiograph.

Silver iodide   Material that makes up 2% of the silver halide crystals in a typical emulsion.

Sine wave   Variation in the movement of photons in electrical and magnetic fields.

Single-target hit model   Model of radiation dose-response relationships for enzymes, viruses, and bacteria.

Sinusoidal   Simple motion; a sine wave.

Skin erythema dose (SED)   Dose of radiation, usually about 200 rad or 2 Gy, that causes redness of the skin.

Slice thickness   The thickness of the tissue that is being imaged.

Slice-acquisition rate (SAR)   Measure of the efficiency of a multislice spiral computed tomographic scanner.

Slip ring technology   Technology that allows the gantry to rotate continuously without interruption, making spiral computed tomography possible.

Sludge   Deposit on the film that results from dirty or warped rollers; causes emulsion pickoff and gelatin buildup.

Sodium carbonate   Alkali compound contained in the developer.

Sodium hydroxide   Alkali compound contained in the developer.

Sodium sulfite   Preservative added to the developer that keeps it clear.

Soft copy   Output on a display screen.

Soft tissue radiography   Radiography in which only muscle and fat structures are imaged.

Soft x-ray   X-ray that has low penetrability and therefore is of low quality.

Software   Computer programs that tell the hardware what to do and how to store data.

Solenoid   Helical winding of current-carrying wire that produces a magnetic field along the axis of the helix.

Solid-state diode   Diode that passes electric current in only one direction.

Solution   Suspension of particles or molecules in a fluid.

Solvent   Liquid into which various solids and powders can be dissolved.

Somatic cells   All cells of the body except the oogonium and the spermatogonium.

Somatic effects   Effects of radiation, such as cancer and leukemia, limited to an exposed individual. *See also* Genetic effect.

Source-to-image receptor distance (SID)   Distance from the x-ray tube to the image receptor.

Source-to-skin distance (SSD)   Distance from the patient's skin to the fluoroscopic tube.

Space charge   Electron cloud near the filament.

Space-charge effect   Phenomenon of the space charge that makes it difficult for subsequent electrons to be emitted by the filament because of electrostatic repulsion.

Spatial distortion   Misrepresentation in the image of the actual spatial relationships among objects.

Spatial frequency   Measure of resolution; usually expressed in line pairs per millimeter (lp/mm).

Spatial resolution   Ability to image small objects that have high subject contrast.

Spatial uniformity   Constancy of pixel values in all regions of the reconstructed image.

Special quantities   Additional quantities designed to support measurement in specialized areas of science and technology.

Spectrum   Graphic representation of the range over which a quantity extends.

Spectrum matching   Use of rare Earth screens only in conjunction with film emulsions that have light absorption characteristics matched to the light emission of the screen.

Speed   Term used to loosely describe the sensitivity of film to x-rays.

Speed index   Step that has an average optical density closest to, but not less than, 1.2.

Sperm   *See* Spermatozoa.

Spermatocyte   Mature spermatogonium.

Spermatogonium   Male germ cell.

Spermatozoa   Functionally mature male germ cell.

Spindle fibers   Fibers that connect a centromere and two chromatids to the poles of the nucleus during mitosis.

Spindles   Poles of the nucleus.

Spinning top   Device used to check exposure timers.

Spiral/helical   Term given to computed tomography because it describes the apparent motion of the x-ray tube during the scan.

Spiral pitch radio   Relationship between patient couch movement and x-ray beam collimation.

Spot film   Static image in a small-format image receptor taken during fluoroscopy.

Square law   Principle that states that one can compensate for a change in the source-to-object distance by changing the mAs by the factor SID squared.

Starch   A plant polysaccharide.

Stationary anode   Anode used in imaging systems in which high tube current and power are not required.

Stator   Stationary coil windings located in the protective housing but outside the x-ray tube glass envelope. It is part of the electromagnetic induction motor.

Stem cell   Immature or precursor cell.

Step-down transformer   Transformer in which the voltage is decreased from the primary side to the secondary side.

Stepping   Computer-controlled capability on a patient table that allows imaging from the abdomen to the feet after a single injection of contrast media.

Step-up transformer   Transformer in which the voltage is increased from the primary side to the secondary side.

Step wedge   Filter used during radiography of a body part, such as the foot, that varies in thickness from one end to the other.

Stereoradiography   Practice of making two radiographs of the same object and viewing through a device that allows each eye to view a different radiograph.

Sthenic Referring to the body habitus of a patient who is strong and active; average body habitus.

Stochastic effects Probability or frequency of the biologic response to radiation as a function of radiation dose. Disease incidence increases proportionally with dose, and there is no dose threshold.

Storage memory Main computer memory in which the program and data files are stored.

Straight-line portion Portion of a sensitometric curve in which the diagnostic or most useful range of density is produced.

Stromal Referring to part of an organ that is composed of connective tissue and vasculature that provides structure to the organ.

Structure mottle Distribution of phosphor crystals in an intensifying screen.

Subatomic particle Particle smaller than the atom.

Subject contrast Component of radiographic contrast determined by the size, shape, and x-ray attenuating characteristics of the subject who is being examined and the energy of the x-ray beam. *See also* Image receptor contrast.

Substance Any drug, chemical, or biologic entity.

Subtraction technique Method of removing all unnecessary anatomic structures from an image and enhancing only those of interest.

Supercomputer One of the fastest and highest-capacity computers; contains hundreds to thousands of microprocessors.

Superconductivity Property by which some materials exhibit no resistance below a critical temperature.

Supporting tissue Tissue that binds tissues and organs together.

Target a. Region of an x-ray tube anode that is struck by electrons emitted by the filament. b. Molecule (DNA) that is most sensitive to radiation.

Target molecules Molecules (DNA) that are few in number yet essential for cell survival; they are particularly sensitive to the effects of ionizing radiation.

Target theory Theory that a cell will die if target molecules are inactivated as a result of radiation exposure.

Technique factors The kVp and mA as selected for a given radiographic examination.

Teleradiology Transfer of images and patient reports to remote sites.

Telophase Final subphase of mitosis that is characterized by the disappearance of structural chromosomes into a mass of DNA and the closing off of the nuclear membrane into two nuclei.

Temperature Measure of heat and cold.

Temporal subtraction Computer-assisted technique whereby an image obtained at one time is subtracted from an image obtained at a later time.

Temporary magnet Magnet that retains the properties of a magnet only while its magnetism is being induced.

Tenth-value layer (TVL) Thickness of an absorber necessary to reduce an x-ray beam to one-tenth its original intensity. 1 TVL = 3.3 half-value layers.

Terminal Input and output device that uses a keyboard for input and a display screen for output.

Terrestrial radiation Radiation emitted from deposits of uranium, thorium, and other radionuclides in the Earth.

Tesla (T) SI unit of magnetic field intensity. An older unit is the gauss (G). 1 T = 10,000 G.

Test object a. Passive device that provides echoes and permits evaluation of one or more parameters of an ultrasound system but does not necessarily duplicate the acoustic properties of the human body. b. Passive device of geometric shapes designed to evaluate the performance of x-ray and magnetic resonance imaging systems. *See also* Phantom.

Thermal energy Energy of molecular motion; heat; infrared radiation.

Thermal radiation Transfer of heat by infrared emission.

Thermionic emission Emission of electrons from a heated surface.

Thermographic Process that uses only heat to produce a visible image on film.

Thermoluminescence dosimetry Emission of light by a thermally stimulated crystal after irradiation.

Thermometer Device that measures temperature.

Thiosulfate Fixing agent that removes unexposed and undeveloped silver halide crystals from the emulsion.

Three-phase electric power Generation of three simultaneous voltage waveforms out of step with one another; thus, voltage never drops to zero during exposure.

Threshold dose Dose below which a person has a negligible chance of sustaining specific biologic damage, or dose at which response to increasing x-ray intensity first occurs.

Thrombocyte Circular or oval disc called a **platelet**; it is found in the blood, and it initiates blood clotting and prevents hemorrhage.

Throughput Number of patients imaged per day. Number of films imaged per hour.

Thymine Nitrogenous organic base that attaches to a deoxyribose molecule.

Time-interval difference (TID) mode Technique that produces subtracted images from progressive masks and the frames that follow.

Time-of-occupancy factor (T) Length of time that the area being protected is used.

Tissue Collection of cells of similar structure and function.

Tissue weighting factor (W_T) Proportion of risk of stochastic effects that result from irradiation of the whole body when only an organ or tissue is irradiated; accounts for the relative radiosensitivity of various tissues and organs.

Tomogram X-ray image of a coronal, sagittal, transverse, or oblique section through the body.

Tomography Imaging modality that brings into focus only the anatomic structure lying in a plane of interest, while structures on either side of that plane are blurred.

Total effective dose (TED) Recommendation by the National Council on Radiation Protection and Measurement that a radiation worker's lifetime effective dose should be limited to the worker's age in years multiplied by 10 mSv.

Total filtration Inherent filtration plus added filtration.

Transaxial Across the body; transverse.

Transcription Process of constructing mRNA.

Transfer Addition of an amino acid during translation.

Transformer Electrical device that operates on the principle of mutual induction to change the magnitude of current and voltage.

Translation Process of forming a protein molecule from messenger RNA.

Translucent Surface that allows light to be transmitted but greatly alters and reduces its intensity.

Transmission Passage of an x-ray beam through an anatomic part with no interaction with atomic structures.

Transparent Surface that allows light to be transmitted almost unaltered.

Transport roller Agent that moves the film through chemical tanks and the dryer assembly.

Transverse Across the body; axial.

Transverse image Image that is perpendicular to the long axis of the body.

Tungsten Metal element that is the principal component of the cathode and the anode.

Turnaround assembly Device in the automatic processor that reverses the direction of film.

Turns ratio Quotient of the number of turns in the secondary coil to the number of turns in the primary coil.

Ultraviolet light Light that is located at the short end of the electromagnetic spectrum between visible light and ionizing x-rays; it is beyond the range of human vision.

Uncontrolled area Area occupied by anyone; the maximum exposure rate allowed in this area is based on the recommended dose limit for the public.

Underexposed Referring to a radiograph that is too light because too little x-radiation reaches the image receptor.

Undifferentiated cell Immature or nonspecialized cell.

Unified field theory Theoretical combination of magnetic, electric, gravitational, and strong nuclear forces, along with weak interaction, to explain the physical laws of magnetism.

Unit Standard of measurement.

Use factor (U) Proportional amount of time during which the x-ray beam is energized or directed toward a particular barrier.

Useful beam Primary radiation used to form an image.

Valence electron Electron in the outermost shell.

Variable aperture collimator Box-shaped device that contains a radiographic beam–defining system. It is the device that is most often used to reduce the size and shape of a radiographic beam.

VDT Abbreviation for video display terminal.

Vector Quantity or measurement that has magnitude, unit, and direction.

Velocity (v) Rate of change of an object's position over time; speed.

Video display terminal Monitor that is similar to a television screen.

Vidicon Television camera tube that is used most often in television fluoroscopy.

Vignetting Reduction in brightness at the periphery of the image.

Visible light Radiant energy in the electromagnetic spectrum that is visible to the human eye.

Volt (V) SI unit of electric potential and potential difference.

Voltage ripple Means of characterizing voltage waveforms.

Voltaic pile Stack of copper and zinc plates that produces an electric current; a precursor of the modern battery.

Voxel Three-dimensional pixel; volume element.

Washing Stage of processing during which any remaining chemicals are removed from the film.

Watt (W) One ampere of current that flows through an electric potential of one volt.

Wave equation Formula that states that velocity equals frequency multiplied by wavelength.

Wave theory Theory that electromagnetic energy travels through space in the form of waves.

Waveform Graphic representation of a wave.

Wavelength Distance between similar points on a sine wave; the length of one cycle.

Wave-particle duality Principle that states that both wave and particle concepts must be retained, because wave-like properties are exhibited in some experiments and particle-like properties are exhibited in others.

Weight Force on a mass that is caused by the acceleration of gravity. Properly expressed in newtons (N), but commonly expressed in pounds (lb). 4.4 lb = 1 N.

Wetting Process that makes the emulsion film swell so that subsequent chemical baths can reach all parts of the emulsion uniformly.

Wetting agent Agent, usually water, that treats the radiograph so that chemicals can penetrate the emulsion.

Whole body For purposes of external exposure, the head, trunk (including gonads), arm above the elbow, and leg above the knee.

Whole-body exposure Radiographic exposure in which the whole body, rather than an isolated part, is irradiated.

Window Thin section of a glass envelope through which the useful beam emerges.

Window level   Location on a digital image number scale at which the levels of grays are assigned. It regulates the optical density of the displayed image and identifies the type of tissue to be imaged.

Window width   Specific number of gray levels or digital image numbers assigned to an image. It determines the grayscale rendition of the imaged tissue and therefore the image contrast.

Windowing   Technique that allows one to see only a "window" of the entire dynamic range.

Word   Two bytes of information.

Work (W)   Product of the force on an object and the distance over which the force acts. Expressed in Joules (J). W = F × d.

Workload (W)   Product of the maximum milliamperage (mA) and the number of x-ray examinations performed per week. Expressed in milliamperes per minute per week (mA/min/wk).

Workstation   Powerful desktop system; often connected to larger computer systems so that users can transfer and share information.

X-axis   Horizontal line of a graph.

X-ray   Penetrating, ionizing electromagnetic radiation that has a wavelength much shorter than that of visible light.

X-ray imaging system   X-ray system designed for radiography, tomography, or fluoroscopy.

X-ray quality   Penetrability of an x-ray beam.

X-ray quantity   Output intensity of an x-ray imaging system; measured in roentgens (R).

X-ray tube rating charts   Charts that guide the technologist in the use of x-ray tubes.

Y-axis   Vertical line of a graph.

Zonography   Thick-slice tomography with a tomographic angle of less than 10 degrees.

Illustration Credits

Figure 1-8

From Eisenberg RL: *Radiology: an illustrated history,* St. Louis, 1992, Mosby.

Figure 14-15

From *Mosby's radiographic instructional series: radiographic imaging,* St. Louis, 1998, Mosby.

Figure 15-9

From Fauber T: *Radiographic imaging and exposure,* St. Louis, 2000, Mosby.

Figure 15-10

From Seeram E: *Computed tomography: physical principalsprinciples, clinical applications, and quality control, ed 2, Philadelphia,* 2000, WB Saunders.

Figure 17-3

From Papp J: *Quality management in the imaging sciences,* St. Louis, 1998, Mosby.

Figure 17-4

From Papp J: *Quality management in the imaging sciences,* St. Louis, 1998, Mosby.

Figure 39-7

From *Mosby's radiographic instructional series: radiographic imaging,* St. Louis, 1998, Mosby.

Figure 39-8

A from Sherer MA: *Radiation protection in medical radiology,* ed 3, St. Louis, 1998, Mosby.

Index

A

AAOO. *See* American Academy of Ophthalmology and Otolaryngology, 553
AAPM. *See* American Association of Physicists in Medicine, 306
Abacus, example, 397f
ABC. *See* Automatic brightness control, 347
ABCC. *See* Atomic Bomb Casualty Committee, 555
Abdomen
   examination, fixed-kVp chart (usage), 262t
   histograms, 493f
   phantom radiographs, 255f
      usage, 263f
   radiograph, 256f, 258f
   serial radiography, aluminum step-wedge (usage), 160f
Abdominal imaging, cathode (superior preference), 131
Abortion. *See* Spontaneous abortion, 564
   recommendation, 610
ABS. *See* Automatic brightness stabilization, 311
Absolute radiation risk, determination, 554
Absolute response, 560
Absolute risk, 554-555
   model, 561f
Absorption, 175
   blur, 291
      reduction, 326
   examples, 65
   process, 175
AC. *See* Alternating current, 81
Acceleration, 19
   calculation, 20
   equation, 20
   example, 20f
   force, requirement, 21
   multiplication. *See* Mass, 21
   SI units, calculation, 20
   usage, 20
   value, 22
Acetic acid, 198
ACP. *See* American College of Physicians, 553
ACR. *See* American College of Radiology, 312f
ACRIN. *See* American College of Radiology Imaging Network, 457

Activator, 198
   atoms. *See* Thallium, 592
   responsibility, 413
Active bone marrow, distribution, 601t
Active matrix array (AMA), detection (usage), 431f
Active matrix array-thin-film transistor (AMA-TFT), photomicrograph, 431f
Active matrix LCD (AMLCD), 469
   ambient light, impact, 470
   digital display devices, difference. *See* Cathode ray tube, 471t
   display characteristics, 469
   grayscale definition, improvement, 470
   image luminance, 469-470
      measurement, aperture ratio (usage), 470
   off-axis viewing, image contrast loss, 471f
   pixel, cross-sectional rendering, 470f
   red-green-blue filters. *See* Color AMLCD, 469
   superiority, 469
Active trace, 356
   series, horizontal retrace (following), 356-357
Acute radiation lethality, 535-538
   nonlinear threshold dose-response relationship, 537
   summary, 536t
Acute radiation syndrome, 535
ADA (computer language), 410
ADC. *See* Analog-to-digital converter, 443
Added filtration, 158, 249
   impact. *See* Half-value layer, 158
Addition
   rounding, usage, 28
   rule, 28
Adenine, 505
Adenine-thymine base, 506
   pairs, 507
Adhesive layer, 181
Adipose tissues, 320
AEC. *See* Automatic exposure control, 108-109
Aerial oxidation, 197
Afterglow. *See* Phosphor, 209b; Radiographic intensifying screens, 210
Age, 515. *See also* Biologic structure, 515
Age-response function, 531

Air-gap technique, 241-243
   disadvantage, 241
   method, 241
   usage, 242f
Al_2O_3. *See* Aluminum oxide, 594
ALARA. *See* As Low As Reasonably Achievable, 12
Algebra
   rules, 28
   usage, 28
Algorithms, usage, 409
Alnico. *See* Aluminum nickel cobalt, 85
Alpha emission, 49. *See also* Radioactive decay, 49
   accompaniment, 49f
   usage, 49f
Alpha particles
   definition, 53
   emission. *See* Radon, 6
   particulate radiation, 52
Alternating current (AC), 81
   explanation, 81
   intensity (change), transformer (impact), 93
   operation. *See* Transformer, 109
   production, 92
   representation, 82f
   waveform, negative portion, 111
Alternating electric current, composition, 57
Alternating voltage intensity (change), transformer (impact), 93
ALU. *See* Arithmetic/logic unit, 401
Aluminum
   nonhygroscopic advantage, 234
   usage, 234
Aluminum chloride (hardener), 199
Aluminum nickel cobalt (alnico), 85
Aluminum oxide (Al_2O_3), usage, 594
Aluminum step wedge (penetrometer), radiographs, 292f
AMA. *See* Active matrix array, 431f
AMA-TFT. *See* Active matrix array-thin-film transistor, 431f
Amber filter, usage, 188
Ambient light
   diffusion/reduction, 336
   impact. *See* Active matrix LCD, 470-474
American Academy of Ophthalmology and Otolaryngology (AAOO), 553
American Association of Physicists in Medicine (AAPM), 306
   AAPM TG 18, 479-480
      measurements/observations, 480

Page numbers followed by f indicate figure; t, table; b, boxes.

American Association of Physicists in Medicine (AAPM) *(Continued)*
five-pin performance test object, 383
test patterns, development, 479-480
TG 18-AD pattern, 482
usage, 482f
TG 18-AFC pattern, usage, 484f
TG 18-CH anatomic image, 479-480
TG 18-CT pattern, 482f
TG 18-CX pattern, 484, 484f
TG 18-LPV/LPH test patterns, usage, 481
TG 18-PX pattern, 484f
TG 18-QC test pattern, 481f
TG 18-UN10/80 test patterns, 483f, 482
American College of Physicians (ACP), intermediate-risk group (representation), 553
American College of Radiology (ACR), 474
accreditation, test object usage, 312
accreditation phantom, 339f
characteristics. *See* Five-pin ACR accreditation phantom, 384t
mammography phantom, analysis, 337f
QC program endorsement, 332
radiologic/fluoroscopic accreditation phantom, 312f
volunteer accreditation program, 319
American College of Radiology Imaging Network (ACRIN), 457
American Registry of Radiologic Technologists (ARRT)
national certification examination, 12
requirement. *See* Radiography, 13b
standard units, adoption (absence), 34
Amino acids, 503
connection. *See* Peptide bond, 503
AMLCD. *See* Active matrix LCD, 469-471
Ammeter, usage, 91
Amorphous selenium (a-Se), 431-432
direct DR process, 432
impact. *See* Digital radiography, 432
usage, 432f
x-rays, incidence, 432
Ampere, equation, 245
Amplitude, 109. *See also* Photons, 57-58
definition, 58
amu. *See* Atomic mass units, 40
Anabolism, 503, 521
impact, 522
relationship, 503
Analog, term (reference), 398f
Analog meters, 399
Analog-to-digital converter (ADC), 443
Anaphase, 508
Anatomically programmed radiography (APR), 265
operating console, 265f
principle, 265

Anatomical structures
artifact interference, 298
imaging, 266
Anatomy, irregularity (impact). *See* Distortion, 287f
Angiography, 347. *See also* Digital subtraction angiography, 443-448
interventional radiologic procedures, usage, 361
reference, 361
Angiointerventional radiology suites, C-arm support system (usage), 121
Angioplasty, 361
Animal
experimentation, 562
Animal glycogen, 504
Animals
chronic irradiation, 552f
Ankylosing spondylitis, 557
Annihilation radiation, 169
Annotation, 472
Annual average radiation dose, percentage, 7
Annual deaths, occupational exposure impact (determination), 555
Anode
angle, decrease, 129
cooling chart, 134-136
definition, 136
time, requirement, 136f
cooling rate, 136
focal-spot blur, 289
heat, 140
dissipation, 133f
overload, example, 128f
rotation
explanation, 127
speed, 134
separation, examples, 128f
temperature, excess, 132
Antennas, usage, 64
Anterior-posterior (AP) abdominal examination, fixed-kVp technique, 251t
Anterior-posterior (AP) cervical spine view, 299f
Anterior-posterior (AP) pelvis examination, variable-kVp technique, 251t
Anteroposterior view, blacked-out spine, 494f
Antibodies, 504
Antigen, 504
Antihalation coating, 188
Antimony trisulfide, photoconductive layer, 354
Antistatic compounds, usage, 219
Aorta-iliac area, DSA, 446f
Aperture diaphragm, 229-230
fixed lead opening, 229f
Aperture ratio, usage. *See* Active matrix LCD, 470
Aplastic anemia, occurrence, 11
Application programs, 407. *See also* Computers, 408-409
APR. *See* Anatomically programmed radiography, 265

Archival quality, 198
reference, 198
silver sulfide stain, impact, 199
Area shielding, 606
Argonne National Laboratory, 551
Arithmetic/logic unit (ALU), 401
arithmetic/logic calculations, 402
Array processor. *See* Computed tomography imaging systems, 373
ARRT. *See* American Registry of Radiologic Technologists, 12
Arterial access, 361-362
Arteriography, risks, 363
Artifacts. *See* Processing artifacts, 300-301
cause, 190
classification, 298f
definition, 298
interference. *See* Anatomical structures, 298
light, impact, 302
occurrence, 300
positioning errors, 299
radiation fog, impact, 302
radiographic characteristic, 273
ASCC. *See* Automatic Sequence Controlled Calculator, 397
a-Se. *See* Amorphous selenium, 431-432
As Low As Reasonably Achievable (ALARA), 457
comparison, 598
consistency, 610, 620
implementation, 571
maintenance, 614
practice, 12, 501, 516, 571
Assemblers, 408
computer program, 408
Asthenic, term (usage), 251
Asymmetric eight-detector array design, 388f
slice thickness, allowance, 389f
Asymmetric screen-emulsion image receptor, front image, 220f
Asymmetric screen-film, 218-219
usage, 218
Asymmetric screens, 219
compensation. *See* X-rays, 219f
emulsion image receptor, characteristic curves, 219f
Atansoff, John, 397
Atomic Bomb Casualty Committee (ABCC), 555-557
Atomic bomb survivors, 555-557
Hiroshima/Nagasaki data, 556f
leukemia, incidence, 556f
Atomic clock, measurement, 18
Atomic configurations, 45f
Atomic mass, 46
atomic mass number, equivalence, 46
Atomic mass numbers, 46
usage, 40
Atomic mass units (amu), 40
Atomic nomenclature, 45
Atomic number. *See* Effective atomic number, 290
dependence, 171-172
increase. *See* Target atomic number, 148

Atomic structure, 41-45
Atoms. *See* Bohr atom, 40; Dalton atom, 38-39; Thomson atom, 39
   building blocks, 3
   combinations, 47-48
   composition, 42f
   definition, 38
   description, isotopes (usage), 47
   discovery. *See* Greek atoms, 38
   disintegration, 54
   electrical neutrality, 42
   Greek perspective, 39f
   ionization, 42. *See also* Carbon atom, 42f
      assumption, 42
   meaning, 38
   precise mass, 46
   radiologic importance, 44
   representation, 39f
   space, 41
Atrophy, 515
   organ/tissue shrinkage, 538
Attenuation
   absorption/scattering, product, 175
   definition, 155
   examples, 65
   pattern, 368-369
   process, 174f
   x-rays, total reduction, 175
Audio input device, analog sound translation, 401
Audio noise, 273
Automatic ball-throwing machine
   bar graph, representation, 144f
   example, 144f
Automatic brightness control (ABC), 347
Automatic brightness stabilization (ABS) system
   adequacy, determination, 311
   control, 439
Automatic exposure basis, 260
Automatic exposure control (AEC), 108-109
   control. *See* X-rays, 108f
   devices, 264, 327
      relative position, 328f
   evaluation, 309
   600-mAs safety override, 264
   systems, commonality, 265
   technique chart, usefulness, 265
   usage, 264
   x-ray imaging system, installation/calibration, 108
Automatic exposure techniques, 263-265
Automatic processing, 194-195
   problem, glutaraldehyde (absence), 198
   revolution, 194
   usage, 199-203
Automatic processor, 314f. *See also* Roller transport automatic processor, 194f
   agitation, necessity, 202
   circulation system, 202
   components, 200t

Automatic processor *(Continued)*
   crossover rack, 201
   cutaway view, 200f
   developer circulation system, filter requirement, 202
   disassembly, 314f
   drive motor, 200
   drive subsystem, 201
   dryer system, 202-203
   entrance rollers, 200
   faults, impact, 203
   feed tray, 200
      guide rail, 200f
   film (shorter dimension), placement, 200
   fixer circulation system, filtration (nonnecessity), 202
   guide shoes, 201
   master roller, 201
      planetary rollers/guide shoes, usage, 201f
   microswitch, engaging, 200
   nonscheduled maintenance, 314
   planetary rollers, 201
   preventive maintenance, 314
   QC program, 314
   replenishment system, 202
   rollers, 200
      subassembly, 201
   scheduled maintenance, 314
   tanks, cleaning, 202
   temperature control system, 201
   transport racks, 200
      power, transfer (means), 202f
      subassembly, 200-201f
   transport rollers, position, 201f
   transport system, 200-201
      cleaning, 202
      speed, control, 202
   turnaround assembly, 201
Automatic processor (Art Haus), 194f
Automatic radiation field recognition, 493
Automatic Sequence Controlled Calculator (ASCC), 397
Automatic systems, exposure chart construction (factors), 264t
Automatic variable-aperture collimator, 231f
Automatic x-ray film processing (advancement), Eastman Kodak Company (involvement), 194
Autotransformer, 95, 104-107
   definition, 95
   function, 104
   law, 105
   secondary voltage, determination, 105
   view, simplification, 105f
   voltage, supply, 104
Average gradient, 280f
   calculation, 281
Average velocity, 20
   calculation, 20
   equation, 20

Axes, graph basis, 31
Axial tomography, 368

B

Babbage, Charles, 397
Background electronic noise, 442
Backscatter radiation, 165, 214
   problem, 490
Baking soda, 48
Bandpass
   impact, 357
   increase, impact. *See* Horizontal resolution, 357
Barcode readers, 401
Barium, atomic number, 46
Barium-based phosphors, 216
Barium fluorohalide, 413, 461-463
   radiographic intensifying screen, similarity, 413
Barium lead sulfate, 208
Barium platinocyanide, 7
   luminescence, 209
Bar pattern, usage. *See* Spatial frequency, 380f
Barrier thickness
   control, 586
   distance, 586
   factors, 586
   occupancy, 586
   use factor, 587
   workload, 586
Basal cells, damage, 539
Base, 181. *See also* Radiographic film, 181-182
   fog OD, addition, 278
Base density, impact, 278f, 278
Baseline mammogram, 320
Base quantities, support. *See* Derived quantities, 18f
BASIC. *See* Beginners All-purpose Symbolic Instruction Code, 409
Basic input/output system (BIOS), 402. *See also* Read-only memory, 402
Battery, cell, 88
Beam. *See* X-ray beam, 8f
Beam-splitting mirror, 355
   retraction, 355
Becquerels (Bq). *See* Curie, 35
Beginners All-purpose Symbolic Instruction Code (BASIC), 409-410
BEIR. *See* Biologic Effects of Ionizing Radiation, 560-561
Bell Telephone Laboratories, 397
   demonstration. *See* Light amplifier tube, 10
Berry, Clifford, 397
Beryllium window, 324
Beta emission, 49
   result, 49
Beta particle
   definition, 53
   emission, 49f
   particulate radiation, 52
BGO. *See* Bismuth germanate, 374
$Bi_4Ge_3O_{12}$. *See* Bismuth germanate, 374

Bilateral wedge filter, 158
Binary digit (bit), 407
    term, usage, 403
Binary notation, 406t
Binary number system, 406-407
    examples, 407
    organization, 406t
Binder, 413
Biochemistry, molecular level, 4
Biologic Effects of Ionizing Radiation
        (BEIR) Committee, 560-561
    determination. *See* Radiation-
        induced malignant disease, 554
    estimated excess mortality. *See*
        Malignant disease, 560t
Biologic specimens
    critical targets, presence, 529
    irradiation, 527
Biologic structure, age, 515
Biologic tissue, ionizing radiation
        (impact), 52
Biopsy, 361
Bipolar field, 83
Bismuth germanate ($Bi_4Ge_3O_{12}$, BGO),
        374
Bit. *See* Binary digit, 407
Blanked electron beam, 356
Blood cells
    radiation response, graphs, 543f
    types, 542f
Blood disorders, occurrence, 11
Blood-forming cells, irradiation, 550
Blue-sensitive film, 187
    usage, 219f
Body
    atomic composition, 503b
    composition, 502
    irradiation, 545
    molecular composition, 503b
    tissue composition, 510b
Body habitus, 251
    states, 251f
Bohr atom, 40
    representation, 39f
Bonds. *See* Covalent bonds 48;
        Ionic bonds, 48
Bone
    cancer, 558
    graphs, vertical displacement, 167
    marrow
        cell proliferation, 543
        dose, 598
    photoelectric absorption, 446f
    x-rays
        Compton effect, relative
            probability, 173
        interaction, likelihood, 171
Bony structures, radiograph, 171f
Bootstrap program, 402, 408-409
Boric acids/salts, usage. *See*
        Sequestering, 199
Bow-tie filters, 159f
    usage, 369
Bow-tie-shaped filters, usage, 158.
        See also Computed tomography
        imaging systems, 158
Bq. *See* Curie, 35

Breast
    architecture, impact. *See* Image
        receptor, 320f; X-ray imaging
        system, 320f
    cancer, 559
    compression (testing), bathroom
        scale (usage), 344f
    examination
        American Cancer Society
            recommendation, 320
        intervals, recommendation, 320t
    shields, contact shield, 606
    tissues, 320
Breast cancer
    incidence, approximation, 321f
    mortality, National Cancer Institute
        report, 319
    risk, 319-320
        factors, 319b
Bremsstrahlung radiation, 142-143
Bremsstrahlung x-rays
    emission spectrum, extension, 145f
    energies, range, 145
    production, 142
        ease, 322
    result, 143f
    spectrum, 145
        change, 148
        shape, 145
    suppression, 325f
Brightness gain, 351
    equation, 351
Brightness level, maintenance, 352
Bromine atoms, migration, 184
Brushes, usage. *See* Multislice spiral
        computed tomography, 375f
Bucky, Gustav, 10, 235
Bucky factor, 235
    equation, 235
    increase. *See* Grid ratio, 235
        indication, 235
        kVp, increase, 235
        radiographic technique/patient
            dose, increase, 235
    values. *See* Grid, 235t
Bucky slot cover, 13f, 583
Buffering agents, 197
Bus (electrical conductor), 401
Byte, 403, 407
    grouping, 407
    representation, 403

C
C++. *See* Visual C++, 410
CAD. *See* Computer-aided diagnosis,
        490
Cadmium tungstate ($CdWO_4$), 374
Calcium fluoride (CaF), activation, 594
Calcium tungstate ($CaWO_4$), 208, 215
    embedding. *See* Crystalline calcium
        tungstate, 208
    screens
        absorption properties, 216
        replacement, 187
        x-ray absorption, probability, 217f
    spectrum, emission, 218f
    usage, 8

Calculus, size, 285
Camera lenses, importance, 355
Cancer, 557-560. *See also* Bone, 558,
        See also, Breast, 559, *See also*
        Liver cancer, 559, *See also,* Lung
        cancer, 559, *See also* Thyroid
        cancer, 558
Candela, 467
Capacitor discharge
    generator, 115
    voltage, decrease, 115
Capture element, 427
Carbohydrates, 504-505
    composition, 504
    function, 505
    hydration, 504
    organic molecules, 503
    structure, difference, 504f
Carbon, element activity, 52f
Carbon atom
    interaction. *See* X-rays, 42
    ionization, 42f
Carbon dioxide, 502-503
Carbon fiber
    material, 215
    usage. *See* Radiographic intensifying
        screens, 215
Carcinogenic risk, 584
C-arm support system, 121. *See also*
        X-ray tube, 121
Carotid computed tomography scan,
        reconstruction, 378f
Carotid flow, evaluation, 444
Cassette-loaded spot film, 357
    positioning, 358f
Cassettes. *See* Radiographic
        intensifying screens, 214
    cross-sectional view, 215f
    spot film
        dependence, 311
        ESE level, assumption, 311
    testing, 343
Cassette spot, photospot (differences),
        358t
Catabolism, 503, 521
    impact, 522
    relationship, 503
Cataracts
    local tissue effects, 551-552
    RBE, 551
Catheters, 362
    shapes, 362f
Cathode. *See* Photocathode 350;
        X-ray tube, 122-124
    components, 10007 # d0030
    electron flow, determination, 246
    electron travel, 140
    focal spot size, 289f
Cathode rays (electrons), 39
    conduction, 7
Cathode ray tube (CRT), 405
    AMLCD digital display devices,
        differences, 471t
    components, 356f
    screen, luminance (measurement),
        311f
$CaWO_4$. *See* Calcium tungstate, 215

CCD. *See* Charge-coupled device, 353
C (computer language), 410
C++ (computer language), 410
CD. *See* Compact disc, 403
CDE. *See* Erasable optical discs, 403
CD-R. *See* Compact disc-recordable, 403
CD-ROM. *See* Compact disc-read-only memory, 404
CD-RW. *See* Erasable optical discs, 403
CdWO$_4$. *See* Cadmium tungstate, 374
CE. *See* Conversion efficiency, 209b
Ceiling support system, 120. *See also* X-ray tube, 120
Celeron microprocessor, photograph, 398f
Cell. *See* Battery, 88
  cloning, 526
  death, occurrence, 525f
  generation time, 530
  phases, G$_1$ (time variation), 530
  population
    synchronization, 531
    usage, 530
  representation. *See* Dry cells, 88
  surviving fraction, estimation, 530
  theory, 503, 502-506
  type, radiation response, 510t
Cell-cycle effects, 530-531
Cell-survival curves, 531f. *See also* Human cell, 532f
Cell-survival kinetics, 526-530
Cellular radiobiology, challenge questions, 532-533
Cellulose nitrate, 182
  substitute, 8
Cellulose triacetate, 182
Celsius
  conversion. *See* Fahrenheit, 25
  scale, usage, 25f
Centering indicators, accuracy, 307
Centimeters grams and seconds (CGS) system, 18
Central electrode, positioning, 589
Central nervous system (CNS) death, 535
Central nervous system (CNS) syndrome, 537
  characterization, 537
  death, cause, 537
Central processing unit (CPU), 400
  components, 401f
  control unit, 401f, 402f
Central ray
  imaginary line, generation, 130
  x-ray beam, 239
Centrifugal force, 44
Centripetal force, 44
CERN, 551
Cervical spine
  examination, 248
  histograms, 493f
Cesium iodide/amorphous silicon (CsI/a-Si), 430-431
  indirect DR process, 430
  pixel detectors, 440

Cesium iodide charge-coupled device, 430
  example, 430f
Cesium iodide (CsI), 350, 427
  crystals, growth/packing, 350f
  phosphor, availability, 430f
CGS. *See* Centimeters grams and seconds, 18
Characteristic curve. *See* Film, 275-277; Radiographic film 276f
  analysis, 283f
  components, 276
  construction, steps, 276f
  gradient, 281f
  position (change), time (increase), 283f
  relationship, 275
  shape, 197f
    change, time (increase), 283f
  straight-line portion, slope, 280f
Characteristic radiation, 140-142
Characteristic x-radiation, 141
Characteristic x-ray emission spectrum, 144
Characteristic x-rays, 140
  fixed/discrete energies, 144
  production, 141f, 142
    photoelectric interaction, impact, 166
    target atom, ionization, 141
  spectrum, 144-145
Charge-coupled device (CCD), 353, 365, 427, 428-430
  advantages. *See* Medical imaging, 441b
  coupling. *See* Image-intensifier tube, 440f
  cross-sectional view, 440f
  dynamic range, 428
  elements, 439f
  image-intensifier tube, coupling, 355f
  light response, 441f
  radiation response, 429f
  sensitivity, 428
    increase, 429
  tilting, 430f
  warm-up, necessity (absence), 440
Charged particle, circular/elliptical path (movement), 84f
Charges
  attraction/repulsion, 75
  production, methods (development), 88
Checklist. *See* Visual checklist, 340f
Chelates, introduction, 198
Chemical agents, 516
Chemical elements, determination, 41
Chemical energy, 4
Chemical fog, 198, 300-301
Chemical symbols, 45
  position, 39
Chemistry runs, excess, 301f
Chernobyl incident, 535
Chest
  examination, trough filter (usage), 159f
  SCR, components, 429f

Chest radiograph. *See* High-voltage chest radiograph, 264f
  100 cm SID, 254f
  overexposure, 253f
  70 kVp, 256f
  simulation, 492f
  usage. *See* High-voltage technique, 294f
Chest radiography
  cathode, inferior preference, 131
  lungs, imaging, 173
Childhood leukemia
  incidence, 563
  relative risk, 563t
Chromium alum (hardener), 199
Chromosomal material, exchange, 509
Chromosome aberrations, 522
  kinetics, 546-547
  production, 546
  types/frequency, 550
  visualization, 546
Chromosomes. *See* Humans, 523f
  damage, 544f
  hit, representation, 545
  local tissue effects, 550
Chronic lymphocytic leukemia, rarity, 557
Ci. *See* Curie, 35
CIE. *See* Commission Internationale de l'Éclairage, 467
Cine cameras, optics requirement, 355
Cine film
  processing, 189
  16mm/35mm, format, 189f
  usage, 189
Cineradiography, 584
Clients, interconnection, 474
Clinical images, processing (avoidance), 334
Clinical tolerance. *See* Radiation, 539
Clinical voltage, workload distribution, 588f
Cloning. *See* Cell, 526
Closed-core transformer, 95
CNS. *See* Central nervous system, 535
COBOL. *See* COmmon Business Oriented Language, 410
Codon, 507
Coherent scattering, 163-164
  importance, absence, 164
  result, 163
Collar-positioned radiation monitor, 618
Collection element, 427
Collimation, 307, 581, 583
  application, 9
  artifacts (cause), vendor algorithm (relationship), 495
  impact. *See* Contrast resolution 224; Patient 224; X-rays, 12
  necessity, 606
  recommendation, 227f
  usage, 12
Collimators. *See* Open collimator, 249f
  filtration, 228
  lamp/mirror, adjustment, 232
  usage, 225

Color AMLCD, red-green-blue filters (usage), 469
Colorimetric evaluation, examples, 480f
Colossus (computer), 397
Commission Internationale de l'Éclairage (CIE), 467
standard photopic spectral response, 480
Common Business Oriented Language (COBOL), 410
Communications. *See* Computers, 405
advances, 405
Compact disc (CD), 403
drive, 403
sizes/capacities, 403f
tracks, 403
Compact disc-read-only memory (CD-ROM), 404
Compact disc-recordable (CD-R), 403
Compass, reaction, 88f
Compensating filters, 158-160, 250
components, 159f
fabrication, 158
usage, 158
Compilers, 408
computer programs, 408
Complete grid cutoff, 235
Compound, 48
Compression. *See* Mammography, 326-327
advantages, 327t
device, 214
impact. *See* Spatial resolution, 327
observation, 344
result, 327
Compton effect, 164-165
calculation, 164
impact. *See* X-rays, 165f
independence, 172
occurrence, 164f
probability, inverse proportion, 165
Compton interaction, 168
probability, graph (usage), 171f
relative frequency, 172
Compton-scattered x-rays
deflection, 165
impact. *See* Image receptor, 170f
information, absence, 170
Compton scattering, 164
features, 165t
impact. *See* Image contrast, 165
Computed radiography (CR), 413
challenge questions, 424-425
collimators, monitoring, 603
computer complement, 421f
contrast resolution, quality, 459
effective dose, 577b
exposure, 416f
optical components/path, 420f
patient characteristics, 422-424
performing, 423
plate, image production, 491f
plates, usage. *See* Spine imaging, 496f
radiation dose, 422
sequence, 416f, 417f, 417f, 418f
terms, 413b
workload, 423-424

Computed radiography (CR) image
noise, 422
sources, 423b
obtaining, 423f
receptor, 413-418
sizes, 494b
Computed radiography (CR) imaging
characteristics, 421-422
dose, 602
glue, residual glue, 488f
plate, 414-415
example, 416f
problem, 489f
Computed radiography (CR) reader, 418-421
computer control, 420-421
drive mechanisms, 419f
example, 419f
mechanical features, 418-420
optical features, 420
Computed tomography (CT), 266, 615
computer, usage, 372-373
contrast resolution, 381
examination. *See* Object organ, 379f
patient dose, 392
gantry, inclusion, 373
generations, 369-371
imaging, x-ray beam (profile) usage, 370f
linearity, 383
acceptability, 384f
noise, 381-383
uniformity, relationship, 390
numbers, 376. *See also* Tissue, 377t
equation, 376
operating console, 371-372
components, 372, 372, 372
operation, principles, 368-369
patient dose, equation, 604
performance measurements, medical physics evaluation, 392f
personnel exposures, 615
physician workstation, 372
quality control, 389-392
spatial resolution, 378-381
limitation, 381
test object, usage. *See* Noise, 390f
uniformity, 383-384
Computed tomography (CT) image
characteristics, 375-377
matrix, 375-376
pixel size
computation, 376
equation, 376
quality, 377-384
evaluation, phantom (usage), 382f
reconstruction, 376-377
illustration, 378f
Computed tomography (CT) imaging systems, 368
array processor, 373
bow-tie-shaped filters, usage, 158
components, 369f, 372f
design, 371-375
laser localizer, 392
SSP, usage, 387f

Computer-aided diagnosis (CAD), 490
Computer-assisted automatic exposure systems, electronic exposure timer (usage), 263
Computers
anatomy, 400-410
application programs, 408
capacity, requirement (determination), 475, 475
classification, 400
communications, 405
hardware, 400-401
history, 397-400
languages, 409-410
output devices, 405
processing
methods, 401-405
speed, measurement, 401-402
programs, 407
software, 407
software, 405-409
storage, 403-405
term, reference, 398
timeline, 399f
transmission speed, 405
Computer science, challenge questions, 411
Concrete
HVL, approximation, 574t
TVL, approximation, 574t
Conduction, 24. *See also* Electrons, 7
definition, 132
observation, 25
relationship, 24
Conductive lines, width. *See* Microprocessor chip, 401f
Conductor
definition, 78
electrical resistance, 78f
electric charge, 77
Cones, 230-231. *See also* Humans, 348
cutting, 231
usage. *See* X-ray beam, 230f
Conic filters, 159f
Connective tissues, 510
Constructive pathology, 252
Contact gonad shield, example, 606, 607f
Contact shield, 606
Continuous charge, region, 591
Continuous ejection spectrum, 143
Continuous quality improvement (CQI), 310f
Continuous spectrum, values, 144
Continuum. *See* Energy, 57
Contrast. *See* High contrast 257; Low contrast, 257
differences, demonstration, 279f
examination, 174
explanation, 279-281
function, 256
gray scale, 257
importance, 228
improvement factor, 234-235
equation, 234

Contrast *(Continued)*
    measurement, 235
    specification, 234
loss, 495f
media, 362
perception, 349
scale, relationship. *See* Kilovolt
        peak, 258t
short scale, demonstration, 257f
x-ray responsibility, 224
Contrast-detail curve, 457-459. *See
    also* Medical imaging 461f
    usage. *See* Digital imaging, 460f;
        Single digital imaging system
        460f
Contrast-detail tool, 459f
    example, 459f
Contrast resolution, 224, 454-457
    definition, 273
    improvement, 326f
        collimation, impact, 224, 231
    limitation, image noise
        (usage), 457
    postprocessing, 455-457
    preservation, 460
    radiographic characteristic, 273
    reference, 212
    relationship, 213
    superiority, 381
Control booth barrier, incidence
        (determination), 586
Control cassette, usage, 336
Control grid, usage. *See* Electron
        beam, 356
Control monitor, measurement, 624
Control panel, exposure conditions
        (indication), 581
Convection
    mechanical transfer, 25
    relationship, 24
Conventional tomograph, obtaining,
        368f
Conventional tomography
    image, result, 369f
    necessity, 265
Conversion efficiency (CE), 209b,
        212. *See also* Radiographic
        intensifying screens, 218
    equation, 212
    improvement, DQE increase
        (combination), 218
    increase. *See* Image noise 212f
Conversion factor, 351
    equation, 351
Coolidge, William D., 9
Coolidge x-ray tube, impact, 10
Cormack, Alan, 368
Cornea, incident light (passage),
        347-348
Cosine law, 468
    importance, 468
Cosmic rays, 6
Coulomb's law
    definition, 76
    equation, 76
Council of Radiation Control
        Program Directors (CRCPD), 306

Coupling element, 427
Covalent bonds, 48
Covering power, 186
CPU. *See* Central processing unit, 400
CQI. *See* Continuous quality
        improvement, 310f
CR. *See* Computed radiography, 413
CRCPD. *See* Council of Radiation
        Control Program Directors, 306
Critical temperature (Tc), 78
    increase. *See* Superconducting
        materials, 79f
Crookes, William, 7
Crookes tube, usage, 7
    example, 7f
Crossed grid, 236-237
    disadvantage, 236
    efficiency, 236
    fabrication, 237f
Cross-linking, 521
    irradiation result, 521f
    process, 521
Crossover, 186. *See also* Film, 344
    control layer, 187f
        light-absorbing dye, addition, 186
    exposure, 186
    occurrence, 187f
    rack. *See* Automatic processor, 201
    reduction/elimination, 186
        dye, addition, 187f
CRT. *See* Cathode ray tube, 311f
Cryogens, usage, 25
Crystal lattice, 183
Crystalline calcium tungstate,
        embedding, 208
CsI. *See* Cesium iodide, 350
CsI/a-Si. *See* Cesium iodide/
        amorphous silicon 430-431
CT. *See* Computed tomography, 266
Cubic grains. *See* Silver halide
        crystals, 186f
Cubic relationships, 168
Cumulative timer, 584
Curie (Ci, Bq), 35
    radioactivity unit, 35
Current. *See* Electric current, 77
    transformer law effect, impact.
        See, 94
    waveforms, secondary side, 112f
Cursor, indication, 400
Curvilinear detector array, source-
        to-detector path length
        production, 370
Cyclotron
    development, 551
    usage, 551f
Cylinders, 230-231
    usage. *See* X-ray beam, 230f
Cytogenetic damage, 522
    radiation dose-response
        relationships, 547
Cytogenetic effects, 544-547
Cytogenetics, 544
Cytoplasm, 506
Cytosine, 505
Cytosine-guanine base, 506
    pairs, 507

D
D_0. *See* Mean lethal dose, 529
Dally, Clarence
    fluoroscope design, 9f
    x-ray burn, 8
Dalton, John, 38
Dalton atom, 38-39
    representation, 39f
DAP. *See* Dose area product, 584
Darkroom
    cleanliness, 333-334
    fog, 342
Data compression, advantage, 489
Daylight processing, 203-204
    system, 204f
        speed, usefulness, 203
DC. *See* Direct current, 81
DDLs. *See* Digital driving levels, 482
Death, annual risk, 561t
Decimals, 27
    conversion. *See* Fractions, 27
    number system. *See* Hexadecimal
        number system 409
    origin, 30f
    places, rounding, 28
    rounding, determination, 28
    system, 29
    usage. *See* Number
Dedicated mammography system,
        features, 322t
Densitometer, 276f
    usage, 276. *See also* Optical density,
        334
Dental radiography, 230
Deoxyribonucleic acid (DNA), 503, 505
    components, 506f
    damage, 523
        types, 523f
    genetic code, 522f
    gross structural radiation response,
        523
    ladder, 506f
    presence, 522
    radiation
        damage, 523f
        effects, 522-523
        response, 523
    radiation-sensitive target molecule, 505
    radiosensitive molecule, 522
    replication, 509
    sugar/phosphate molecules,
        alternation, 505f
    synthesis, 522
        phase, 508
    target molecule, 525
Derived quantities, 17
    base quantities, support, 18f
    representation, 18
Desquamation, 539
    early effects, 550
Destructive pathology, 252
Detail. *See* Image detail, 212;
        Radiographs, 258; Recorded
        detail 258
    term, imprecision, 273
    visibility, 212, 224
        reference, 273

Detective quantum efficiency (DQE), 209b, 212, 461-463
  analysis, 463
  equation, 212
  increase, 212
  relative value, 463
  usage, 440. *See also* X-rays, 463
Detector rows, combination, 604f
Detector size, decrease, 388
Deterministic radiation responses, 516
Developer
  components/function, 196t
  temperature, control, 334
Developing, 196
  agent, 196
  occurrence, 197
  processing stage. *See* Film 195
Development fog, 197
DF. *See* Digital fluoroscopy, 437
Dg. *See* Glandular dose, 602
Diagnosis, distortion (interference), 286
Diagnostic imaging systems, characteristics, 306t
Diagnostic imaging team, 12
Diagnostic mammography, 320
Diagnostic radiology, pregnancy (impact), 627t
Diagnostic ultrasound, exclusion. *See* Electromagnetic spectrum, 61
Diagnostic x-ray exposures, 564
Diagnostic x-ray imaging
  performing, 514
  system, types, 101f
Diagnostic x-ray procedures, radiation quantities, 598t
Diagnostic x-rays, 6
  beams, partial-body exposure, 535
  LET, approximation, 513
  RBE levels, 513
  tube, target, 146
Diagnostic x-ray tube, anode classification, 125f
Diamagnetic materials, 85
Diaphragm
  position, 132f
  usage, 8
Dichroic stain, 300
DICOM. *See* Digital Imaging and Communications in Medicine, 474
Differential absorption, 169-173
  characteristics, 173t
  increase, kVp (decrease), 164
  occurrence, 169
    reasons, 173f
  x-ray interaction, difference, 171
Diffuse reflection, 481f
Digital, term (usage), 399
Digital chest radiograph, simulation, 492f
Digital computers, analog computer replacement, 398
Digital CRT, soft copy viewing, 469
Digital display, quality control
  challenge questions, 485
  technologist, impact, 485

Digital display devices
  display noise, 484
  display resolution, 483-484
  luminance response, 482-483
  photometric evaluation, 480
  quality control, 480-484
  viewing, 468f
Digital driving levels (DDLs), 482
  luminance, 482
Digital file sizes. *See* Imaging modalities 491t
Digital fluoroscope, FPIR (usage), 441f
Digital fluoroscopy (DF), 437
  advantages, 437
  CCD
    light sensitivity, increase, 440
    usage, 440, 439-440
  challenge questions, 448
  examinations, advantages, 443
  high-resolution systems, importance, 357
  image capture, 439-442
  image display, 442-443
  imaging system, 437-439
  operating console, 438f
  pixel size, equation, 437
  system. *See* Remotely controlled DF system, 438f
    components, 438f
  video system, 442
Digital image artifacts
  alignment, 497
  collimation/partition, 493-496
  image compression, 489-490
  image histogram, 491-493
  preprocessing, 488
Digital image receptor
  artifacts, uniqueness, 487
  exposure, 463f
  irradiation, 488
  response, 461f
Digital images, 407. *See also* Foot phantom, 462f
  artifacts, challenge questions, 497
  challenge questions, 465
  dynamic ranges, 472
  inversion, 473f
  PACS, combination, 476f
  partitioning, 495
  postprocessing, 472-473
    list, 472t
    operator manipulation, requirement, 472
  preprocessing, 471-472, 471t
  viewing
    challenge questions, 477
    optimum, 483
Digital imaging
  advantage, 455-456
  artifacts classification scheme, 487f
  systems
    contrast-detail curve, 460f
    dynamic range, 456f
Digital Imaging and Communications in Medicine (DICOM), 474
  standard, 479

Digital mammographic imaging system, 433f
Digital mammography (DM), 432-434
  technique, acceptance, 602
Digital Mammography Imaging Study Trial (DMIST), 432-433, 457
Digital mammography tomosynthesis (DMT), 433
  projection/reconstruction scheme, 433f
  view, 433f
Digital medical imaging systems, dynamic range, 456t
Digital meters, 399
Digital radiographic (DR) image receptors, speed, 606
Digital radiographic images (production), CsI phosphor light (usage), 431f
Digital radiographic imaging system, MTF curve, 455f
Digital radiography (DR), 413. *See also* Direct DR, 431
  challenge questions, 434-435
  efficiency, 427
  image receptor
    debris, 487f
    sizes, 494b
  MTF curve representation, 454
  organizational scheme, 427f
  processing artifacts, usage, 301
  spatial resolution, a-Se (impact), 432
  underexposure, 493f
Digital recording (DR), 487
Digital subscriber lines (DSLs), 405
Digital subtraction angiography (DSA), 443-448
  image formation, 443-444
  patient dose, 447-448
  roadmapping, 447
  switch, 471
  usage. *See* Aorta-iliac area 446f
Digital thermometer, 276f
Digital versatile disc-read-only memory (DVD-ROM), 403
Dimensional stability, 182
DIN 2001, 479
Dipolar field, 74
Direct current (DC), 81
  electric motor, 92f
  explanation, 81
  representation, 82f
Direct DR, 431
Direct effects. *See* Ionization, 525
  hits, occurrence, 526
Direct-exposure film (nonscreen film, special application film), 183
  availability, 185
  explanation, 188
  speed, 185
  function, 185
Direct film exposure
  screen-film exposure, difference, 215-216
  x-rays/light photons, relative numbers (comparison), 215t

Direct square law, 248
    calculation, 248
Disaccharides, 504
Disc drive, example, 404f
Discrete emission spectrum, shift, 148f
Discrete spectrum, values, 143
Dissociation, 523
    equation, 524
Distance, 248, 571
    assumption, 573
    excess, 573
    impact. *See* Image receptor 248;
        Optical density, 248
        absence. *See* Radiation, 248
    indicators, accuracy, 307
    maximization, 573
Distortion, 259-260, 286-287
    anatomy/object irregularity, impact,
        287f
    dependence, 286
    interference. *See* Diagnosis, 286
    object thickness, impact, 286f
    reduction, 260
Division, rounding (usage), 20
DLs. *See* Dose limits, 616
DM. *See* Digital mammography, 432
DMIST. *See* Digital Mammography
    Imaging Study Trial, 432-433
DMT. *See* Digital mammography
    tomosynthesis, 433
DNA. *See* Deoxyribonucleic acid, 503
Dose. *See* Patient dose, 459-463
    creep, 459
        replacement, technique creep
            (usage), 461
    dependence, 608
    fractionation, 514
    protraction, 514
Dose area product (DAP), 584
    quantity, 584
Dose limits (DLs)
    emphasis, 627
    establishment, 616
    historical levels, 618f
    linear nonthreshold dose-response
        relationship, basis, 617
    NCRP recommendation, 619t
    specification, 617
Dose-response relationship. *See*
        Radiation, 518f
    construction, 517
    determination. *See* Whole-body
        response, 517
    example, 554
    extrapolation, 518
    form, 564
    production, 518f
Dosimeters, usage, 588
Dosimetry, application, 588
Double-capacity processors, 313
Double emulsion. *See* Screen-film, 185
Double-emulsion film, 181
    availability, 8
    processing, 188
    usage, 208
Double exposures, avoidance, 299
Double-helix configuration, 506

Doubling dose, 565
DQE. *See* Detective quantum
    efficiency, 209b
DR. *See* Digital radiography 301;
    Digital recording, 487
DRAM. *See* Dynamic RAM, 402
Drosophila, irradiation, 564
Dry cells
    carbon rod, usage, 88
    representation, 89f
Drying. *See* Film, 199
Dry processing, 204-206
    photothermic method, 204f
DSA. *See* Digital subtraction
    angiography, 443-448
DSLs. *See* Digital subscriber lines, 405
Dual-filament cathode, 123f
Dual filament x-ray tube, filament
    circuit, 106f
Dual-focus x-ray tube, focal spot size
    (control), 125f
Dual-source multislice spiral CT
    imaging system, 389f
Duty cycle, involvement, 439f
DVD-ROM. *See* Digital versatile
    disc-read-only memory, 403
Dwell time, 206
    reduction. *See* Photothermography,
        205f
Dynamic RAM (DRAM), 402
Dynamic range, 454. *See also*
        Charge-coupled device, 428
Dynodes, 592
    gain, 593

E

Early age (exposure), cancer
    development, 560f
Early effect of radiation. *See*
    Radiation, 502
Eckert, J. Presper, 397
Edge enhancement, 319
    effectiveness, 473
Edge response function (ERF), 379
Edison, Thomas A., 8, 209
    fluoroscope, usage, 9f
EEPROM. *See* Electronically erasable
    programmable read-only memory,
    402
Effective atomic number, 290
    differences, absence, 383f
Effective dose, 575. *See also*
        Patient, 575 *See also* Radiologic
        technologist, 575
    assumption. *See* Occupational
        effective dose, 576
    equation, 618
    formula, 575
Einstein, Albert. *See* Mass-energy
    equivalence, 4
Ejected electron, energy, 164
Elective booking, 608
    instituting. *See* Patient, 608
Electrical conductor, 125
Electrical energy, 4
Electrical resistance. *See* Conductor, 78f
    determination, 74

Electric charges. *See* Conductor 77
    association. *See* Electrons, 73;
        Protons 73
    potential energy, 77
    unit, 74
Electric circuits, 78-81
Electric current (electricity), 77
    elements, symbols/functions, 80t
    measurement, 78
    occurrence, 78
    result, 112
Electric energy, conversion, 75f
Electric fields
    radiation, 76f
    sinusoidal change, 57
Electric forces, magnetic forces
    (joining), 88
Electric generator, output waveform,
    92f
Electric ground, 74
Electricity. *See* Electric current, 77
    challenge questions, 97
Electric potential, 77
    measurement, 87
Electric power, 81-83
    equation, 83
    measurement, 81
Electric resistance, increase, 78
Electrification. *See* Objects, 73
    creation, 73
Electrified clouds, lightning source,
    75f
Electrodynamics, 77-83
    definition, 78
Electromagnetic energy, 4, 57
    attenuation, 64
    challenge questions, 70-71
    frequency/wavelength, inverse
        proportion, 60
    intensity, inverse relation, 67
    properties, 57
    wave-particle duality, 57
Electromagnetic induction, 91
Electromagnetic radiation, 5, 52
    Maxwell's field theory, 88
    usage, 53
    visualization, 69f
Electromagnetic relationship
    triangle, 64f
Electromagnetic spectrum, 60-63
    definition, 60
    diagnostic ultrasound,
        exclusion, 61
    measurement, 61-62
    representation, 61f
    segments, ranges, 61
Electromagnetic wave
    equation, 60
Electromagnetism, 88-95
    challenge questions, 97
Electromagnets
    closed iron core, incorporation,
        94f
    current-carrying wire coil, 90
    magnetic field lines, 91f
    usage, 85f
Electromechanical devices, 88-95

Electron beam. *See* Blanked electron
   beam, 356
  intensity modulation, control grid
   (usage), 356
  modulation, 357
Electron gun, 354
Electronically erasable programmable
  read-only memory (EEPROM),
  402
Electronic computer, development, 397
Electronic Numerical Integrator And
  Calculator (ENIAC), 397
  photograph, 398f
Electronic preprocessing, failure, 490f
Electronic signal, obscuration, 442
Electronic timers, 108
Electrons, 40. *See also* Cathode
  rays, 39
  arrangement, 43-44
   definition, 43
   shell notation, 43
  attachment, strength, 44
  binding energies/levels, 41
   approximation, 45f
   designation, 44-45
  conduction, 7
  configuration, complexity, 42
  electric charges, association, 73
  electrostatic charge, determination, 74
  existence, shells, 41
  flow, 82f
   reversal, problem, 110
  interaction, number, 153
  maximum number per shell, 43
   summary, 43t
  migration. *See* Sensitivity center, 184f
  orbits/shells, 41
  outer shell number, determination, 43
  reflection, 131
  release, 184f
  revolution, 44f
  target, interactions, 139-143
  total number, 42
   mAs measurement, 153
  transition, 166
  usage, requirement, 153
Electrostatic charge
  concentration, 77f
  determination. *See* Electrons, 74
  excess, 77f
Electrostatic focusing lenses, 351
Electrostatic force, 75
  inverse square relationship, 76
Electrostatic grids, 354
Electrostatic laws, 74-77
Electrostatics, 73-77
  definition, 73
Elemental mass, 46
Elements, 38. *See also* Transitional
  elements, 43
  characteristics, 46t
  chemical properties, 45
  determination. *See* Chemical
   elements, 41
  particle, size, 48b
  periodic table, 39
   representation, 40f

Elements *(Continued)*
  radiation, self-absorption
   (impossibility), 324
  radiological importance, atomic
   number, 166t
  representation, protocol, 47f
Elongation. *See* Image 259; Scapula,
  260f
Embolization, 361
Emergency room CT, 605
EMI imaging system, translations
  (requirement), 369
Emissions. *See* X-ray emissions, 140
Employee notification, form, 626f
Emulsion, 181. *See also* Radiographic
  film, 182-183
  gelatin portion, hardening, 195
  pick-off, 300
Encode, process, 407
Endocrine glands, 504
Endoplasmic reticulum, 506
Energy, 23
  conservation, law, 69
  continuum, 57
  definition, 4
  equation, 5
  equivalence. *See* Mass-energy
   equivalence, 4
  explanation, 3
  forms, 70f. *See also* Mechanical
   energy, 23
  frequency, proportion. *See*
   Photons, 62
  levels, 40
  measurement, 4
  reflection, 65f
  relationship. *See* Temperature, 26
  thermometer, 26f
  transformation, 23
  work ability, 23
Energy subtraction, 445-447
  comparison. *See* Temporal
   subtraction, 444t
  disadvantage, 446-447
  techniques, involvement, 447f
Engineering prefixes, 34t
ENIAC. *See* Electronic Numerical
  Integrator And Calculator, 397
Entrance exposures. *See* Radiographic
  examinations, 610t
Entrance skin dose, usage. *See* Pelvic
  examination, 241t
Entrance skin exposure (ESE), 599.
  See also Photofluorospot imagers,
  312t
  average, 311
  calculation, 600
  cassette-loaded spot film,
   combination, 311t
  determination, 29, 246, 248
  effect, 583b
  estimation, 599
  identification, 599
  level, assumption. *See* Cassettes, 311
  rate, 311
  reduction, 582
  report, 598

Environmental radiation, usage.
  See Ghost artifacts, 487
Enzymes, 504
Epidemiologic studies, 550
  requirement, 550
Epithelium, 510
EPROM. *See* Erasable programmable
  read-only memory, 402
Equivalent Planck's equation, 68
Erasable optical discs
  (CDE, CD-RW), 403
Erasable programmable read-only
  memory (EPROM), 402
Erase (sequence), 418f
ERF. *See* Edge response function 379
Ergonomically designed digital image
  workstation, 471f
Erythema, 539
  early effects, 550
  intermediate radiation doses,
   impact, 540
Erythrocytes, 542f
ESE. *See* Entrance skin exposure, 29
Essences, 38
  symbolic representation, 39f
Europium (Eu), presence, 413
Examination
  Necessity, absence, 605
  repetition, 605
Examination repeat analysis form, 341f
Excess risk, 554
  equation, 554
Excited energy states, range, 210
Exit beam, 181
Exponential attenuation, 174-175
Exponential form, expression.
  See Number, 30
Exponential x-ray attenuation data,
  linear/semilog plots, 175f
Exponents
  division, 31
  multiplication, 31
  rules, 31
   application, 31
  value, determination. *See* Positive
   exponent 30
Exposure
  artifacts, 298-300
   list, 300t
  control, 583
  doubling, 277. *See also* Radiation,
   277
  formula, 573
  latitude, 185
  level, straight-line portion, 276
  linearity, 309
   accuracy, 309
   assessment method, 309
   determination, 309
  mAs equivalence, 247
  rate, 311
  reduction, maximum, 624
  reproducibility, 309-310
Exposure factors, 245-248
  change, absence, 254f
  control, 245
  types, 245

Exposure technique
  charts, 260-263
  factors, 251
    impact. *See* Radiographic
      contrast, 258t
  usage, 263
Exposure time, 246-248. *See also*
  Radiographic exposure times,
  246-248
  determination, 247
  electronic basis, 108
  fractional seconds, expression, 246
  impact. *See* Motion, 246
  mA combinations, 310t
  range, 337
  shortness, 293
  units, relationship, 246t
Exposure timer, 107-109
  accuracy, 309, 308-309
    measurement device, 309f
Extended processing, 203
  improvements, 203
External filtration, 146
Extinction time, 113, 438
  involvement, 439f
Extrafocal radiation, reduction, 132f
Extrafocal x-rays, result, 132f
Extrapolation number (target
  number), 529
Extremities
  imaging, trauma radiographic
    imaging system (usage), 230f
  radiation, 619
  radiographs, sharpness, 227f
Extremity monitoring, 615
Eyes. *See* Humans, 349f
  responses, 467

F

Fahrenheit
  Celsius conversion, 25
  scale, usage, 25f
Falling load generator, 106
Faraday, Michael, 91
  experiment
    application, 91
    schematic description, 91f
Faraday's law, 91
Fast scan, 418
Fatal accident rates, 616t
Fatal cancers, expectation
  (determination), 554-555
Fatty acid, 504
Ferromagnetic material, 84f
  inclusion, 85
Ferromagnetic objects, 87
Fertility
  low-dose chronic irradiation, impact
    (absence), 561
  radiation, impact, 561
Fetal doses. *See* Radiographic
  examinations, 610t
Fetal irradiation, effects, 502b
Fiber interspace grids, warping, 234
Fiber optics, usage, 355
Fibrous tissues, 320
Field of view (FOV), 375-376

Field size. *See* X-ray beam, 225-226
  radiographic exposure factors,
    comparison, 226
Fifteen percent rule, 254
Filament
  circuit, 106
  current, 123-125
    increase, 127
  definition, 122
  temperature, 106
  thoriated tungsten, usage, 122
  transformer, 106
    high-voltage generator
      component, 109
    primary coil current,
      determination, 107
Filament Heating Isolation Step-down
  Transformer, 107
File, term (usage), 403
Fill factor, 431. *See also* Picture
  element 431f
Film
  badges
    disadvantages, 621
    wearing, requirement, 621
  characteristic curve, 275-277
  combinations. *See* Radiographic
    intensifying screens, 214-219
  compression, necessity, 344
  contrast, relationship, 279
  crossover, 344
  cross-section. *See* Radiographic film,
    181f
  drying, 195, 199
  emulsion surface, proximity, 328
  factors, 275-284
  fixer retention, analysis, 342, 342f
  flashing, 276
  format, size increase (benefit), 358
  graininess, 274
  illuminators, 310-311
  OD, 573
  processing, 194-195, 283-284
  screen, specks (production), 333f
  selection, limitation, 279
  shorter dimension, placement.
    See Automatic processor, 200
  washing, 195, 199
Film development
  chemical reaction, 198
  processing stage, 195
  temperature, 284
  time, 283
Film-loaded cassettes, insertion, 232
Film-screen PA chest radiography,
  158
Filtered back projection, 376
Filtration, 9, 249-250, 306-307.
  See also Added filtration, 158;
    External filtration, 146; Inherent
    filtration, 157
  addition (hardening), 147
    impact. *See* X-ray emission
      spectrum, 147
  amount, 581
  necessity, absence. *See* Automatic
    processor 202

Filtration *(Continued)*
  relationship. *See* X-ray quantity,
    154-155
  selective usage. *See* Low-energy
    x-rays, 157f
  types, 157-160
  usage, 12
Final velocity, 20
  equation, 23
  example, 20f
Fine-detail radiography, focal spots
  (impact), 248
Fingernail marks, film kinking, 302f
Firmware, 402
First-generation computers, 398
First-generation CT imaging systems,
  369
First-generation imaging system,
  components, 369
First Law of Newton. *See*
  Newton, 20
Five-minute reset timer, 572
Five-pin ACR accreditation phantom,
  characteristics, 384t
Five-pin test object, design version,
  383f
Fixed kilovoltage, 260
Fixed-kVp chart, usage. *See*
  Abdomen, 262t
Fixed SID, usage. *See* Trauma system,
  230
Fixer
  circulation system, filtration
    (necessity, absence), Automatic
    processor, 202
  components/functions, 198t
  pH, constancy, 199
  preservative, 199
  retention, analysis. *See* Film 342
Fixing, 198-199. *See also* Silver
  halide, 195
  processing, 198
Flash drive (jump drive, jump stick),
  403
  example, 404f
Flatfielding, 471
  performing, 488
  preprocessing, 490f
  software connection, 488
Flat Panel Display Measurement
  (FPDM) standard, 479
Flat panel displays, 405
Flat panel image display, 442-443
Flat panel IR (FPIR), 440
  advantages, 442b, 441
  composition, 440
  digital signal, 443
  fluoroscopy, 442f
  image capture, 441
  size/weight, reduction, 440-441
  usage. *See* Digital fluoroscope, 441f
Flies, irradiation, 564f
Floor-to-ceiling support system,
  120-121. *See also* X-ray tube,
  120-121
Floppy disc, 403
Fluorescence, 7, 210

Fluoroscope
  components, 348f
  development, 8
  usage, 347
Fluoroscopic contrast agents, 44
Fluoroscopic examination
  isoexposure contours, 573f
  patient dose, approximation, 448t
Fluoroscopic foot switch, training, 572
Fluoroscopic image
  monitoring, 353-358
  television monitoring system, 353
Fluoroscopic kVp, 350t
Fluoroscopic mA, level (comparison), 116
Fluoroscopic protection features, 582
Fluoroscopic table
  head position, 103
  identification, 103f
Fluoroscopic technique, 349
Fluoroscopist, pregnancy, 626f
Fluoroscopy, 614
  challenge questions, 359
  conducting, 8
  demands, 347-349
  image intensification, 349-353
  imaging chain, 437f
  overview, 347
  quality control, 311
  x-ray examination, 8
Flux gain, 351
  equation, 351
  product, 351
Focal point, change, 352
Focal-spot blur, 288-289. *See also*
    Anode, 289
  cause, 288f
  equation, 288
  geometry, 365f
  importance. *See* Spatial resolution, 288
  occurrence, 288
  phenomenon, 288
  region, calculation, 288
  size, 289f
Focal-spot cooling algorithms, 373
Focal spots. *See* Mammography, 323-324
  change, 248
  impact. *See* Fine-detail radiography 248
  production, 130f
  range, 124
  reduction, heel effect (impact), 131
  shape, 130f
    change, 132f
  usage, 269
  x-ray source, 128b
  x-ray tube tilt, impact, 324f
Focal-spot size, 128, 248, 307-308.
    See also Cathode, 289f
  change, 132f
  comparison. *See* Nominal focal spot size, 130
  difference, 248
  measurement, 308f
  variation, 289

Focused grid, 237-238
  design, 237
  fabrication, 237f
  misalignment, 238t
  off-center positioning, 239f
  positioning, absence, 239f
  upside-down positioning, 240f
Focusing cup, 123
  absence, beam spreading, 124f
  filament, embedding, 123
  illustration, 123f
  usage, beam condensation, 124f
Fog. *See* Chemical fog, 198;
    Development fog 197;
    Radiation 198
  density
    impact, 278, 278f
    increase, 278
  level. *See* Radiographic film 190
  excess, 342
Football kick, example, 17
Foot examination, wedge filter (usage), 159f
Foot phantom
  digital images, 462f
  screen-film radiographs, 462f
Foot tomographs (usage), x-ray tube motion (usage), 269f
Force. *See* Weight, 22
  calculation. *See* Mass, 21
  imaginary lines, 85f
  magnetic lines, demonstration, 87f
  requirement. *See* Acceleration, 21
Force, equation, 21
Foreshortening, 259. *See also* Image, 259; Scapula 260f
FORmula TRANslation (FORTRAN), 409
4:1 ratio grid, usage, 327
4% voltage ripple, 115
Four-slice spiral CT, 388f
14-bit dynamic range, gray (shades), 456f
14% voltage ripple, 115
Fourth-generation CT imaging systems, 371f
Fourth-generation imaging systems, components, 371
FOV. *See* Field of view, 375-376
FPDM. *See* Flat Panel Display Measurement, 479
FPIR. *See* Flat panel IR 440-442
Fractionation, 514. *See also* Dose, 514
  levels, 514
Fractions, 26. *See also* Improper fraction 26; Proper fraction, 26
  addition, 26
    value, determination, 26, 26
  application, 27
  decimal conversion, 27
  definition, 26
  division, 27
    value, determination, 27, 27
  multiplication, 27
    value, determination, 27, 27

Free radical, 524
  energy, 525
  formation. *See* Organic free radical formation, 525
Frequency, 58-60
  definition, 58
  importance, 58
  increase/decrease, 58
  inverse proportion. *See* Electromagnetic energy, 60
  radiographer usage, 110
  relationship. *See* Sine waves, 59f
  velocity/wavelength, inverse proportion, 59
  wavelength, inverse proportion. *See* Electromagnetic energy, 60
  wave parameters, 59
Friction, presence, 21
Frontal sinus, radiograph, 231f
Frost, E.B., 9f
Frost, G.D., 9f
Fulcrum, object plane/tomographic angle (relationship), 267f
Full-wave rectification, 112-113
  advantage, 113
  definition, 112
  usage, 115
  voltage waveform, 250
Full-wave-rectified circuit
  diodes
    conduction, 113f
    presence, 112f
    positive voltage, 113f
Full width at half maximum (FWHM), 387
Fundamental laws of motion.
    See Motion, 20
Fundamental particles, 40-41
  characteristics, 41t
  definition, 40
FWHM. *See* Full width at half maximum, 387

G

Gadolinium, 208
  screen, 216
Gadolinium oxysulfide (GdOS), 427, 461-463
  usage, 431
Gain images, 471
Galvani, Luigi, 88
Gametogenesis, 540
Gamma rays
  contrast. *See* X-rays, 63
  existence, 53
  ionizing electromagnetic radiation, form, 53
  ionizing radiation, capability, 5
  production. *See* Nucleus, 63f
Gamma spectrometry, 593
Gantry, 373-375
  components. *See* Multislice spiral computed tomography, 375f
  inclusion. *See* Computed tomography, 373
Gas, ionization, 589

Gas-filled detectors, 589
components, 589f
impact. *See* Signal amplitude 589f
proportional region, 590
recombination, region, 589
Gastrointestinal (GI) death, 535
occurrence, 537
Gastrointestinal (GI) syndrome,
536-537
doses, consistency, 537
GB. *See* Gigabyte, 403
GdOS. *See* Gadolinium oxysulfide, 427
Geiger counters, usage, 591
Geiger-Muller (G-M) region, 590
Gelatin
buildup, 300
mixture, 182
similarity, 182
Generator functions, evaluation, 308f
Genetically significant dose (GSD),
601, 601
equation, 601
estimates, 601
diagnostic x-ray examination,
usage, 601t
gonad dose, 601
Genetic cells, 507
Genetic effects, 564-565
linear-nonthreshold dose-response
relationship, 517
Geometric distortion, 481
appearance, 481
Geometric factors, 284-289
Germ cell, 505
progression, 541f
Ghost artifacts (contribution),
environmental radiation
(usage), 487
Ghost images, appearance, 487
GI. *See* Gastrointestinal, 535
Gigabyte (GB), 403
Glandular dose (D_g), 602
Glandular tissues, 320
radiation sensitivity, 321
Glass envelope, 354
usage, 592
Glass/metal enclosure. *See* X-ray
tube, 122
Glitterblende, 10
Glow curve, 594
Glutaraldehyde, absence, 198
Glycerol, 504
Glycogen. *See* Animal glycogen, 504
G-M. *See* Geiger-Muller, 590
Gonadal dose, importance, 598
Gonadal shielding, usage, 4
Gonads, effects, 540-542
Gonad shielding, 607b
Gradient, 281
slope, 281f
Granulocytes, 542f, 543
Graph
semilogarithmic scale, usage, 32
x-axis/y-axis, intersection, 32f
Graphing, 31
Gravitational field, impact.
See Mass, 57

Gravity, explanation, 3
Gray scale, 454. *See also* Long gray
scale 282; Short gray scale, 282
consideration, 456
displays, 480
Gray Scale Display Function (GSDF),
479
Gray shades (visualization),
postprocessing (usage), 456
Greek atoms, discovery, 38
Green-sensitive film, 187
usage, rare Earth screens
(combination), 218
Grenz rays, 540
Grid, 232-234
Bucky factor values, 235t
cutoff, 235. *See also* Complete grid
cutoff 235; Partial grid cutoff,
235
equation, 236
design, 232
frequency, 233-234
equation, 234
increase, 233
strips per centimeter, 233
lines
presence, 238
production, 238
performance, scatter radiation
(impact), 234-235
problems, 238-240
radiographic technique, change,
241t
selection, 240-243
clinical considerations, 242t
factors, 241
strips, 232, 234
surface x-ray absorption, 233
term, usage, 123
types, 235-238
usage, 225. *See also* Tomography,
268
Grid ratio, 233-234
calculation, 233
definition, 233f
equation, 233
increase, 240f
Bucky factor, increase, 235
Grids
usage, 327
Gross artifacts (cause), processor
rollers (impact), 339f
GSD. *See* Genetically significant dose,
601
GSDF. *See* Gray Scale Display
Function, 479
Guanine, 505
Guide shoe marks, 300
turnaround assembly, impact, 301f
Guidewires
J-tip, usage, 362
usage. *See* Interventional radiology,
362
Guillotine blade, potential/kinetic
energy (demonstration), 4f
Gy_a. *See* Roentgen, 34
Gy_t. *See* Radiation absorbed dose, 34

H
Halation, effect, 188
Half-life ($T_{1/2}$). *See* Radioactive
half-life, 50
definition, 50-52
number, 51
representation, 50f
Half-value layer (HVL), 51
approximation. *See* Concrete, 574t;
Lead, 574t
determination
data, illustration, 156f
experimental arrangement, 155f
methods, 155
steps, 156
estimation, 574
experimental determination, 155
increase, added filtration (impact),
158
measurement, 245, 307
relationship. *See* Kilovolt
peak, 157t
usage, 155-156. *See also* X-rays,
156
Half-wave rectification, 111-112
illustration, 112f
radiation quality, 250
Half-wave-rectified circuit, diodes
(presence), 112f
Half-wave-rectified generator, 100%
voltage ripple, 250
Halide ions, 183
Handling artifacts, 302
list, 302t
Hard copy, medical images, 468
Hard copy-soft copy, 468-469
Hard discs (memory), 403
Hardener, usage, 197, 199
Hardening. *See* Emulsion 195;
Filtration, 147
Hardware, 400. *See also* Computers,
400-401
Health physics, challenge questions,
579
Heart, volume-rendering display, 379f
Heat, 24. *See also* Thermal energy, 4
kinetic energy, defining, 24
production, 142
transfer, 24. *See also* Thermal
radiation, 25
Heat units (HUs), 134
generation, determination, 135
Heel effect, 129-131, 289
demonstration. *See* Postanterior
chest images, 131f
impact. *See* Focal spots, 131
result, 130f
Hematologic death, 535
Hematologic effects, 542-544
Hematologic syndrome, 536
characterization, 536
radiation doses, 536
Hemopoietic cell survival, 543-544
Hemopoietic system, 542-543
Hermetic seal, usage, 592
Hexadecimal number system, 409
list, 409t

High anode heating (allowance), line-focus principle (usage), 129f

High atomic number. *See* Phosphor, 209b

High contrast, 257

High-contrast radiographs, gray scale production, 257

High-energy electrons, interaction, 351

High-energy particle accelerators, 40

High-energy particles, beam (extraction), 551

High-energy x-rays, nucleus (interaction), 170f

Higher-energy bremsstrahlung x-rays, reduction, 324

High-frequency generation, result, 250

High-frequency generator, 114
    advantage, 114
    development, 250
    1% ripple, 115

High-frequency grids (usage), radiographic technique (requirement), 233

High-frequency voltage, usage, 115

High-frequency voltage waveform, 114f

High-frequency wire mesh phantom, images, 343f

High-frequency x-ray generator
    characteristics, 115t
    grouping, 114

High kilovoltage, 260

High-kVp technique, 172
    advantage, 294
    charts
        kVp selection, 263
        preparation, 245

High-LET radiation, usage, 526

High-level control, option, 584

Highlighting, effectiveness, 473

High-quality radiograph, 273

High-ratio grids
    effectiveness, 234f
    impact. *See* Patient, 233
    positioning latitude, reduction, 237
    usage. *See* Scatter radiation, 233

High spatial frequency, object representation, 379

High-transmission cellular (HTC) grid, 327
    design. *See* Mammography, 327f

High-voltage chest radiograph, 264f

High-voltage functions, evaluation, 308f

High-voltage generation, 321

High-voltage generator, 109, 250-251
    adjustment, 247
    characteristics, 250t
    components, 109
    cutaway view, 109f
    housing, 103
    inverter circuit, 114f
    power, determination, 116
    usage, 103. *See also* Interventional radiology, 365
    voltage supply, determination, 106

High-voltage power supply, substitute, 9

High-voltage step-up transformer, secondary winding (voltage induction), 110f

High-voltage technique (demonstration), chest radiographs (usage), 294f

High-voltage transformer, 109
    high-voltage generator component, 109
    primary side, 108

Hip radiograph, quantum mottle (demonstration), 273f

Histogram, 492f
    analysis errors, sampling, 494f
    error prevention, collimation/ centering (usage), 494
    occurrence, frequency (graph), 491
    plotting, example, 491

Hoff, Ted, 398

Holes, 110

Hollerith, Herman, 397

Homeostasis, 503

Horizontal resolution
    determination, 357
    improvement, bandpass (increase), 357

Horizontal retrace, 356

Hormesis, 516. *See also* Radiation, 516

Hormones, 504

Horsepower (hp), 23

Hospital admission, 605
    chest x-ray examinations, performing (avoidance), 605

Hounsfield, Godfrey, 368

Hounsfield unit (HU), 375
    nomenclature, 376

HTC. *See* High-transmission cellular, 327

Human biology
    challenge questions, 511
    input devices, usage, 401

Human cell, 506-509
    cell-survival curves, 532f
    cycle phases, identification, 508
    division, completion, 508
    function, 507
    nucleus, metaphase (photomicrograph), 545f
    progress, 508f
    proliferation, 507
        process, 507
    recovery, 515
    schematic view, 507f
    sensitivity, 509, 531

Human peripheral lymphocytes, usage, 545

Humans
    chromosomes, 523f. *See also* Radiation-damaged human chromosomes, 523f
    eye, appearance, 349f
    fibroblasts, age response, 531f
    lens, 347-348
    natural environmental radiation, impact, 6

Humans *(Continued)*
    populations, radiation effects (observation), 502t
    radiation
        early effects, 535t
        exposure, levels (estimation), 611f
    radiation exposure, events sequence, 501f
    radiation response, 501-502
    threshold dose, 535t
    vision, 347-349
        photometric response curves, 467f
        range, 348f

Humans, cones
    color perception, 349
    number, 348
    sensation, 347-348
    usage, 348

Hurter and Driffield (H&D) curve, 275
    response, 429

HUs. *See* Heat units, 134

HVL. *See* Half-value layer, 51

Hybrid subtraction, 443, 447
    involvement, 447f

Hydrogen ions, concentration (control), 197

Hydrogen peroxide, formation, 524, 525

Hydroperoxyl formation, equation, 524

Hydroquinone, 196
    phenidone, combination, 196

Hygroscopic scintillation crystals, 592

Hyperbaric oxygen, 514

Hypersthenic, term (usage), 251

Hypo retention, 199, 302

I

ICRU. *See* International Commission on Radiation Unites and Measurement, 34

ICs. *See* Integrated circuits, 398

IF. *See* Intensification factor, 210

Illuminance, 467
    example, 468t
    meter, 480

Illumination, 347
    levels, 347

Image
    acquisition rates, 438, 443
    artifacts
        challenge questions, 303
        reduction, darkroom cleaning (impact), 334
    blur, off-focus radiation (impact), 231
    brightness, increase, 347
    buffer, 421
    characteristics, 224
    elongation, 259
    flip, 472
    foreshortening, 259, 287
        result, 287f
    histogram, 495
    integration, 444
    interpretation (improvement), PACS (usage), 473

Image *(Continued)*
  inversion, 473
  lag, 471
  magnification, calculation, 352
  matrix
    description, 437
    size, 443
  recording, 357-358
  superimposition, 445
Image contrast
  electronic enhancement, 443
  impact, 254
  loss. *See* Active matrix LCD, 471f
  reduction, 228
    Compton scattering, impact, 165
  scatter radiation, impact, 228-229
Image detail, 212, 224
  determination, 457
  relationship, 213
  sharpness, 258
  visibility, 258
    description, 259
    measurement, 259
Image-forming x-rays, 181
  beam, 181
  description, 459f
  effect (amplification), radiographic
    intensifying screen (usage), 208
  illustration, 224f
  x-ray interaction, 224
Image-intensified fluoroscopy, 347
  television monitor, weakness, 357
Image intensifier
  coupling, 354-355
  location, 13f
  TV system spatial resolution,
    impact, 357
Image-intensifier tube, 349-352
  CCD coupling, 440f
  contrast (reduction), veiling glare
    (usage), 353f
  incident x-ray, interaction, 351f
  input phosphor, constancy, 312
  operation modes, 352f
  25/17/12 tube, 354f
  x-ray beam pattern conversion, 350f
Image noise, 170. *See also*
    Radiographic intensifying screens,
    212-214
  increase, CE (increase), 212f
  sources. *See* Computed radiography
    423b; Screen-film radiography,
    423b
  usage. *See* Contrast resolution, 457
Image quality
  challenge questions, 295
  contrast characteristic, 228
  definitions, 273-275
  factors, 251, 252-260
Image receptor (IR), 181, 293, 365,
    606
  artifacts, 487-488
  atomic number, 463t
  characteristic curve, 279
    usefulness, 281
  Compton-scattered x-rays, impact,
    170f

Image receptor (IR) *(Continued)*
  contrast, 185, 279
    equation, 280
  exposure
    determination, 154
    distance, impact, 248
    factors, 152t
    latitude, 185
  image covering, 236
  K-shell binding energy, 463t
  latitude, 283f
  requirements, breast architecture
    (impact), 320f
  response, 422f, 460-461
    analysis, 463
    curve, usage, 423f
    function, 421-422
  selection, 606
  speed, 282f
    equation, 282
  types, 328
  x-ray, arrival, 224
  x-ray beam exposure, 490f
Imaginary lines of force. *See* Force,
    85f
Imaging modalities, digital file sizes,
    491t
Imaging plate (IP), 414. *See also*
    Computed radiography, 414-415
  cassette, relationship, 418-420
  documentation form, 488f
  erasure, completion (absence), 489f
  multiple fields, collimation
    (problems), 496f
  usage, 416
Imaging system
  characteristics, 248-251
  contrast resolution, improvement,
    380f
  spatial frequency, increase, 451
  spatial resolution, 453
    improvement, 451
Impact printers, 405. *See also*
    Nonimpact printers, 405
Improper fraction, 26
  examples, 26
Improvised nuclear device (IND), 577
IND. *See* Improvised nuclear
    device, 577
Indirect effects. *See* Ionization, 525
  amplification, oxygen (impact), 526f
  hits, occurrence, 526
Induced current, constancy
  (absence), 92
Induction, 86
  magnetic lines, 86
Induction motor, 127-128
  function, 127
  parts, 93f
  usage, 127. *See also* X-ray tube, 93
Inertia, 21
  law, 21
Infrared radiation, emission, 25
Inherent filtration, 157-158, 249
  approximation, 157
Initial velocity, 20
  example, 20f

Initiation time, 113
Ink-jet printers, 405
  images, formation, 405
Input, 400-402
  hardware, data conversion, 400
  power, conduction, 104
Input/output (I/O) device, 405
Input phosphor, 350
Insulator
  definition, 78
  service, 122
Integrated circuits (ICs), 398
Integrated services digital network
    (ISDN), 405
Integrate mode, usage, 588
Integration process, 145
Intensification factor (IF), 210
  assumption, 215
  calculation, 211
  impact. *See* Spatial resolution, 213
  kVp variation, graph, 211f
Intensifying screen, 12
  characteristics. *See* Radiographic
    intensifying screens, 210-214
  phosphors, x-ray absorption, 218f
Intensity profile (projection),
    formation, 368-369
Interlaced mode, progressive mode
    (differences), 442
Intermediate radiation doses, impact.
    See Erythema, 540
Internal carotid artery, iodinated
    compound (filling), 174
Internally deposited radionuclides, 6
International Commission
    on Radiation Unites and
    Measurement (ICRU), standard
    units (issuance), 34
International System (SI, Le Système
    International d'Unités), 4
  standard units, adoption, 34
Interphase, 507, 508
  death, 515
    occurrence, 515
  synthesis phase, 508f
Interpolation, 384-385
  algorithms, 385. *See also* Multislice
    spiral computed tomography,
    384-385
  estimates, 385f
  usage. *See* Z-axis resolution, 385
Interpreters, 408
  computer programs, 408
Interrogation time, 438
  involvement, 439f
Interrupterless transformer, 9
Interspace material, 232, 234
  primary beam x-rays, incidence, 233
Interstitial silver ions, positive charge,
    183
Interventional procedures, types, 361
Interventional radiology, 347, 614
  challenge questions, 366
  contrast media, 362
  equipment, usage, 363-365
  guidewires, usage, 362
  high-voltage generator, usage, 365

Interventional radiology *(Continued)*
  patient
    couch, 365f, 365
    preparation/monitoring, 362
  personnel, involvement, 363, 614
  principles, 361-363
  procedures, x-ray tube (usage), 364
  spatial resolution, approximation,
    364
  suite, 363-365
    layout, 363f
    representative procedures, 361t
    x-ray imaging apparatus, usage,
     364f
Interventional x-ray tube,
  specifications, 364t
Intracellular recovery, repair
  mechanism, 515
Intracellular repair/repopulation,
  processes (combination), 515
In utero irradiation, 561-564
  effects, summary, 564t
  human level, 563
  level, 562f
In utero radiation
  effects, 562
  exposure, 563
Inverse square law, 66-68, 154
  application, 67
  definition, 66
  description, 66f
Inverter circuit. *See* High-voltage
  generator, 114f
  DC power, 321
In vitro radiation, 521
In vivo radiation, 521
I/O. *See* Input/output, 405
Iodine
  atoms, migration, 184
  photoelectric absorption, 446f
  x-ray interaction, probability, 174
Ion chamber configuration, 591f
Ion chamber dosimeter, usage, 590f
Ion chamber region, 589
Ion chamber survey instrument,
  590f
Ionic bonds, 48
Ionization
  definition, 5
  direct/indirect effects, 525
  equation, 523, 524
  event, occurrence, 525
  explanation, 5f
  potential, 44
Ionizing radiation, 5
  classification, 52t
  human responses, 502b
  impact. *See* Biologic tissue, 52;
    Radiographic film, 190
  sources, 5
    NCRP estimate, 6
  types, 52
    characteristics, 54t
Ion pair, 5f
Ions, 183
IP. *See* Imaging plate, 414
IR. *See* Image receptor, 181

Irradiation, 5. *See also* In utero
  irradiation 561-564; Matter, 5
  dose-response relationship, 528f
  effects, summary, 564
ISDN. *See* Integrated services digital
  network, 405
Isobar, 47
Isobaric radioactive transitions, 47
Isoeffect curves, 540f
Isoexposure contours. *See*
  Fluoroscopic examination, 573f
Isoexposure lines, 573
Isoexposure profile. *See* Unshielded
  fluoroscope 584f
Isomer, 47b
Isotone, 47
Isotopes. *See* Radioactive isotopes, 49
  definition, 46
  neutrons, number, 41
  usage. *See* Atoms, 47
Isotropic emission, 209

J

Joules
  usage, 4
  work unit, 22
Joystick, usage, 437
Jukeboxes, 404
  model, 404f
Jump drive (jump stick). *See* Flash
  drive, 403

K

K absorption edge, 446
Karyotype, 545
kB. *See* Kilobyte, 407
K-characteristic x-rays, usefulness.
  See Tungsten, 141
KE. *See* Kinetic energy, 17
Kelvin, scale (usage), 25f
Kidneys ureter and bladder (KUB)
  examination, exposure time
    (determination), 107
  radiographic technique, 153
Kilobyte (kB), 407
Kilogram, mass, 17
Kilo (prefix), usage, 3
Kilovoltage. *See* Fixed kilovoltage
  260; High kilovoltage 260;
  Variable kilovoltage, 260
Kilovolt peak (kVp), 245, 291-292
  adjustment, 106
  calibration, 308
  change, impact, 146
  contrast scale, relationship, 255f
  decrease. *See* Differential
    absorption, 171
  exposure technique factor, 245
  15% increase, 254
  HVL, relationship, 157t
  impact. *See* X-ray beam quality,
    106b; X-ray emission spectrum
    146-147
    importance. *See* Subject contrast,
     292
  increase, 294
  measurement

Kilovolt peak (kVp) *(Continued)*
  accuracy, 308
  usage, 8
  meter. *See* Prereading kVp meter, 106
  optimum, 262
  peak, increase. *See* X-ray beam
    quality, 157
  selection, 308
  variation, 261
Kinetic energy (KE), 4
  calculation, 139
  conversion. *See* Projectile electrons,
    140
  definition. *See* Photoelectrons, 166
  equation, 23, 139
  equivalence, 139
  increase, 24
  magnitude, determination, 139
  motion energy, 139
  proportion, 139f
Kink marks, 302
Knee
  examination, variable-kVp chart
    (usage), 262t
  histogram, 493f
  phantom, radiographs, 262f
Krypton, isotope (usage), 17
K-shell absorption edge, 217
K-shell binding energy. *See* Image
  receptor, 463t
  matching, 463
K-shell electron
  binding energy, 166t
  ionization, 141f
KUB. *See* Kidneys ureter and bladder,
  107

L

Lanthanum, 208
  screen, 216
Lanthanum oxysulfide (LaOS),
  461-463
Large-grain emulsions, 185
Large-scale integration (LSI), 398
Laser beam
  deflection, 420
  diameter, impact, 415
  raster writing, 188f
  size, importance, 420
Laser discs. *See* Optical discs, 404
Laser film, 188-189
Laser printers, 405
Late-developing carcinoma, 550
Late effect of radiation. *See* Radiation,
  502
Latent image, 183, 184-185
  amplification, development
    (impact), 196f
  center, 184. *See also* Metallic silver,
    182
  change, invisibility, 183
  formation, 183-185
  invisibility, 194
  production, 184f
  stimulation, 417f
  storage, challenge questions, 206
  visible image conversion, 199f

Latent period, 535, 536
  manifest illness, following, 537
  postexposure time, 536
Lateral cerebral angiogram, exposure
  time (determination), 107
Lateral cervical spine, P. Diddy starter
  set, 299f
Lateral chest technique, intensity
  (determination), 153
Lateral decentering, 239
Lateral dispersion, reduction, 356
Latitude
  contrast, inverse proportion, 282
  definition, 282
Law of Beronie and Tribondeau, 513
  explication, 513b
  verification, 513
Law of conservation of energy. See
  Energy, 69
Law of conservation of matter. See
  Matter, 69
Law of inertia. See Inertia, 21
Lawrence, E.O., 551
Layered anode, components, 126f
LCDs. See Liquid crystal displays, 204
LD$_{50/60}$. See Lethal dose, 537-538
Lead
  HVL, approximation, 574t
  TVL, approximation, 574t
Lead attenuator, pinhole images, 313f
Lead bar patterns, 454f
Leaded apron/gloves, usage, 13f
Lead protective aprons, lead
  equivalence, 625
Leakage radiation
  intensity (reduction), protective
    housing (usage), 122f
  secondary radiation type, 585
LEDs. See Light-emitting diodes, 204
Left cerebral angiogram, performing,
  364
Length, 17
  base quantity, 17
Lens. See Humans, 347-348
  radiation, 619
  shield, contact type, 606
Lens-coupling system, example, 441f
Leonard, Charles L., 8
LET. See Linear energy transfer, 44
Lethal dose (LD$_{50/60}$), 537-538. See
  also Mice, 562f
  approximation, 538t
Leukemia, 555-557
  atomic bomb survivors, summary,
    555t
  cases, occurrence, 557
  incidence. See Atomic bomb
    survivors 556f; Childhood
    leukemia, 563
  elevation, 550t
  linear-nonthreshold dose-response
    relationship, 517
  observations, results, 557f
  occurrence, 11
  rarity. See Chronic lymphocytic
    leukemia, 557
LiF. See Lithium fluoride, 594

Life expectancy, 572f
Life span, reduction (expectation),
  552
Life-span shortening, 552-552
  risk, 552t
Light
  absorption, 66f
  localization, 232
  phenomenon, 64
  refraction. See White light, 62f
  stimulation-emission, 415
  travel, 20
  velocity, 20
Light-absorbing dyes, 211b
Light amplifier tube, Bell Telephone
  Laboratories demonstration, 10
Light-emitting diodes (LEDs), 204
Like charges, 75
  repulsion, 76f
Linear anatomical structure, imaging,
  267
Linear dose-response relationships,
  516-517
  nonthreshold/threshold types, 516f
Linear energy transfer (LET), 513,
  531-532
  approximation. See Diagnostic
    x-rays, 513
  dependence. See Oxygen
    enhancement ratio, 515
  description, 44
  increase, 514f
  levels. See Radiation doses, 514t
  measure, 513
  radiation, OER level, 515f
Linear graph, usage, 50f, 51f
Linear graphic scales, 168f
Linear interpolation, usage. See Z-axis
  resolution, 385
Linearity, 582
  maximum acceptable variation, 582
Linear nonthreshold dose-response
  relationship, 518
  conformance, 523
  slope, 555f
Linear-nonthreshold dose-response
  relationship, 517
Linear nonthreshold radiation dose-
  response relationship (LNT), 571
Linear scale, equal lengths (equal
  value), 33f
Linear threshold, 517
Linear tomographic examination,
  aspects, 266
Linear tomography, section thickness
  (value approximation), 268t
Linear tomography techniques, 266t
Line-focus principle, 128-129
  usage. See High anode heating, 129f
Line pair (lp), 379
  high-contrast line, 451f
  pattern, imaging, 453f
  spatial frequency, 452f
Line-pair test pattern, 213
  radiographic image, usage, 308f
Line spread function, 432
  example, 432f

Lipids, 504
  organic molecules, 503
  presence, 504
  structural configuration, 504f
Liquid crystal displays (LCDs), 204,
  405
Liquid crystals, random orientation,
  469f
Liquid scintillation detectors, usage,
  592
Lithium fluoride (LiF)
  sensitivity, 594
  thermoluminescence glow curve,
    594f
  TLD usage, 594
Liver cancer, 559
LNT. See Linear nonthreshold
  radiation dose-response
  relationship, 571
Local tissue damage, 538-542
Local tissue effects, 550-552
Lodestone, 83
Logarithmic graphic scales, 168f
Logic functions, 399-400
LOGO (computer language),
  410
Log relative exposure (LRE)
  increase, 277
  mAs, relationship, 277f
  scale, presentation, 277
  usage, 277
Long bone, cross section
  (radiographs), 229f
Long gray scale, 282
  contrast, 292
Lossless compression, 490
Lossy compression, 490
Low contrast, 257
Low-contrast CT test object,
  schematic drawing, 391f
Low-contrast objects (resolution), CT
  imaging system noise (limitation),
  383
Low-energy bremsstrahlulng x-rays,
  result, 142
Low-energy x-rays
  absorption, likelihood, 146
  atoms, interaction, 163f
  removal, filtration (selective usage),
    157f
Lower extremities, serial radiography
  (aluminum step-wedge usage),
  160f
Low-kVp radiography, disadvantages,
  292
Low-ratio grids, usage, 241
Low spatial frequency, object
  representation, 379
lp. See Line pair, 379
LRE. See Log relative exposure, 277
LSI. See Large-scale integration, 398
L-to-K transition, occurrence, 166
Lucency, 182
Lumbar spine radiography,
  recommendation, 227f
Lumen, basis. See Photometric
  units, 467

Luminance
   intensity, 467
   NIT level, requirement, 335
   quantity, 467
   response, uniformity (maximum
      deviation), 483
Luminescence, 210. *See also*
   Photostimulable luminescence,
   413-414; Radiographic
   intensifying screens, 210
   types, 210
Luminescent material, 210
   stimulation, 210
Luminous flux, 467
Lung cancer, 559
   incidence, 559
Lymphocytes, 542f, 543
   production, 543
   radiosensitivity, 543
Lymphocytic stem cells, radiation
   damage, 550
Lymphopenia, 543
Lysosomes, 506

M
mA. *See* Milliamperage, 106-107;
   Milliampere, 8
Macromolecular cellular components,
   irradiation, 506
Macromolecular synthesis, 521-522
Macromolecules, 503
   incorporation, 507
   irradiation, 521-523
      results, 521f
   synthesis, 521
Macros, 410
   design (recording), 410
   writing, 410
Magnesium oxide, usage, 209
Magnetic dipole, 83
   random orientation, 84f
Magnetic domain, 83
Magnetic field lines. *See*
   Electromagnets, 91f
   closed loops, 83
   concentric circles, formation, 90f
   overlap, 89
Magnetic fields
   creation, 83
   imaginary lines, 87f
   induction
      charge, movement (usage), 89
      moving charged particle, usage, 83f
      spinning charged particle, usage,
         84f
   intensity, variation, 91
   linesd
      direction, determination, 89
   oscillation, 91
   production, 90
   sinusoidal change, 57
   strength, SI unit, 88
Magnetic force, proportion, 88
Magnetic induction, 86-88
Magnetic laws, 86
Magnetic lines of force,
   demonstration. *See* Force, 87f

Magnetic lines of induction.
   See Induction, 86
Magnetic permeability, 84
Magnetic resonance imaging (MRI),
   266
   contrast resolution, quality, 459
   introduction, 63
   usage, 25
Magnetic steering, possibility, 442f
Magnetic susceptibility, 86
Magnetism, 83-88
   challenge questions, 97
   etymology, 83
Magnets
   breakage, 87f
   classification, 85
   poles, 86
Magnification, 284-286, 472
   calculation. *See* Image, 352
   image size/object size ratio, 285f
   inequality, 287
   mammography, 327-328
   minimization, 285
   mode, 352
   radiography, 284
   similarity, 285f
Magnification factor (MF), 284
   equation, 269, 284, 285
Magnification radiography, 269-270
   disadvantage, 270
   principle, 270f
Magnitude, 18
Main-chain scission, 521
   irradiation result, 521f
   long-chain macromolecule,
      breakage, 521
Mainframe computers, 400
Main memory, 402
Major organogenesis, period, 563-607
Male gametogenesis, self-renewing
   system, 542
Malignancy, total risk, 560-561
Malignant disease, BEIR Committee
   estimated excess mortality, 560t
Mammalian cell lines, doses, 530t
Mammogram
   masking, 335
      example, 337f
   processing/viewing, 328
   view, 433f
Mammographer, 332, 333
   responsibility. *See* Quality control,
      333
Mammographic exposures, total
   glandular dose, 602f
Mammographic imaging system,
   321-328
Mammographic QC program,
   elements, 333t
Mammographic screen-film contact
   (evaluation), wire mesh test tool
   (usage), 343f
Mammographic technique chart, 323t
Mammography, 615. *See also*
   Diagnostic mammography, 320;
   Digital mammography 432-434;
   See also Xeromammography 319

Mammography *(Continued)*
   AEC, 327
   basis, 319-321
   challenge questions, 329-330
   compression, 326-327, 344
      advantages, 326f
   dose, 601
   film, 188
      emulsions, cubic grains
         (photomicrograph), 328f
      loading, correctness, 329f
   filtration, 324-325
   focal spot, 323-324
   grids, usage, 327, 327
   heel effect, 325-326
      importance, 325
      usage advantage, 326f
   high-voltage generation, 321-322
   HTC grid, design, 327f
   imaging systems, dedication, 322f
   midgradient, importance, 281
   personnel exposures, 615
   QA program, radiologist
      responsibility, 332
   screen position, 213
   shoulder gradient, importance,
      281
   single screen, placement, 214f
   soft tissue radiography,
      example, 319
   system, features. *See* Dedicated
      mammography system, 322t
   test images, masking, 335
   tubes, focal spots, 248
   types, 320
   x-ray tube
      circular focal spot, pinhole
         camera image, 324f
      design, 131
Mammography quality control
   challenge questions, 345
   program, 333-345
      daily tasks, 333-334
      monthly tasks, 339-340
      nonroutine tasks, 344
      quarterly tasks, 340-342
      semiannual tasks, 342-344
      weekly tasks, 334
   team, 332-333
      members, 332f
Mammography Quality Standards Act
   (MQSA), 319
   accreditation phantom, 336
   mandate, 332
   QC program endorsement, 332
Mammomat (Siemens), 322f
Manifest illness, 536-537
   period, 536
Man-made radiation, 5
   sources, 7
Mark I, 397
mAs. *See* Milliampere seconds, 32
Mask image, 444
   inadequacy, 445
Mask mode
   result, 444
   usage, 443-444

Mask-mode DF
  imaging sequence, control, 444
  schematic representation, 444f
Mass, 17. *See also* Elemental
      mass, 46
  acceleration
      force, calculation, 21
      multiplication, 21
  base quantity, 17
  counting, 339
  definition, 3
  energy equivalence, 3
      formula, 5
  form, 70f
  gravitational field, impact, 57
  measurement, 3
  transformation, capability, 4
  weight, equivalence, 22
Mass density
  dependence, 172-173
  differences, absence, 383f
  equation, 19
  materials, 173t
  OD, relationship, 172
  report, 19
Mass-energy equivalence
      (Einstein), 4
Master rollers. *See* Automatic
      processor, 201
Matter
  characteristic, 3
  classification, 85
  conservation, law, 69
  definition, 3
  discovery, 38
  electrical states, 79t
  energy, relationship, 69-70
  exposure/irradiation, 5
  forms, 4
  ionization
      capability, 5
      efficiency, degrees, 54f
  magnetic states, 86t
  organization, levels, 48f
  structure, challenge questions,
      54-55
  substances, composition, 38
  transformation, 4
  x-ray interactions
      challenge questions, 177
      delineation, 163-169
Mauchly, John, 397
Maxillary sinus, radiograph, 231f
Maximum intensity projection
      (MIP), 377
  image reconstruction, 377
  reconstruction, example, 378f
  three-dimensional imaging
      form, 377
Maxwell, James Clerk, 57
MD. *See* Mid-density, 334
Mean lethal dose (D_0), 529
  cell recovery, 529
  indication, 529
Mean marrow dose, 601
Mean survival time, 538. *See also*
      Radiation exposure, 538f

Measurement
  components, 18
  requirement, 17
  standard units, 17
Mechanical energy, forms, 23
Mechanical support, providing, 121,
      125
Mechanics, 19
  equations, usage, 25t
  quantities, usage, 25t
  units, usage, 25t
Mediastinal tissue, enhanced
      rendering, 220f
Medical flat panel digital display
      devices
  monochrome AMLCDs, 469
  standard sizes, 470t
Medical images, digital file size, 476t
Medical imaging, 185
  CCD, advantages, 441b
  film, types, 185t
  systems
      contrast-detail curves, 461f
      spatial resolution, 453t
Medical physicist, 332, 332-333
  annual QC evaluation, performing,
      332b
  responsibility, 333
  role, 332
Medical radiation exposure, 7
Meiosis, 509
  process, 509
  reduction division, process, 509f
Memory, 402-403
  locations, sequence, 402
  storage, 403-404
Mendeleev, Dmitri, 39
Messenger RNA (mRNA), 505, 507
  transcription, 522
Metabolism, 503
  components, 522
Metal filters, usage, 12. *See also* X-ray
      imaging system, 154
Metallic silver
  formation, 184
  latent image center, 182
  reduction, 196
Metaphase, 508, 508
Metastable electrons, ground state
      (return), 415f
Meter
  English-speaking country standard,
      17
  light basis, 17
Meters kilograms seconds (MKS)
      system, 18
Metol, 196
MF. *See* Magnification factor, 284
mGy$_a$. *See* Milliroentgens, 152
Mice, LD$_{50/60}$, 562f
Microcalcifications
  deposits, 321
  x-rays, differential absorption, 173
Microcomputers, 400
  hard disc drives, 404
Microcontrollers, 400
Microfocus tubes, 248

Microprocessor, 401
  chip, conductive lines (width), 401f
Microswitch, engaging. *See* Automatic
      processor, 200
Microwave radiation, 63
  interaction, 64
Mid-density (MD), 334
Midgradient, importance. *See*
      Mammography, 281
Milliamperage (mA), control, 106-107
Milliampere (mA), 245-246
  calculation, 247
  change, 146
      impact, 146f
  impact. *See* X-ray emission
      spectrum, 146
  measurement, usage, 8
  meter, location, 107f
  products, 247t
  station, 245
      calibration, accuracy, 309
Milliampere seconds (mAs)
  calculation, 246
  change, 146
  control. *See* Optical density, 246
  expression, 107
  impact. *See* X-ray emission
      spectrum, 146
  increase, 225, 458-459
  OD, contrast, 32
  range, 337
  relationship. *See* X-ray quantity,
      153
  timers, 108
  value
      change, 254, 255f
      determination, 247
  x-ray quantity, proportion,
      152-153
Millions of instructions per second
      (MIPS), 401-402
Milliroentgens (mR, mGy$_a$), 152
Minification gain, 351
  equation, 351
  product, 351
MIP. *See* Maximum intensity
      projection, 377
MIPS. *See* Millions of instructions per
      second, 401-402
Misregistration, 445
  artifacts, 445
      examples, 446f
Mitochondria, 506
Mitosis, 507-508
  cell cycle phase, 508f
MKS. *See* Meters kilograms seconds,
      18
Mobile radiography, conducting, 154
Mobile radiology, 615
  exposure, 615
Mobile x-ray imaging system, 101f,
      582
Mobile x-ray unit, protective apron
      (assignation), 620
Modem (modulator/demodulator),
      405
Modulation data, plot, 454f

Modulation transfer function (MTF), 379, 452-454
  application, 452
  complexity, 380
  construction, 454f
  curves, 380f
    display, 453
    image differences, 455f
    photographic representations, 454
  evaluation, purpose, 452
  image fidelity/spatial frequency, plot, 380f
  impact, 458, 459
  perspective, 452
Modulator/demodulator. *See* Modem, 405
Molecular composition, 503
Molecular radiobiology, challenge questions, 532-533
Molecules
  building blocks, 3
  definition, 47
  random motion, 24
Molybdenum
  mammography usage, 148, 322
  target x-ray tube
    usage, 325
    x-ray emission spectrum, 323f
  x-ray absorption, probability, 325f
Momentum. *See* Total momentum, 22
  Conservation, example, 22f
  definition, 22
  mass/velocity, product, 22
  representation, 22
Monoenergetic x-ray beam, 172
  usage, alternative, 446
Monosaccharides, 504
Motherboard (system board), 402
Motion
  fundamental laws, 20
  Newton's laws, 20
Motion blur, 292-293
  impact, 293
  patient motion, impact, 293
  reduction
    exposure time, impact, 246
    procedures, 293t
  result, 292
Mouse, usage, 400, 437
Moving charged particle, usage. *See* Magnetic fields, 83f
Moving grid, 238
  device, 238
  disadvantage, 238
  installation, 238f
MPR. *See* Multiplanar reformation, 377
MQSA. *See* Mammography Quality Standards Act, 319
mR. *See* Milliroentgens, 152
MRI. *See* Magnetic resonance imaging, 266
mRNA. *See* Messenger RNA, 505
MTF. *See* Modulation transfer function, 379
Muller, H.J., 564, 564f
  studies, basis, 565

Multidetector array, detectors (number), 374f
Multifield image intensification, 352
Multi-hit chromosome aberrations, 546
  postirradiation, 546f
Multiplanar reformation (MPR), 377. *See also* Three-dimensional MPR, 377
Multiplication
  rounding, usage, 20
  rule, 28
Multislice detector array, 387-388
Multislice spiral computed tomography
  brushes, usage, 375f
  challenge questions, 392
  collimation, 374
  contrast resolution, 391
  couch incrementation, 391
  data acquisition rate, 388-389
  detector array, 373-374
  excellence, 377
  features, 390t
  focal-spot size, importance, 373
  high-speed rotors, usage, 373
  high-voltage generator, usage, 374
  horizontal/vertical planes, isoexposure profiles, 616f
  image data, sampling, 385f
  imaging principles, 384-387
  imaging system
    gantry, components, 375f
    prepatient collimator/predetector collimator, usage, 374f
  imaging techniques, 387-389
  interpolation algorithms, 384-385
  object size, representation, 381
  operator console, 373f
  patient positioning, 374-375
  photodiodes, convergence, 374
  pitch, 385-387
  slice thickness, 391
  slip rings, usage, 375f
  spatial resolution, 391
  SSD, 387f
  support couch, usage, 374-375
  x-ray tube
    size, 373
    usage, 373
Multislice value, increase, 603
Multislice width, increase, 388
Multitarget, single-hit model, 528-529
  biologic system application, 526
Muscle, 510
  photoelectric absorption, 446f
  x-ray interaction, likelihood, 171

N

NaI. *See* Sodium iodide, 374
National Academy of Science (NAS) determination. *See* Radiation-induced malignant disease, 554
National Committee on Radiation Protection (NCRP), tissue/organ identifications, 575

National Council on Radiation Protection, 565
National Council on Radiation Protection and Measurements (NCRP)
  dose limits, recommendation, 571
  estimate. *See* Ionizing radiation, 5
National Electrical Manufacturers Association (NEMA), 474
  focal spot size standards/variances, 129
  standard, 479
National Institute of Standards and Technology (NIST) calibration method, 480
National Institutes of Health (NIH), 457
Natural environmental radiation, 5
  components, 6
  impact. *See* Humans, 6
  source, 6
  result, 6
Natural magnet, example, 85
NCRP. *See* National Committee on Radiation Protection 575; National Council on Radiation Protection and Measurements, 571
Near-range evaluation, example, 480f
Negative electrification, region (production), 184
NEMA. *See* National Electrical Manufacturers Association, 129
Nervous tissue, 510
Neutrons, 40
  mass, 41
  number. *See* Isotopes, 41
Newton, Isaac, 20
  First Law, 20
    example, 21f
  laws. *See* Motion, 20
  Second Law, 21
    example, 21f
  Third Law, 21
    definition, 21
    example, 21f
Newton, SI unit, 21
NIH. *See* National Institutes of Health, 457
NIST. *See* National Institute of Standards and Technology, 480
NMR parameters proton density, 459
Noise. *See* Audio noise, 273; Background electronic noise 442; Image noise 170
  definition, 273-274
  radiographic characteristic, 273
  reduction, 604
  spatial resolution (evaluation), CT test object (usage), 390f
Nominal focal spot size, comparison, 130t
Nomogram
  type, 600f
  usage, 599
Nonimpact printers, 405

Nonlinear dose-response
    relationships, 517
    shapes, variation, 517f
Nonlinear nonthreshold dose-response
    relationship, 517
Nonscreen film. See Direct-exposure
    film, 183
N-type semiconductors, 110
Nuclear arrangements, characteristics,
    47t
Nuclear energy, 4
Nucleic acids, 505-506
    macromolecules, size/complexity,
        505
Nucleolus, 506
Nucleons, 41
    arrangement, 47
Nucleotide, 505
Nucleus, 506
    components, 41
        representation, 41f
    gamma rays, production, 63f
    projectile electron, proximity, 142
    x-rays, production, 63f
Nuclides, 48. See also Radionuclides,
    48
Number
    exponential form
        expression, 30
        handling, rules, 31t
    representation, decimal system
        (usage), 30t
    systems, 29
Numeric prefixes, 33

O
Objective lens, light acceptance, 355
Object organ, CT examination, 379f
Object plane
    anatomical structure distance,
        blurring (increase), 267
    image plane, distortion
        (occurrence), 287
    object imaging, 267f
    relationship. See Fulcrum, 267f
Objects
    artifacts, 490-497
    distortion, 286
    electrification, 73
    elongation, 287
    foreshortening, 287f
    image, test, 268f
    inclination, lateral positioning, 287f
    irregularity, impact. See Distortion,
        287f
    lateral positioning, 286
    magnification, inequality, 286f
    positioning, spatial distortion
        (occurrence), 288f
    resolution, determination, 450
    shape, 290-292
    thickness, 286-287
        impact. See Distortion, 286f
Object size
    determination, 285
    representation, 381
    variation, 38f

Object-to-image distance (OID), 289f
Occupancy exposure, dose limits
    (historical review), 617t
Occupancy factor, time, 586
Occupancy levels, 587t
Occupational effective dose,
    assumption, 576
Occupational exposure, calculation,
    571
Occupational radiation
    dose management, challenge
        questions, 629
    monitor, protection (absence), 620
Occupational/radiation effective dose,
    578b
Occupational radiation exposure, 614
    effective dose, 577f
    reduction, 620
    unit. See Radiation equivalent man,
        34
Occupational radiation monitoring,
    620
    report, 623
        illustration, 623f
OD. See Optical density, 31
OER. See Oxygen enhancement ratio,
    503
Oersted, Hans, 89
    experiment, 89f
        application, 91
Off-center grid, 239-240
    off-focus grid, combination, 240
Off-focus grid, 239
Off focus radiation, 131
    problem, 131
Off-focus radiation
    control, 232
    impact. See Image, 231
Off-level grid, 239
    central axis, nonperpendicularity,
        239f
Offset images, 471
Offset voltage, 471
Ohm's law
    definition, 79
    equation, 79
OID. See Object-to-image distance,
    289f
1% voltage ripple, 115
100% voltage ripple, 115
One-on-one exposure, 357
Oocytes, 541
Oogonia, 540
Open collimator, 249f
Open filament, production, 133-134
Operating console, 103
    circuit diagram, 105f
    usage, 103. See also Overhead
        radiographic imaging system
Operator shield, 582
Optical coupling, providing, 592
Optical density (OD), 31, 252-256
    blackening, 252
    calculation, 277, 278
    constancy, maintenance, 248
    contrast. See Milliampere seconds, 32
    control, 294

Optical density (OD) (Continued)
    decrease, 255f. See also Parallel
        grid, 236f
    determination, 255f
    distance, impact, 248
    equation, 277
    establishment, 262
    mAs control, 246
    maximum, 235
    measurement/recording,
        densitometer (usage), 334
    milliampere seconds, relationship, 32f
    overexposure, impact, 253
    production, 147
    radiation exposure, relationship, 275
    range, 278
        extension, 421
    relationship. See Mass density, 172
    technique factors, impact, 256t
    underexposure, impact, 253
    x-ray responsibility, 224
Optical discs (laser discs), 404
Optically stimulated luminescence
    (OSL), 415, 594, 620, 622
    dosimeters, 622
    dosimetry, 594
        multistep process, 595f
    usage, 588
Optical step wedge (sensitometer),
    276f
    usage, 276
Orange light, wavelength (usage), 17
Orbital electrons, projectile electron
    (avoidance), 142
Ordered pairs, form, 31
Organic free radical formation, 525
Organic molecules, 503
Organogenesis. See Major
    organogenesis, 607
Organs, 503
    dose limits, 618
    formation, 509
    radiosensitivity, 510t
    systems, 509
Origin, axes (meeting), 31
Orthochromatic film, 187
Orthovoltage x-rays, 539
Oscillating grid, 238
OSL. See Optically stimulated
    luminescence, 415
Outcome analysis, 305
Outer-shell electron, vacancy (filling),
    141f
Output, 405
    devices. See Computers, 405
    hardware, components, 405
    intensity, determination, 600
    phosphor, 350
    x-ray intensity (estimation),
        nomogram (usage), 599f
Ovaries, 541
    irradiation, 541
    radiation response, 541t
Overcoat, 181
Overhead radiographic imaging
    system, operating consol
    (usage), 104f

Over-table tube, usage, 438f
Oxford Survey, 563
  data, 563
Oxidation, 196. *See also* Aerial
    oxidation, 197
  opposite. *See* Reduction, 196
Oxygen effect, 514-515, 526
Oxygen enhancement ratio (OER),
    514, 531-532
  equation, 514, 532
  LET dependence, 515
  level. *See* Linear energy transfer,
    515f

P
PACS. *See* Picture Archiving and
    Communication Systems 372
Pair production, 69, 168-169
  occurrence, 169f
  process, 168
Pako, x-ray film processor
    introduction, 194
Panchromatic film, 187
Pan movement, 473
Panoramic tomogram, usage, 270f
Panoramic tomography, 267
  x-ray source-to-image receptor
    motion, usage, 269f
Parallel circuit, 80
  rules, 80
    representation, 81f
Parallel grid, 235-236
  construction, parallel grid strips
    (usage), 236f
  disadvantage, 234f
  OD, decrease, 236f
  usage. *See* Tomography, 268
Paramagnetic materials, 85
Parenchymal tissue, 510
Par speed, 282
Par-speed screen-film combination,
    215
Partial grid cutoff, 235
Particles. *See* Fundamental particles,
    40-41
  accelerators. *See* High-energy
    particle accelerators, 40
  model, 68-69
Particulate radiation, 52
  types, 52
  usage, 52-53
Pascal (computer language), 410
Passbox, cleaning, 334
Pathology. *See* Constructive
    pathology, 252; Destructive
    pathology 252
  appearance, radiolucency/
    radiopacity (increase), 252
  classification, 253b
  type, 252
Patient
  composition, 252
  couch. *See* Interventional radiology,
    365
    computer-controlled stepping
      capability, 365
  effective dose, 575

Patient *(Continued)*
  elective booking, instituting, 608
  ESE, 583f
  examination, principles
    (consideration), 293
  factors, 251-252
    inclusion, 251
  holding, 625
  information, 608
  pathology, 252
  positioning, 293, 606
    heel effect, advantage
      (usage), 290t
    importance, 260
  posting, 609
  pregnancy
    impact, 607
    radiobiologic considerations, 607
    responsibility, 609
  preparation, 298
  questionnaire, 608
  thickness, 226-228, 251-252,
    290-292
    guessing, avoidance, 251
    impact. *See* Scatter radiation, 226
  x-ray interaction, 224f
Patient dose
  calculation, 352
    prepatient collimation, usage, 374
  collimation, impact, 224, 231
  considerations, 459-463
  descriptions, 598
  distribution. *See* Step-and-shoot
    multislice spiral computed
    tomography, 603f
  estimation, 598
  necessity, absence (reduction), 605
  reduction, 326f, 327
    x-ray detector array, impact, 374
  trends, 610
  usage. *See* Special examinations, 601
Patient examination table, 103f
Patient radiation
  challenge questions, 611
  dose
    increase, high-ratio grid (usage),
      233
    reduction, 604f
PBL. *See* Positive-beam-limiting, 232
PE. *See* Potential energy, 4
Pelvic examination
  entrance skin dose, usage, 241t
  performing, 211
Pelvis
  phantom, radiographs, 257f
  radiographs, 258f
Pen-based systems, usage, 401
Penetrability. *See* X-rays, 155
  description, 155
  reference, 155
Penetrometer. *See* Aluminum step
    wedge, 292f
Peptide bond, 503
  amino acid connection, 503
Perceptual linearization, principle, 479
Performance assessment standards,
    479-480

Periodic blood examination, 542
Permanent magnet
  design, developments, 86f
  example, 85
Personal computer, advantages, 399f
PET. *See* Positron emission
    tomography, 551
pH
  constancy. *See* Fixer, 199
  impact, 197
Phantom cassette, usage, 336
Phantom images, 336-339
  control chart, 338f
  scoring, 337
Phantom knee, thickness
    measurement, 261
Phenidone, 196
  combination. *See* Hydroquinone,
    196
Phosphor, 208-209, 210. *See also*
    Input phosphor, 350; Output 350
  afterglow, 209b
  availability, 218
  composition, 211b
  constancy. *See* Image-intensifier
    tube, 312
  crystals
    concentration, 211b
    size, 211b
  high atomic number, 209b
  impact. *See* X-ray beam, 208
  thickness, 211b
  usage. *See* Radiographic intensifying
    screens, 208
Phosphorescence, 210
Photocathode, 350, 592
  electrons, emission, 350, 592
Photodiode, 427
Photodisintegration, 169
  interactions, 170f
  occurrence, absence, 169
Photoelectric absorption, 321
Photoelectric effect, 165-168
  equation, 166
  features, 168t
  occurrence, 166f
  probability
    graph, usage, 171f
    inverse proportion, 166, 167
  process, 165
  total x-ray absorption, 166
Photoelectric interaction, relative
    probability, 168f
Photoelectrons
  escape, 166
  kinetic energy, determination, 166
Photoemission, 350, 592
Photofluorospot imagers, ESE, 312t
Photofluorospot images
  dependence, 311
  usage, 311
Photographic effect, 183
Photography, origins, 181
Photometer, 310
Photometric evaluation, examples,
    480f
Photometric quantities, 467-468, 468t

Photometric units, 467-468, 468t
  lumen, basis, 467
Photomultiplier tubes (PMTs), 415
  gain, formula, 593
  plancet assembly, 593
Photons, 54, 57-60. *See also* X-ray
      photons, 57
  amplitude, 57-58
  energy, frequency (proportion), 62
  energy disturbances, 57
  interaction, 63. *See also* Silver
      halide crystals, 184
  naming, 57
  radiation, intensity (loss), 53
  velocity, 57-58
Photopic vision, 348
Photospot cameras, 357-358
  optics requirement, 355
Photospot differences. *See* Cassette
      spot, 358t
Photostimulable luminescence (PSL),
      413-414
  process, 413
  signal beam, production, 415
  signal production, final stage, 416
Photostimulable phosphor (PSP), 413
  cross section, 415f
  processing, stimulation portion, 416
  screen, 414
  stimulation
    laser light, usage, 418
    monochromatic laser light, usage,
        419f
  x-ray interaction, 414f
Photothermic method. *See* Dry
      processing, 204f
Photothermography (PTG), 204
  advantages, 206
  dwell time, reduction, 205f
  low-power modulated laser beam,
      usage, 206
Physicians, death (groups), 553t
Picture Archiving and Communication
      Systems (PACS), 473-474
  combination. *See* Digital images,
      476f
  components, 473-474
  implementation, 473
  justification, 475
  network, 372, 474-475
    impact, 475f
  storage system, 475-477
  usage. *See* Image, 473
  workstations, 474. *See also* Remote
      PACS workstations, 474
Picture element (pixel), 407
  dynamic range, 443
  failure, 487
  fill factor, 431f
  shift, 473
  size. *See* Computed tomography
      image, 376
  values, variation, 382
Pi lines, 300
  artifacts, 301f
Pinhole camera, 308f
  usage, difficulty, 308

Pitch. *See* Multislice spiral computed
      tomography, 385-387
  change. *See* Tissue, 386t
  determination, 386. *See also* X-ray
      beam, 386
  patient couch movement/x-ray beam
      width, division, 387f
Pixel. *See* Picture element, 407
Planck's constant (h), 30, 68
  relationship. *See* X-ray energy, 30
Planck's equation. *See* Equivalent
      Planck's equation, 68
Planck's quantum equation, 68
Planck's quantum theory, 68
Planetary rollers. *See* Automatic
      processor, 201
Plant starches, 504
Plastic fiber, usage, 234
Platelet depletion. *See*
      Thrombocytopenia, 543
Pleural spaces, enhanced rendering,
      220f
Plotters, usage, 405
Plumbicon, 353-354
Pluripotential stem cell, 542
PMTs. *See* Photomultiplier tubes, 415
P-n junction semiconductor, 111f
Point lesions, 521
  cellular radiation damage,
      consideration, 521
  irradiation result, 521f
Point mutations, 523
  result, 524f
Poisson distribution, 527
Poles, 86. *See also* Magnets, 86
Polyenergetic x-rays, 172
Polysaccharides, 504
Population sample, requirement, 550t
Portable fluoroscopy, scatter
      radiation, 615f
Positioning errors. *See* Artifacts, 299
Positive-beam limitation, 581
Positive-beam-limiting (PBL)
      collimators, 307
Positive-beam-limiting (PBL) devices,
      232
Positive exponent, value
      (determination), 30
Positron, 168
Positron emission tomography (PET),
      551
Postanterior chest images, heel effect
      (demonstration), 131f
Posterior-anterior chest radiography,
      effective dose, 577f
Posteroanterior (PA) chest digital
      radiographs, characteristic, 491
Posteroanterior (PA) chest
      radiography, effective dose, 577b
Postinjection image, 445f
Postmenopausal breasts,
      characteristics, 321
Postprocessing. *See* Contrast
      resolution, 455-457
  tool, 457f
  usage. *See* Gray shades, 456
Potassium, natural metabolites, 6

Potassium alum (hardener), 199
Potassium bromide, 197
Potassium iodide, 197
Potential energy (PE), 4, 23
  decrease, 24
  determination, 24
  equation, 24
  result, 24f
  stored energy, 24
Potter, Hollis E., 10, 238
Potter-Bucky diaphragm, 238
Power, 23. *See also* Single-phase
      power, 113; Three-phase power
      113-114
  ampere/volt, product, 117
  equation, 23, 116
  exertion, determination, 23
  rating, 116-117
    determination, 117
    equation, 117
  requirement, 23
  SI unit, 23
  work, rate, 23
  work/time, quotient, 23
Power of ten, 406t
Power of two, 406t
Preamplifier, electron pulse
      (conduction), 593
Precursor cells, 509
Predetector collimator, 374
  usage. *See* Sensitivity profile, 374;
      Slice thickness, 374
Preemployment physicals, 605
Preferred detent position, 120
Prefixes. *See* Engineering prefixes, 34t;
      Scientific prefixes, 34t
Pregnancy
  counseling, 627
  first trimester, radiosensitivity, 562
  impact. *See* Patient, 607
  radiation
    response, 563
    risk, acknowledgment form, 628f
    warnings, posters, 610f
  relationship. *See* Radiation, 561-
      565
  second/third trimesters, responses,
      608
Preinjection mask, 445f
  subtraction, 445f
Preneoplastic incidence, 558
Prepatient collimation, usage. *See*
      Patient dose, 374
Prepatient collimator, 374
Preprocessing actions, 471
Preprocessing pressure artifacts, 302f
Prereading kVp meter, 106
Presentation values (p-values), 482
Preservative, 197. *See also* Fixer, 199
Primary beam x-rays, incidence. *See*
      Interspace material, 233
Primary connections, 104
Primary protective barrier, 583
  lead/concrete equivalents, 585t
Primary radiation, 585
Primary side. *See* High-voltage
      transformer, 108

Primordial follicles, 541
Principal quantum number, 43
Printers, 405
 toner, usage, 405
Processing. *See* Automatic processing,
  194-195; Daylight processing,
  203-204; Dry processing, 204-
  206; Extended processing, 203;
  Rapid processing 203
 chemistry, 195-199
 importance, 194
 methods, alternates, 203-206
 sequence, 195
 sludge, impact, 313
 term, application, 185
 wetting, involvement, 195
Processing artifacts, 300-301
 elimination, 300
 list, 300t
Processor. *See* Automatic processor,
  314f
 cleaning, 313-314
 maintenance, 314
 monitoring, 314-315
 QC, 334
  kit, 335f
  record, example, 336f
 quality control, 313-315
Prodromal period, 535, 536
 radiation sickness, response, 536
Programmable read-only memory
  (PROM), 402
Programming languages, list, 409t
Projectile electrons, 140
 acceleration, 146
 kinetic energy
  conversion, 140, 140f
  loss, 142
Projection. *See* Intensity profile, 368-369
PROM. *See* Programmable read-only
  memory, 402
Prompt emission, 415
Proper fraction, 26
 examples, 26
Prophase, 508, 508
Proportion, 29
 equation, cross-multiplication/
  solution, 28
Proportional region. *See* Gas-filled
  detectors, 590
Protective apparel, 624
 radiographing, 310
 usage, 12
Protective aprons, radiographs, 310f
Protective barriers
 design, 584
 usage, 12
 window, necessity, 103
Protective coating, 208. *See also*
  Radiographic intensifying screens,
  208
Protective curtain, 583
Protective housing. *See* X-ray tube,
  121-122
 guard purpose, 121
 usage. *See* Leakage radiation
  intensity, 122f

Protective lead
 aprons, physical characteristics,
  624t
 requirement, 575
Protective viewing window, 13f
Protective x-ray tube housing, 581
Proteins, 503-504
 amino acids, peptide bonds
  (linkage), 504f
 manufacture, genetic code
  translation, 522
 organic molecules, 503
 synthesis, 503
  cellular function,
   necessity, 507
  process, complexity, 507f
Protons, 40
 electric charges, association, 73
 mass, 41
Protraction, 514. *See also* Dose, 514;
  Radiation doses, 514
PSL. *See* Photostimulable
  luminescence, 413-414
PSP. *See* Photostimulable phosphor,
  413
PTG. *See* Photothermography, 204
P-type semiconductors, 110
Pulse height analysis, usage, 593
Pulse mode, usage, 587
Pulse-progressive fluoroscopy, 439f
Pupin, Michael, 8
P-values. *See* Presentation
  values, 482
Pyrimidines, 505

Q
Quality assurance (QA), 305, 332
 image interpretation,
  involvement, 305
 team effort, requirement, 306
 usage, 305
Quality control (QC), 298,
  305-306, 487
 challenge questions, 315
 mammographer, responsibility,
  333
 measurements, preparation, 307f
 program
  elements. *See* Radiographic
   systems, 306t
  steps, 306
 team effort, requirement, 306
 usage, 305
Quantization, 421
Quantum, 57
 theory, 68-69
Quantum chromodynamics (QCD),
  39
Quantum mottle, 212, 274
 control, 274
 demonstration. *See* Hip radiograph,
  273f
 effect, 216
 reduction, 274
Quarks, binding, 41f
Quenching agent, addition, 591
QuickBASIC, 410

R
Rad. *See* Radiation absorbed dose, 34
Radiation, 5. *See also* Electromagnetic
  radiation, 5 *See also* Ionizing
  radiation, 5; Man-made radiation,
  5; Natural environmental
  radiation 5
 administration, 552
 damage. *See* Sublethal radiation
  damage, 515
 definition, 132
 dose-response relationships, 516
  applications, 516
 early effect, 502b, 502
  challenge questions, 547-548
  cytogenetic effects, 544-547
  hematologic effects, 542-544
 educational considerations, 620
 effect, 525
 emission. *See* Infrared radiation, 25
 employee training, 625
 explanation, 5
 fog, 198
  impact. *See* Artifacts, 302
 genetics, conclusions, 565b
 health, relationship, 571
 hormesis, 516
  dose-response relationship,
   518f
  principle, support, 554
  theory, 554
 injury, reports, 11
 in-service training, 627
 interaction, 184f
 internal source, 53
 inverse relation, 67
 late effect, 502, 502b
  challenge questions, 567
  risk estimates, 553-555
 management principles, 625
 matter, random interaction, 527
 measurement, 587
  device characteristics/uses, 588t
  equipment, 578
  units, usage, 33
 monitors, representation, 621f
 output, proportionality, 29
 pregnancy, relationship, 561-565
 public exposure, 619
 quality. *See* Radiographic
  intensifying screens, 211-212
  change, absence, 250
  distance, impact (absence), 248
  expression, 513
 radioactive material, emission, 34f
 relationship, 24
 sickness, response, 536
 source, distance (determination), 67
 therapy, 557
  clinical tolerance, 539
 types, 54f, 584
  illustration, 585f
  weighting factors, 619t
 worker, radiation dose excess, 616
Radiation absorbed dose
  (rad, Gy_t), 34
 usage, 34

Radiation-damaged human
    chromosomes, 523f
Radiation detection, 587
    accomplishment, 371
    device characteristics/uses, 588t
    equipment, 578
    instrument, design, 578f
Radiation doses, 550t
    estimation, 538
    fractionation, 514
    LET/RBE levels, 514t
    limits, 616
    protraction, 514
Radiation Effects Research
    Foundation (RERF), 555
Radiation equivalent dose, scales, 35f
Radiation equivalent man (rem, Sv),
    occupational radiation exposure
    unit, 34
    usage, 34
Radiation exposure, 152
    absence, 608
    doubling, 277
    mean survival time, 538f
    measurements, 587
    necessity, absence (avoidance), 618
    repair/recovery, 501
    reproducibility, 309
Radiation exposure device (RED), 577
Radiation-induced breast cancer, risk,
    320
Radiation-induced cancer,
    linear-nonthreshold dose-response
    relationship, 517
Radiation-induced cataracts,
    occurrence, 551
Radiation-induced chromosome
    damage, 544
    analysis, 508
Radiation-induced congenital
    abnormalities, 563
Radiation-induced leukemia, 556
    linear nonthreshold dose-response
    relationship, 556
    relative risk, determination, 554
Radiation-induced life span
    shortening, 552
Radiation-induced malignancy,
    555-559
Radiation-induced malignant disease,
    absolute risk (NAS/BEIR
    determination), 554
Radiation-induced preneoplastic
    thyroid nodularity, 558f
Radiation-induced reciprocal
    translocations, 546f
    result, 546
Radiation-induced skin cancer, 558
Radiation protection, 11
    cardinal principles, 572b
    design, challenge questions, 595
    features, 581
    guidance, 578
    guides, 550
    practices, 11
    principles, 576f
    rules, 12b

Radiation weighting factor (W_R),
    value, 513
Radioactive combination, life threat
    (rarity), 578
Radioactive decay, 48
    alpha emission, 49
    definition, 51
    impact, 51
    law, 50
    result, 49b
Radioactive disintegration, 48
Radioactive half-life, 50
Radioactive isotopes (radioisotopes), 49
    decay, calculation, 49
Radioactivity, 48-52
    definition, 49
    estimation, 51f
        linear graph, usage, 50f
        semilog graph, usefulness, 50f
Radiobiologic studies, design, 516
Radiobiology, 502
    challenge questions, 518-519
Radiodermatitis, 550
Radiofrequency (RF), 62-63, 405
    emissions, 62
    frequency identification, 63
Radiographic cones/cylinders, usage.
    See X-ray beam, 230f
Radiographic contrast, 279, 290-292
    agents, 44
    control, kVp (impact), 256, 294
    determination, 290
    equation, 290
    exposure technique factors, impact,
        258t
    impact, 279
    relationships, 278
Radiographic examinations
    entrance exposures, 610t
    fetal doses, 610t
Radiographic exposure times, 246
Radiographic film
    base, 181-182
        characteristics, 182
        density, 281
    blue sensitivity, 187f
    boxes, storage, 191
    challenge questions, 191
    characteristic curve, 276f
    construction, 181-183
    cross-section, 181f
    emulsion, 182-183
    fog
        density, 281
        level, 190
    green sensitivity, 187f
    handling/storage, 189-191
    heat/humidity, impact, 190
    ionizing radiation, impact, 190
    light, impact, 190
    manufacture, 183
    OD, light transmission
        (relationship), 277t
    radiation, impact, 190
    safelights, usage, 188
    sensitivity, 190
    shelf life, 190-191

Radiographic film (Continued)
    sizes, standards, 186t
    speed/contrast/resolution,
        differences, 182
    storage time, 191
    tabular grains, usage, 182
    types, 185-189
Radiographic/fluoroscopic (R&F)
    imaging system, example, 13f
Radiographic grids, usage, 602
Radiographic image
    contrast, 456f
        reduction, 278
    photographic effect/Compton
        scattering, combination, 225f
Radiographic image-quality factors,
    260t
Radiographic intensifying
    screens, 310
    active layer, phosphor (usage), 208
    base, 209
        properties, 209b
    carbon fiber, usage, 215
    care, 219-221
    cassettes, 214-215
        usage, 214-215
    CE, 218-219
    challenge questions, 222
    characteristics, 210-214, 211t
    cleaning, 219, 220
    composition/emulsion, 216
    construction, 208-209
    cross-sectional view, 208f
    film, combinations, 214-219
    image noise, 210, 212
    image processing, 212
    lag (afterglow), 210
    luminescence, 210
    periodic cleaning, 219
    phosphor, 208-209
        high-z elements, atomic number/
            K-shell electron binding
            energy, 217t
        properties, 209b
    properties, radiologic technologist
        (noncontrol), 211b
    protective coating, 208
    radiation quality, 211-212
    radiologic technologist control,
        absence, 211
    rare Earth materials, usage, 217
    reflective layer, 209, 211b
        absence, 209f
    safelights, usage, 218-219
    spatial resolution, 210, 212-214
    speed, 210-212
    temperature, 212
    usage, 188, 213, 257. See also
        Image-forming x-rays, 208
Radiographic noise
    components, 274
    definition, 273
Radiographic output intensity, 153
Radiographic procedures, equipment
    (involvement), 8
Radiographic processor,
    QC program, 313t

Radiographic quality
  anatomical structure, fidelity, 273
  characteristics, interrelationships, 274f
  definition, 273
  factors, organization chart, 275f
  improvement, tools (usage), 293
  rules, 274
  technique factors, selection, 293-295
Radiographic quality control, 306-311
Radiographic rating chart, 134
  application, 134
  illustration, 135f
  series, usage, 134
Radiographic systems, QC program elements, 306t
Radiographic technique, 605
  application, absence, 133
  challenge questions, 271
  chart, 261, 260
    preparation, 261
    usage, 261
  description, 245
  problems, 422f
  specifications, 154
Radiographs. *See* High-quality radiograph, 273
  completion, 203
  copying, 189
  double-emulsion film, usage, 293
  example, 8f, 291f
  image detail visibility, reduction, 259f
  light, transmission (amount), 253f
  making
    factors, 295t
    x-ray types, usage, 170f
  obtaining, 368f
  OD, change, 253
  1-mm focal-spot x-ray tube, usage, 259f
  permanence, 198
  processing, event sequence, 195t
  6:1 parallel grid, 237f
  underdevelopment, result, 197f
Radiography
  high-quality glass, usage, 8
  task inventory, ARRT requirement, 13b
  x-ray examination, 8
Radioisotopes. *See* Radioactive isotopes, 49
Radiological Society of North America (RSNA), 553
Radiologic device, usage, 577
Radiologic dispersal device (RDD), 577
Radiologic science
  challenge questions, 15
  fundamentals, challenge questions, 36
  materials, importance, 167t
  mathematics, 26
  special quantities, 18f
    representation, 19t
    special units, association, 35t
  terminology, 33
  units, representation, 13-14

Radiologic technologist
  effective dose, 575
  occupational radiation exposure, origin, 620
  patient distance, 573
  specialization, 361f
Radiologic technology, safety, 552
Radiologic terrorism, 576
Radiologic units, 33
Radiologist, 332
  leukemia, appearance, 557
  mammography QC responsibility, 332
  pregnancy, 625
  responsibility. *See* Mammography
Radiology
  development, 8
    dates, 10b
  safety, 11
Radiology, emergence, 10
Radiology Information System (RIS), 474
  workstations, 474-475
Radiolucency
  degree, 252
  increase. *See* Pathology, 252
  relative degrees, 252t
Radiolucent, term, 66
Radiolucent patient, 298
Radionuclides, 48
  low-energy beta particles, emission, 592
Radiopacity
  increase. *See* Pathology, 252
  term, usage, 252
Radiopaque, term, 66
Radioprotectors, 516
Radio reception, basis, 92f
Radioresistant cells, indication, 529
Radiosensitive cells, indication, 529
Radiosensitivity
  biologic factors, 514-516
  physical factors, 513-514
  variation, 515f
Radiosensitizers, 516
Radium salts, usage, 558
Radon, 6
  alpha particles, emission, 6
  uranium decay product, 559
RAID. *See* Redundant array of inexpensive discs, 404
Random access memory (RAM), 402
  built-in chips, 405
  chips, manufacture, 402
  contents, 402
  types, 402
Rapid processing, 203
Rapid processors, usefulness, 203
Rare Earth, description, 216
Rare Earth elements, 208
Rare Earth phosphors, CE, 218
Rare Earth radiographic intensifying screens
  manufacture, 216
  speed advantage, 216

Rare Earth screens, 186, 216-219
  identification, 216
  usage, 209
  x-ray absorption probability, calcium tungstate screen (comparison), 217f
Raster pattern, 356
Rate mode, usage, 587
Ratio
  determination, 27, 27
  usage, 27
RBE. *See* Relative biologic effectiveness, 503
RDD. *See* Radiologic dispersal device, 577
Reaction, equal/opposite, 21
Read-only memory (ROM), 402
  basic input/output system (BIOS), 402
  built-in chips, 405
Read (sequence), 417f
Reciprocating grid, 238
Reciprocity law, 187
  equation, 187
  explanation, 278-283
  failure, 187, 309. *See also* Screen-film, 278
    approximation, 188t
  statement, 278
Recombination region. *See* Gas-filled detectors, 589
Recorded detail, 258
  term, imprecision, 273
Recording. *See* Macros 410
Recovery, 515, 530. *See also* Human cell, 515
  equation, 515
Rectification, 110. *See also* Voltage, 110
Rectifiers
  assembly, 111
  high-voltage generator component, 109
  type, 111f
  usage, 110
RED. *See* Radiation exposure device, 577
Red filter, usage, 188
Redox. *See* Reduction/oxidation, 196
Reducing agent, 196
Reduction. *See* Metallic silver, 196
  oxidation, opposite, 196
Reduction/oxidation (redox) reactions, 196
Redundant array of inexpensive discs (RAID), 404
Reflection, 65, 481-482. *See also* Diffuse reflection, 481f; Specular reflection, 481
Reflective layer. *See* Radiographic intensifying screens, 209
Region of interest (ROI)
  identification, 473
  manipulation, 437
  viewing, 372
Registers (high-speed circuitry), 402

Relative biologic effectiveness (RBE), 513-514, 531-532. *See also* Cataracts, 551
  determination, 514, 530
  equation, 513, 531
  levels. *See* Diagnostic x-rays 513; Radiation doses, 514t
Relative radiolucency, 252f
Relative response, 560
Relative risk, 553-554. *See also* Childhood leukemia, 563t
  equation, 553
  model, 561f
Relativity, definition, 69
Rem. *See* Radiation equivalent man, 34
Remnant x-rays, scattering, 228
Remote fluoroscopy, 614
Remotely controlled DF system, 438f
Remote PACS workstations, 474
Removable hard disc system, 404
Repair mechanism. *See* Intracellular recovery, 515
Repeat analysis, 340-342
  equation, 342
  form. *See* Examination repeat analysis form, 341f
Replenishment tanks, checking, 314
Repopulation, 515
Reproducibility, 582
Reregistration, usage, 445
RERF. *See* Radiation Effects Research Foundation, 555
Residual chemicals, washing, 199
Residual metastable electrons, movement, 418f
Resolution, definition, 273
Resolving time, 591
Retina, light (focus), 347-348
RF. *See* Radiofrequency, 62-63
R&F. *See* Radiographic/fluoroscopic
Rhodium
  mammography usage, 148
  target x-ray tube, x-ray emission spectrum, 323f
Ribonucleic acid (RNA), 505
  copies, presence, 522
Ring artifacts, occurrence, 371f
Ripple, reduction, 149
RIS. *See* Radiology Information System, 474
Risk. *See* Absolute risk, 554-555; Excess risk 554; Relative risk, 553-554
  estimates. *See* Radiation, 553-555
  usage, 553
RNA. *See* Ribonucleic acid, 505
Roadmapping. *See* Digital subtraction angiography, 447
  DSA application, 447
  neurovascular image, 447f
Rods
  color blindness, 349
  number, 348
  sensation, 347-348
  sensitivity, 348

Roentgen, Wilhelm, 7
  Nobel Prize, 7
Roentgen (Gy$_a$), radiation exposure/ intensity unit, 34
ROI. *See* Region of interest, 372
Roller marks, 300
Roller transport automatic processor, 194f
Rollins, William, 8
ROM. *See* Read-only memory 402
Rongelap Atoll, radiation fallout (exposure), 558
Rotating anode, 125
  appearances, comparison, 128f
  illustration, 125f
  power, 127
  tube, target
    location, 126f
    power, 128f
  usage, 126
Rotating anode x-ray tube
  components, 120f
  filaments, mounting, 123
RSNA. *See* Radiological Society of North America, 553

S

Saccharides, 504
Safelights
  filters, checking, 342
  fog, 259f
  usage. *See* Radiographic film, 188
Sampling, 421
SAR. *See* Slice acquisition rate, 388-389
Saturation current, 124
  illustration, 125f
Scanned projection radiograph (SPR), 428
  components. *See* Chest, 429f
  example, 428f
  obtaining, 428f
Scanned projection radiography, 428
Scanners, 401
Scapula
  elongation, 260f
  foreshortening, 260f
  projection, 260f
Scattered x-ray
  beam, energy (reduction), 463
  energy, 164
  photoelectric absorption, 165
  relative intensity, 227
Scattering. *See* Coherent scattering, 163; Compton scattering 164; Turbid scattering, 413
  interaction, 163f
Scatter radiation, 274. *See also* Portable fluoroscopy, 615f
  cleanup, 232
    effectiveness, high-grid ratio (usage), 233
  control, 228-234
    challenge questions, 243
  impact. *See* Grid, 234-235; Image contrast, 228-229
  patient thickness, impact, 226

Scatter radiation *(Continued)*
  production, 224-228
  reduction, 227f. *See also* Tissue, 228f
    x-ray beam collimation, impact, 226f
  relative intensity, increase, 228f
  secondary radiation type, 585
Schaetzing, Ralph, 420
Scientific prefixes, 34t
Scintillation, light emission intensity (proportion), 591f
Scintillation detector, 591
  arrays, 373-374
  assembly, 592
    characteristics, 592f
  x-ray detection efficiency, 374
Scintillation phosphors, types, 592
Scotopic vision, 348
Screen
  blur (improvement), spatial resolution (usage), 273
  cassette combination, label clarity, 335
  characteristics. *See* Radiographic intensifying screens, 210-214
  cleanliness, 334-339
  drying, procedure, 337f
  fluoroscopy, red goggles (usage), 349f
Screen-film, 185-188
  combination, 293
  compatibility, 214
  contact, 342
    causes, 221b
    evaluation, wire mesh test tool (usage). *See* Mammographic screen-film contact, 343f
    testing, 221
  contact, checking, 220
    wire mesh radiographs, usage, 221f
  developing time, excess, 212
  double emulsion, 185
  exposure
    difference. *See* Direct film exposure, 215-216
    reciprocity law, failure, 278
    x-rays/light photons, relative numbers (comparison), 215t
  image receptors, 487
  imaging, exposures (usage), 455
  IR, image unacceptability, 422f
  mammography, 328
    display, 458f
    MTF, increase, 454f
    technique, acceptance, 602
  radiographs. *See* Foot phantom, 462f
  response, 461f
  use, advantages, 215b
Screen-film radiography
  activity, sequence, 414f
  exposure factor-related repeat rate, 460
  image noise, sources, 423b
  spatial resolution, determination, 460
  transition, 424f, 423
Screening mammography, 320

Scroll movement, 473
SCRs. *See* Silicon-controlled rectifiers, 114
Secondary barriers, material thicknesses (equivalence), 586t
Secondary coil, winding, 94
Secondary connections, 104
Secondary electrons
  emission, 592
  formation, 184
Secondary memory, requirement, 402-403
Secondary protective barriers, 585
Secondary quantities, 17
Secondary radiation, types, 585
Secondary voltage, determination. *See* Autotransformer, 105
Second-generation computers, 398
Second-generation CT imaging systems, operation, 370f
Second-generation imaging systems, 369
  components, 370
Second Law. *See* Newton, 21
Second-stage collimator shutter, leaves (composition), 232
Section sensitivity profile (SSP), 387. *See also* Multislice spiral computed tomography, 387f
  usage. *See* Computed tomography 387f
Section uniformity, evaluation, 312
SED$_{50}$. *See* Skin erythema dose 540
Seldinger, Sven Ivar, 361
Selectable added filtration, examples, 249f
Semiconduction, demonstration, 78
Semiconductor. *See* N-type semiconductors, 110; P-type semiconductors, 110
  definition, 78
  electricity, conduction, 110
Semilogarithmic graph
  explanation, 167-168
  usage, 51f
  usefulness, 50f
Semilogarithmic paper, usage, 33f, 527f
Semilogarithmic scale, usage. *See* Graph, 32
Senograph (General Electric), 322f
Sensitivity, accuracy (nonequivalence), 589
Sensitivity center, 182
  electrons, migration, 184f
Sensitivity measurement, 281
Sensitivity profile, 374
  determination, predetector collimator (usage), 374
Sensitometer. *See* Optical step wedge, 276
Sensitometric strip, usage, 314
Sensors, usage, 401
Sequential radiation exposure, reproducibility, 310
Sequestering
  agents, introduction, 198
  boric acids/salts, usage, 199

Serial radiography, aluminum step wedge (usage). *See* Abdomen, 160f; Lower extremities, 160f
Series circuit, 80
  rules, 80
    representation, 81f
Shaded surface display (SSD), 377
  computer-aided technique, 377
Shaded surface image, obtaining, 378f
Shaded volume display (SVD), 377
Shadowgraph, 284f
Shadow shield, 606
  example, 606, 607f
  suspension, 607f
Shell-type transformer, 95
Shielding, 571. *See also* Area shielding, 606
  formula, 574
  usage, 574
Shockley, William, 78, 397
Short gray scale, 282
  contrast, 292
Short wavelength waves, production, 65f
Shoulder, characteristic curve component, 276
  gradient, 281
    importance. *See* Mammography, 281
  OD, result, 280f
SID. *See* Source-to-image distance, 18
Sigmoid-type (S-type) dose-response relationship, 517
Sigmoid-type (S-type) radiation dose-response relationship, 517
Signal amplitude (increase), gas-filled detector (impact), 589f
Signal plate, 354
Signal-to-noise ratio (SNR), 442, 457
  high level, 443f
  impact, 459
  importance, 457
  increase, 374, 440
  insufficiency, 442
Significant figures, 27
  example, 27
Silicon-controlled rectifiers (SCRs), 114
Silver bromide, 182
Silver halide, fixing, 195
Silver halide crystals, 182, 183-184
  cubic grains, 186f
  formation, 182
  lattice, 183f
  model, 184f
  negative electrostatic charge. *See* Unexposed silver halide crystal, 197
  photon interaction, 184
  rigidity, 183
  size, irregularity, 186f
  size/distribution, 185
  tablet-like grains, 186f
Silver iodide, 182
Silver ion, reduction, 196
  bromide ion, liberation, 197

Silver sulfide stain, impact. *See* Archival quality, 199
SIMMs. *See* Single-line memory modules, 402
Sine waves, 57
  amplitude, variation, 58, 58f
  associations, 58f
  motion, 59f
  similarity, 58f
  velocity/frequency/wavelength, relationship, 59f
  wavelength
    relationship, 59f
    variation, 59f
Single cells, planting, 526f
Single digital imaging system, contrast-detail curve, 460f
Single-emulsion film, processing, 188
Single-emulsion laser film, cross-section, 189f
Single-emulsion mammography film, cross-section, 189f
Single-hit aberrations, dose-response relationships, 547f
Single-hit chromosome aberrations, 545-546
  postirradiation, representation, 546f
Single-hit effects, radiation production, 546
Single-line memory modules (SIMMs), 402
Single phase, 135
Single-phase generators 100% voltage ripple, 117
Single-phase kVp, usage, 261
Single-phase power, 113
  100% voltage ripple, 115
Single-target, single hit model, 526-528
  biologic target application, 526
  equation, 528
Sinusoidal change. *See* Electric fields, 57; Magnetic fields, 57
16-detector array, 387f
Skin
  anatomic structures, sectional view, 539f
  cancer, 558-559
    production, determination, 554
  chronic irradiation, 550
  dose, determination, 600
  exposure, radiation therapy, 539
  local tissue effects, 550
  responses, high-dose fluoroscopy, 540t
Skin effects, 539-540
  high-dose fluoroscopy, impact, 517
Skin erythema dose (SED$_{50}$), 540
Skull
  imaging, trauma radiographic imaging system (usage), 230f
Skull radiographs, quality (acceptability), 226f
Slice acquisition rate (SAR), 388

Slice thickness. *See* Multislice spiral
    computed tomography, 391
  allowance. *See* Asymmetric
    eight-detector array, 389f
  determination, predetector
    collimator (usage), 374
Slip rings
  electromechanical devices, 375
  impact, 375
  technology, 375
  usage. *See* Multislice spiral
    computed tomography, 375f
Slit camera, 308f
  measurement tool, 308
Slow scan, 418
Sludge deposits, result, 300
SMPTE. *See* Society of Motion Picture
  and Television Engineers, 479
Smudge static, 303f
Snook, H.C., 9
Snook interrupterless transformer, 368
Snook transformer, 9
  impact, 10
SNR. *See* Signal-to-noise ratio, 442
Society of Motion Picture and
  Television Engineers (SMPTE),
  479
  display systems resolution
    standards, 479
  pattern, development, 479f
SOD. *See* Source-to-object distance, 19
Sodium carbonate, 197
Sodium hydroxide, 197
Sodium iodide (NaI), imaging system
  crystal (usage), 374
Sodium sulfite, 197
  hardener, 199
Soft copy. *See* Hard copy-soft copy,
  468-469
  viewing. *See* Digital CRT, 469
Soft tissue
  Compton scattering, 321
  differences, imaging, 172
  differential absorption, 171f
  graphs, vertical displacement, 167
  interaction, 168
  radiography, 319
    contrast resolution, importance,
    433
    example, 319
    x-rays, Compton effect (relative
    probability), 173
Software. *See* Computers, 405-409
  artifacts, 488-490
  invisibility, 400
  manipulations, sequence, 408f
  term, usage, 406
Solenoid, 90
Solid-state diode, 110
  electronic symbol, 111f
Solid-state p-n junction, electricity
  conduction, 110
Solid-state radiation detectors, usage,
  109f
Solution
  definition, 521
  viscosity, reduction, 521

Somatic cells, 507
Source data entry devices, 401
Source-detector assembly, sweep,
  368-369
Source-to-image distance (SID)
  approximation, 599
  determination, 31
  increase, 242, 242f
  indicator, accuracy, 581
  level, 325
  measurement, 19
  76 mm (specification), 237f
  standard, 18, 285
  usage, 152
  variation, 120
Source-to-image receptor distance
  indicator, 581
Source-to-object distance (SOD), 19
Source-to-skin distance (SSD), 582
  approximation, 599
  effect, 583b
  intensity, determination, 599
Source-to-tabletop distance (STD),
  indicator, 240
Space charge, 124
  effect, 106
    phenomenon, 124
Spatial distortion, occurrence, 287
Spatial frequency, 379, 450-452
  determination, 450, 451, 452
  increase, bar pattern
    (usage), 380f
Spatial resolution (SR), 224,
  450-454. *See also* Radiographic
    intensifying screens, 212-214
  description, 450
  determination, focal-spot blur
    (importance), 288
  equation, 381
  example, 451f
  imaging system ability, 450
  improvement, 213, 326f, 327
    compression, impact, 327
    higher-megapixel digital display
    devices, usage, 469
  lines per frame, impact, 357
  measurement, 213
  pixel size, relationship, 379
  radiographic characteristic, 273
  reduction, 214f
    IF, impact, 213
  reference, 212
  relationship, 213
  usage. *See* Screen, 273
Spatial uniformity, 383
Special application film.
  See Direct-exposure film, 185
Special examinations, patient dose
  (usage), 601
Special quantities, 17. *See also*
  Radiologic science, 18f
  representation. *See* Radiologic
    science, 19t
Special units, representation, 18
Speck
  group, counting, 339
  production. *See* Film, 333f

Spectral matching, 186-188
  importance, 216f
  usage, 209b
Spectrum. *See* Characteristic x-rays,
  144-145; Continuous ejection
    spectrum 143
  term, usage, 143
  values. *See* Continuous spectrum,
    144; Discrete spectrum 143
Specular reflection, 481
  illustration, 481f
Speed. *See* Par speed, 282
  ability, 281-283
  characteristic, 274
  definition, 274
  index, 334
  mAs, difference, 282
  velocity equivalence, 19
Spermatid, 541
Spermatocyte, 541
Spermatogonia, 541
  radiosensitivity, 543
Spermatozoa (sperm), 541
Sperry-Rand Corporation, 397
S phase, 522f
Spindles, 508
  fibers, 508
Spine imaging
  CR plates, usage, 496f
  trauma radiographic imaging
    system, usage, 230f
Spinning charged particle, usage. *See*
  Magnetic fields, 84f
Spiral computed tomography. *See*
  Multislice spiral computed
    tomography, 384-387
  x-ray tube, design, 373f
Spiral pitch ratio, equation, 385
Split-dose irradiation, 530
  result, 530f
Spontaneous abortion, 564
  post-irradiation, 608
Spot film, 189. *See also* Cassette-
  loaded spot film, 357
  105 mm, format, 189f
  processing, 189
Spot-film exposures, 311
Spot-film kVp, 350t
SPR. *See* Scanned projection
  radiograph, 428
SPSs. *See* Storage phosphor screens,
  413
Square law, 154. *See also* Direct
  square law, 248, *See also* Inverse
    square law, 66-68
  calculation, 154
SR. *See* Spatial resolution, 224
SRAM. *See* Static RAM, 402
SSD. *See* Shaded surface display, 377;
  Source-to-skin distance, 582
SSP. *See* Section sensitivity profile, 387
Starches. *See* Plant starches, 504
Star pattern, 308f
  measurement, usage, 308
Static. *See* Smudge artifact 303f; Tree
  static, 303f
  artifact, 300

Static RAM (SRAM), 402
Stationary anode, 125
  illustration, 125f
  target, 126
  tube, target (embedding), 126f
STD. *See* Source-to-tabletop distance
    240
Stem cells, 509. *See also* Pluripotential
    stem cell, 542
  cytogenetic damage, 545
  phase, 541f
  sensitivity, 509
Step-and-shoot multislice spiral
    computed tomography, patient
    dose distribution, 603f
Step-down transformer, 94
Step-up transformer, 94
  operation, 95
  secondary winding, voltage
    (induction). *See* High-voltage
    step-up transformer, 110f
Step-wedge filter, 158
Step wedge images, 257f
Sthenic, term (usage), 251
Stickiness, 546
Stochastic effect, 584
Stochastic responses, 516
Stop bath, 198
Storage artifacts, 302
  list, 302t
Storage (memory form), 403
Storage phosphor screens (SPSs),
    413-414
  mechanical stability, 413
  phosphors, incorporation, 415f
Stored program computer,
    development, 397
Straight-line portion. *See* Exposure, 276
Stromal tissue, 510
Structure mottle, 274
Subcutaneous fat, 504
Subdiaphragmatic tissue, enhanced
    rendering, 220f
Subject contrast, 290-292, 279
  anatomical thickness, contribution,
    291f
  enhancement, 290
  kVp, impact (importance), 292
  tissue mass density variations,
    contribution, 292f
Subject factors, 290-293
  components, 290b
Sublethal damage, 530
Sublethal radiation damage, 515
Substances, 38
  identification, 38
  symbolic representation, 39f
Subtraction, rounding (usage), 28
Sugar-phosphate molecules,
    alternation, 505f, 505
Supercomputers, 400
Superconducting materials, 78
  critical temperature, increase, 79f
Superconductivity, 78
  discovery, 78
Superimposition. *See* Image, 445
Supporting tissues, 510

Surgery, 615
  nursing personnel, radiation
    exposure, 615
Surroundings, classification, 3
Sv. *See* Radiation equivalent man, 34
SVD. *See* Shaded volume display, 377
Synchronous timers, 108
Synergism, 196
System dynamic range, 443
SystÉme International d'UnitÉs, Le.
    See International System, 4
System noise, 381
System of units. *See* Units, 18t
Systems software, 407-408

T
$T_{1/2}$, definition. *See* Half-life, 50
Tabular grain emulsions, 186
  replacement, 328
Tabular silver halide crystals, 182
  example, 183f
Target
  area, 128
  assembly, 354
  definition, 126
  material, impact. *See* X-ray emission
    spectrum, 148
  number. *See* Extrapolation number,
    529
  theory, 525-526
    basis, 525
Target atomic number, increase, 147
TB. *See* Terabyte, 403
Tc. *See* Critical temperature, 78
Technique chart. *See* Radiographic
    technique, 260; Variable-kVp
    radiographic technique chart,
    261; Variable-kVp technique
    chart, 261-262
Technique compensation, 258
Technique creep, usage. *See* Dose, 461
Technologist, pregnancy, 625
Teleradiology, 405, 474
Telescopic evaluation, examples, 480f
Television
  camera, usage, 353-354
  field, 356-357
  image, 356-357
  picture tube, 356
    components, 356f
Television camera tubes
  image-intensifier tubes, coupling,
    355f
  target, electron conduction, 355f
Television monitoring, 353-357
  advantage, 353
  image storage, allowance, 353
  system. *See* Fluoroscopic image, 353
  target, 354
  window, 354
Telophase, 508
  characterization, 508
Temperature
  conversion, 25
  determination, 26
  energy, relationship, 26
  measurement, 25

Temperature *(Continued)*
  scales, 25
    usage, 25f
Temporal subtraction, 443-444
  contrast media, change, 445
  energy subtraction, comparison, 444t
  techniques, involvement, 447f
Tenth-value layer (TVL)
  approximation. *See* Concrete, 574t;
    Lead, 574t
  estimate, 574
Terabyte (TB), 403
Terbium activation, 218
Terminal, 405
Terrestrial gamma-ray exposure, 6f
Testes, 541
  atrophy, 541
  radiation response, 541t
TFT. *See* Thin-film transistor, 427
TG. *See* Thermography, 204
TG 18. *See* American Association of
    Physicists in Medicine, 479-480
Thallium, activator atoms, 592
The Joint Commission (TJC), QA
    program, 305b
Thermal cushion, 122
Thermal dissipator, 125
Thermal energy (heat), 4
Thermal radiation, heat transfer, 25
Thermionic emission, 106, 350
  phenomenon, 122
  space charge limitation, 124
Thermionic television camera tube,
    353
Thermographic process, heat (usage),
    205f
Thermography (TG), 204
  technology, heat source (usage), 206
Thermoluminescence dosimeters, 621
  availability, 622f
Thermoluminescence dosimetry
    (TLD), 588, 593, 621
  analyzer, 593
  light emission, 593
  material, types, 594
  multistep process, 593f
  occupational radiation monitor, 621
  properties, 594
  wearing, 622
Thermoluminescence glow curve. *See*
    Lithium fluoride, 594f
Thermoluminescent dosimetry (TLD),
    415
Thermoluminescent phosphors,
    characteristics/uses, 595t
Thermometer. *See* Energy, 26f
  usage, 25
Thin film digitizer, laser beam (usage),
    474f
Thin-film transistor (TFT), 427, 469
  embedding, 430
  requirement, 470
Third-generation computers, 398
Third-generation CT imaging
    system, 370
  disadvantages, 370
  operation, rotate-only mode, 370f

Third-generation imaging system, components, 371

Third Law of Newton. *See* Newton, 21

Thomson, J.J., 39

Thomson atom, 39-40
representation, 39f

Thoriated tungsten, usage. *See* Filament, 122

Thorium, deposits, 6

Thorotrast, usage, 559

Three-dimensional data points, usage, 377

Three-dimensional MPR, 377

Three Mile Island, 560
incident, 535
radiation-induced deaths, prediction, 560

Three-phase high-frequency, 135

Three-phase operation
efficiency, 149f
kVp reduction requirement, 116

Three-phase power, 113-114
efficiency, 114f
result, 246
six-pulse power14% ripple, 115
twelve-pulse power4% ripple, 115
usage, 116
voltage, constancy, 113

Three-phase six-pulse power, three-phase twelve-pulse power (contrast), 148

Three-phase x-ray apparatus, disadvantage, 116

Threshold dose (D$_Q$), 529
measurement, 530

Threshold representation, 528

Thrombocytes, 542f, 543

Thrombocytopenia (platelet depletion), 543

Thrombolysis, 361

Thymine, 505

Thyroid cancer, 558

Thyroid nodularity, incidence, 558

TID. *See* Time-interval difference, 443-444

Time, 18
base quantity, 17
equation, 571
example, 20f
minimization, 571

Time-interval difference (TID) mode, 443-444
subtracted images, production, 445

Time-interval difference (TID) study, sequentially obtained images (subtraction), 445f

Time of occupancy factor. *See* Occupancy factor, 586

Tinea capitis, 540

Tissue, 509-510
compression, scatter radiation (reduction), 228f
Compton scattering, 165
CT number, 377t
differences, CT imaging (usage), 383f

Tissue *(Continued)*
dose, effective dose (relationship), 576f
dose limits, 618
imaging, amount, 386
mass density, 290
variations, contribution. *See* Subject contrast, 292f
pitch, change, 386t
radiosensitivity, 510t
structures, superimposition (reduction), 326
weighting factors, 576t
list, 619t
x-ray interactions, 172
proportion, 172

Titanium dioxide, usage, 209

TJC. *See* The Joint Commission, 305b

TLD. *See* Thermoluminescent dosimetry, 415; Thermoluminiscence dosimetry, 588

Toe, characteristic curve component, 276
gradient, 281
OD result, 280f

Tomogram, geometric characteristics, 312

Tomographic angle
function, 268t
increase, 267
relationship. *See* Fulcrum, 267f

Tomographic examination, design, 265

Tomographic x-ray imaging system, 101f
features, 265

Tomography, 265-268. *See also* Panoramic tomography, 267
advantage, 266, 267
grid, usage, 268
image system, arc movement design, 266f
necessity. *See* Conventional tomography, 265
parallel grids, usage, 268
quality control, 312
system, linear movement (design), 265f
techniques. *See* Linear tomography techniques, 266t

Toner, usage. *See* Printers, 405

Total beam filtration, level, 324

Total filtration, 232
components, 158f

Total momentum, 22

Total projectile electrons, 247

Total risk. *See* Malignancy, 560-561

Touchpads, usage, 400

Trackball, usage, 400, 437

Tracks. *See* Compact disc, 403

Transaxial image (transverse image), 368
reconstruction, 385f

Transbrachial selective coronary angiography, 361

Transfer RNA (tRNA), 505, 507

Transformer, 93. *See also* Interrupterless transformer 9 *See also* Snook transformer, 9
alternating current operation, 109
law, 94
effect, impact. *See* Current, 94
type, 95f

Transistor, development, 397

Transitional elements, 43

Translation, 368-369

Transmission, examples, 65

Transverse image. *See* Transaxial image, 368

Trauma radiographic imaging system, usage. *See* Extremities 230f; Skull imaging 230f; Spine imaging 230f

Trauma system, fixed SID (usage), 230

Trauma x-ray imaging system, 101f

Tree static, 303f

Trifield tubes, size variation, 352

tRNA. *See* Transfer RNA 505

Trough filter, 159f
usage. *See* Chest, 159f

Tube. *See* X-ray tube, 13f

Tuberculosis
mass screening, 605
treatment, 559

Tungsten
alloying, 126
atom, K-shell electron replacement, 141
atomic configuration, 142f
characteristic x-rays
effective energies, 142t
emissions, 145f
electron binding energies, 142f
K-characteristic x-rays, usefulness, 141
L-shell x-rays, value (absence), 322
radiography usage, reasons, 126
target x-ray tube
emission spectrum, molybdenum/rhodium filtration, 325f
x-ray emission spectrum, 323f
x-ray target tube, usage, 324

Tungsten vaporization, impact. *See* X-ray tube, 122

Turbid scattering, 413

TVL. *See* Tenth-value layer, 574

Two-on-one exposure, 357

U

Ultraviolet light, ionizing radiation (capability), 5

Uncontrolled area, occupation, 586

Underdevelopment, result. *See* Radiographs

Under-table IR, usage, 438f

Under-table x-ray tube, radiographic mode (operation), 437

Undifferentiated cells, 509

Unexposed silver halide crystal, negative electrostatic charge, 197

Unfiltered molybdenum beam, 325

Unfiltered molybdenum x-ray emission spectrum, 325f

Uniform interaction, 527
Units, 18
  representation. *See* Radiologic
    science, 19t
  system, 18t
    dimensions, 19
    usage, 19
  usage, 18
UNIVersal Automatic Computer
  (UNIVAC), development, 397
Unlike charges, 75
  attraction, 76f
Unrectified voltage, 111
  secondary side, 112f
Unshielded fluoroscope, isoexposure
  profile, 584f
Upside-down grid, 240
Uranium, natural radioactive decay, 6
Urologic x-ray imaging system, 101f
U.S. population radiation dose,
  sources, 5f

V

Valve tubes, 110
van Leeuwenhoek, Anton, 502-503
Variable aperture collimator, 231-232
Variable-aperture light-localizing
  collimator, schematic, 231f
Variable kilovoltage, 260
Variable kVp, 261
Variable-kVp chart, usage. *See* Knee,
  262t
Variable-kVp radiographic technique
  chart, 261
Variable-kVp technique chart, result,
  261
Vascular stents, 361
VDT. *See* Video display terminal, 405
Veiling glare, 352
  usage. *See* Image-intensifier tube 353f
Velocity, 19. *See also* Average
    velocity, 20 *See also*
    Electromagnetic radiation 57 *See
    also* Final velocity, 20 *See also*
    Initial velocity, 20 *See also* Light,
    20 *See also* Photons, 57-58
  change, rate, 20
  constancy, 20
  determination, 19
  equation, 19
  increase, 22
  maximum, 20
  measurement, 19
  relationship. *See* Sine waves, 59f
  square, computation, 23
  wavelength/frequency, inverse
    proportion, 59
  wave parameters, 59
Vertical chest Bucky, AEC sensors
  (position), 264f
Vertical resolution, determination, 357
Very large-scale integration (VLSI),
  398
Video display terminal (VDT), 405
Video Electronics Standard
    Association (VESA), 479
  standard, 479

Video frame, formation, 356f
Videography, 584
Video monitoring, frames per second
    rate, 357
Video signal
  electron beam modulation, 356
  modulation, 356
  reading, progressive mode, 442f
Video system, information content,
    443f
Vidicon television camera
  tube, components, 354f
  variations, 354f
Viewboxes
  maintenance, 335
  visual inspection, 335
Viewing conditions, maintenance, 335
Vignetting, 352
Virtual colonoscopy, 378f
Visible image, 183
Visible light, 62
  behavior, 64
  definition, 64
  interaction, 64
    result, 184
  photon, 63
  physics, 57
  wavelength
    identification, 63
    measurement, 64
  wave model, 64-66
Visual acuity, 349
Visual C++, 410
Visual checklist, 340f
  usage, 339-340
VLSI. *See* Very large-scale integration,
  398
Voice-recognition systems, usage, 401
Volta, Alessandro, 88
Voltage, 77
  determination, 74
  rectification, 110
  ripple, 115-116. *See also* 4%
    voltage ripple; 115 *See also*
    14% voltage ripple; 115 *See
    also* 1% voltage ripple; 115 *See
    also* 100% voltage ripple; 115
  selection, 172
Voltage waveform. *See* High-
    frequency voltage waveform, 114f
  impact. *See* X-ray emission
    spectrum 148-149
  result, power supplies (impact), 115f
  smoothing, long high-voltage cables
    capacitance (impact), 116f
Voltaic pile, 88
  representation, 89f
Volt (joule/coulomb), 77
Volume
  equation, 19
  imaging, equation, 386
Volume element (voxel), 376
  size, 376
    determination, 376
Volume rendered, 377
Volume-rendering display. *See*
    Heart, 379f

W

Washing. *See* Film, 199
Wash water temperature, 313
Wasted hits, absence, 527
Water, 503
  abundance, 501
  radiolysis, 523-525
    action, 523
    result, 524, 524f
Waters view, 299f
Watt (W), 23
  equation, 82, 116, 136
  usage, 81
Wave equation, 60
Waveform, 81
Wavelength, 58-60
  creation. *See* Short wavelength
    waves, 65f
  distance, 59
  importance, 58
  relationship. *See* Sine waves, 59f
  velocity/frequency, inverse
    proportion, 59
  wave parameter, 59
Wave model. *See* Visible light,
  64-66
Wave parameters, 59
Wave-particle duality, 63-64. *See also*
    Electromagnetic energy, 57
Wedge filter, 159f. *See also* Bilateral
    wedge filter; 158 *See also*
    Step-wedge filter; 158
  usage, 158. *See also* Foot
    examination, 159f
Weight, 22
  equivalence. *See* Mass, 22
  force, 22
  mass/acceleration, product, 22
  term, usage, 3
  variation, 22
Wet-pressure sensitization, 301
  processor dirt, impact, 301f
Wetting, 196
  involvement. *See* Processing, 195
White light, refraction, 62f
Whole-body dose limits, 616
Whole-body radiation exposure,
    538t
Whole-body response, dose response
    relationship (determination), 517
Window, 592. *See also* X-ray tube,
    592
Window/level adjustment, 472
Window/level postprocessing tool,
    457f
Wire mesh radiographs, usage. *See*
    Screen-film, 221f
Wirth, Nicklaus, 410
Women (childbearing age), x-ray
    consent (form), 609f
Words, 407
Work, 22
  determination, 23
  equation, 22
  force/distance, product, 23
  unit, 22
  usage, 22

Workload (W). *See* Barrier thickness, 586
  characteristic, 587
  distribution, 587. *See also* Clinical voltage, 588f
Workstations, 400. *See also* Ergonomically designed digital image workstation, 471f *See also* Radiology Information System, 474-475
W_R. *See* Radiation weighting factor, 513
Wrist
  images, signal intensity, 496f
  X-light exposure, 9f

X
X-axis, 31
  intersection. *See* Graph, 32f
Xeromammography, 319
X-light
  exposure. *See* Wrist, 9f
  term, usage, 7
X-radiation, photon, 63
X-ray beam
  alignment, 581
  aperture diaphragm, 229-230
  average energy, increase, 147
  circular shape (production), radiographic cones/cylinders (usage), 230f
  collimation, 224, 494
    impact. *See* Scatter radiation, 226f
  conversion, phosphor (impact), 208
  exposure, 472f
  field size, 225-226
    control, 225
  filtration, importance, 306
  incidence, 464f
  intensity
    determination, 156
    estimation, nomogram, 152f
    measurement, 582f
  intensity/penetrability, increase, 116
  light field, coincidence (monitoring test tool), 307f
  penetrability, 245
  pitch, determination, 386
  profile, usage. *See* Computed tomography, 370f
  providing, 8f
  quantity, change, 149t
  restriction, 229-232
    collimation, impact, 12
  size, excess (control), 232
  width, reduction, 604
X-ray beam quality, 145
  change, 149t
  determination, kVp (impact), 106b
  increase, 158
    filtration, increase, 157
    kVp peak, increase, 157
  voltage/filtration identification, 156
X-ray beam-restricting devices, 229f
X-ray emissions, 140
  challenge questions, 160-161

X-ray emission spectrum, 144, 143-145
  amplitude
    change, 146f
    increase, kVp (change), 147f
  factors, 145-149
  factors, impact, 149t
  filtration, addition (impact), 147
  kVp, impact, 146-147
  mA/mAs, impact, 146
  rhodium target, 322
  shape, 142
    factors, 146
  size/relative position, factors, 146t
  target material, impact, 148
  voltage waveform, impact, 148-149
X-ray energy
  calculation, 141
  DQE, 464f
  identification, 63
  increase, 224
    voltage waveform, increase, 116f
  K-shell electron binding energy, equivalence, 216
  maximum/minimum, association, 145
  Planck's constant, relationship, 30
X-ray film, introduction, 194
X-ray-generated signal, transfer, 427
X-ray imaging system, 11
  challenge questions, 118
  electrical energy, conversion, 74f
  emission spectrum, expectation, 145
  image receptor, 266f
  metal filters, usage, 154
  patient-supporting examination table, requirement, 101
  requirements, breast architecture (impact), 320f
  schematic circuit, 117f
  tube head, 266f
X-ray-induced image-forming signal, 416f
X-ray intensity, 67, 152
  reduction
    requirement, 32
    result, 130f
  result, 155
X-ray interaction
  absorption/scatter, impact, 174f
  percentage, photoelectric/Compton processes, 225t
  probability, 461
    Compton effect, impact, 165f
  relationship, 173f
X-ray linear attenuation coefficients, 377t
X-ray mammography, impact, 320
X-ray photons, 57
X-ray quality
  factors, impact, 157t, 245t
  fixed value, 246
X-ray quantity, 152-155
  definition, 152
  distance, inverse proportion, 154
  distance, relationship, 154
    calculation, 154

X-ray quantity *(Continued)*
  factors, 152-155, 152t
    impact, 157t, 245t
  filtration, relationship, 154-155
  impact, 247
  kVp, relationship, 153
  low level, 148
  mAs, relationship, 153
  variation, kVp (relationship), 153-154
X-rays. *See* Diagnostic x-rays, 6
  absorption
    asymmetric screens, compensation, 219f
    efficiency, DQE measure, 463
  annual dose, acceptance, 6
  application, benefits, 6
  attenuation, 66f
  behavior, 64
  biologic effects, control, 11
  burn, reduction (possibility), 8
  carbon atom, interaction, 42
  circuit, 117
  diagnostic range, bremssrahlung x-rays (equivalence), 143
  discovery, 7, 62
    characterization, 7
  examination
    performing, avoidance, 605
    room, plan drawing, 104f
  existence, 53
  exposure
    determination, 158
    termination, AEC control, 108f
  fatality, occurrence, 11
  gamma rays, contrast, 63
  generator, capability, 438
  ionizing electromagnetic radiation, form, 53
  ionizing radiation, capability, 5
  light photons, relative numbers (comparison). *See* Direct film exposure, 215t; Screen-film, 215t
  number
    emission, 149
    increase, voltage waveform (increase), 116f
  pair production, absence, 169
  penetrability, 155
  photoelectric interaction, 171, 218
    relative probability, 167f
  photon, 68
    consideration, 68
  production, 63. *See also* Nucleus, 63f
    challenge questions, 150
    efficiency, increase, 140
    electrons, number (determination), 247
    range, examples, 69t
  quality, 155-160
    specification, HVL (usage), 156
  scattering, 165
  targets, characteristics, 127t
  test pattern, radiographs, 213f
  transmission, 172, 232f
  types, usage. *See* Radiographs, 170f
  velocity, determination, 31
  voltages, measurement, 8

X-ray source-to-image receptor
  distance, explanation, 8
X-ray source-to-image receptor
  motion, usage. *See* Panoramic
  tomography, 269f
X-ray tube, 103, 364-365
  anode, thermal stress, 133
  C-arm support
    method, 121f
    system, 121
  cathode, 122-125
  ceiling support
    method, 121f
    system, 120
  challenge questions, 122
  design, 122
  external components, 120-122
  fabrication, 308
  failure, 131-134
    cause, frequency, 133
    cause, tungsten vaporization
      (impact), 122
  filtration, addition, 147f
  floor-to-ceiling support
    method, 121f
    system, 120-121
  focal-spot size, 307
  glass/metal enclosure, 122

X-ray tube *(Continued)*
  heat dissipation, 129f
  housing cooling chart, 136
  internal components, 122-131
  life
    heat, excess, 132
    length, 132
  metal enclosure tubes, 122
  motion, usage. *See* Foot
    tomographs, 269f
  movement, appearance, 384f
  output, description, 144
  protective housing, 121-122
  radiation cooling, 25
  rating charts, 134-136
  rotating anode (powering),
    induction motor (usage), 93
  secondary voltage, determination,
    109
  support methods, 121f
  tilt, impact. *See* Focal spots, 324f
  usage, 13f
  voltage
    decrease, capacitor discharge
      generator (usage), 115f
    increase, 148f
  voltage/current, supply, 8
  window, 592

X-ray tube current, 106
  adjustment, 123
  exposure, product, 106
  increase, 124f
    possibility, 126
  monitoring, 107

Y

Y-axis, 31
  intersection. *See* Graph, 32f
Yttrium, 208
  screen, 216

Z

Z-axis coverage
  determination, 389
  equation, 389
Z-axis resolution (improvement),
  linear interpolation
  (usage), 385
Zinc-based phosphors, 216
Zinc cadmium sulfide, usage, 8
Zinc sulfide, 208
Zonography, 267
Zoom movement, 473
Z-related photoelectric effect,
  172-173